FOUNDATIONS OF NORMAL AND THERAPEUTIC NUTRITION

D1365942

v

BOOKS OF RELATED INTEREST

Bodinski: **The Nurse's Guide to Diet Therapy,** 1982, 0-471-08167-1

Burke: **Human Anatomy and Physiology for the Health Sciences,** 2nd edition, 1985, 0-471-80686-2

Mason: **The Dynamics of Clinical Dietetics,** 2nd edition, 1982, 0-471-06088-7

FOUNDATIONS OF NORMAL AND THERAPEUTIC NUTRITION

T. Randall Lankford, M.S.

Instructor
Department of Biology
Galveston Community College
Galveston, Texas

Paula Marie Jacobs-Steward, M.S., R.D., L.D.

Dietary Director
Memorial Hospital—Southwest
Memorial Care Systems
Houston, Texas
Clinical Instructor
Dietetic Internship Program
Department of Foods and Nutrition
Houston Medical Center Branch
Texas Woman's University
Denton, Texas

A WILEY MEDICAL PUBLICATION
JOHN WILEY & SONS
New York ● Chichester ● Brisbane ● Toronto ● Singapore

Interior design: Wanda Lubelska
Cover design: Raphael Hernandez
Cover: Photomicrograph of iodine, Roland Birke, Peter Arnold, Inc.

The following figures were drawn by Masako Herman:
Figures 2-2, 3-4, 3-7, 3-9, 3-12, 3-16, 3-17, 4-8, 4-10, 4-11, 4-12, 5-6, 5-9, 5-10, 6-7, 6-8, 6-20, 6-21, 6-22, 6-24, 6-25, 7-1, 7-5, 7-6, 7-8, 7-9, 7-10, 8-1, 8-3, 8-4, 9-4, 10-1, 10-6, 10-7, 10-8, 17-1, 17-3, 17-4, 18-2, 18-5, 19-3, 19-6, 19-7, 19-8, 19-10, 19-13, 19-15, 19-16, 20-1, 20-3, 20-4, and 23-3.

Library of Congress Cataloging in Publication Data:

Lankford, T. Randall, 1942–
   Foundations of normal and therapeutic nutrition.

   (A Wiley medical publication)
   Includes bibliographies and index.
   1. Diet therapy.   2. Nutrition.   I. Jacobs-Steward, Paula Marie.   II. Title.   III. Series.
   RM216.L26   1986   615.8′54   85-22664
   ISBN 0-471-88815-X

Printed in the United States of America

10 9 8 7 6 5 4 3 2

To my parents for their encouragement

To my wife, Billie Jo, whose sacrifices and support made completion of this text possible

To my sons, Christopher and Nicholas, whose nutritional state, I hope, will always be optimal

T. R. L.

To my parents, Frank and Jessie Jacobs

P. M. J.-S.

PREFACE

Nutrition is a complex, dynamic field in which new information is being discovered almost daily. Knowledge and application of nutritional principles by health professionals are essential in averting the occurrence of disease, protecting the general health and well-being of the public, diagnosing diseases, and preventing further complications of illnesses. To accomplish these goals, health professionals need a sound nutritional background composed of a knowledge of the chemical principles of nutrients, the ability to integrate nutritional concepts to the functioning of the organ systems, and the application of this information to clinical situations.

Foundations of Normal and Therapeutic Nutrition is written for students in nursing, nutrition, and allied health programs for use in either a separate course or in an integrated curriculum that includes a nutrition component. Our primary goal is to present the study of normal and therapeutic nutrition in as clear and informative a manner as possible that will, in turn, encourage maximum retention of the material by students and help them to effectively apply the concepts to daily practice. With this purpose in mind, the book is organized so as to illustrate the relationship of basic science principles (chemistry and anatomy and physiology) to nutrition and give students the opportunity to measure their progress in learning the material. This goal is achieved in the following ways.

First, the book provides students with a thorough knowledge of the chemical principles of nutrients. These principles are of primary importance to health professionals whether counseling patients about how to cope with all the nutritional information they are being bombarded with or helping them to recover from an illness. This material is presented on a level that assumes the student has no prior chemistry background. Many explanatory figures have been specially prepared to help students in learning these concepts.

Second, it helps students relate the chemical principles of nutrients to the normal and abnormal functions of the organ systems. The clinical applications in Part I are unique tools that integrate chemistry with nutritional therapy examples and are designed to attract and increase student interest.

Third, students learn how to apply nutritional concepts to clinical situations. By first discussing the normal functioning of various body systems and then presenting explanations of diseases and disorders that can affect these systems and the role therapeutic diets play in patient recovery, a logical cause-and-effect relationship is established so that students can see the association between illness and nutrition. In particular, the case studies in each of the therapeutic chapters reinforce the concepts learned earlier in the book and help students apply the principles to actual clinical situations.

Finally, the inclusion of numerous and well-designed pedagogical aids is the book's single most important feature and one that should prove to be extremely valuable to students. These aids include the following:

- *Objectives.* Appear at the beginning of each chapter so that students are aware of the important concepts they should study. They also help instructors in planning and organizing lectures.

- *Definition of terms.* Important terms and their definitions are placed in the margins next to the terms in the text.

- *Detailed chapter outlines.* Provide reviews of the chapter in a succinct format. This feature aids students in studying the chapter for exams and is useful to instructors as a source of lecture notes.

- *Chapter review questions.* True-false, multiple choice (answers given at the end of the book for both types of questions), and discussion questions are presented at the end of each chapter as opposed to being contained in a separate study guide.

- *Clinical applications.* Highlighted throughout most of Part I. This material helps students apply nutritional concepts to the clinical setting.

- *Case studies.* Provided at the end of Chapters 18–26. The case studies are presented in a logical format that consists of a general description of a clinical disorder followed by laboratory, anthropometric, and drug data (with normal values given in parentheses) as they might appear on a patient's hospital chart. Objective questions are then presented so as to help students analyze the data and use information learned from previous chapters. (Please note that, in order for instructors and students to obtain the maximum benefit from these questions, the answers are given in the instructor's manual for this book.) This format is very similar to the one in which case studies appear on nursing board exams.

- *Explanatory figures.* Many of the figures in the book are prepared specifically to explain certain difficult concepts or a series of interrelated changes.

- *Glossary.* Presents a comprehensive summary of the important terms in the book. All glossary terms are identified in boldface in the text.

The book is divided into three parts: Principles of Nutrition, Nutrition Throughout the Life Cycle, and Therapeutic Nutrition. Part I discusses dietary planning, the four-food group system, the food exchange system, and the six basic nutrients (carbohydrates, lipids, proteins, vitamins, minerals, and water).

Part II discusses the measurement of and types of energy; causes and treatment of obesity, underweight, anorexia nervosa, and bulimia; presents nutritional requirements for the different phases of the life cycle from pregnancy through the elderly years; and explains the importance of nutrients in physical activity.

Chapter 15 presents the steps in the clinical process (assessment, planning, implementation, and evaluation) and how they are applied to the nutritional care of the patient. Chapter 16 provides examples of many common drugs and their interactions with foods (nutrients). This information is reinforced throughout the remaining chapters in Part III.

Due to the importance of the topic, enteral-parenteral nutrition (Chapter 17) is presented in a separate chapter, as opposed to a few pages scattered throughout the text. Chapters 18 through 23 discuss diseases and disorders of organ systems and the use of therapeutic nutrition in alleviating the symptoms of these illnesses. Chapters 24 through 26 contain material on nutrition and cancer, pre- and postoperative nutrition, and nutrition and mental health. Throughout these chapters, sample menus of therapeutic diets with analysis and comments are provided.

We believe that the approach used in presenting normal and therapeutic nutrition in this book will be an instructive and interactive one. We hope that, by becoming familiar with the concepts and examples in this book, students will gain the knowledge and confidence to plan and implement effective nutritional care for their clients.

T. Randall Lankford
Paula Marie Jacobs-Steward

ACKNOWLEDGMENTS

This textbook lists two authors on the title page; however, as with any book, there are actually many dedicated and talented people who are responsible for the final product. It is impossible to name all these individuals, but several groups are especially deserving. We wish to express our appreciation to the following:

To the reviewers who provided so many suggestions for improving the manuscript: Linda Fern, R.N., Gardner–Webb College; Pamela Fletcher, M.A., Albuquerque Technical Vocational Institute; Dale J. Gordon, R.N., M.Sc.N., Northern Maine Vocational Technical Institute; and Beverly Hatrock, R.N., M.S., North Idaho College.

To John Wiley & Sons, Inc., and all the people there who were involved in this project. A special note of thanks goes to Andrea Stingelin, Executive Editor, for her keen perception of the importance of this project. Our very special gratitude goes to Janet Walsh Foltin, Associate Editor, who worked very closely with us through all the stages of writing, designing, and editing; to Denise Watov, Production Supervisor, for her coordination of the production stage of the book; and to Masako Herman, for both her excellent illustrations and suggestions for the book.

To Glenda Counts, John Fortune, Jayme Hesson, Frank and Jessie Jacobs, Linda James, Cynthia McCreight, Brenda Meadows, Ron Russell, Linda Schnur, William Steward, Ellen Toelke, and many other friends and family for their interest, support, and encouragement during this project.

And, finally, to a computer, printer, and two word processing programs that made this whole process much more manageable and enjoyable.

T. Randall Lankford
Paula Marie Jacobs-Steward

CONTENTS

PART I PRINCIPLES OF NUTRITION 1

1 Introduction to Nutrition 3
Introduction 4
Definition of Nutrition 5
Four Main Components of the Study of Nutrition 5
Important Nutritional Terms 7
Health Team 8
Cultural Influence on Food Habits and Importance to Health Professionals 10
Food Fallacies, Controversies, and Facts: A Challenge for the Health Professional 11
Dietary Goals for the United States 13
Outline 16
Review Questions 16
References 17

2 Dietary Planning 19
Introduction 20
Food Guides for Planning Nutritious Diets 20
Recommended Dietary Allowances (RDAs) 30
U.S. RDAs 34
Outline 35
Review Questions 36
References 37

3 Carbohydrates 38
Introduction 39
Chemistry of Carbohydrates 39
Carbohydrates Found in Foods 39

Functions of Carbohydrates 53
Digestion and Absorption of Carbohydrates 54
Metabolism of Carbohydrates 56
Amounts and Food Sources of Carbohydrates in Diets of Different Cultures 60
Carbohydrates and the Exchange Groups 61
Outline 65
Review Questions 66
References 68

4 Lipids 69
Introduction 70
Chemistry of Lipids 70
Phospholipids 76
Sterols 77
Lipoproteins 78
Functions of Lipids 81
Digestion and Absorption of Lipids 82
Storage of Fat 84
Problems Associated with Digestion and Absorption of Fats 85
Fat and the Exchange Groups 86
Outline 91
Review Questions 92
References 94

5 Proteins 95
Introduction 96
Chemistry of Proteins 96

Functions of Proteins   102
Digestion and Absorption of Proteins   105
Metabolism of Proteins   107
Protein Digestibility, Quality, and
   Recommended Dietary Allowance
   (RDA)   108
Food Sources of Protein   112
Protein-Calorie Malnutrition (PCM)   113
Distribution of Protein Kilocalories in
   Balanced and Typical American
   Diets   115
Outline   117
Review Questions   118
References   120

6   Vitamins   121
Introduction   122
General Description   122
Fat-Soluble Vitamins   122
Water-Soluble Vitamins   140
Outline   162
Review Questions   166
References   167

7   Major Minerals   168
Introduction   169
Major Minerals   169
Outline   185

Review Questions   187
References   188

8   Trace Minerals   190
Introduction   191
Iron (Fe)   192
Iodine (I)   199
Zinc (Zn)   201
Trace Minerals with Estimated Safe and
   Adequate Daily Dietary Intake   203
Outline   206
Review Questions   208
References   209

9   Water   210
Introduction   211
Percentage of Body Weight as Water and
   Location   211
Functions of Water in the Body   212
Movement of Water between Fluid
   Compartments   213
Diarrhea: Example of the Shift of Water Out
   of Fluid Compartments   220
Outline   221
Review Questions   221
References   223

PART II   NUTRITION THROUGHOUT THE LIFE CYCLE   225

10   Energy, Obesity, and
     Underweight   227
Introduction   228
Measurement of Energy   228
Energy Balance   229
Energy Expenditure   231
Calculating Total Energy
   Requirements   234
Ideal or Desirable Body Weight and Body
   Composition   236
Overweight and Obesity   242
Nonrecommended Treatments
   of Obesity   250

Recommended Treatments of Obesity   250
Underweight, Anorexia Nervosa, Bulimia,
   and Bulimarexia   256
Outline   258
Review Questions   260
References   261

11   Nutrition During Pregnancy and
     Lactation   263
Introduction   264
Nutritional Requirements during Pregnancy
   and Lactation   264

Proper Diet for Pregnancy and
Lactation   269
Problems and Complications of
Pregnancy   270
Outline   273
Review Questions   274
References   276

12   Nutrition During Infancy, Childhood, and Adolescence   277
Nutrition During Infancy   278
Nutrition During Childhood   284
Nutrition during Adolescence   287
Childhood and Adolescent Problems Related to Nutrition   290
Outline   291
Review Questions   293
References   294

13   Nutrition and the Elderly   295
Introduction   296
Nutrient Needs of the Elderly   296
Common Nutritional Problems of the Elderly   300

Dietary Planning for the Elderly   303
Nutrition Programs for the Elderly   304
Outline   306
Review Questions   307
References   308

14   Nutrition and Physical Fitness   310
Introduction   311
Importance of Protein in Muscle Development and Athletic Performance   311
Importance of Fat in Physical Activity   312
Importance of Carbohydrates in Physical Activity   313
Fluid and Electrolytes in Physical Activity   316
Prevent Meal   317
Weight-Gain Diet   318
Weight-Loss Diet   319
Outline   320
Review Questions   321
References   323

PART III   THERAPEUTIC NUTRITION   325

15   Introduction to Diet Therapy   327
Introduction   328
Principle and Purpose of Diet Therapy   328
Identifying and Providing Nutritional Care to Patients   329
Clinical Care Process   329
Problem-Oriented Medical Record (POMR)   351
Outline   355
Review Questions   356
References   358

16   Drug–Food (Nutrient) Interactions   359
Introduction   360
Ways in Which Drugs and Foods (Nutrients) Interact   360

Drugs + Foods (Nutrients) = Altered Drug Effects   360
Drugs + Foods (Nutrients) = Altered Nutritional Balance   364
Food (Nutrients)–Drug Interaction in the Elderly   368
Outline   371
Review Questions   373
References   374

17   Enteral-Parenteral Nutrition   375
Introduction   376
Enteral Nutrition   376
Parenteral Nutrition   379
Transitional Feedings   387
Outline   388

Review Questions   389
References   390

18   **Diabetes Mellitus and
     Hypoglycemia   392**
Introduction   393
Diabetes Mellitus   393
Hypoglycemia   418
Case Study: Insulin-Dependent
     Diabetes   422
Case Study: Non-Insulin-Dependent
     Diabetes   425
Outline   427
Review Questions   430
References   432

19   **Diseases of the Gastrointestinal
     Tract   434**
Introduction   435
Esophagus   435
Stomach   437
Small Intestine   453
Large Intestine (Colon)   463
Case Study: Peptic Ulcer and the Dumping
     Syndrome   469
Outline   473
Review Questions   475
References   477

20   **Disorders of the Liver, Gallbladder,
     and Pancreas   478**
Introduction   479
Liver   479
Gallbladder   491
Pancreas   493
Case Study: Liver Disease   499
Outline   502
Review Questions   503
References   505

21   **Diseases of the Cardiovascular
     System   506**
Introduction   507
Atherosclerosis   507
Hypertension   519

Myocardial Infarction   530
Congestive Heart Failure   531
Case Study: Hyperlipoproteinemia   532
Outline   536
Review Questions   538
References   540

22   **Diseases of the Respiratory
     System   541**
Introduction   542
Chronic Obstructive Pulmonary
     Disease   542
Pneumonia   547
Tuberculosis   547
Lung Cancer (Bronchiogenic Cancer)   548
Cystic Fibrosis   550
Case Study: COPD in a 45-Year-Old
     Man   551
Outline   554
Review Questions   555
References   556

23   **Diseases of the Kidneys   558**
Introduction   559
Functions of the Kidneys   559
Nephron: Functional Unit of the
     Kidney   560
Kidney Diseases   562
Dialysis Treatment   570
Renal Calculi (Kidney Stones)   573
Case Study: Chronic Renal Failure   573
Outline   579
Review Questions   580
References   582

24   **Nutrition and Cancer   583**
Introduction   584
Diet and Possible Causes of Breast and
     Colon Cancers   584
Dietary Recommendations to Reduce the
     Risk of Cancer   585
Nutritional Problems and Diet Therapy for
     Cancer Patients   585
Case Study: Cancer Patient   588

Outline   590
Review Questions   590
References   591

**25   Pre- and Postoperative
        Nutrition   592**
Introduction   593
Preoperative Nutrition   593
Preoperative Diet   594
Postoperative Diet   594
Diet Therapy for Burn Patients   599
Case Study: Severe Burn Patient   602
Outline   605
Review Questions   606
References   606

26   Nutrition and Mental Health   607
Introduction   608
Malnutrition and Behavior   608
Hyperkinesis (Hyperactivity) and Its
    Relation to Food Additives and High
    Sugar Intake   609
Vitamin Therapy and Mental
    Disorders   609
Alcoholism and Nutrition   610
Dementia   612
Eating Disorders   613
Case Study: Alcoholic Patient   613
Outline   615
Review Questions   616
References   616

Appendixes   617
A   Exchange Lists for Meal Planning   619
B   Dietary Fiber in Selected Foods
      (g/100g)   626
C   Cholesterol Content of Foods   628
D   Supplemental Food Choices for
      Calorie-Controlled Diets   630
E   Alcoholic Beverages in
      Calorie-Controlled Diets   632
F   Drug-Nutrient Interactions   633
G   Nutritive Values of the Edible Part of
      Foods   636
H   Relative Ratios of Polyunsaturated Fat
      and Saturated Fat (P/S Ratio) in
      Representative Foods   710
I   Sodium and Potassium Content of
      Foods   711
J   Physical Growth NCHS
      Percentiles   717
K   Mid-Upper-Arm Circumference
      Percentiles (cm)   725

L   Triceps Skinfold Percentiles (mm)   726
M   Recommended Energy Intake   727
N   Conversion Tables   728
O   Recommended Food Intake for
      Good Nutrition for Children and
      Adolescents   729
P   Levels of Nutritional Assessment for
      Infants and Children   731
Q   Nutrition History: Birth to 24
      Months   733
R   Range of Average Water Requirement
      of Children at Different Ages Under
      Ordinary Circumstances   735

Glossary   737

Answers to Review Questions   757

Index   761

PART I

PRINCIPLES OF NUTRITION

1. INTRODUCTION TO NUTRITION

2. DIETARY PLANNING

3. CARBOHYDRATES

4. LIPIDS

5. PROTEINS

6. VITAMINS

7. MAJOR MINERALS

8. TRACE MINERALS

9. WATER

1 INTRODUCTION TO NUTRITION

OBJECTIVES

Upon completion of this chapter, you should be able to:

1. Define nutrition and describe the four main components of the study of nutrition.

2. List the energy nutrients.

3. Define an organic compound and list the four classes of organic nutrients.

4. List the two inorganic nutrients and two of their functions.

5. Identify the members of a health team and describe, in sequences, the four steps they follow in providing nutritional care to a patient.

6. Define culture and describe four ways in which culture relates to food and eating habits.

7. Explain two ways in which cultural influence is important to health professionals.

8. List three ways in which food faddism may adversely affect a person.

9. Define food fad, natural food, organically grown food, and megadose.

10. State the Senate Select Committee's recommended dietary goals in terms of percentages of fat, protein, and carbohydrates.

INTRODUCTION

Primary level Health care that is aimed at averting the occurrence of disease and protecting the health of the general public.

Secondary level Health care that is utilized for early diagnosis of disease and prevention of further complications.

Tertiary level Health care that is designed to educate a patient for the maximum use of his or her remaining capacities.

Nutrition is a human need and is recognized by consumers as essential to life itself. Food and eating are among the great pleasures of life. In the last few years, the public has become more concerned about the relationship of nutrition and general health. As a result, the public is being bombarded with nutritional information and claims in books, magazines, newspapers and even grocery stores. As a result, many consumers are confused by conflicting food and health claims. Food manufacturers are providing more information about nutrients on labels, but many consumers do not understand how to read or analyze it.

To help consumers understand nutritional information they read and to explain the relationship of nutrition to normal health and disease are two reasons why health professionals need to study nutrition. In addition, health professionals must study nutrition in order to provide preventive health care on the **primary, secondary,** and **tertiary** levels. Knowledge of nutrition is important in primary prevention because it prevents the occurrence of disease and protects the general health and well-being of the public. To do this, health professionals must be knowledgeable about nutritious diets, foods, and exercise. In addition, they need to be aware of government primary prevention programs such as Head Start preschool programs, breakfast programs, and food stamp programs.

Nutritional information is important in secondary preventive health care in that it can be utilized for early diagnosis of diseases and prevention of further complications. Specifically, the health professional frequently alerts the medical service or physician to abnormal laboratory values and is aware of the patient's tolerance of the prescribed therapeutic diet.

Tertiary preventive health care involves the health professional in retraining and educating patients for the maximum use of their remaining capacities. For example, this involves advising paraplegics and quadriplegics about the possible dietary side effects of their immobility, such as constipation, kidney stones, and dietary measures to help prevent or alleviate such problems.

In summary, nutritional information is increasing at a rapid rate. This challenges health professionals to be knowledgeable about nutrition so that they can provide competent health care on all three levels. Nutritional knowledge will enrich a health professional's personal life.

DEFINITION OF NUTRITION

Nutrition The combination of processes by which the body receives and utilizes the materials necessary to maintain homeostasis.

Nutrition is the combination of processes by which the body receives and utilizes the materials necessary to maintain homeostasis. These processes are also important in their relationship to health and disease. In addition, nutrition is concerned with the social, economic, cultural, and psychological implications of food and eating.

FOUR MAIN COMPONENTS OF THE STUDY OF NUTRITION

The study of nutrition involves four main components (see Fig. 1-1):

Nutrients. Substances that are necessary for the metabolic processes of the body.

Body processes. Physiological activities (e.g., digestion and absorption) that interact with nutrients to maintain homeostasis.

Nutrient requirements. Individual nutritional requirements to maintain homeostasis depend upon various factors (age, sex, and physical condition).

Homeostasis. The maintenance of organ systems, such as the respiratory and cardiovascular systems, in a dynamic state. The above three components are essential for homeostasis, as shown in Figure 1-1.[1]

NUTRIENTS

There are six classes of nutrients:

Carbohydrate	Vitamins
Lipid (Fat)	Minerals
Protein	Water

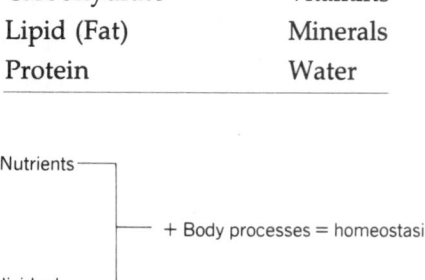

FIGURE 1-1   Interaction of four components of the study of nutrition.

These classes are subdivided into energy, organic, and inorganic nutrients.

Energy Nutrients

Oxidation A chemical
reaction in which an atom
or molecule either loses
hydrogen atoms and electrons or accepts oxygen.

Carbohydrate, fat, and protein are designated as energy nutrients, since they release energy when **oxidized** (chemical reaction). The maintenance of homeostasis depends upon continual input of energy.

Organic Nutrients

Organic compounds
Substances that contain
carbon atoms.

Carbohydrate, fat, protein, and vitamins (see Table 1-1) are composed of **organic compounds.** Vitamins are the only type of organic nutrients that do not provide energy. Organic nutrients have many functions, such as building, maintaining body tissues and regulating body processes, which will be discussed in detail in later chapters.

Inorganic Nutrients

Inorganic nutrients Substances that do not contain carbon atoms.

Minerals and water are **inorganic nutrients** (see Table 1-1). Minerals are required in minute amounts and are essential for many body functions such as bone formation, conduction of nerve impulses, and synthesis of red blood cells. Water is the most prevalent nutrient, as well as the most important. This is evidenced by the fact that a person can live for about 40 days in a fasting state, but can live for only about 3 days without taking in water. Examples of body functions for which water is important are as a medium for chemical reactions, in transporting materials, and in helping to maintain body temperature.[2]

TABLE 1-1 SUMMARY OF CLASSES OF NUTRIENTS

Description	Classes	Functions
Energy nutrients	Carbohydrate Fat Protein	Release energy for maintenance of homeostasis
Organic nutrients	Carbohydrate Fat Protein Vitamins	Build and maintain body tissues Regulate body processes
Inorganic nutrients	Water Minerals	Medium for chemical reactions Transport materials Maintain body temperature
		Bone formation Conduction of nerve impulses

IMPORTANT NUTRITIONAL TERMS

A meaningful discussion of nutrition must contain words and terms that are clearly defined. The following list of terms will appear in many places throughout the text; therefore, knowledge of them is essential.

Health. State of optimal physical, mental, and social well-being, not just the absence of illness.

Nutritional status. An individual's condition of health in relation to the digestion and absorption of nutrients.

Nutritional care. Application of the science of nutrition in nourishing the body regardless of health problems or potential problems.[1]

Malnutrition. A condition of the body that arises from a prolonged lack or excessive intake or impaired utilization of food. This condition is often evidenced by the appearance of specific clinical conditions such as **anemia, goiter,** and **rickets.**[3]

Nutritious. Food in a diet that provides needed nutrients for maintenace of homeostasis. A food cannot be determined to be nutritious when considered by itself, but rather in relation to the total diet.

Junk food. A term for which there is no acceptable scientific definition, but in popular usage refers to foods that are harmful, for example, foods high in salt, sugar, or fat content[4] (see Fig. 1-2).

Anemia A condition in which the total quantity of red blood cells and hemoglobin is less than normal. See iron deficiency anemia (Chapter 8) and pernicious anemia (Chapter 6).

Goiter Abnormal enlargement of the thyroid gland due to an inbalance in the amount of the mineral iodine (see Chapter 8).

Rickets A condition caused by a deficiency of vitamin D that leads to decreased absorption of calcium by the bones.

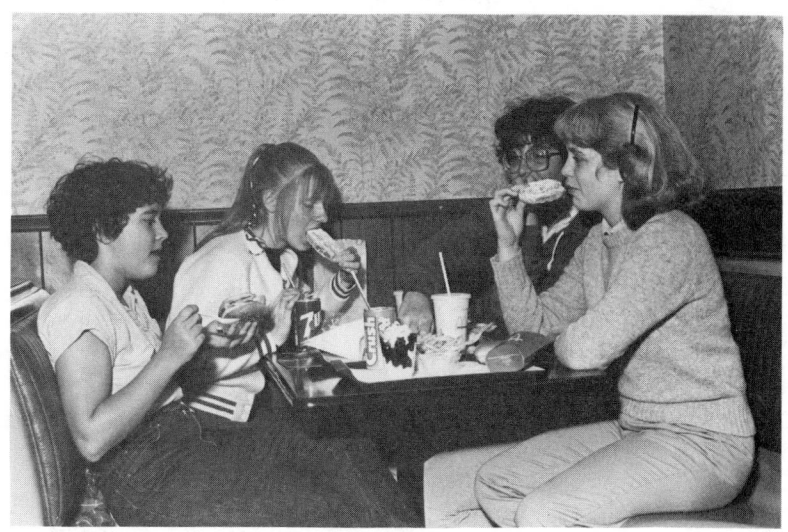

FIGURE 1-2 Teenage girls eating junk food. (Courtesy of Nancy Conroy.)

Health food. Another term for which there is no scientifically accepted definition; however, it usually refers to foods that have been subjected to less processing than usual (for example, hydrogenated nut butter and whole grain flour).

HEALTH TEAM

The provision of nutritional care involves a health team—a physician, nurse, dietitian or nutritionist, social worker, and occupational or physical therapist (see Fig. 1-3). A team approach with interaction of the members and the patient is necessary as a result of increasing complexity in providing health care.

Notice in Figure 1-3 that the patient is the central figure in the health team. Also notice the interaction of the members of the health team with each other (in reality, arrows should be drawn between every member of the team and every other member).[5]

UNIQUE ROLE OF THE NURSE ON THE HEALTH TEAM

A person might ask, "Why is the nurse bothered with nutritional care of the patient? I thought that the dietitian and the physician were responsible for this." The basic answers to this question focus on the fact that a staff nurse has more contact with a patient that any other member of the team. Some of the roles of the nurse as a member of the nutritional health team are as follows:

- Providing liaison service between the patient and dietitian and between the dietitian and physician.

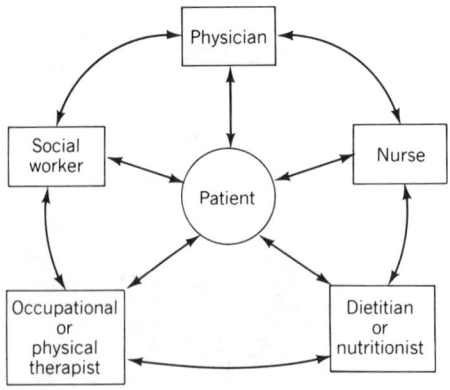

FIGURE 1-3 Health team interacting with a patient.

- Interpretation and transmittal of diet prescriptions.
- Assessment of the patients' response to the diet.
- Monitoring patients for food and drug interactions.
- Monitoring food intake of patients.
- Informing the dietitian of the food and nutrient concerns of patients.
- Alerting physicians to either maintenance or changes in the health status of patients in relation to nutrition.
- Teaching or reinforcing nutritional concepts to patients and their families.
- Reminding the health team that a patient has emotional as well as physical needs.[6]

STEPS FOLLOWED BY THE HEALTH TEAM IN PROVIDING NUTRITIONAL CARE

The provision of nutritional care in a clinic or hospital is a problem-solving process. There are four steps to this process: (1) assessment, (2) planning, (3) implementation, and (4) evaluation (see Fig. 1-4). A brief description of each step is presented below, and detailed information on this process is presented in Chapter 14.

Assessment

This step involves the collection of subjective and objective nutritional data on the patient, analysis of information, and diagnosis of the problem. The nurse plays a key role in this step, since much information is gathered while she completes the standard admitting nursing notes. The physician relies greatly on these notes, together with laboratory values on blood, urine, and stool specimens, to help diagnose the patient's problem.

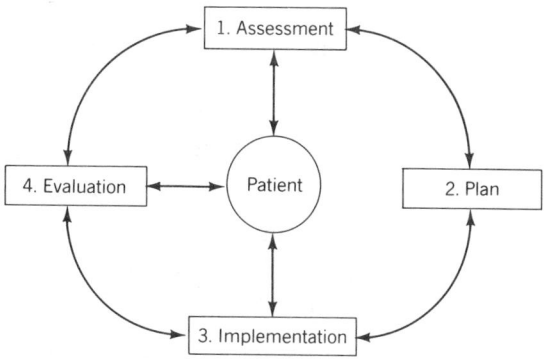

FIGURE 1-4   Problem-solving process for providing nutritional care.

Planning

Information gathered in the previous step is used to write a nutritional care plan. Since the plan is a written record of the care given a patient, it provides good communication among the members of the team. Some dietary departments may use a specific form for recording and implementing the plan.

Implementation

This step involves carrying out the nutritional orders. Members of the health team help by giving supportive care, providing a consistent approach, and facilitating communication between the doctor and patient. This stage also involves teaching and counseling patients.

Evaluation

In this final step, the effectiveness of the nutritional care plan objectives is assessed. If the objectives have not been met, the team will start the cyclical problem-solving process again, assessing new data on the patient and proceeding through the rest of the process.[6,7]

CULTURAL INFLUENCE ON FOOD HABITS AND IMPORTANCE TO HEALTH PROFESSIONALS

Food habits are the result of many influences such as personal, cultural, social, and psychological factors. A full discussion of each is beyond the scope of this text. However, we will discuss the cultural influence on food habits and why it is important for health professionals to understand it.

Culture The concept, skills, and broad-based characteristics of a given population.

    Culture relates to food and eating habits in a variety of ways.[8] Culture determines:

• Acceptable foods

• Appropriate methods of food handling, preparation, and storage

• Table manners

• Attitudes toward eating

• Attitudes toward obesity and other aspects of body size

• Attitudes about the relationship of food and health[9]

One might ask, of what importance is cultural influence on food habits to a health professional? The answer is related essentially to the roles of health team members in teaching nutrition concepts to patients and their families, as well as in assessment of patient responses to diets. In order to perform these roles effectively, a health professional needs to separate his or her own cultural background and apply the patient's cultural food patterns to the task at hand. Food patterns of two major U.S. cultures are given in Table 1-2.

FOOD FALLACIES, CONTROVERSIES, AND FACTS: A CHALLENGE FOR THE HEALTH PROFESSIONAL

Food fallacies False, deceptive ideas about food and its effects in the body.

If a health professional is to teach nutrition concepts effectively to patients and their families, it is not enough to have only a good scientific foundation of nutritional knowledge. The professional needs to be informed about **food fallacies** and controversies in order to respond accurately and authoritatively to patients who have questions about food fallacies.

HEALTH DANGERS OF FOOD FALLACIES

There are three basic ways that food fallacies may adversely affect a person.

Increase the Risks of High-Risk People

People who are in high-risk health groups can be adversely affected by food fallacies. For example, people with a chronic illness (such as cancer, arthritis, or diabetes) may turn to food fads to alleviate their symptoms, since conventional treatments have not produced dramatic results. Teenagers can be harmed by food fallacies that promise to improve physique and figure development.[10]

Rebound scurvy A condition that occurs when a pregnant woman takes megadoses of vitamin C, causing the fetus to adapt to the massive doses. After birth, without continued ingestion of vitamin C, the infant shows signs of scurvy.

Malnutrition

Some people may actually suffer from malnutrition as a result of a food fad. Vitamin A poisoning (see Chapter 6) can occur following consumption of large doses of vitamin A for acne. Excessive intake of vitamin C has been found to cause kidney stones, impaired ability of white blood cells to kill bacterial, and **rebound scurvy** in infants born to mothers who take megadoses of vitamin C.[11]

TABLE 1-2 CULTURAL FOOD HABITS

Culture	Milk	Meat	Vegetables and Fruit	Bread and Cereals
Southern United States food habits	Limited amount consumed Cheese is consumed in sandwiches	Chicken Beef in stews Eggs are usually fried Legumes—black eyed peas Peanut butter	Few vegetables raw leafy green, turnip greens and mustard greens, and collards are popular Little citrus fruit eaten; watermelon and lemonade are popular in summer	Few whole grain cereals are eaten Hominy grits with gravy Cornbread Dumplings and pancakes White rice combined with ham, tomatoes, onions, and okra
Spanish American and Mexican food habits	Limited due to availability Cheese can be limited due to certain financial conditions (poverty)	Chicken, pork chops, weiners and cold cuts Eggs are usually fried Beans usually eaten with each meal	Fried potatoes are basic Green and red peppers are popular for all meals Pumpkin, corn, field greens, onions, and carrots Bananas, melons, peaches, and canned fruit	Tortillas from enriched wheat flour Breakfast cereals with sugar coating are popular Oatmeal used occasionally Fried macaroni is popular

Source: Adapted with permission from *Cultural Food Patterns in the USA,* Chicago, American Dietetic Association, 1976.

Economics

People spend large sums of money on food fads:

$105 million on weight fads in 1980

$2 million on vitamin fads

70% higher food prices for "organic," "natural," or "health foods"[11]

Consumers are frequently confused by claims made for organic, natural, and health foods. As a result, they tend to buy these more expensive foods in the belief that if it costs more, it must be better. Often the consumer who spends excessively on food fads cannot afford to do so.

DEFINITIONS

Some terms and their definitions are necessary to discuss food fallacies and controversies.

Food fad. Any dietary concept that remains scientifically unproven.

Natural food. A term for which there is little agreement on meaning. It is marketed as a food that is produced with minimal processing and without the use of preservatives, additives, or other artificial ingredients.

Organically grown food. Food fertilized with manure rather than chemical fertilizers and processed without additives or chemicals.[12]

Megadose. A quantity that exceeds by 10 times or more the normal recommended amount of a vitamin.

Table 1-3 briefly presents examples of various fallacies; details are given in later chapters.

DIETARY GOALS FOR THE UNITED STATES

Calorie A measure of the energy value of substances; defined as the amount of heat required to raise the temperature of 1 g of water 1° Celsius (C).

In the 1960s, the Senate Select Committee on Nutrition and Human Needs was formed to study the nutritional status of the public. The committee held hearings for several years before publishing a number of recommendations in its publication entitled *Dietary Goals for the U.S.* (1977). The seven goals stated in the revised edition are:

1. To avoid becoming overweight, consume only as much energy (**calories**) as is expended. If you are overweight, decrease energy intake and increase energy expenditure.

TABLE 1-3 FOOD FALLACIES VERSUS FACTS

Fallacy	Facts
1. Grapefuit causes the body to burn fat more rapidly than other foods.	1. No foods actually cause fat to be burned up. Bulky, low-calorie foods cause a feeling of fullness and, therefore, less food is eaten.[13]
2. Vitamin C prevents common colds.	2. Extensive research shows that megadoses of vitamin C do not prevent common colds, but can be toxic when taken over a long period (see Chapter 6 for details).[14]
3. Vitamin A can help reduce acne.	3. Megadoses of vitamin A for acne caused many toxic problems. A derivative of vitamin A (accutane) has shown success in reducing acne when given in megadose amounts. People are carefully monitored for toxic effects.[10]
4. Oysters increase sexual potency.	4. No foods have been shown to increase sexual potency (affected by levels of hormones).[15]
5. Red wine and beets are good for increasing the amount of blood.	5. Increased production of blood requires protein and iron. Neither of these foods are rich in these nutrients.[16]
6. Orange juice is too acid for infants.	6. Citrus fruits are not acid formers in the body of an adult or an infant, but rather are base formers.
7. Eating two eggs per day can double the blood cholesterol level.	7. Increasing blood cholesterol is not a simple matter of eating two eggs per day.[15]
8. Cheese can cause constipation.	8. Low-residue foods in general can cause constipation. Cheese is essentially milk and therefore an excellent food.[15]
9. Adolescent acne is caused by eating too much chocolate and junk foods.	9. Acne in adolescents is a result of an increase in sex hormones and their interaction with oil-producing (sebaceous) glands.
10. Bread and potatoes are especially fattening and should be eliminated from weight loss diets.	10. Any food eaten in excess can cause a person to become fat. Both of these foods contain complex carbohydrates that are very beneficial for the body (see Chapter 3 for details).[18]
11. Natural vitamins and minerals are superior to synthetic ones.	11. The body cannot distinguish between synthetic and natural vitamins and minerals. Chemically they are identical.[13]
12. Honey is a better nutritional source of sugar than refined sugar.	12. Refined white sugar and honey contain the same sugars (carbohydrates). Honey also contains a very small amount of vitamins and minerals (for details see Chapter 3).[13]
13. Food grown with natural organic fertilizers is superior to that grown with chemical fertilizers.	13. Natural organic and chemical fertilizers essentially contain the same nutrients necessary for plant growth.[17]
14. Fad weight loss diets (for example, the Beverly Hills Diet, Cambridge Diet, Dr. Atkins Diet) are equal to or better than medically prescribed and supervised diets.	14. Best-seller fad diets will help some people lose weight, but 80–90% of them regain the weight. These diets do not attack the psychological problems that cause overeating. A medical diet is designed to help a person lose weight permanently by changing the person's eating habits.[10]

Naturally occurring sugars Sugars found naturally in foods, such as glucose and fructose, as opposed to artificial sugars, such as sorbital and xylitol (see Chapter 19).

2. Increase the consumption of complex carbohydrates and **naturally occurring sugars** from about 28% to about 48% of energy intake.

3. Reduce the consumption of refined and processed sugars by about 45% to about 10% of total energy intake.

4. Reduce overall fat consumption from approximately 40% to about 30% of energy intake.

5. Reduce saturated fat consumption to about 10% of total energy intake and balance that consumption with polyunsaturated and monounsaturated fats, which should each account for about 10% of energy intake.

6. Reduce cholesterol consumption to about 300 mg a day.

7. Limit the intake of sodium by reducing the intake of salt to about 5 g a day.

The Senate Select Committee compared the current American diet with its recommended diet as set forth in its dietary goals:

Current Diet	Dietary Goals
Fat: 42%	Fat: 30%
Protein: 12%	Protein: 12%
Carbohydrates: 46%	Carbohydrates: 58%
Complex carbohydrate: 22%	Complex carbohydrate: 48%
Sugar: 24%	Sugar: 10%

It should be emphasized that the committee's dietary goals were criticized by many groups. Other dietary reports have been published by other committees, such as the joint committee of the U.S. Department of Agriculture and the former Department of Health, Education and Welfare. They published a set of dietary guidelines for Americans called "Nutrition and Your Health" (1980), which recommended the following:

1. Eat a variety of foods.

2. Maintain ideal weight.

3. Avoid too much fat, saturated fat, and cholesterol.

4. Eat foods with adequate starch and fiber.

5. Avoid too much sugar.

6. Avoid too much sodium.

7. If you drink alcohol, do so in moderation.

OUTLINE

DEFINITION OF NUTRITION

Nutrition is the combination of processes by which the body receives and utilizes the materials necessary to maintain homeostasis.

FOUR MAIN COMPONENTS OF THE STUDY OF NUTRITION

Nutrients
Body processes
Nutrient requirements
Homeostasis

Nutrients
There are six classes: carbohydrates, fats, proteins, vitamins, minerals, and water.

Energy Nutrients
Carbohydrates, fats, and proteins release energy when oxidized.

Organic Nutrients
Carbohydrates, fats, proteins, and vitamins are composed of compounds that contain carbon atoms; they provide energy, build tissues, and regulate body processes.

Inorganic Nutrients
Minerals and water are inorganic nutrients or are composed of compounds that do not contain carbon. Minerals: bone formation and conduction of nerve impulses. Water: medium for chemical reactions and transports materials.

IMPORTANT NUTRITIONAL TERMS

Seven terms are defined on p. 7.

HEALTH TEAM

A health team is composed of a physician, nurse, dietitian, social worker, and occupational or physical therapist.

Unique Role of the Nurse on the Health Team
The nurse has a great deal of contact with the patient and, as a member of the health team, has several roles: provides liaison service between the patient and dietitian and between the dietitian and physician; interprets and transmits diet prescriptions; assesses the responses of patients to diets; and monitors patients for food and drug interaction.

Four Steps Followed by the Health Team in Providing Nutritional Care

1. Assessment: collection and analysis of data on the patient, followed by diagnosis.
2. Planning: patient data are used to write a nutritional care plan.
3. Implementation: carrying out of the nutritional orders.
4. Evaluation: assessment of the effectiveness of the plan. If it is ineffective, then the process starts over again.

CULTURAL INFLUENCE ON FOOD HABITS AND IMPORTANCE TO THE HEALTH PROFESSIONAL

Culture is the concept, skills, and broad-based characteristics of a given population.
   Importance to the health professional of cultural influence on food habits:

1. Aids in teaching nutrition concepts to patients and families.
2. Assessment of patients' responses to diets.

FOOD FALLACIES, CONTROVERSIES, AND FACTS: A CHALLENGE FOR THE HEALTH PROFESSIONAL

Health Dangers of Food Fallacies

Increase the risks of high-risk people
Malnutrition
Economics

REVIEW QUESTIONS

TRUE (A) OR (B) FALSE
Questions 1–8

1. Nutrition is defined as the maintenance of organ systems (respiratory and cardiovascular) in a dynamic state.
2. The four main components of the study of nutrition include nutrients, body processes, nutrient requirements, and homeostasis.
3. Energy nutrients include carbohydrate, fat, and vitamins.
4. Organic nutrients do not contain carbon atoms and function only to release energy.
5. Inorganic nutrients contain carbon atoms and include water and minerals.

6. The four steps followed by a health team in providing nutritional care are assessment, planning, implementation, and evaluation.
7. Cultural influence is important to health team members in teaching nutrition concepts and assessment of patient responses to diets.
8. Food fallacies may adversely affect a person by increasing the risks of high-risk people, causing malnutrition, and causing people to spend excessive amounts of money.

MATCHING
Questions 9–13

9. __ Homeostasis
10. __ Minerals
11. __ Energy nutrients
12. __ Culture
13. __ Food fad

A. dietary concept that remains scientifically unproven.
B. conduction of nerve impulses.
C. concepts, skills, and broad-based characteristics of a given population.
D. maintenance of organ systems in a dynamic state.
E. carbohydrate, fat, and protein.

14. The components of the study of nutrition are
   1. nutrients
   2. organic compounds
   3. body processes
   4. inorganic compounds
   A. 1, 2, 3 B. 1, 3 C. 2, 4 D. 4
   E. all of these
15. Inorganic nutrients include:
   A. minerals
   B. vitamins
   C. water
   D. A, C
   E. B, C
16. The steps followed by a health team (in sequence) in providing nutritional care are:
   A. assessment, implementation, planning, and evaluation.
   B. assessment, evaluation, implementation, and planning.
   C. assessment, planning, evaluation, and implementation.
   D. assessment, planning, implementation, and evaluation.
17. Which of the following is (are) *incorrectly* paired?
   A. food fad—dietary concept that remains scientifically unproven.
   B. natural food—foods fertilized with manure rather than chemical fertilizers.

C. fallacy—a false, deceptive idea.
D. none of these.

DISCUSSION QUESTIONS

1. Define nutrition and describe the four main components of the study of nutrition.
2. Define culture and list four ways in which it relates to food and eating habits.
3. Define food fad, natural food, health food, and megadose.
4. Give the Senate Select Committee's recommended dietary goals in terms of percentages of fat, protein, and carbohydrates.

REFERENCES

1. D.F. Tver and P. Russell. *The Nutrition and Health Encyclopedia.* New York: Van Nostrand Reinhold, 1981.
2. M. Green and J. Harry. *Nutrition in Contemporary Nursing Practice.* New York: John Wiley & Sons, Inc., 1981, pp. 56–79.
3. S.J. Wickham. *Human Nutrition.* Bowie, Md.: Robert J. Brady, 1982, p. 4.
4. H.A. Guthrie. "Junk foods: A scientific evaluation." *The Professional Nutritionist,* 12(12), 251–253 (1980).
5. W.A. Krehl. "Nutrition: Does the physician know enough?" *The Professional Nutritionist,* 8(3), 3 (1976).
6. M. Gordon. "Nursing diagnosis and the diagnostic process." *American Journal of Nursing,* 76, 1298 (1976).
7. A. Henneman and J.F. Haufek. "Teaching nutritional assessment to nursing students." *Journal of the American Dietetic Association,* 78, 498–500 (May 1981).
8. American Dietetic Association. *Cultural Food Patterns in the U.S.A.* Chicago: American Dietetic Association, 1976.
9. C.W. Suitor and M.F. Hunter. *Nutrition: Principles and Application in Health Promotion,* 2nd ed. Philadelphia: J.B. Lippincott, 1984, p. 92.
10. T. Beaudette. "Food fads, facts and controversies: A challenge for the dietitian." *Nutrition in Practice,* (April–May 1982), p. 20.
11. V. Herbert. "The Health Hustlers," in V. Herbert, ed., *Nutrition Cultism: Facts and Fiction.* Philadelphia: George F. Stickley Co., 1980, pp. 36–45.
12. M. Stephenson. "The confusing world of health foods." *FDA Consumer,* 12(18) (1978), pp. 11–14.

13. L.E. Poplin. "Practical knowledge of nutrition in the health sciences." *Journal of the American Dietetic Association*, 77, 576–580 (November 1980).

14. W.T. Jarvis. "Coping with food faddism." *Nutrition and the M.D.*, 6, 3 (October 1980).

15. D. Roe. *Clinical Nutrition for the Health Scientist*. Boca Raton, Fla.: CRC Press, Inc., 1979, pp. 4–6.

16. S.R. Williams. *Nutrition and Diet Therapy*, 4th ed. St. Louis: C.V. Mosby Co., 1981, pp. 228–229.

17. E.M. Hamilton and E.N. Whitney. *Nutrition: Concepts and Controversies*, 2nd ed. St. Paul: West Publishing, 1982, p. 307.

18. V. Aranson and B. Fitzgerald. *Guidebook for Nutrition Counselors*. North Quincy, Mass.: Christopher Publishing House, 1980, p. 31.

2 DIETARY PLANNING

OBJECTIVES

Upon completion of this chapter, you should be able to:

1. Define the four components of a nutritious diet.

2. List the four food groups and the major nutrients contributed by each one.

3. List the number of daily servings for each food group appropriate for adults.

4. Describe five ways in which the Modified Four-Food Group Plan is different from the Traditional Four-Food Group Plan.

5. Describe the difference between a vegan and a lacto-ovo vegetarian diet.

6. Discuss three possible deficiencies of a vegetarian diet.

7. Discuss four advantages of a vegetarian diet.

8. Name the six exchange lists.

9. Give the grams of carbohydrate, protein, and fat and the kilocalories for one exchange on each list.

10. Take a meal and calculate the grams of carbohydrate, fat, protein, and kilocalories for each food, as well as the total kilocalories.

11. Utilize information from objective 10 to calculate the percentage of the total kilocalories in the meal due to carbohydrate, fat, and protein.

12. Utilize information from objective 11 to determine whether the meal is balanced in regard to the distribution of carbohydrate, fat and protein.

13. Distinguish between RDAs and U.S. RDAs.

14. Name the nutrients that have established RDA values.

INTRODUCTION

The maintenance and restoration of good health are objectives with which consumers and health professionals are concerned. One way to achieve these objectives is by eating a nutritious diet. Four components of a nutritious diet are:

Essential nutrients
Compounds that the body cannot synthesize.

Adequacy. Foods that provide all of the **essential nutrients** and calories in the proper amounts.

Nutrient density (calories control). Refers to the content of specific nutrients in relation to kcal. High nutrient density foods are those that have a high level of nutrients with a low level of kcal. An example is skim milk compared to whole milk (see Table 2-5 for details).

Balance. Distribution of daily calories among fat, protein, and carbohydrate in a certain ratio. The normal ratio is: fat 30%, carbohydrate 55–60%, and protein 10–15% of calories.

Variety. Inclusion of a variety of foods in the daily diet.

FOOD GUIDES FOR PLANNING NUTRITIOUS DIETS

Two commonly used guides in planning nutritious diets are the Four-Food Group System and the Food Exchange System. These two guides allow one to plan a diet and achieve the four dietary components.

THE FOUR-FOOD GROUP SYSTEM

The Four-Food Group System was developed in 1954 by the United States Department of Agriculture (USDA). It converts quantitative nutrient data into food-related information that can be used by both consumers and health professionals in diet planning to achieve adequacy (see Clinical Application Importance of the Four-Food Group System to Health Professionals").

Recommended Dietary Allowances (RDAs)
Recommended allowances of certain nutrients that are established by the Food and Nutrition Board of the National Academy of Sciences–National Research Council (NAS–NRC).

Foods are placed into one of four groups (Table 2-1) depending on their composition and nutrient value. The four groups are: milk and milk products, meat (and meat substitutes), fruit and vegetables, and bread and cereal. The Four-Food Group Plan allows a person to achieve the nutrient needs specified in the **Recommended Dietary Allowances** (RDA) and, in so doing, also achieve adequacy. Each group specifies the major nutrients that it provides, along with serving sizes of foods

---

CLINICAL APPLICATION; IMPORTANCE OF THE FOUR-FOOD GROUP SYSTEM TO HEALTH PROFESSIONALS

---

1. Tool for Nutritional Assessment and Screening

A brief dietary history can quickly disclose inadequate intake from any of the four food groups. This information could be the first clue that the patient may be at high risk of developing a nutrition-related disorder or is compounding an existing health problem.

2. Tool for Nutritional Counseling

The dietary history and the simplicity of the Four-Food Group System allow members of the health team to counsel effectively or to teach a patient about nutrition.

3. Basis for Explaining Therapeutic Diets to Patients

Therapeutic diets are scientifically based on RDA values. However, use of the Four-Food Group System helps to explain the diet to a patient. For example, when instructing a patient placed on a mild sodium-restricted diet (2 to 3 g), a health professional can easily explain the diet by discussing foods allowed and foods to be avoided in each group.

The meat group can be discussed first by telling the patient that salted or smoked meats (bacon, luncheon meats, sausage, etc.) are to be avoided and baked, broiled, or stewed meats are allowed. Discussed next can be the vegetable group, with most fresh or frozen vegetables allowed and canned vegetables not allowed because of added salt. The other groups can be discussed in the same way.[1]

Kilocalorie (kcal) A unit of energy measurement that is calculated and expressed in relation to nutrition. A *calorie* is often called a *small calorie*, since 1,000 small calories equal 1 kilocalorie. Although it is not technically correct, some nutritional books and consumer literature refer to energy units in food as calories. To avoid confusion between the small physical calorie and the nutritional calorie, the unit *kcal* will be used throughout this book.

from that group. The number of servings required from each group for an adequate diet varies for adults, adolescents, infants and children, and pregnant or lactating women. These servings are presented in Table 2-2.

If an adult follows the Four-Food Group Pattern (two-two-four-four), his or her caloric intake would be about 1200 **kilocalories (kcal).** Additional kilocalories for people who require more than 1,200 can be obtained from the fifth group, known as the "Other" group (Table 2-1), which includes fats, sweets, and alcohol. A person can also consume additional servings from the Basic Four Food Groups.

TABLE 2-1 THE FOUR FOOD GROUPS

Group	Major Nutrients	Foods and Nutritional Service Sizes
Milk and milk products	Calcium Riboflavin (vitamin B$_2$) Protein	8 oz milk 1½ oz cheese 8 oz yogurt 2 cups cottage cheese 1 cup custard/pudding 4 scoops ice cream
Meat (and meat substitutes)	Protein Niacin Iron Thiamin (vitamin B$_1$)	2 oz cooked meat, poultry, fish 2 eggs 1 cup dried beans 4 tbsp peanut butter
Fruits and vegetables	Vitamin A Vitamin C	½ cup cooked fruit or vegetable ½ cup juice 1 cup raw whole fruit A citrus fruit is recommended daily for vitamin C
Bread and cereal	Carbohydrate Thiamin (vitamin B$_1$) Iron Niacin	1 slice bread 1 cup ready-to-eat cereal ½ cup cooked cereal, rice, or pasta
Other	—	Fats, sweets, and alcohol Foods from this group should not replace any from the four groups. Amounts consumed should be determined by individual caloric needs.

TABLE 2-2 RECOMMENDED SERVINGS FROM EACH FOOD GROUP

Food Group	Adult	Adolescents	Infants and Children	Pregnant and Lactating Women
Milk	2	4	3	4
Meat (and meat substitutes)	2	2	2	3
Fruit/vegetable	4	4	4	4
Bread/cereal	4	4	4	4

Source: S.J. Wickham: *Human Nutrition: A Self-Instructional Text.* Bowie, Md.: Robert J. Brady Co., 1982, p. 22.

MODIFIED FOUR-FOOD GROUP PLAN

Research has found that if a person follows the Four-Food Group Plan, the diet will be adequate except for the following nutrients: vitamin B_6, magnesium, zinc, and vitamin E.[2] In order to solve these deficiencies, a Modified Four-Food Group Plan (see Table 2-3 for a comparison of the Modified Four-Food Group Plan with the Traditional Four-Food Group Plan) was devised and published in 1978. Essentially, the modified features of the diet are as follows:

• The serving size of meat is increased to three ounces.
• A daily source of vegetable protein from legumes or nuts is recommended.
• One serving of fat or oil is recommended to provide vitamin E.
• One serving of dark green vegetables is recommended.
• One serving of a vitamin C fruit is recommended.

VEGETARIAN DIETS AND MODIFICATION OF THE FOUR-FOOD GROUP SYSTEM

Some people choose to follow a vegetarian diet for religious reasons, health concerns, environmental considerations, humanitarian issues, or economic or political reasons. There are two major classes of vegetarians (approximately four other variations exist):

Vegan Pure vegetarian diet that uses no animal or dairy products.

Vegan (pure vegetarian). A strict vegetarian diet, using no animal or dairy products. This diet may be inadequate in vitamins B_{12} and D,

TABLE 2-3 MODIFIED FOUR-FOOD GROUP PLAN COMPARED TO TRADITIONAL PLAN

Food Group	Number of Adult Servings for Modified Diet	Number of Adult Servings for the Traditional Diet
Milk and milk products	2	2
Meat and meat substitutes	4 2 servings (3 oz) of animal protein 2 servings ($\frac{3}{4}$ cup) of legumes and/or nuts	2
Fruit/vegetable	4 1 serving vitamin C–rich fruit 1 serving dark green vegetable	4
Bread/cereal	4	4
Fat	1	0

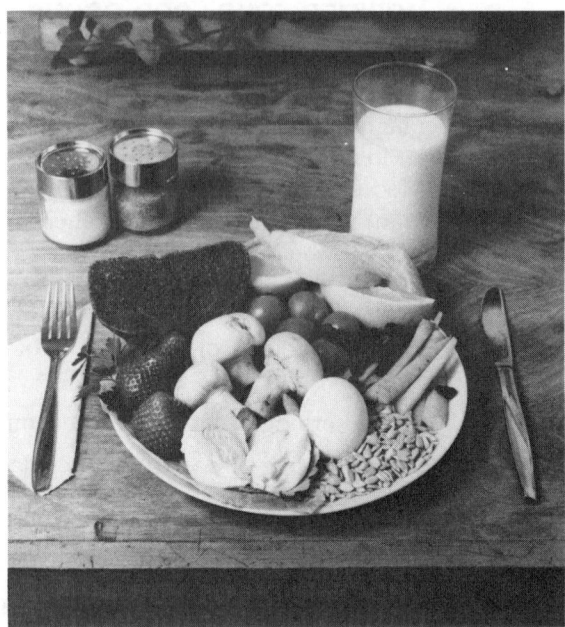

FIGURE 2-1 A lacto-ovo vegetarian meal.

riboflavin, calcium, iron, and zinc. Supplements of each are recommended.

Lacto-ovo vegetarian A
vegan diet that includes
milk, eggs, and other
dairy products.

Lacto-ovo vegetarian (lacto-milk, ovo-egg). This diet is a vegan diet,
except that milk, eggs, and other dairy products are included (see Fig.
2-1). This diet may be inadequate in iron, since meats are a good
source of iron.

Disadvantages and Advantages
of Vegetarian Diets

As indicated above, vegetarian diets can be deficient in certain nutrients.
A large quantity of food must be consumed in vegetarian diets in order
to meet calorie needs and can be difficult for some people to do, especially children. A person needs to know how to combine protein foods
in order to obtain all of the essential amino acids, a process known as
complementary protein supplementation (discussed in Chapter 5). Some
adaptations to the Four-Food Group Plan that help to overcome the
disadvantages in vegetarian diets (see Table 2-4) are as follows:

**Complementary protein
supplementation** A
strategy that involves eating two or more foods
that are complementary
to each other in amino
acids.

• Whole grain breads, cereals, and legumes. Make these foods the basis
  of the diet. Increase the number of servings from the grain group,
  including nuts and seeds.

TABLE 2-4 FOUR-FOOD GROUP PLAN FOR THE VEGETARIAN

Food Group	Number of Servings and Description
Milk and milk products	2–8-oz glasses (or soy milk fortified with vitamin B_{12}).
	Eggs can be used on the lacto-ovo diet as a substitute for dairy products.
Meat and meat substitutes	2 cups legumes daily; count 4 tbsp peanut butter as 1 serving.
Fruit	1 to 4 servings; include a raw source of vitamin C like citrus fruits, strawberries, or cantaloupe.
Vegetable	4 servings; include one or more servings of dark green vegetables.
Bread/cereal	4 servings of whole-grain foods.

Source: Reprinted by permission from *Laurel's Kitchen: A Handbook for Vegetarian Cookery and Nutrition,* by Laurel Robertson, Carol Flinders, and Bronwen Godfrey. Copyright 1976, Nilgiri Press, Petaluma, Calif.

- Milk and eggs. The recommended servings of milk and dairy products for the age group should be consumed. These are the only sources of vitamin B_{12} unless eggs are eaten.
- Vegetables and fruits. Eat a wide variety of vegetables and fruits daily.

Advantages of Vegetarian Diets

While there are several disadvantages to a vegetarian diet, there also are some advantages, such as these:

It increases fiber. Vegetables are high in fiber compared to meat, which is eliminated in this diet. Increased fiber aids in bowel movements and possibly helps to prevent problems like **diverticulitis** and colon cancer.

Diverticulitis Inflammation of diverticuli (outpouching of the colon lining) (see Chapter 19).

It decreases daily caloric intake. Vegetables tend to be low in calories; therefore, a vegetarian diet should be beneficial to people on a low-kilocalories weight-loss diet.

It decreases total fat, saturated fat, and cholesterol. Vegetables are low in fat and cholesterol compared to meat. This diet can be beneficial to people who have **hyperlipidemia** (elevated level of lipids in blood) and decreases the chances of developing **atherosclerosis.**

Hyperlipidemia Elevated level of lipids in the blood (see Chapter 21).

It provides a more economical source of protein than meat. For some societies, especially those of developing countries, meat is not readily available and can be very expensive. A vegetarian diet provides an affordable source of protein; however, it lacks some essential nu-

Atherosclerosis Accumulation of fatty plaques within medium-sized and large arteries (see Chapter 21).

trients, and protein supplementation has to be practiced to overcome this deficiency.[3]

The Traditional Four-Food Group System provides an average of about 1,200 kcal per day, whereas the Modified Four Food Group Plan provides adequacy and an average of about 2,200 kcal. The high level of kilocalories provided by the modified group is a problem for people whose kilocalorie allowance is not this high and therefore can cause them to gain weight. A person can plan a nutritious diet and can control the caloric intake by combining a second food guide, the Food Exchange System, with the Four-Food Group Plan.

THE FOOD EXCHANGE SYSTEM

The Food Exchange System is important in planning a nutritious diet, since two components, nutrient density and balance, are achieved when the guide is utilized. Essentially, the Food Exchange System can be used to select foods that are high in nutrient content but low in kilocalories. In order to make these calculations, one needs to know that:

1 g of carbohydrate = 4 kcal

1 g of lipid (fat) = 9 kcal

1 g of protein = 4 kcal

As an example, compare whole milk with skim or nonfat milk:

	Carbohydrate (g)	Protein (g)	Fat (g)	Total kcal
Whole milk	12	8	10	170
Skim milk	12	8	0	80

As we can see, whole milk and skim milk contain the same amounts of carbohydrate and proteins; however, whole milk also contains 10 g of fat, which contributes 90 kcal more than skim milk. Therefore, skim milk is a better nutrient density choice than whole milk.

In order to understand how the Food Exchange System allows one to choose foods high in nutrient density, a person must know the following important points about the system:

• Foods in the Four-Food Group System are separated into six exchange lists (see Table 2-5).

• Each list consists of foods of specific serving sizes that are equal in kilocalories, protein, fat, and carbohydrate (see Appendix A).

TABLE 2-5 THE SIX EXCHANGE LISTS

Exchange List	Serving Size	Carbohydrate (g)	Protein (g)	Fat (g)	Energy (kcal)
Milk	1 cup	12	8	0	80
(skim or nonfat)					
1% low-fat	1 cup	12	8	2.5	102.5
(add ½ fat exchange)					
2% low-fat	1 cup	12	8	5	125
(add 1 fat exchange)					
Whole milk	1 cup	12	8	10	170
(full fat; add 2 fat exchanges)					
Vegetable	½ cup	5	2	0	28
Fruit	varies	10	0	0	40
Bread	1 slice	15	2	0	68
(includes bread, cereal and starchy vegetables; serving sizes for cereal and starchy vege-tables are given in Appendix A)					
Meat					
(lean)	1 oz	0	7	3	55
(medium fat, add ½ fat exchange)	1 oz	0	7	5	75
(high-fat meat)	1 oz	0	7	8	100
Fat	1 tsp	0	0	5	45

- A food is placed on a list not because of the group it is in but because of its kilocalorie and nutrient contents (for example, corn and lima beans are not on the vegetable list but on the bread list because their kilocalorie and carbohydrate contents are similar to those of bread).
- Individual foods on the same list may be exchanged for each other, but not for foods on different lists.

Some important points about each exchange list are as follows:

1. *Milk list: one milk exchange is one cup of skim milk = 80 kcal.* A person using this exchange should think of skim milk as "milk" and whole milk as "milk plus two fat exchanges." See Table 2-5 for the calories and fat content of 1% and 2% low-fat milk.

2. *Vegetable list: one vegetable exchange is one-half cup = 25 kcal.* The vegetable list includes only low-calorie vegetables; therefore, higher-calorie vegetables (for example, corn, potatoes, and lima beans) are not included on this list but rather on the bread list.

3. *Fruit list: one fruit exchange serving size varies = 40 kcal.* Serving sizes of fruits vary, but always equal 40 kcal. This exchange list specifies "no added sugar or sugar syrup."

4. *Bread list: one bread exchange serving size varies = 70 kcal.* This list includes breads, cereals, and starchy vegetables. The serving sizes vary, but all equal 70 kcal. The list also indicates which foods contain added fat exchanges (see appendix A).

5. *Meat list: one meat exchange is 1 oz lean meat = 55 kcal.* This list separates meats, cheeses, and peanut butter into three groups (lean, medium-fat, and high-fat) depending upon the amount of fat present.

6. *Fat list: one fat exchange serving size varies = 45 kcal.*[4] This list informs users about foods that contain almost nothing but fat and indicates which foods contain saturated and polyunsaturated fats. Appendix A summarizes information about each exchange list.

USE OF THE FOOD EXCHANGE SYSTEM TO ACHIEVE BALANCE

The Food Exchange System can be used to achieve the balance component of a nutritious diet. Previously, it was stated that a balanced diet is one that distributes kilocalories among fat, protein, and carbohydrate in the following proportions:

fat: 30% of total kilocalories

carbohydrate: 55–60% of total kilocalories

protein: 10–15% of total kilocalories

Since the number of grams of carbohydrate, fat, and protein within each food exchange is known, it can then be calculated how many grams and kilocalories are present in a meal. Also, meals can be planned to achieve these or modified percentages of fat, carbohydrate, and protein.

An example of a meal in which these calculations can be made is shown in Figure 2-2. The calculations for the foods in Figure 2-2 are shown in Table 2-6 and explained below.

1. Total kilocalories = 440

2. Calculations of carbohydrate
   a. Total grams of carbohydrate = 32
   b. Total kilocalories due to carbohydrate $= \frac{32\cancel{g}}{1} \times \frac{4 \text{ kcal}}{\cancel{g}} = 128$ kcal
      (1g = 4 kcal)
   c. Percentage of total kilocalories due to carbohydrate $= \frac{128 \text{ kcal}}{440 \text{ kcal}} \times 100 = 29\%$

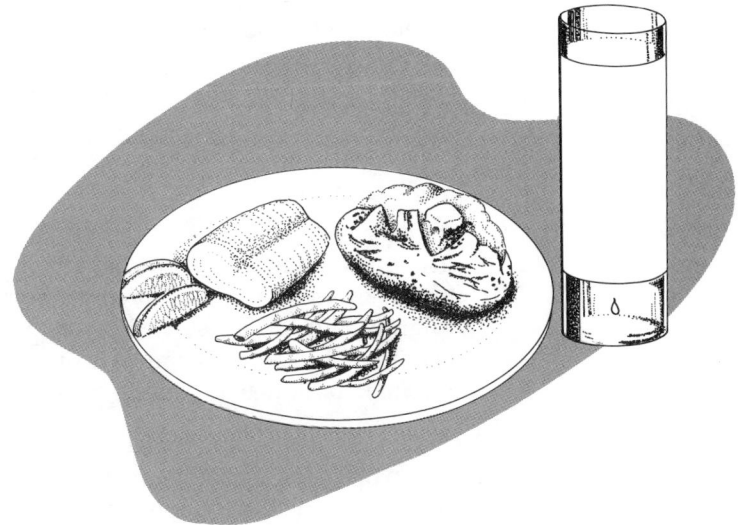

FIGURE 2-2 This meal consists of 1 cup skim milk, $\frac{1}{2}$ cup green beans, 1 small potato, 1 pat of margarine, and 4 oz of fish. See the text for determining the number of grams of carbohydrate, fat, protein, and kilocalories.

3. Calculation of fat
   a. Total grams of fat = 17
   b. Total kilocalories due to fat = $\dfrac{17\cancel{g}}{1} \times \dfrac{9 \text{ kcal}}{\cancel{g}}$ = 153 kcal
      (1g = 9 kcal)
   c. Percentage of total kilocalories due to fat = $\dfrac{153 \text{ kcal}}{440 \text{ kcal}} \times 100 =$ 35%

4. Calculations of protein
   a. Total grams of protein = 40

TABLE 2-6

	Exchange(s)	Carbohydrate (g)	Fat (g)	Protein (g)	Kcal
1 cup skim milk	milk	12	0	8	80
$\frac{1}{2}$ cup green beans	vegetable	5	0	2	25
1 small potato	bread	15	0	2	70
1 pat margarine	fat	0	5	0	45
4 oz fish	4 meat (lean)	0	12	28	220 (4 × 55)
		32	17	40	440

b. Total kilocalories due to protein $= \dfrac{40 \ g}{1} \times \dfrac{4 \ \text{kcal}}{g} = 160$ kcal

(1g = 4 kcal)

c. Percentage of total kilocalories due to protein $= \dfrac{160 \ \text{kcal}}{440 \ \text{kcal}} \times$

100 = 36%

5. Summary of calculations

The meal in Fig. 2-2 is low in carbohydrate, since 29% of the total kilocalories are due to carbohydrate compared to 55–60%. The meal is slightly high in fat, since 35% of the total kilocalories are due to fat compared to 30%. The meal is quite high in protein, since 36% of the total kilocalories are due to protein compared to 10–15%.

This meal is not exactly balanced, but the next two meals can be planned so that carbohydrates are increased (possibly by including fruits) and proteins are decreased (possibly by decreasing the serving sizes of high-protein foods) to achieve the recommended percentages.

Health professionals use the Food Exchange System in planning diets for hospitalized patients (see the Clinical Application "Planning a Hospital Diet Using the Food Exchange System").

The fourth component of a nutritious diet is variety. People should eat a variety of foods rather than the same ones each day. A variety of foods enables a person to achieve adequacy more easily than by consuming only a few foods. The adherence of hospital patients to their diets is increased if a variety of foods are served. Most foods contain some additives, some of which can be toxic at high levels; by eating a variety of foods, the possibility of developing a toxic condition is reduced.

RECOMMENDED DIETARY ALLOWANCES (RDAS)

Nutritionists and health professionals frequently refer to Recommended Dietary Allowance (RDA) values when planning an adequate diet. The recommendations are established by the Food and Nutrition Board of the National Academy of Sciences–National Research Council (NAS–NRC) and published by the U.S. government.[5] Approximately every 5 years, the Committee on RDA meets to reexamine and revise these recommendations on the basis of new evidence regarding people's nutrient needs. The most recent recommendations were published in 1980 (see inside front cover).

CLINICAL APPLICATION: PLANNING A HOSPITAL DIET USING THE FOOD EXCHANGE SYSTEM

In planning a diet for a hospitalized patient, health professionals utilize the Food Exchange System. First, the total kilocalories for a day is established; then the percentage of protein, carbohydrate, and fat that is to make up the total kilocalories is calculated. The amount of carbohydrate, fat, and protein in grams can then be determined. A calculation of the total number of exchanges for each list necessary to meet the above requirements has to be made. Then the distribution of these exchanges into actual recommended foods for breakfast, noon, evening, and bedtime meals is planned.

The following example illustrates these points. The patient has been prescribed a 1,500 kcal/day diet.

25% protein	375 kcal	94 g	$4 \dfrac{\text{kcal}}{\text{g}}$
50% carbohydrate	750 kcal	188 g	$4 \dfrac{\text{kcal}}{\text{g}}$
25% fat	375 kcal	42 g	$9 \dfrac{\text{kcal}}{\text{g}}$

Exchange List	Number of Exchanges
1. Milk	2
2. Vegetable	5
3. Fruit	5
4. Bread (starch)	6
5. Meat	8
6. Fat	2

Exchange	Foods
Breakfast	
1 Milk (skim) exchange	1 cup skim milk
1 fruit exchange	½ grapefruit
2 Bread (starch) exchange	1 serving all-bran cereal 1 slice whole wheat bread
2 Meat exchange (med.-fat)	2 poached eggs
0 Fat exchange	

Noon

<u>0</u> Milk (skim) exchange	
<u>2</u> Vegetable exchange	1 whole tomato
	2 medium carrots
<u>2</u> Fruit exchange	$\frac{1}{2}$ cantaloupe
<u>2</u> Bread exchange	2 slices whole wheat bread
<u>3</u> Meat exchange (lean)	3 oz white tuna
<u>1</u> Fat exchange	1 tsp. mayonnaise

Evening

<u>0</u> Milk exchange	
<u>3</u> Vegetable exchange	$1\frac{1}{2}$ cup broccoli
<u>1</u> Fruit exchange	1 small apple
<u>1</u> Bread exchange	1 small baked potato
<u>3</u> Meat exchange (lean)	3 oz lean roast beef
<u>1</u> Fat exchange	1 tsp margarine

Bedtime Snack

<u>1</u> Milk exchange	1 cup skim milk
<u>1</u> Fruit exchange	$\frac{1}{2}$ banana
<u>1</u> Bread exchange	1 serving all-bran cereal

If you add up the total kilocalories for all of the meals (420 + 480 + 395 + 190 = 1,485) and the number of exchanges for each list, you will see that the meals have achieved all of the original nutritional objectives.

Assuming that the 25% protein, 50% carbohydrate, and 25% fat of the total kilocalories does not change, a diet planner uses different patterns of exchanges for different kilocalorie levels. The following example illustrates this for 1,500-, 1,800-, and 2,000-kcal diets.

Energy Level (kcal)—25% Protein, 50% Carbohydrate, 25% fat.

Number of Exchanges	1,500	1,800	2,000
Milk	2	2	2
Vegetable	5	5	5
Fruit	5	7	7
Bread	6	7	9
Meat	8	10	11
Fat	2	2	2

NUTRIENTS RECOMMENDED AND DIVISION OF RDA INTO AGE AND SEX GROUPS

The main RDA table contains recommendations for protein, 10 vitamins, and 6 minerals. In addition to the main table, there is the Estimated Safe and Adequate Daily Dietary Intake (ESADDI) table (see inside back cover) of recommended values for three vitamins and nine more minerals. These nutrients are listed in a separate table, since there is less information on which to base the allowances, and the figures are in the form of ranges of recommended intakes.

The revised 1985 RDA publication also separates the kilocalorie recommendations or the Recommended Energy Intake (Appendix M) from the main table.

The recommendations are made for different groups—infants, children, men, women, and pregnant and lactating women. Each grouping is further subdivided into age groups.

Important points about the RDAs are as follows:

- They are recommendations, not requirements.

- They include a substantial margin of safety; therefore, two-thirds of the RDA is often deemed adequate, except for energy.

- The recommendations are for health people only; therefore, for ill people, the values could be higher or lower.

- There is a recommendation for protein but not for carbohydrate and fat.

U.S. RDAs

U.S. RDAs Nutrient
recommendations estab-
lished by the U.S. Food
and Drug Administration
(FDA) that are used as a
standard for nutritional
labeling.

The **U.S. RDAs** are used as a standard for nutritional labeling. For example, a food label on a cereal box might state that one serving provides about 25% of the U.S. RDA for iron.

There are four different sets of U.S. RDAs:

• Baby food set. These recommendations are for infants 12 months of age or under and are used with baby foods.

• Junior food set. These recommendations are for children between the ages of 1 and 4 years and are used with junior foods.

• Pregnant and lactating women. These recommendations are for increases in certain nutrients for women in these special situations.

• Adults and children over the age of 4. This is the set that is used on the majority of food labels that a person reads.

Although the 1980 revised RDA tables included a few changes for certain nutrients, the rest of the recommendations are based on 1968 RDAs. The U.S. RDA values were chosen from among the highest amounts recommended for each nutrient in the 1968 RDA table. Therefore, most of the U.S. RDA values are the same as the RDAs for a man, since they have the greatest nutrient requirements of any group. The exceptions to this statement are iron, thiamin, niacin, iodine, and magnesium. Women have a greater need for iron then men and, as a result, the woman's RDA for iron is used for the U.S. RDA. The RDAs for thiamin, niacin, iodine, and magnesium are based on the needs of an adolescent boy, since they are even higher than adult RDAs.

The highest RDA values are used for each nutrient to ensure that the nutrient needs of all persons are met. Therefore, when a person reads that a label provides 25% of the U.S. RDA for iron, whether the person is a 7-year-old boy or a 60-year-old woman, he or she can be assured that the need for iron is being met.

OUTLINE

INTRODUCTION

Four components of a nutritious diet:

1. Adequacy—foods that provide all essential nutrients and calories in the proper amounts.
2. Nutrient density—foods high in nutrient content but low in kilocalories.
3. Balance—distribution of calories—fat 30%, carbohydrate 55–60%, and proteins 10–15%.
4. Variety—eating a variety of foods to achieve adequacy and avoid possible toxic buildup of additives.

FOOD GUIDES FOR PLANNING A NUTRITIOUS DIET

Two guides for planning nutritious diets: Four-Food Group System and Food Exchange System

1. The Four-Food Group System
   a. Foods are placed into four groups depending on their composition.
   b. The system is adequate except for vitamin B_6, magnesium, zinc, and vitamin E.
   c. The Modified Four-Food Group Plan was designed to eliminate the above deficiencies.
   d. Vegetarian diets and modifications of the Four-Food Group System
      Two major classes of vegetarians:
      • Vegan—strict vegetarian, using no animal or dairy products.
      • Lacto-ovo vegetarian—vegan diet, except that milk, eggs, and other dairy products are included.
      (1) Disadvantages—the diet can be deficient in vitamins B_{12} and D, riboflavin, calcium, iron, and zinc; a large quantity of food must be consumed to meet calorie needs; protein supplementation must be practiced.
      (2) Advantages—the diet increases fiber; decreases daily calorie intake; decreases total fat, saturated fat, and cholesterol; and provides a more economical source of protein.
2. The Food Exchange System
   a. This guide can be used to achieve nutrient density and balance.
   b. Foods of the Four-Food Group System are separated into six exchange lists.
      (1) Foods are placed on a list because of their kilocalorie and nutrient contents.
      (2) Each food on a list is equal in kilocalories, protein, fat, and carbohydrate.
      (3) Individual foods on the same list may be exchanged for each other but not for foods on different lists.
   c. Use of the Food Exchange System to achieve balance.
      (1) A balanced diet is one that distributes daily kilocalories in the following proportions: carbohydrates 55–60%, fat 30%, and protein 10–15%.
      (2) The system can distribute kilocalories in the above proportions, since the exact number of grams for each nutrient is known and using 1 g carbohydrate = 4 kcal, 1 g lipid = 9 kcal and 1 g protein = 4 kcal.
   d. Variety
      This is the fourth component of a nutritious diet. A variety of foods should be consumed in order to achieve adequacy and to reduce the possibility of toxicity from additives.

RECOMMENDED DIETARY ALLOWANCES (RDA)

Recommendations for certain nutrients that are used by nutritionists and health professionals when planning an adequate diet; recommendations established by the Food and Nutrition Board of the National Academy of Sciences–National Research Council (NAS–NRC); approximately every 5 years, the committee meets to re-examine and revise these recommendations on the basis of new evidence on nutrient needs.

Nutrients Recommended and Division of RDA Into Age and Sex Groups

Main RDA table has recommendations for protein, 10 vitamins, and 6 minerals; in addition, nutrient values for 3 more vitamins and 9 more minerals are in the Estimated Safe and Adequate Daily Dietary Intake (ESADDI) table.

Recommendations are made for infants, children, men, women, and pregnant and lactating women.

Important points about the RDAs are as follows:

• They are recommendations, not requirements.
• Two-thirds of the RDA is often deemed adequate except for energy.
• Recommendations are for healthy people only; for ill people, the values may be higher or lower.
• RDAs are given for protein, but not for carbohydrate and fat.

U.S. RDAs
Nutrient values that are used as a standard for nutritional labeling
Four different sets of U.S. RDAs:

• Baby food set
• Junior food set
• Pregnant and lactating women
• Adults and children over the age of 4

U.S. RDA values are chosen from the highest amount recommended for each nutrient in the RDA table; the highest RDA values are chosen to ensure that the nutrient needs of all persons are met.

REVIEW QUESTIONS

TRUE (A) OR (B) FALSE
Questions 1–19

1. The four components of a nutritious diet are adequacy, nutrient density, balance, and high fiber.
2. An adequate diet is defined as a diet that is composed of foods that provide all of the essential nutrients and calories in the proper amounts.
3. A balanced diet is one that distributes daily kilocalories in to the following proportions: fat 55–60%, carbohydrate 30%, and protein 10–15%.
4. Two diet planning guides that help people achieve a nutritious diet are the Four-Food Group System and the Cambridge Diet.
5. The Four-Food Group System includes milk, meat, fruit/vegetable, and bread/cereal.
6. If one followed the traditional Four-Food Group Plan, one's diet would be adequate except for vitamin B_6, magnesium, zinc, and vitamin E.
7. The two most common vegetarian diets are vegan and lacto-ovo vegetarian.
8. The only disadvantage of vegetarian diets is that a person does not receive an adequate amount of kilocalories without consuming a large amount of food.
9. The Modified Four-Group Plan is a low-kilocalorie plan and decreases the intake of nutrients above those of the Traditional Four-Food Group Plan.
10. The Food Exchange System is most valuable in achieving adequacy.
11. Any food on any exchange list can be exchanged for any food on any other list.
12. A user of the Food Exchange System should think of skim milk as milk and whole milk as milk plus two fat exchanges.

13. Based upon the Food Exchange System, all meats are in the same group.
14. If a person consumes 2,000 kcal/day, approximately 55–60%, or 1,100–1,200 kcal, should come from carbohydrate.
15. RDA values are established for energy (kcal), protein, (g), vitamins (10), and minerals (6).
16. RDAs are very valuable for planning therapeutic diets.
17. RDAs are not expressed in group by age, sex, and weight.
18. U.S. RDAs differ from RDAs in that they appear on food labels.
19. Each U.S. RDA for persons aged 4 years or older was chosen from the highest amount for each RDA.

MATCHING

These questions and answers are based on information in Table 2-1. Match each group on the left with major nutrients on the right.

Group	Major Nutrients
20. Milk	A. Fats, sweets, and alcohol
21. Meat	B. Vitamins A and C
22. Fruit and vegetables	C. Carbohydrate
23. Bread and cereal	D. Calcium
24. Other	E. Protein

MATCHING

These questions and answers are based on information in Table 2-5. Match each exchange on the left with nutritional information on the right.

Exchange List	Carbohydrate (g)	Protein (g)	Fat (g)	Energy (kcal)
25. Milk	A. 10	0	0	40
26. Vegetable	B. 0	7	3	55
27. Fruit	C. 15	2	0	70
28. Bread	D. 12	8	0	80
29. Meat	E. 5	2	0	25

Questions 30–35 are based on the following meal. An example of how to make the calculations necessary to answer these questions is given in Table 2-6. The values for the foods below are found in Appendix A.

½ cup spinach
1 cup whole milk
1 small potato
1 pat margarine
6 oz fish

30. The total kilocalories for the meal are _____.
    A. 550
    B. 1,040
    C. 640
    D. 440

31. The total grams of carbohydrate in the above meal are _____.
    A. 32
    B. 17
    C. 25
    D. 62

32. The total grams of fat in the above meal are _____.
    A. 17
    B. 22
    C. 35
    D. 33

33. The total grams of protein in the above meal are _____.
    A. 40
    B. 54
    C. 45
    D. 65

34. The percentages of kilocalories due to carbohydrate (C), fat (F), and protein (P) in the above meal are:
    A. C—20%
       F—46%
       P—34%
    B. C—46%
       F—20%
       P—34%

35. In evaluating the balance of the meal, one could say that it is:

A. about normal in carbohydrate, normal in fat, and high in protein.
B. low in carbohydrate, high in fat, and high in protein.

DISCUSSION QUESTIONS

1. Name and define the four components of a nutritious diet.
2. Give the four food groups and major nutrients contributed by each one.
3. Give the grams of carbohydrate, protein, fat, and kilocalories for one exchange on each of the six lists.
4. Distinguish between RDAs and U.S. RDAs.

REFERENCES

1. D. Derebian and D. Shaefer. "Clinical use of the four food groups." *Nutrition and the M.D.*, 7, 1–4 (1981).
2. E.M. Hamilton and E.N. Whitney. *Nutrition: Concepts and Controversies*, 3rd ed. St. Paul, Minn.: West Publishing Co., 1985, p. 20.
3. Chicago Dietetic Association. *Manual of Clinical Dietetics*, 2nd ed. Philadelphia: W.B. Saunders Co., 1981, pp. 3–6.
4. B.W. Wipe and R.G. Hansen. "Nutrient analysis of exchange lists for meal planning." *Journal of the American Dietetic Association*, 75(9), 242–249 (1979).
5. Food and Nutrition Board, Committee on Recommended Allowances. *Recommended Dietary Allowances*, 9th ed. Washington, D.C.: National Academy of Sciences, 1980.

3 CARBOHYDRATES

OBJECTIVES

Upon completion of this chapter, you should be able to:

1. List the names of the monosaccharides commonly found in food.

2. Describe two clinical applications of monosaccharides.

3. List the disaccharides found in foods and their monosaccharide components.

4. Give two reasons why honey is not nutritionally better than table sugar.

5. State where glycogen is stored and its function.

6. Identify the polysaccharide composing fiber and distinguish between crude and dietary fiber.

7. Describe two functions of fiber.

8. List the food groups rich in fiber together with the amount in a serving.

9. Describe two functions of carbohydrates.

10. Describe the digestion of starch in terms of location, enzymes, and products.

11. List the two phases of metabolism.

12. Describe three important events that occur during glycolysis.

13. Describe three important functions of a citric acid cycle.

14. Describe two important facts about an electron transport system.

15. Differentiate between glycogenesis and glycogenolysis, and give the functions of each process.

16. Compare the current U.S. diet with the recommended diet in regard to percentages of polysaccharides and disaccharides (sugar).

17. Give the type(s) and grams of carbohydrates in each of the six exchange lists.

INTRODUCTION

Dental caries Decay or cavities of the teeth.

Diabetes mellitus Disease of the pancreas that causes inadequate secretion of insulin, thereby resulting in an inability to regulate blood glucose level normally (see Chapter 18).

Galactosemia A genetic disease in which galactose is not properly metabolized due to the lack of an enzyme.

Carbohydrates are important for both the normal functioning of the body and their possible cause–effect relationship with certain disorders. Studies are being done to determine the relationship of low-fiber diets and diseases of the large intestine such as colon cancer. Other studies are examining excessive sugar intake and **dental caries.** Health professionals need a knowledge of carbohydrates, their functions, metabolism, and food sources to help prevent these problems, as well as to treat **diabetes mellitus** and inborn errors of carbohydrate metabolism such as **galactosemia.** A knowledge of carbohydrates is also essential in order for a health professional to educate a patient effectively about quick-weight-loss fad diets.

CHEMISTRY OF CARBOHYDRATES

Carbohydrate Organic compound composed of carbon, hydrogen, and oxygen, with a 2:1 ratio of hydrogen to oxygen atoms.

Each **carbohydrate** molecule is composed of three basic atoms: **carbon** (C), hydrogen (H), and oxygen (O). The hydrogen and oxygen atoms occur in the same 2:1 ratio as water.
For example:

$C_6H_{12}O_6$—glucose

$C_{12}H_{22}O_{11}$—sucrose

Health professionals frequently write the word *carbohydrate* in a shorthand way as CHO; however, it is more accurate to write it as CH_2O due to the 2:1 ratio of hydrogen to oxygen.

CARBOHYDRATES FOUND IN FOODS

Saccharide Sugar unit.

Monosaccharide Simple sugar.

Disaccharide Double sugar.

Polysaccharide Complex sugar.

The carbohydrates found in foods are divided into three classes according to the number of **saccharides** composing the molecule:

Monosaccharide. Each molecule in this class is composed of a simple sugar.

Disaccharides. Two monosaccharides bonded together compose each disaccharide molecule.

Polysaccharides. These complex molecules are composed of many monosaccharides bonded together.

MONOSACCHARIDES (SIMPLE SUGARS, $C_6H_{12}O_6$)

Three monosaccharides are commonly found in food: glucose, galactose, and fructose (see Fig. 3-1). Notice that they all have the same chemical formula, $C_6H_{12}O_6$, but differ slightly in the geometrical arrangement of their atoms. This class of carbohydrate is absorbed into the blood from the intestines as a result of their small size. Table 3-1 summarizes information about carbohydrates.

Glucose

Glucose is found free in foods such as honey and fruits. It is the major chemical building block of disaccharides and polysaccharides and is transported by the blood to the cells, where it is oxidized for energy. Glucose is present in the blood in a concentration of 70–120 mg/dl.* (See the Clinical Application "Clinical Importance of Monosaccharides").

Galactose

Galactose (Fig. 3-1) is not found in nature as a monosaccharide, but rather as a part of the disaccharide, *lactose* (Fig. 3-3). Lactose is broken down into glucose and galactose; is then converted to glucose by the liver (see Fig. 3-4).

Milk is the primary food source of galactose. Mammary tissue in human breasts converts glucose to galactose and then synthesizes lactose. The presence of galactose in milk is a dietary planning problem for

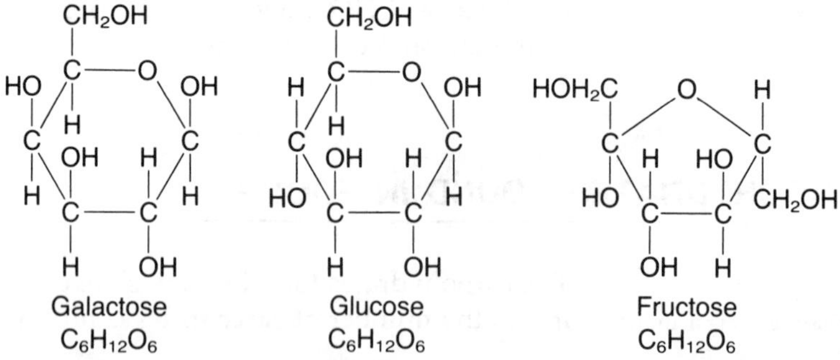

FIGURE 3-1 The three monosaccharides commonly found in food. (From T. Randall Lankford, *Integrated Science for Health Students*, 3rd ed., 1984. Reprinted by permission of Reston Publishing Company, a Prentice-Hall Company, 11480 Sunset Hills Road, Reston, Va. 22090.)

*Note: dl (deciliter) (*deci*: one-tenth); a deciliter is one-tenth of a liter, or 100 ml.

TABLE 3-1 SUMMARY OF INFORMATION ABOUT CARBOHYDRATES

Class	Composition	Food Sources	Comments
Monosaccharide ($C_6H_{12}O_6$)			
Glucose		Found free in honey and fruits	Important as a primary source of energy; used as carbohydrate source in IVs
Galactose		Not found free in nature; found in human breast milk	Galactosemia, the inability to digest galactose, is an inherited trait
Fructose		Fruits and honey	Sweetest-tasting of the monosaccharides
Disaccharide ($C_{12}H_{22}O_{11}$)			
Sucrose	Glucose and fructose	Found naturally in sugar cane, maple syrup, bananas, green peas, and sweet potatoes	Commonly called *table sugar;* found in many convenience and fast foods
Lactose	Glucose and galactose	Milk is the main food source	Main source of carbohydrate for infants; some infants and adults develop the inability to digest lactose
Maltose	Glucose and glucose	Not found free in nature	Used in candy flavor and brewing beer
Polysaccharide ($C_6H_{10}O_5)_n$			
Glycogen	Many glucose molecules	Not found in foods	Synthesized in liver and muscles; important as a reserve source of blood glucose
Cellulose	Many glucose molecules	Found in many vegetables	Human body cannot digest it due to inability to synthesize enzymes; important to the body in increasing motility, attracting water into intestines, and possibly preventing certain health conditions
Starch	Many glucose molecules	Plant seeds, cereal grains, and some vegetables	Major source of carbohydrate in many countries; for example, corn and rice

CLINICAL APPLICATION: CLINICAL IMPORTANCE OF MONOSACCHARIDES

Some clinical conditions can be helped by the use of certain monosaccharides; other conditions require regulation and monitoring of the kinds and amounts of simple sugars. A few examples will be presented here, with more details presented in Part 3.

1. Use of glucose (dextrose) in intravenous therapy

Many clinical conditions (for example, inability to ingest fluids orally or severe burns, in which patients lose large amounts of fluids) require that a patient be given fluids directly into the veins or *intravenous (IV) therapy*. The most common type of IV contains dextrose (glucose used by hospitals) in a 5% concentration along with 0.9% saline. It is commonly referred to as *D-5-W*. Each liter (1,000 ml) of 5% IV fluid provides only about 170 kcal. (See Chapter 16 for the kilocalorie values of dextrose infused parenterally.)

The reason why dextrose (a monosaccharide) is used in IVs instead of sucrose (a disaccharide) is that glucose is in a form that can be readily absorbed into the body's cells. Sucrose (a disaccharide) must undergo digestion before glucose and fructose can be absorbed.

2. Use of fructose by diabetics in the control of blood glucose

Some studies show that if fructose is used as a table sugar substitute, it can reduce the level of blood glucose and insulin, following meals, in insulin-treated diabetics.[1] These studies have been short-term in duration and, therefore, the use of fructose on a continual basis for diabetics cannot definitely be recommended.

3. Galactosemia

In this rare genetic disease, an infant lacks the enzyme necessary to convert galactose to glucose (see Fig. 3-2). The result is that the galactose in the body increases to toxic levels, possibly resulting in mental retardation, liver damage, and cataracts. Treatment requires that all forms of milk and lactose (source of galactose) be removed from the infant's diet. Milk substitutes such as Nutramigen can be fed to infants. (More details on galactosemia can be found in Chapter 19).

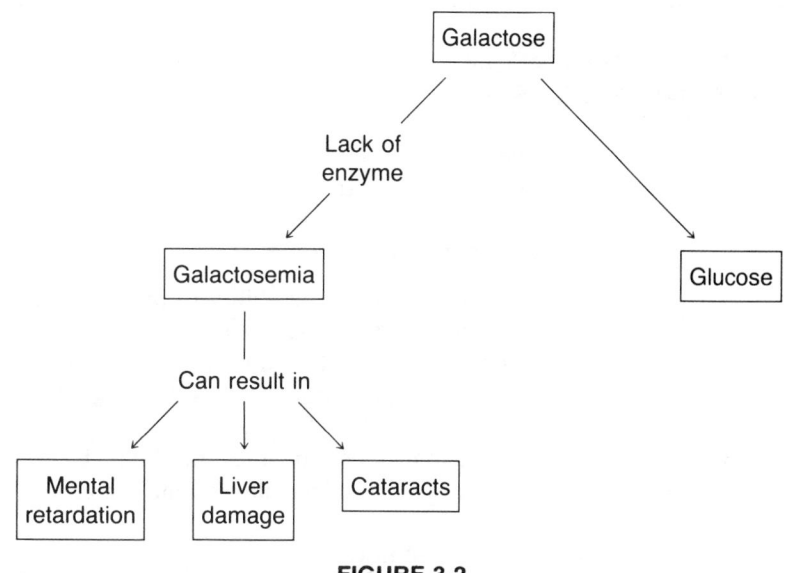

FIGURE 3-2

children who have galactosemia (see the Clinical Application "Clinical Importance of Disaccharides").

Fructose

Fructose   Fruit sugar.

Fructose (Fig. 3-1) is found in many fruits as well as in honey. It is also a component of sucrose (see Fig. 3-5). Fructose can be absorbed into the blood from food, but the majority of it is converted to glucose in the

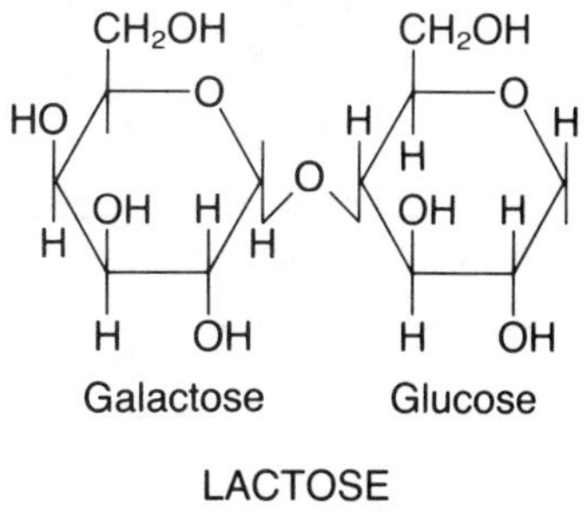

CH_2OH CH_2OH

Galactose   Glucose

LACTOSE

FIGURE 3-3 Lactose is composed of galactose and glucose. (From T. Randall Lankford, *Integrated Science for Health Students,* 3rd ed., 1984. Reprinted by permission of Reston Publishing Company, a Prentice-Hall Company, 11480 Sunset Hills Road, Reston, Va. 22090.)

CLINICAL APPLICATION: CLINICAL IMPORTANCE OF DISACCHARIDES

Some human disorders and diets used in tube feedings are important in relation to certain disaccharides.

1. Lactose intolerance

Some people lack the ability to produce the enzyme lactase, which is necessary to digest lactose into glucose and galactose. There are three types of lactose intolerances: congenital, primary, and secondary. Each of these types is discussed further in Chapter 19. This condition results in lactose not being digested, thereby passing intact into the intestines. The intestines then absorb large amounts of water, which causes bloating, abdominal discomfort, nausea, and vomiting.

2. Tube feedings

Some hospitalized patients cannot ingest food through the mouth (for example, comatose patients or those with neck or facial surgery); therefore, they may require tube feeding. Usually the tube is inserted through the nasal openings down to the stomach. Liquid commercial formulas containing different carbohydrate sources are delivered through the tube. Many of these formulas contain disaccharides, as the following examples show:

Tube Formula Product	Carbohydrate Source
Ensure	sucrose and glucose
Sustacal	sucrose and glucose
Sustagen	lactose and glucose
Nutri-1000	lactose, sucrose, dextrose, and maltose

When choosing a particular product, it is important to know which disaccharides, if any, it contains, since some people cannot digest certain disaccharides; lactose intolerance is a common example.

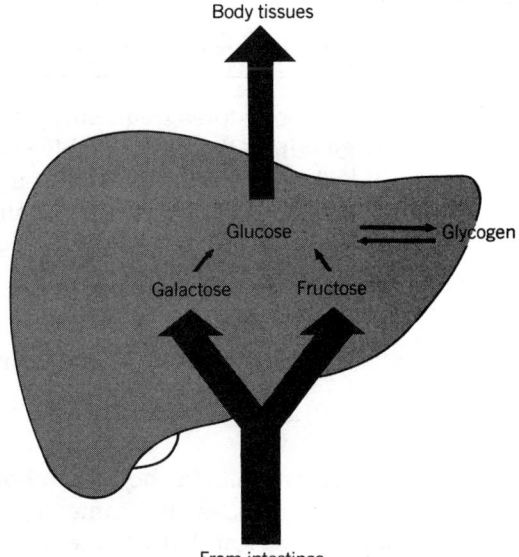

Body tissues

Glucose ⇌ Glycogen

Galactose   Fructose

From intestines

FIGURE 3-4   Conversion of galactose and fructose to glucose in the liver.

liver (see Fig. 3-4), most of which is stored in glycogen.[1] Fructose is the sweetest-tasting of the monosaccharides.

DISACCHARIDES (DOUBLE SUGAR, $C_{12}H_{22}O_{11}$)

A disaccharide is composed of two monosaccharides. Three disaccharides commonly found in foods are sucrose, lactose, and maltose.

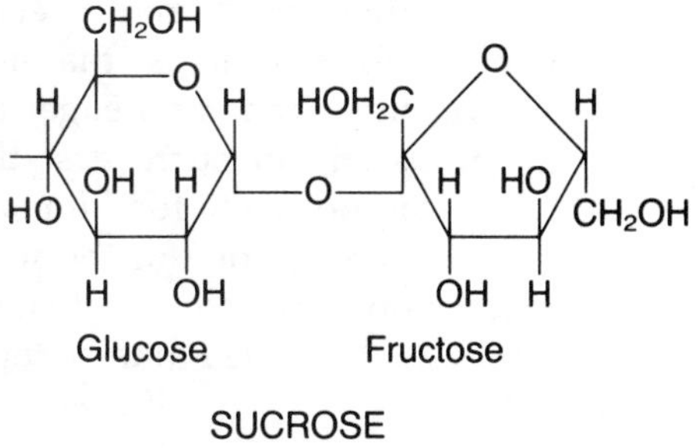

Glucose   Fructose

SUCROSE

FIGURE 3-5   Sucrose is a disaccharide composed of glucose and fructose. (From T. Randall Lankford, *Integrated Science for Health Students,* 3rd ed., 1984. Reprinted by permission of Reston Publishing Company, a Prentice-Hall Company, 11480 Sunset Hills Road, Reston, Va. 22090.)

REFINED SUGAR VERSUS HONEY FALLACY

Health food stores frequently advocate honey as a better source of carbohydrate than white table sugar (sucrose). Their reasoning essentially is that honey is a natural pure product, whereas table sugar is a refined product. The information below shows the carbohydrate content of each.

	Types of Sugars Present	kcal/tsp
Honey	Glucose and fructose	22
Table sugar	Sucrose (glucose-fructose)	13

This information shows that honey contains glucose and fructose monosaccharides, the same sugars that compose sucrose, a table sugar. It is clear that whether a person ingests honey or table sugar, the bloodstream will absorb the same monosaccharides. In addition, the body's cells cannot determine whether the glucose came from honey or table sugar. Honey advocates also point out that it contains nutrients (proteins, calcium, iron, and five vitamins) that table sugar does not have. This information is true, but it should also be pointed out that the amount of each nutrient is so minimal that its presence in honey is not considered important to a person's diet.[3]

Sucrose

Sucrose Table sugar.

Sucrose is composed of glucose and fructose (see Fig. 3-5). This disaccharide occurs naturally in foods such as sugar cane, maple syrup, bananas, green peas, and sweet potatoes. The sugar that is bought in supermarkets is sucrose that has been produced by purifying and granulating sugar cane and sugar beets. Many convenience and fast foods are prepared with sucrose, so that it comprises about 15–20% of the total calories in our daily food intake.[2]

In Chapter 1, one of the food fallacies presented is that honey is a better nutritional source of sugar than refined sugar. Details about this fallacy are presented in the entitled material "Refined Sugar versus Honey Fallacy."

Lactose

Lactose Milk sugar.

Lactose contains glucose and galactose bonded together (see Fig. 3-3). It is found in cow's milk and can be synthesized by women during lactation. Lactose in cow's milk is the energy source for bacteria that converts it to lactic acid which is the source of the taste in spoiled milk.

Newborn infants obtain the majority of their carbohydrates from lactose, since milk is their main food source. However, some children become unable to digest lactose at about 4 years of age and experience a variety of difficulties when they drink milk (see the Clinical Application "Clinical Importance of Disaccharides").

Maltose

Maltose Malt sugar.

Maltose is composed of two glucose molecules (see Fig. 3-6) and is not found naturally in foods. The maltose in beer is produced by the partial digestion of starch.

Maltose itself has no dietary significance in humans. After it is ingested, it undergoes digestion to release its two glucose molecules.

POLYSACCHARIDES (COMPLEX SUGAR $C_6H_{10}O_5)_n$

A polysaccharide is composed of many monosaccharides. The n in the above formula refers to the number of saccharide units composing the molecule, it varies from several hundred to over one-half million. Three polysaccharides will be discussed: glycogen, cellulose (fiber), and starch.

Glycogen

Glycogen Branched-chain polysaccharide composed of glucose molecules.

Glycogen (see Fig. 3-7) is synthesized and stored in the liver and skeletal muscles. Approximately 100 g of glycogen are stored in the liver and 200 g in skeletal muscle tissue.[3]

Glycogen is important as a source of glucose for the blood whenever

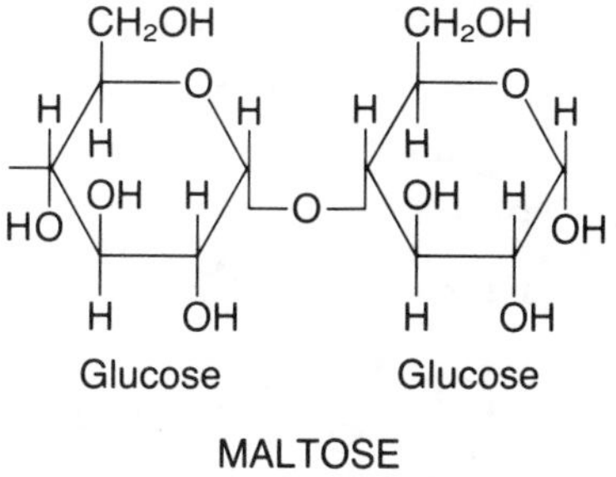

MALTOSE

FIGURE 3-6 Two glucose molecules bonded together compose maltose. (From T. Randall Lankford, *Integrated Science for Health Students,* 3rd ed., 1984. Reprinted by permission of Reston Publishing Company, a Prentice-Hall Company, 11480 Sunset Hills Road, Reston, Va. 22090.)

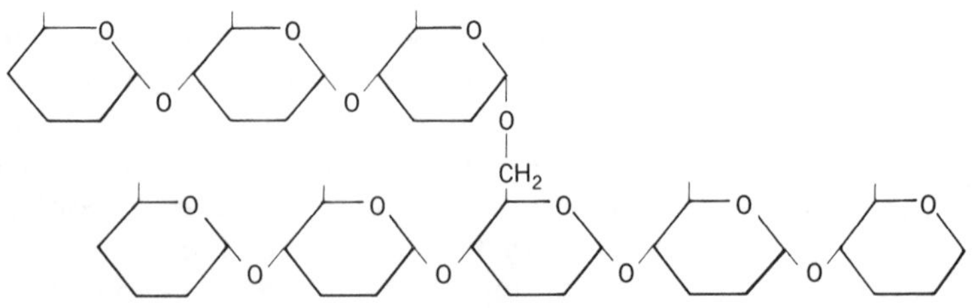

Glycogen

FIGURE 3-7   Glycogen is a branched chain polysaccharide composed of glucose molecules.

the level drops too low. It can be quickly decomposed to glucose in time of need (details of this process are presented later in this chapter).

Cellulose

Cellulose   Fiber

Crude fiber   The residue left after laboratory treatment of food with acid and alkali.

Dietary fiber   Fiber resistant to the human digestive enzymes.

Hemicellulose   A polysaccharide that is similar to cellulose.

Lignin   A noncarbohydrate substance that functions as a structured bonding agent in plants.

Pectin   A water-soluble, nonstructural polysaccharide.

Gum   A water-soluble, nonstructural polysaccharide.

Cellulose is composed of many glucose molecules but is different from glycogen in that it is a straight-chain polysaccharide (see Fig. 3-8). It is found in plants, where it provides strength and support to cell walls.

The human body does not synthesize any enzymes that will break down cellulose; therefore, it passes through the small intestine undigested. However, when fiber from fruits and vegetables reaches the large intestine, bacteria digest (see Fig. 3-9) or ferment these molecules. The end result is an increase in the bacterial mass, fatty acids, methane gas (or flatulence), and fiber residue. Two kinds of fiber are important in the study of nutrition: **crude fiber** and **dietary fiber.**

A crude fiber measurement is thought to be too restrictive in measuring the total fiber content, since it measures very little of the **hemicellulose** or **lignin** and only about 50% of the cellulose present in food. Dietary fiber measures five different components:

Cellulose

Hemicellulose

Lignin

Pectin

Gums[4]

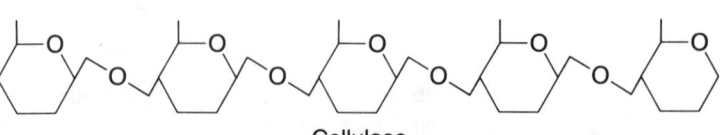

Cellulose

FIGURE 3-8   Cellulose is a straight chain polysaccharide.

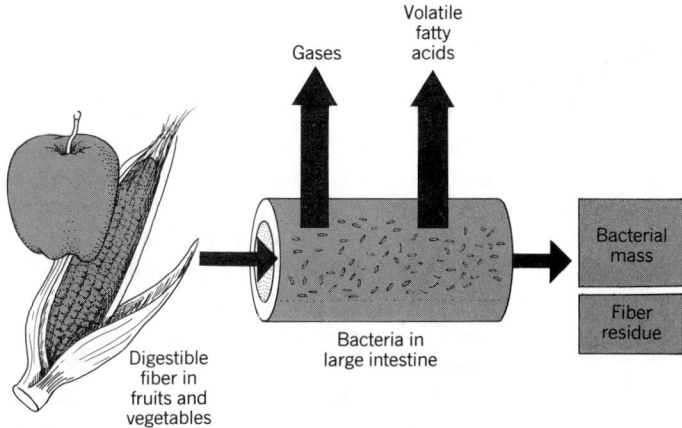

FIGURE 3-9   Breakdown of fiber by bacteria in the large intestine.

Functions of Fiber.   The functions (see Fig. 3-10) of dietary fiber in the body are:

• To increase intestinal motility. Undigested fiber increases the peristaltic contractions of the intestines and thereby decreases the transit time of feces.

• To attract more water into the intestines. Increased attraction of water tends to soften stools and thereby helps prevent constipation.

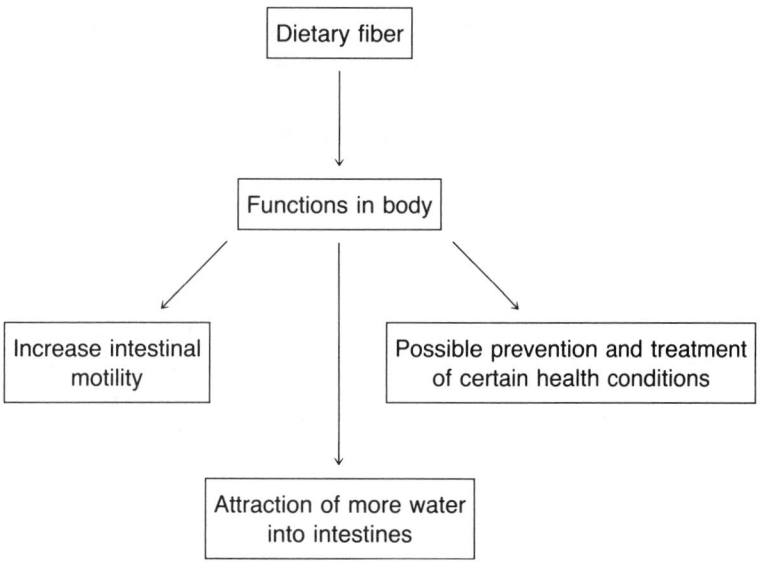

FIGURE 3-10   Functions of dietary fiber.

CLINICAL APPLICATION: CLINICAL IMPORTANCE
OF DIETARY FIBER

Hypoglycemia Abnormally low level of blood glucose (see Chapter 18).

Hypercholesterolemia High level of cholesterol in the blood.

Much research has been done on the beneficial effects of high-fiber diets in preventing certain disorders: constipation, diverticulosis, colon cancer, obesity, **hypoglycemia,** and **hypercholesterolemia** (high level of cholesterol in the blood). Insulin-dependent diabetics can control their blood glucose levels more effectively and lower their insulin needs with an increased intake of fiber. Details concerning the relationship of fiber to these disorders will be presented in later chapters.

What is a high-fiber diet? Are there any disadvantages of increasing the fiber content of a person's diet? Most nutritional authorities define a high-fiber diet as one in which dietary fiber exceeds 40 g/day.[5] The average American now eats about 10–20 g of dietary fiber per day. This does not mean that the average person needs to double or quadruple the dietary fiber intake to help prevent the disorders discussed above. Ideal or desirable dietary fiber intakes range from 25 to 50 g/day.[5] One does not have to sprinkle bran on all foods to achieve this intake. The average amounts of fiber in the fruit, bread and cereal, and vegetable groups are presented in this chapter. An example of three meals that contain a total of more than 40 g of dietary fiber is presented below.

Some of the disadvantages of increasing fiber in the diet are abdominal fullness, increased flatulence, nausea, and vomiting. These problems can be reduced or will disappear (except flatulence) by gradually decreasing the fiber content.

Three Typical Meals That Contain 40 g of Dietary Fiber

		Dietary fiber (g)
Breakfast	¾ cup All-Bran	11.2
	½ cup milk	0
	2 slices whole wheat toast with margarine	4.3
Lunch	2 slices whole wheat bread	4.3
	1 tomato (small)	1.4
	2 tbsp peanut butter	2.2
	1 apple	1.4

		Dietary fiber (g)
Dinner	3 oz beef	0
	1 baked potato with skin	7.0
	1 stalk broccoli	8.2
	1 cup of lettuce	1.6
	½ cup peas (canned)	5.3
Total fiber content		46.9

- Possibly to prevent and treat certain health conditions (see the Clinical Application "Clinical Importance of Dietary Fiber").

Food Source of Fiber.   The amount of fiber in the fruit, bread and cereal, and vegetable groups is given below.

Fruit groups: Each serving (varies) has approximately 2 g of fiber:

Apple	Strawberries	Orange
Banana	Cherries	Peach

Bread and cereal group: Each serving (varies) has approximately 2 g of fiber (see Fig. 3-11):

Whole wheat bread	All-Bran
Rye bread	Corn Flakes
Shredded wheat	

Vegetable group: Each serving (½ cup) has approximately 2 g of fiber:

Broccoli	Corn on the cob
Carrots	Green beans
Celery	Tomato, raw

Meat group: Meats are low in fiber.

Diverticulosis Presence of diverticula (outpouching of the colon wall) (see Chapter 19).

Since the turn of the century, Americans have decreased their fiber consumption. This is the result of consuming more low-fiber foods such as meat, dairy products, and highly refined carbohydrate processed foods. Some scientists have attributed the increases in colon and rectum cancer, hemorrhoids, and **diverticulosis** to the low-fiber diet. Information on high-fiber diets and possible prevention of diseases is presented in the Clinical Application "Clinical Importance of Dietary Fiber."

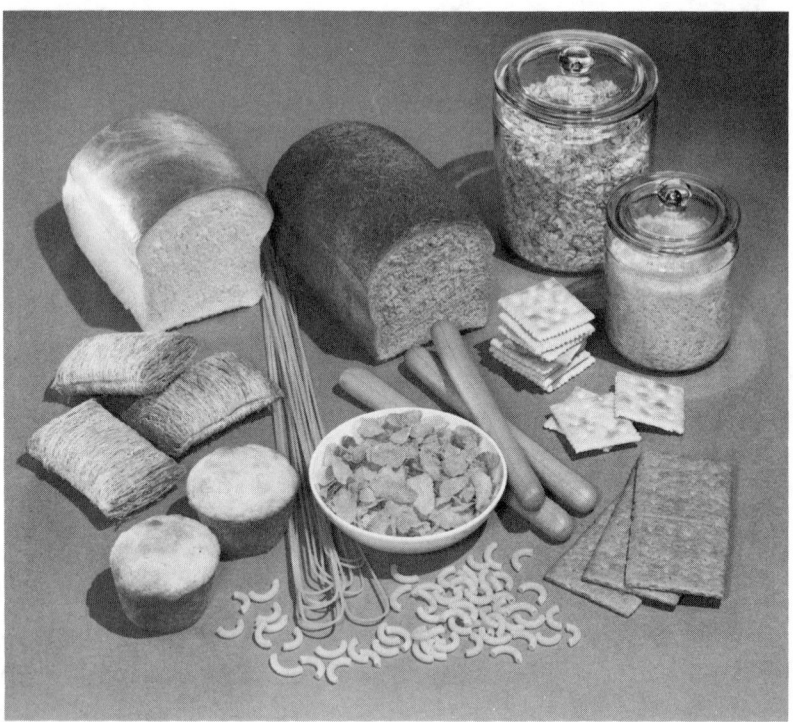

FIGURE 3-11   Each serving from the bread and cereal group contains approximately 2 g of fiber. (Courtesy of the National Dairy Council.)

Starch

Starch is similar in structure to glycogen in that it is a branched polysaccharide molecule composed of glucose units. It is a storage form of glucose but is found only in plants. Starch is found in plant seeds, cereal grains, fruits, and roots. **Legumes** and nuts also contain large amounts of starch.

Starch is a major source of carbohydrate and total energy intake in many countries. In the United States, wheat, oats, rye, barley, corn, potatoes, and rice are the primary food sources of starch. People in South American countries obtain most of their starch from corn, whereas Orientals use rice.

The digestion of starch begins in the mouth and is described later in this chapter.

Legumes Seeds of plants such as kidney beans, soybeans, garden peas, and lima beans.

FUNCTIONS OF CARBOHYDRATES

SOURCE OF ENERGY

Glucose is the prime source of energy (see Fig. 3-12) for physiological activities (for example, muscle contractions and nerve impulse transmission). Each gram of glucose yields 4 kcal of energy when metabolized.

The brain tissue normally uses glucose as a source of energy. However, glycogen is not stored in nerve tissue; thus, the blood must continually bring glucose to the brain cells. Therefore, a low-calorie, low-carbohydrate diet can impair the normal functions of the brain.

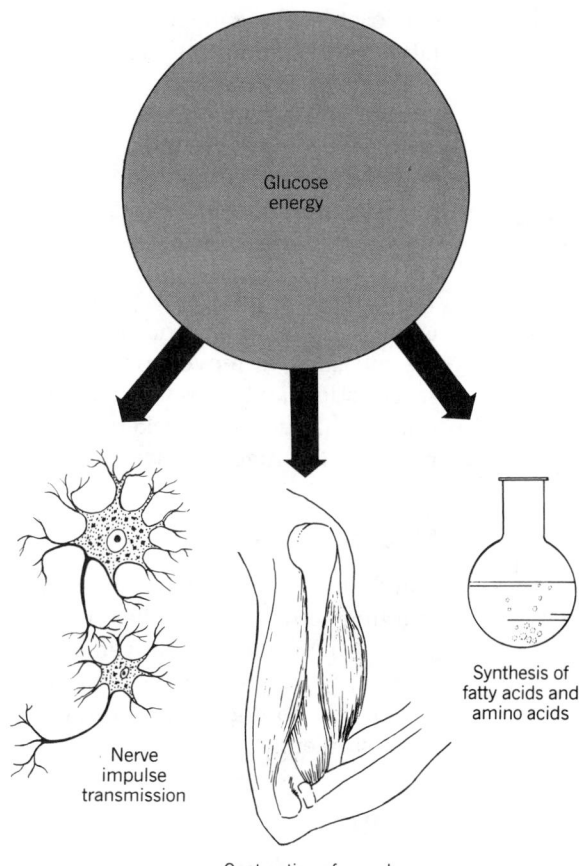

Nerve impulse transmission

Contraction of muscles

Synthesis of fatty acids and amino acids

Glucose energy

FIGURE 3-12 Glucose as a source of energy for physiological activities such as nerve impulse transmission and contraction of muscles, plus starting material for synthesis of other compounds.

Triglyceride A lipid compound composed of three fatty acids attached to a glycerol molecule.

Ketones Products of incomplete metabolism of fats (acetone is an example of a ketone).

Blood acidosis A condition in which blood pH is below 7.35. This condition can result from an excess amount of ketones.

If a person does not ingest an adequate amount of carbohydrates, **triglycerides** and proteins will be used as a source of energy. A danger in using triglycerides for energy is the release of **ketones,** which are acids. A high level of ketones can result in **blood acidosis,** which, if prolonged, can result in brain failure. Body proteins have many important functions (discussed in Chapter 5). If an adequate amount of carbohydrate is ingested, proteins are spared; therefore, carbohydrates are described as having "protein-sparing" action. A person must ingest a minimum of 100–125 g (400–500 kcal) of carbohydrate per day in order to spare proteins as a source of energy.

STARTING MATERIAL FOR THE SYNTHESIS OF OTHER COMPOUNDS

Glucose can be converted into other molecules, such as nonessential fatty acids and some amino acids, whenever their levels are inadequate.[5]

DIGESTION AND ABSORPTION OF CARBOHYDRATES

The carbohydrates in the foods we eat are usually disaccharides (sucrose is the most common) and polysaccharides (starch). These carbohydrates are too large to move from the intestines into the blood. Only monosaccharides can be absorbed into the blood; therefore, disaccharides and polysaccharides are broken down into their monosaccharide components by the digestive system.

Salivary amylase An enzyme secreted in the mouth that splits starch into smaller fragments.

Dextrins Products of starch digestion in the mouth.

Peristalsis Wavelike, muscular contractions that propel food and wastes through the gastrointestinal tract.

Hydrochloric acid Acid secreted by cells in the stomach that changes pepsinogen to pepsin.

MOUTH

Starch digestion begins in the mouth with the enzyme **salivary amylase** splitting starch into smaller fragments, disaccharide, and **dextrins** (see Fig. 3-13). Swallowing movements and **peristalsis** function to pass these fragments through the esophagus into the stomach.

There is no digestion of disaccharides in the mouth due to a lack of necessary enzymes.

STOMACH

Starch digestion continues for a short time before the **hydrochloric acid (HCl)** in gastric juice denatures (changes salivary amylase) into a nonfunctional state. No additional carbohydrate digestion occurs in the stomach due to its acidity and lack of enzymes.

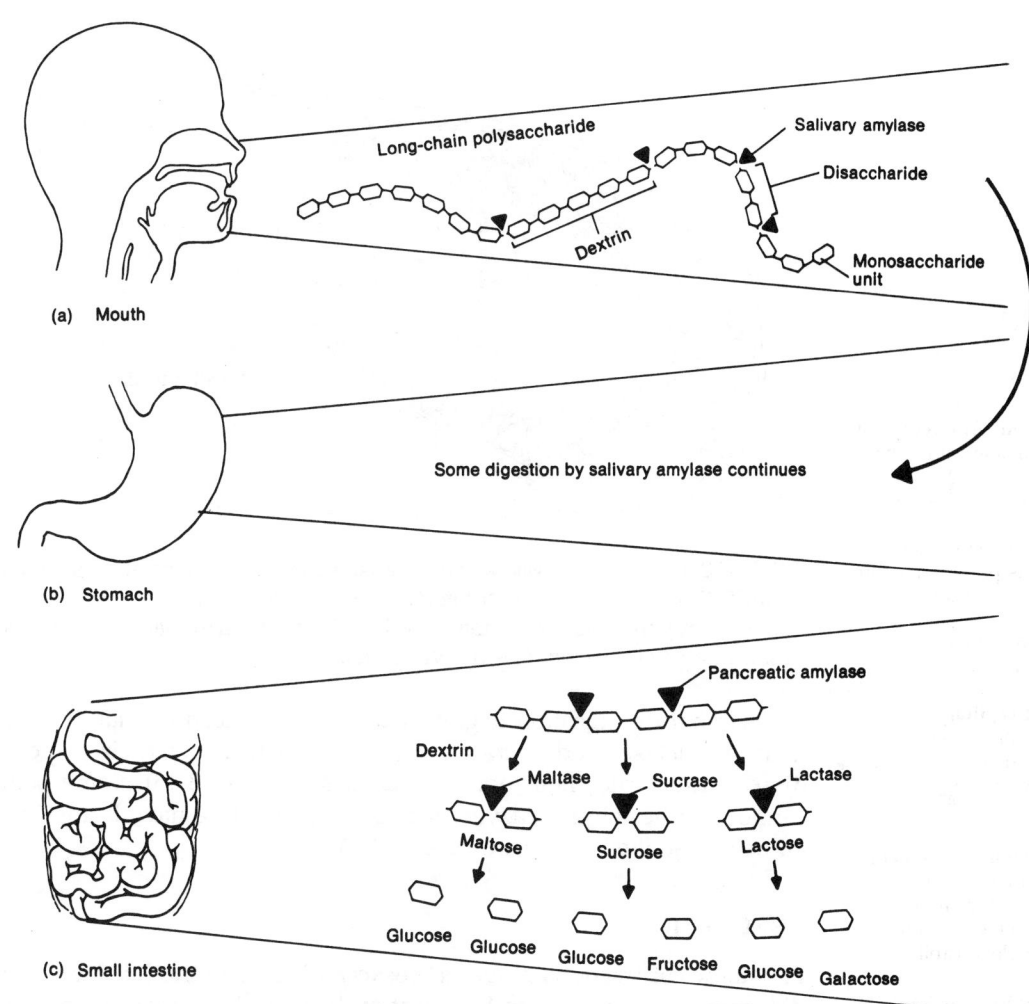

(a) Mouth

(b) Stomach

(c) Small intestine

FIGURE 3-13 Digestion of carbohydrates in the mouth, stomach, and small intestine. (From *Principles of Anatomy and Physiology*, 2nd ed., by Gerard J. Tortora and Nicholas P. Anagnostakos. Copyright © 1975, 1978 by Gerard J. Tortora and Nicholas P. Anagnostakos. Reprinted by permission of Harper & Row, Publishers, Inc.)

Duodenum First region of the small intestine.

Pancreatic amylase An enzyme secreted by the pancreas that breaks down dextrins into maltose.

SMALL INTESTINE

Rhythmic contractions (*peristalsis*) of the stomach move maltose, dextrins, and other disaccharides that a person may have ingested into the **duodenum.** The pancreas secretes the enzyme **pancreatic amylase** into the duodenum, breaking down dextrins into maltose (see Fig. 3-13).

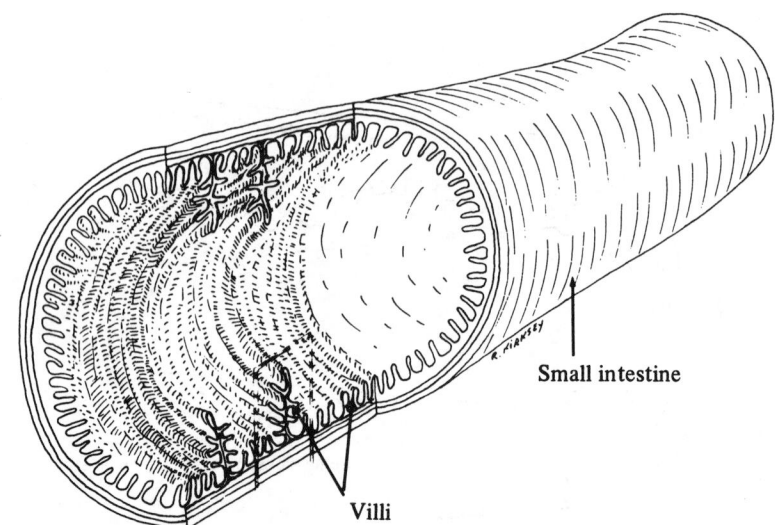

Small intestine

Villi

FIGURE 3-14   Intestinal villi, which increase absorption surface area, are shown. (From T. Randall Lankford, *Integrated Science for Health Students*, 3rd ed., 1984. Reprinted by permission of Reston Publishing Company, a Prentice-Hall Company, 11480 Sunset Hills Road, Reston, Va. 22090.)

Jejunum The region of the small intestine that extends from the duodenum to the ileum.

Intestinal villi Small mucous projections lining the small intestine.

Lumen The opening of the intestine.

Blood capillary Microscopic blood vessels through which nutrients and wastes are exchanged.

Diffusion Movement of molecules from high concentration in the intestines to low concentration in the blood capillary.

Active transport Movement of molecules from a low concentration in the intestine to a high concentration in the blood. Energy is required and involves carrier molecules.

Disaccharide digestion begins at this point. Intestinal glands secrete maltase, lactase, and sucrase enzymes, which digest their respective disaccharides into their monosaccharides (see Fig. 3-13). Some people cannot synthesize the enzyme lactase and therefore have lactose intolerance (described earlier in the chapter).[7]

ABSORPTION

Peristaltic contractions move monosaccharides into the **jejunum** where digestion is completed and absorption begins. Absorption is increased as a result of **intestinal villi** (see Fig. 3-14) projecting into the **lumen**. Each villus contains a **blood capillary** (see Fig. 3-15) into which the monosaccharides pass via **diffusion** and **active transport**.

Monosaccharides are absorbed at different rates; galactose, glucose, and fructose have decreasing rates of absorption.

METABOLISM OF CARBOHYDRATES

Metabolism All chemical reactions that absorbed molecules undergo inside cells.

Metabolism is divided into two phases, **catabolism** and **anabolism**.

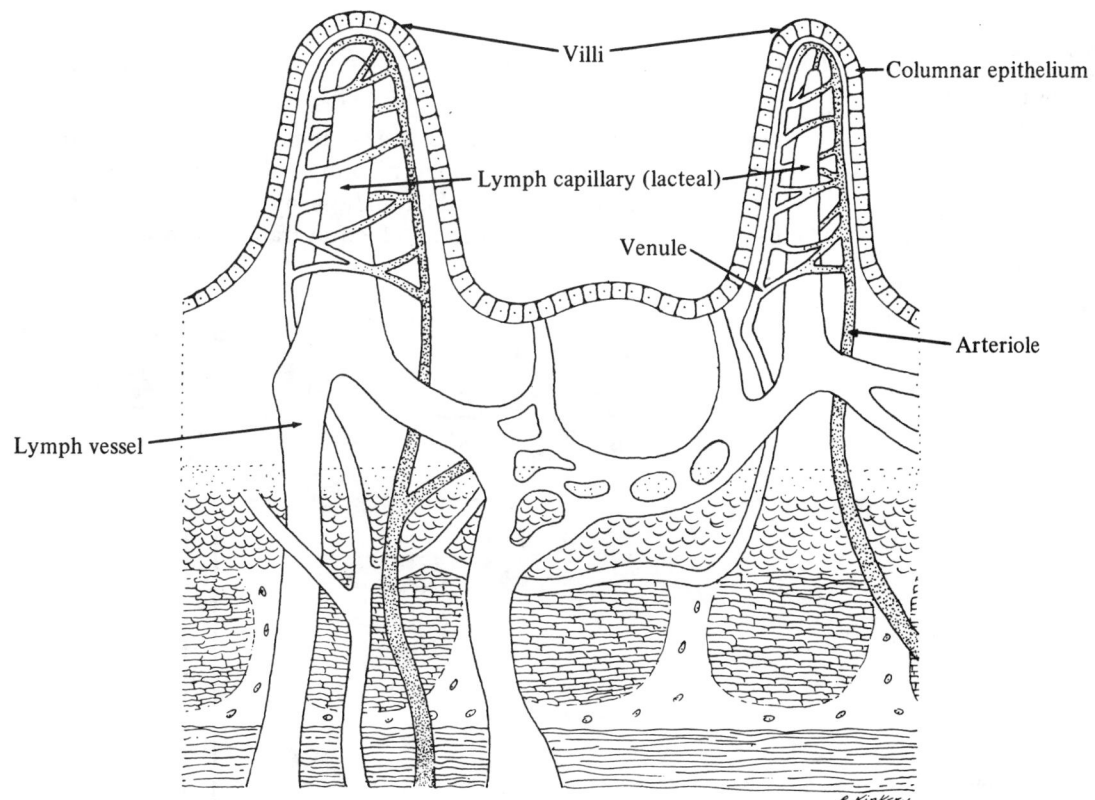

FIGURE 3-15 Blood and lymph capillaries, which transport absorbed nutrients in villi, are shown. (From T. Randall Lankford, *Integrated Science for Health Students,* 3rd ed., 1984. Reprinted by permission of Reston Publishing Company, a Prentice-Hall Company, 11480 Sunset Hills Road, Reston, Va. 22090.)

ATP Adenosine triphosphate. A high-energy compound that supplies energy for body processes.

Anaerobic (glycolysis) respiration A process in cell respiration in which ATP molecules are synthesized and oxygen is not required.

Aerobic respiration A process in cell respiration in which ATP molecules are synthesized and oxygen is required.

Pyruvic acid An end product of anaerobic respiration.

CATABOLISM

Catabolism of glucose is important, since it results in the synthesis of the high-energy compound **ATP.**

Oxidation of Glucose and Synthesis of ATP

Two main processes are involved in the oxidation of glucose to synthesize ATP: **anaerobic (glycolysis)** and **aerobic respiration.** In anaerobic (glycolysis) respiration:

Glucose (6C) is oxidized (loses four hydrogen atoms) and splits into two pyruvic acid (3C) molecules (see Fig. 3-16). This process releases enough energy to form ATP.

Hydrogen transport molecules Molecules in cell respiration that transport hydrogen atoms from glucose to cytochrome molecules.

Electron transport system Composed of cytochrome molecules by which the pairs of hydrogen electrons released from glycolysis and citric acid cycles are carried.

Two ATP molecules are used up.

Four ATP molecules are synthesized (see Fig. 3-16). Since two ATP are used up, there is a net gain of two ATP.

Two hydrogen transport molecules are synthesized. The four hydrogen atoms combine in pairs with two nicotinamide adenine dinucleotide (NAD) molecules to form $NADH_2$. These hydrogen transport molecules carry their hydrogens to an **electron transport system.**

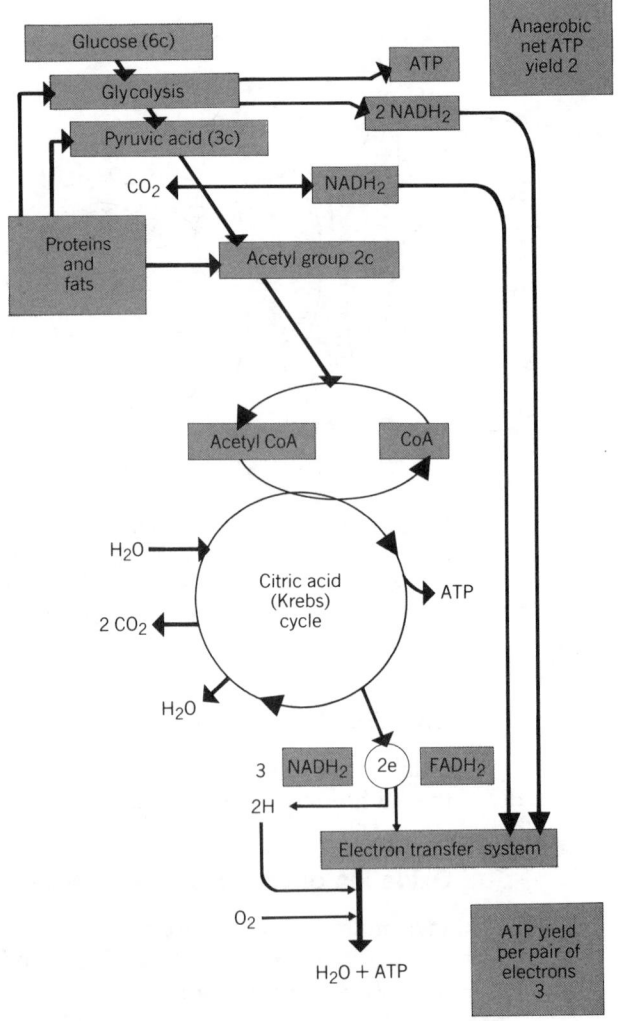

FIGURE 3-16 Metabolism of glucose resulting in the synthesis of ATP molecules. (From Lankford, T.R. *Cell Respiration Made Easy.* Copyright © National Teaching Aids, Inc., 1982.)

Citric acid cycle (Krebs Cycle) A series of aerobic respiration reactions that result in the release of hydrogen atoms and CO_2 molecules and the synthesis of one ATP molecule.

Aerobic respiration involves the **citric acid cycle (Krebs cycle)** and the *electron transport system.* Two citric acid cycles occur for each glucose molecule oxidized. Due to space limitations, Figure 3-15 shows only one cycle. The important points about one citric acid cycle are as follows:

Four pairs of hydrogen atoms are released. Three pairs combine with NAD molecules to form three $NADH_2$ molecules. One pair combines with flavin adenine dinucloetide (FAD) molecules to form $FADH_2$, another hydrogen transport molecule.

Two CO_2 molecules are released.

One ATP molecule is synthesized.

After the two citric acid cycles are completed, the electron transport system (see Fig. 3-16):

Synthesizes three molecules for each pair of hydrogen electrons. Each pair of hydrogen electrons transported through the system results in the synthesis of three ATP molecules.

Produces oxygen (O_2), the final electron and hydrogen ion acceptor (see Fig. 3-16). The citric acid cycle and the electron transport system are aerobic because of the role of oxygen. Without O_2, the transfer of electrons and the citric acid cycle would cease. Most importantly, though, ATP synthesis would stop.

ANABOLISM AND INTERACTION OF GLYCOGENESIS AND GLYCOGENOLYSIS

Insulin A hormone secreted by the pancreas that aids in both the diffusion of glucose into the liver and muscle cells and the synthesis of glycogen.

Glycogenesis Synthesis of glycogen.

Hyperglycemia A condition that pertains to high blood glucose.

Glycogenolysis The catabolism of glycogen.

Glucagon A hormone secreted by the pancreas.

Epinephrine A hormone secreted by the adrenal gland in times of stress.

A carbohydrate example of anabolism is the synthesis of glycogen (see Fig. 3-17) by liver and muscle cells. Figure 3-17 shows that **insulin** aids in both the diffusion of glucose into the liver and muscle cells and the synthesis of glycogen, which is called **glycogenesis.** It occurs whenever the blood glucose level becomes high. The normal blood glucose range is 70–120 mg per deciliter of blood. Whenever this upper limit is exceeded, a **hyperglycemia** condition exists. Persistent hyperglycemia can result in *diabetes mellitus* and other serious problems (see Chapter 18). The body normally corrects a hyperglycemic condition by glycogenesis.

Whenever the blood glucose level drops below 70 mg/dl, a **hypoglycemic** condition exists. The liver cells correct this condition by **glycogenolysis** (see Fig. 3-17). This breakdown process releases glucose and, therefore, blood glucose increases into the normal range. **Glucagon** and **epinephrine** (Fig. 3-17) stimulate the liver cells to undergo glycogenolysis. A continuous hypoglycemic condition is abnormal; its cause, symptoms and diet are discussed in Chapter 18.

Glycogenesis (anabolism) and glycogenolysis (catabolism) interact to maintain a normal blood glucose range. In other words, the liver tissue

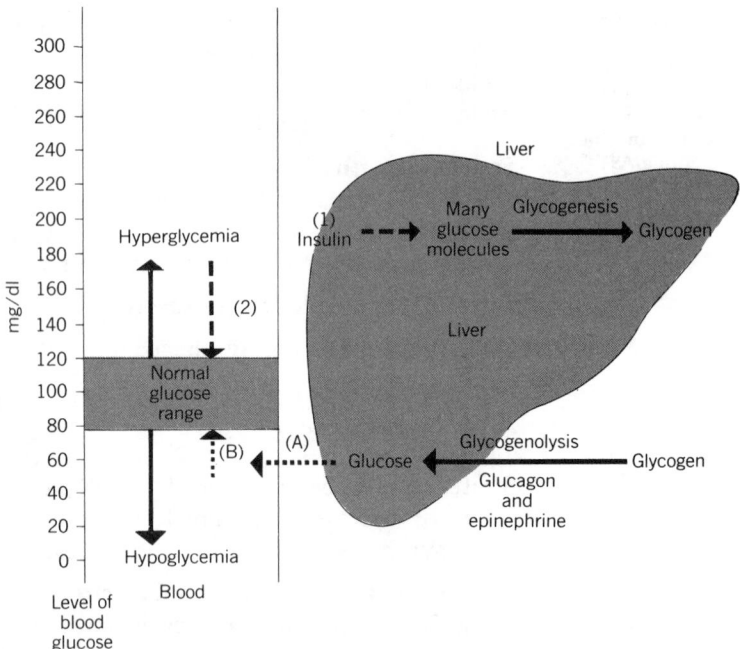

FIGURE 3-17 Interaction of glycogenesis and glycogenolysis to maintain the normal blood glucose range. Hyperglycemia results in excess glucose moving into liver, shown as (1). This action results in a lowering of blood glucose, shown as (2). The glucose is synthesized into glycogen by glycogenesis. Hypoglycemia results in release of glucose, supplied by glycogenolysis, into blood, shown as (A). This results in blood glucose rising to normal range, shown as (B).

alternates between anabolic and catabolic reactions with carbohydrates to regulate the blood glucose level.[7]

AMOUNTS AND FOOD SOURCES OF CARBOHYDRATES IN DIETS OF DIFFERENT CULTURES

In the United States, a person currently obtains about 46% of the daily kilocalories from carbohydrates, with the amount of polysaccharides (complex carbohydrates) and disaccharides (sucrose) shown below. The Select Committee on Nutrition and Human Needs of the U.S. Senate has recommended that we increase from 46 to 58% the number of kilocalories derived from carbohydrates in the daily diet. The recommended amount of polysaccharide and disaccharide in the diet are compared to the current diet:

	Current U.S. Diet (%)	Recommended U.S. Diet (%)
Polysaccharide (complex carbohydrate)	22	48
Disaccharide (sucrose)	<u>24</u>	<u>10</u>
	46	58

These figures show that the recommended diet suggests an approximate doubling of the amount of complex carbohydrates consumed compared to the current diet. It is also recommended that the amount of disaccharides be cut approximately in half.[8]

It was mentioned in Chapter 2 that the bread and cereal food group contributes the bulk of carbohydrates. The specific foods in this group consumed to obtain carbohydrates vary from culture to culture. Table 3-2 specify the foods consumed by various groups in obtaining their carbohydrates. For each culture, the table also suggests foods that will enable a person to comply better with the recommended carbohydrate guidelines.

As discussed in Chapter 1, it is important for health professionals to be knowledgeable about the food habits of different cultures. This knowledge of carbohydrates is important in order to counsel patients about achieving greater consumption of complex carbohydrates and reducing their intake of disaccharides (sugar).

CARBOHYDRATES AND THE EXCHANGE GROUPS

In Chapter 2, the exchange groups and the six exchange lists were discussed. These six lists are presented in this chapter for the purpose of discussing carbohydrate information for each list and for use in dietary planning to achieve recommended percentages of the nutrients.

MILK GROUP

One milk exchange is a serving of food equivalent to one cup of skim milk and 80 kcal. Table 3-3 shows that each milk exchange contains 12 g of carbohydrate and that disaccharide (lactose) is the primary type of carbohydrate.

As discussed in Chapter 2, one cup of whole milk is milk plus two fat exchanges, for a total of 170 kcal. However, whole milk does not contain more carbohydrate or protein than skim milk.

TABLE 3-2 FOODS CONSUMED FROM THE BREAD AND CEREAL GROUP IN VARIOUS CULTURES

Culture	Examples of Foods Consumed from the Bread and Cereal Group	Suggestions
Chinese	Millet (whole grain) and rice predominant; wheat products include noodles and steamed bread.	Use brown rice.
Italian	Pasta (noodles of various shapes and sizes) and rice are staples eaten at each meal. Use of oatmeal and farina (cream-colored breakfast cereal) has increased.	Encourage use of whole-grain bread.
Japanese	Polished white rice is a staple. Consumption of wheat products is a post–World War II practice.	Encourage use of restored rice and whole-grain breads.
Jewish	Water rolls (bagels), rye bread, and pumpernickel are often used, since these do not have milk or milk solids and therefore can be eaten with meat or dairy meals.	Encourage use of whole wheat bread at dairy meals.
Polish	Bread eaten with each meal. Pumpernickel, sour rye bread, and white bread are well liked. Oatmeal, rice, noodles, dumplings, cornmeal, and porridge are prominent.	Encourage whole grains.
Southern United States	Few whole-grain cereals are used. Hominy grits with gravy, hot biscuits with molasses, and cornbread are eaten.	Encourage consumption of whole-grain breads and cereals. Stress use of cooked cereals such as oatmeal.
Spanish-American, Mexican	Tortillas from enriched wheat flour; sweet rolls and breakfast cereals tend to be sugar coated. Fried macaroni is prepared and served with beans and potatoes.	In some areas where corn tortillas are used encourage use of enriched flour or whole wheat tortillas.

Source: Adapted with permission from *Cultural Food Patterns in the USA*, Chicago, the American Dietetic Association, 1976.

TABLE 3-3 CARBOHYDRATE CONTENT IN EXCHANGE GROUPS

Exchange Group	Grams of Carbohydrate	Type(s) of Carbohydrate(s)	Total kcal
Milk (1 cup)	12	Disaccharide (lactose)	80
Vegetable ($\frac{1}{2}$ cup)	5	Complex (starch); 2 g of fiber in some vegetables	25
Fruit (serving varies)	10	Monosaccharide (fructose); 2 g of fiber in some fruit servings	40
Bread and starchy vegetables	15	Complex (starch); 2 g of fiber in some servings	70

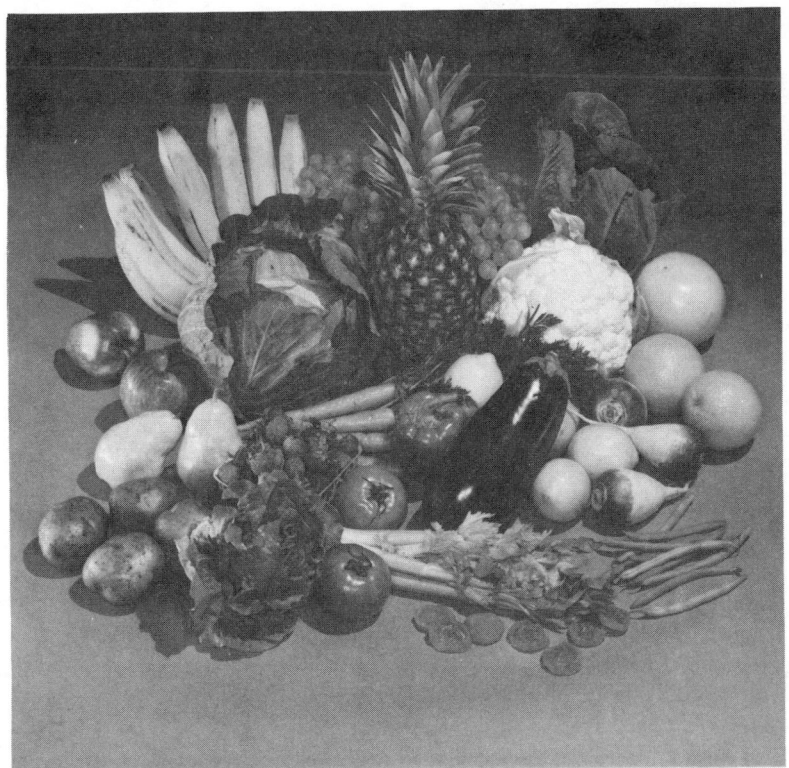

FIGURE 3-18 Servings from the vegetable and fruit groups provide starch and fructose. (Courtesy of the National Dairy Council.)

VEGETABLE GROUP

A vegetable exchange is one-half cup of a low-calorie vegetable and provides 24 kcal (see Fig. 3-18). One-half cup of some vegetables contain 2 g of fiber (listed on p. 51).

This group is important, since it contains complex carbohydrates (starch) and fiber (Table 3-3). Increasing daily servings of vegetables will help one achieve the recommended 48% of the total kilocalories from complex carbohydrates. Eating the vegetables listed on p. 51 helps one achieve a high fiber diet.

FRUIT GROUP

A fruit exchange varies from fruit to fruit in order that the exchange provides 10 g of carbohydrate and 40 kcal. Some fruit exchanges (listed on p. 51) have approximately 2 g of fiber.

This exchange group is a good source of monosaccharides, especially fructose (Table 3-3), but it is a poor source of dietary complex carbohydrates (starch). However, some fruits are good sources of fiber.

BREAD AND STARCHY
VEGETABLE GROUP

A bread and starchy vegetable exchange varies, so that a serving provides 15 g of carbohydrate (Table 3-3). Some foods in this group (listed on p. 51) contain 2 g of fiber per serving.

More complex carbohydrate, starch, and fiber are contributed by this group that any of the others. It is important to point out that some vegetables, such as corn and potatoes, are on this list rather than the vegetable list, since starchy vegetables contain 15 g of carbohydrate per serving compared to 5 g for those on the vegetable list.

FAT AND MEAT GROUPS

The fat and meat groups contain no dietary carbohydrates or fiber per exchange serving.

SUGAR

The exchange lists do not include one that gives the amount of concentrated sugar found in various foods. Dietary planning cannot be realistically done unless this information is available. Each food presented below contains the equivalent of 5 g of pure white sugar.

Serving Size (1 tsp; 20 Kcal; 5 g)	*Food*
Brown sugar	Jam
Molasses	Jelly
Corn syrup	Candy
Honey	Maple syrup

Catsup lovers should be aware that each tablespoon contains 1 tsp of sugar. Also, people who drink regular 12-oz cans of soft drink beverages, as opposed to the diet drinks, ingest about 9 tsp of sugar per can.[3]

OUTLINE

INTRODUCTION

Carbohydrates are important for normal body functioning and because of the cause–effect relationship in certain disorders: diseases of the large intestine, colon cancer, and dental caries.

CHEMISTRY OF CARBOHYDRATES

Molecules of carbohydrates are composed of carbon (C), hydrogen (H), and oxygen (0); hydrogen and oxygen atoms occur in a 2:1 ratio.

Carbohydrates Found in Foods
Monosaccharides $(C_6H_{12}O_6)$

1. Glucose: Found in foods like honey and fruits. Function: oxidized for energy; only monosaccharide is transported by the blood.
2. Galactose: Not found free, but rather as part of lactose, which is found in milk; converted to glucose by the liver.
3. Fructose: Found in fruits and honey; converted to glucose by the liver.

Disaccharides $(C_{12}H_{22}O_{11})$

1. Sucrose: Composed of glucose and fructose; found in sugar cane, maple syrup, bananas, sweet potatoes and table sugar.
2. Lactose: Composed of glucose and galactose; found in cow's milk and human breast milk; some people lack the enzyme (lactase) to digest lactose.
3. Maltose: Composed of two glucose molecules; not found naturally in foods.

Polysaccharides $(C_6H_{10}O_5)_n$
Composed of many glucose molecules

1. Glycogen: Branched chain; synthesized and stored in liver and skeletal muscles. Function: source of blood glucose.
2. Cellulose (fiber): Straight chain; found in plant cell walls; the body cannot digest it due to a lack of the necessary enzymes. Functions: increase intestinal motility, attract water into the intestines, and possibly prevent certain health conditions.
3. Starch: Branched chain; composed of glucose but found only in plants; found in seeds, cereal grains, fruit, roots, legumes, and nuts; the major source of carbohydrate in many countries, with corn and rice being two main examples.

FUNCTIONS OF CARBOHYDRATES
Source of Energy
Glucose is the prime source of energy for physiological activities. Inadequate intake of carbohydrates results in metabolism of triglycerides and release of ketones (acids). High level of ketones results in blood acidosis. From 100 to 125 g of carbohydrates must be consumed daily to prevent proteins from being used as a source of energy.

Starting Material for the Synthesis of Other Compounds
Nonessential fatty acids and amino acids can be synthesized from glucose.

DIGESTION AND ABSORPTION OF CARBOHYDRATES

Mouth
Salivary amylase digests starches to disaccharides and dextrins.

Stomach
Starch digestion continues until HCl denatures salivary amylase.

Small Intestine
Intestinal enzymes digest disaccharides to their respective monosaccharides.

Absorption
Intestinal villi in the jejunum and ileum increase absorption of nutrients by diffusion and active transport.

METABOLISM OF CARBOHYDRATES

Metabolism is divided into catabolism (breakdown phase) and anabolism (build-up phase).

Catabolism
Breakdown of glucose by oxidation reactions; important since it results in synthesis of ATP molecules.

Anaerobic Glycolysis
Two pyruvic acid molecules are produced together with two hydrogen transport molecules. Four ATP molecules are synthesized but two are used up.

Aerobic Respiration
Consists of the citric acid cycle and the electron transport system.

1. Citric acid (Krebs) cycle. Four pairs of hydrogen atoms are released, resulting in the synthesis of

three $NADH_2$ molecules and one $FADH_2$ molecule. Two CO_2 molecules are released; one ATP molecule is synthesized.

2. Electron transport system. Three ATP molecules are synthesized for each pair of hydrogen electrons transported through the system. Oxygen (O_2) is the final electron and hydrogen ion acceptor.

Anabolism and Interaction of Glycogenesis and Glycogenolysis

Glycogenesis: synthesizes glycogen and decreases blood glucose. Glycogenolysis: breaks down glycogen and releases glucose.

AMOUNTS AND FOOD SOURCES OF CARBOHYDRATES IN DIETS OF DIFFERENT CULTURES

1. Approximately 46% of the kilocalories in the U.S. diet come from carbohydrates: polysaccharides, 22%; disaccharides (sucrose), 24%.
2. The U.S. Senate Select Committee on Nutrition recommends that the kilocalories from carbohydrates be increased to 58%: polysaccharide, 48%; disaccharide, 10%.
3. Carbohydrates and the exchange groups. Each exchange contains:
   a. Milk: 12 g of carbohydrate; lactase is the primary carbohydrate.
   b. Vegetable: 5 g of carbohydrate; complex carbohydrate; 2 g of fiber in some vegetables.
   c. Fruit: 10 g of carbohydrate; fructose is the primary carbohydrate; some fruits contain 2 g of fiber.
   d. Bread and starchy vegetables: 15 g of carbohydrate; some foods contain 2 g of fiber.
   e. Fat and meat groups: These two groups contain no dietary carbohydrates or fiber per exchange.

REVIEW QUESTIONS

TRUE (A) OR (B) FALSE

Questions 1–26

1. Glucose, galactose, and sucrose are monosaccharides.
2. The body uses all of the monosaccharides as a source of energy.
3. Conversion of galactose and fructose to glucose occurs in the liver.
4. Glucose is the type of carbohydrate used in intravenous (IV) solutions.
5. Disaccharides include sucrose, lactose, and maltose.
6. Sucrose is composed of glucose and galactose.
7. Lactose is found only in cow's milk.
8. Lactose intolerance occurs only in people in their thirties.
9. Sucrose is also known as table sugar.
10. Honey is a better source of carbohydrate than refined sugar.
11. Polysaccharides important in the body are glycogen, cellulose, and starch.
12. Glycogen is important as a reserve source of blood glucose.
13. Most glycogen is stored in the liver.
14. Cellulose is second only to glycogen as a reserve source of blood glucose.
15. Glucose is a source of energy and a starting material for the synthesis of other compounds.
16. In order for carbohydrates to have a "protein-sparing" action, one must ingest 400–500 g/day.
17. Carbohydrate digestion begins in the mouth, with all types initially being broken down.
18. Disaccharide digestion begins in the small intestine with enzymes secreted by the pancreas.
19. Absorption of monosaccharides is increased by the intestinal villi.
20. Catabolism of glucose is important because it results in the synthesis of ATP molecules.
21. Glycogenesis or synthesis of glycogen occurs when a hyperglycemic condition exists.
22. Whenever the blood glucose level is above 120 mg/dl, glycogenolysis occurs to reduce it to normal.
23. A milk exchange contains more grams of carbohydrate than any other exchange.
24. The U.S. Senate Select Committee recommended that Americans reduce their intake of carbohydrates to 10–15% of their daily kilocalorie intake.
25. Each gram of carbohydrate yields 4 kcal of energy.
26. A meal that contains one exchange of milk, bread, and fruit has a total of 37 g of carbohydrate and 148 kcal.

MULTIPLE CHOICE

27. The shorthand way that health professionals write *carbohydrate* is:
    A. CHON.
    B. CARBO.
    C. CHO.
    D. none of these.
28. Two clinical applications of monosaccharides are the following:

A. Glucose is a source of carbohydrate in intravenous (IV) therapy.
B. Monosaccharides help reduce the chance of developing diverticulosis.
C. Short-term studies have shown that fructose can reduce the need for insulin for diabetics.
D. A, B.
E. A, C.

29. Two reasons why honey *is not* nutritionally better than sucrose are that:
A. honey contains no monosaccharides that sucrose does not contain.
B. honey does not contain appreciably higher amounts of proteins, calcium, iron, and vitamins.
C. honey is lower in kilocalories per teaspoon than sucrose.
D. A, B.
E. A, C.

30. The polysaccharide composing fiber is _____ _____ and dietary fiber is _____.
A. glycogen—the residue left after the laboratory treatment of food with acid and alkali.
B. starch—fiber resistant to human digestive enzymes.
C. cellulose—the residue left after digestion.
D. none of these.

31. Two functions of carbohydrates are _____ _____ and _____.
A. a source of energy—amino acids.
B. the starting material for the synthesis of other compounds—source of vitamins.
C. a source of energy—starting material for the synthesis of other compounds.
D. none of these.

Questions 32–37 apply to the meals below. The information necessary to answer them is found in Table 3-3.

	Exchanges	Grams of Carbohydrate	kcal
Breakfast			
1 egg	1 meat and ½ fat		75 70
1 slice toast	1 bread		45
1 tsp margarine	1 fat		
Lunch			
1 cup skim milk	1 milk		80
2 slices bread	2 bread		140
1 oz cottage cheese	1 lean meat		55
1 banana	2 fruit		80

	Exchanges	Grams of Carbohydrate	kcal
Dinner			
6 oz fish	6 oz lean meat		330
½ cup green beans	1 vegetable		25
½ cup carrots	1 vegetable		25
1 plain roll	1 bread		70
1 tsp margarine	1 fat		45
1 cup skim milk	1 milk		80

32. The breakfast meal contains _____ g carbohydrate and _____ kcal.
A. 25—190
B. 0—250
C. 15—190
D. none of these

33. Lunch contains _____ g of carbohydrate and _____ kcal.
A. 82—215
B. 62—355
C. 37—215
D. none of these

34. The dinner meal contains _____ g of carbohydrate and _____ kcal.
A. 37—575
B. 25—425
C. 45—635
D. none of these

35. The three meals contains a total of _____ g of carbohydrate and _____ kcal.
A. 124—1,250
B. 114—1,120
C. 105—955
D. none of these

36. For all three meals, the number of kilocalories contributed by carbohydrates is _____ kcal, which is _____% of the total kilocalories.
A. 496—65
B. 420—49
C. 456—41
D. none of these

37. In reference to adequacy, the total kilocalories contributed by the carbohydrates is _____.
A. higher than the recommended 55–60% of total kilocalories per day.
B. within the recommended 55–60% of total kilocalories per day.
C. lower than the recommended 55–60% of total kilocalories per day.

DISCUSSION QUESTIONS

1. Give two examples of how monosaccharides can be used clinically.

2. Discuss how much fiber is necessary to have a a high-fiber diet and describe two functions of fiber.
3. Discuss the digestion of starch in terms of location, enzymes, and products.
4. Differentiate between glycogenesis and glycogenolysis, and state the functions of each.

REFERENCES

1. P.A. Crapo and J.M. Olefsky. "Fructose—its characteristics, physiology, and metabolism." *Nutrition Today*, (July–August 1980).
2. R.B. Howard and N.H. Herbold. *Nutrition in Clinical Care*, 2nd ed. New York: McGraw-Hill, 1981, pp. 54–55.
3. E.M. Hamilton and E.N. Whitney. *Nutrition, Concepts and Controversies*, 2nd ed. St. Paul, Minn.: West Publishing Co., 1982, pp. 94–95.
4. J.W. Hole. *Human Anatomy and Physiology*, 2nd ed. Dubuque, Iowa: William C. Brown Co., 1981, p. 456.
5. "On fiber, dietary and Crude." *Nutrition and the M.D.*, *10*(10), 2 (October 1984).
6. G.J. Tortora and N.P. Anagnostakas. *Principles of Anatomy and Physiology*, 3rd ed. New York: Harper & Row, 1981, pp. 628–630.
7. T.R. Lankford. *Integrated Science for Health Students*, 2nd ed. Reston, Va.: Reston Publishing Co., 1979, pp. 53, 513, 567–572.
8. Food and Nutrition Board, Committee on Recommended Allowances. *Recommended Dietary Allowances*, 9th ed. Washington, D.C.: National Academy of Sciences, 1980.

4 LIPIDS

OBJECTIVES

Upon completion of this chapter, you should be able to:

1. Describe the structure of a triglyceride molecule.

2. Distinguish between saturated and unsaturated fatty acids and name three polyunsaturated fatty acids.

3. Describe what an iodine number of fatty acids is and why vegetable fats have greater iodine numbers than animal fats.

4. List two functions of saturated and unsaturated fats.

5. Distinguish between essential and nonessential fatty acids and give an example of a polyunsaturated essential fatty acid.

6. Describe the structure of phospholipids and name two phospholipids that are important in the body.

7. Describe three functions of phospholipids and two food sources.

8. Recognize the structure of a cholesterol molecule and name the origin of the majority of cholesterol in the body.

9. Give the functions of cholesterol and three food sources.

10. Differentiate between low-density lipoproteins (LDL) and high-density lipoproteins

(HDL) in terms of their functions and correlation with increased heart attack.

11. Give six functions of lipids.

12. Describe what emulsification and digestion to globules accomplish.

13. Discuss what happens to glycerol and fatty acids when they pass into intestinal wall cells.

14. Discuss what transports short chain and long chain fatty acids.

15. Describe the basic symptom that indicates the inability to digest and absorb fats and give three conditions that can cause this symptom.

16. List three reasons why medium chain triglycerides (MCTs) can compensate for fat malabsorption problems.

17. Differentiate between low-, medium-, and high-fat meats in terms of their fat content.

18. Analyze different diets in terms of which ones are higher in fat and be able to calculate the total kilocalories and percentage due to fat.

INTRODUCTION

Lipid A biological substance that has an oily or
greasy touch and is insoluble in water. Lipids are
soluble in organic sol-
vents such as ether and
alcohol.

Lipids are a very diverse group of organic compounds that includes oils,
fats, resins, and waxes that originate in plants and animals. Subclasses
of lipids that are important in the body are **glycerides, phospholipids,
sterols,** and **lipoproteins.**

CHEMISTRY OF LIPIDS

GLYCERIDES

Triglyceride A molecule
that is composed of a
glycerol molecule to
which is attached three
fatty acids.

Glycerides compose about 95–98% of the fats in food and in the body.
Triglyceride is the most common example in this subclass (see Fig.
4-1). A triglyceride molecule is composed of a glycerol to which is attached three fatty acids. A fatty acid is a straight, even-numbered carbon

chain. One end of the chain is a carboxyl acid radical $\left(-C\overset{\displaystyle O}{\underset{\displaystyle OH}{\diagup}}\right)$, which

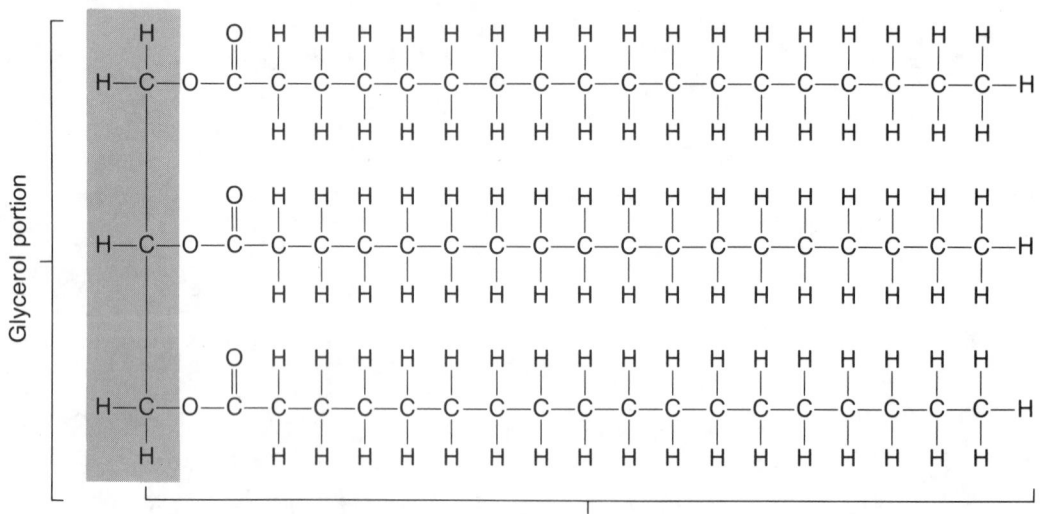

Fatty acid portions

FIGURE 4-1 A triglyceride molecule is composed of a glycerol molecule that is
attached to three fatty acids (FA). (From Hole, John W., Jr., *Human Anatomy and
Physiology,* 3d ed. (c) 1978, 1981, 1984 Wm. C. Brown Publishers, Dubuque,
Iowa. All rights reserved. Reprinted by permission.)

Fatty acid Chain of carbon and hydrogen atoms that functions as a building block of fat molecules.

Long chain fatty acids Fatty acids that are 18 to 20 carbon atoms in length.

Medium chain fatty acids Fatty acids that contain 14 to 16 carbon atoms.

Short chain fatty acids Fatty acids that contain 8 to 12 carbon atoms.

Saturated fatty acid A fatty acid whose carbon atoms are linked by single bonds, and are bonded to as many hydrogen atoms as possible.

Unsaturated fatty acid A fatty acid whose carbon atoms are linked by double or triple bonds, and therefore are not bonded to as many hydrogen atoms as possible.

Monounsaturated fatty acid A fatty acid that contains one double bond.

Polyunsaturated fatty acid A fatty acid that contains two or more double bonds.

Hydrogenation A process by which an unsaturated fat is changed to a solid saturated fat by forcing hydrogens into the substance.

PUFA Polyunsaturated fatty acids.

Cholesterol A lipid that is produced by the body and used in the synthesis of steroid hormones and excreted in bile.

gives off hydrogen ions (H^+) and therefore is the source of the acid part of the **fatty acid.**

Fatty acids vary in length from 4 to 24 carbon atoms. The more common fatty acids in dietary fat are called **long chain fatty acids. Medium chain fatty acids** contain 14 to 16 carbon atoms, whereas **short chain fatty acids** contain 8 to 12. Triglycerides are named long, medium or short chain triglycerides, depending on the number of fatty acids present in the three chains.[1]

SATURATED AND UNSATURATED FATTY ACIDS

Double bonds may or may not be present between carbon atoms in fatty acids. There are two types of fatty acids: **saturated** and **unsaturated.** The term *saturated* comes from the fact that the fatty acid contains as many hydrogen atoms as possible (Fig. 4-2). Unsaturated fatty acids contain fewer hydrogen atoms due to the double bonds. For every double bond in a fatty acid, there are two fewer hydrogen atoms (Fig. 4-2). A **monounsaturated fatty acid** has one double bond, whereas a **polyunsaturated fatty acid** has two or more.

The dietary sources of saturated fatty acids are animal fat, beef, butter, chicken eggs, and whole milk. Unsaturated fatty acids are obtained from vegetable oils: corn, olive, soybean, peanut, and safflower.

The more saturated a fat is, the harder it is at room temperature. Likewise, unsaturated fats are more liquid at room temperature. As a rule of thumb, a person who wanted to buy unsaturated fatty acids would buy the more liquefied ones, which are generally the vegetable and fish oils.

Margarine is an example of a fat that must be somewhat hard in order to be spread. To make a margarine from a polyunsaturated oil such as corn oil, the producer will put it through **hydrogenation.**[2]

POLYUNSATURATED FATTY ACIDS (PUFA)

The ratio of **PUFA** to saturated fatty acids (i.e., the P/S ratio) in the total diet concerns nutritionists because of the potential health benefits of the unsaturated plant–derived PUFA. Research shows that polyunsaturated fat can reduce the **serum cholesterol** level.

Three PUFA that are important in the body are **linoleic, arachidonic,** and **linolenic** acids (See Fig. 4-3). Table 4-1 presents the number of carbon atoms, double bonds, and food sources of these PUFA.

IODINE NUMBER OF FATTY ACIDS

One way to determine the degree of unsaturation of a fat is to measure how much iodine combines with fatty acids at their double bonds. The

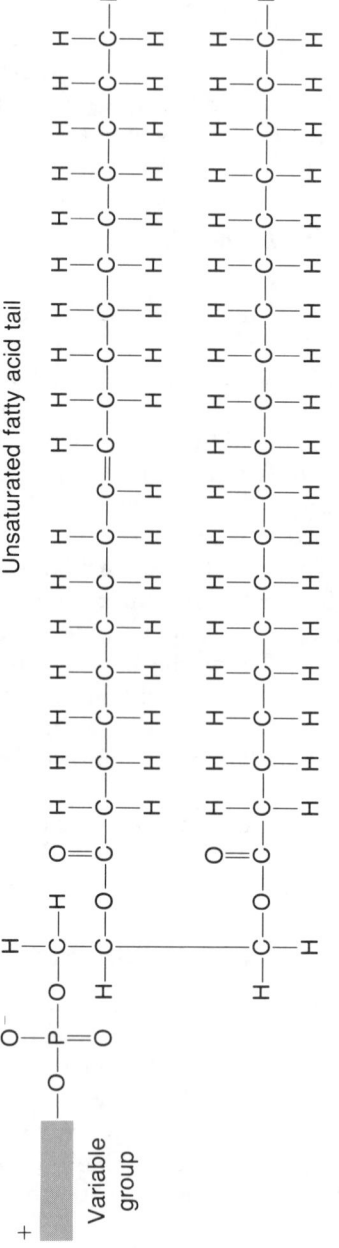

Unsaturated fatty acid tail

Saturated fatty acid tail

Variable group

(a)

FIGURE 4-2 (a) A phospholipid is composed of two fatty acids and a phosphate group, with an attached nitrogen group in place of the third fatty acid. (b) Lecithin and cephalin are two important phospholipids in the body. (From T. Randall Lankford, *Integrated Science for Health Students*, 3rd ed., 1984. Reprinted by permission of Reston Publishing Company, a Prentice-Hall Company, 11480 Sunset Hills Road, Reston, Va. 22090.)

H—C—O—C—R₁ (structure)

Cephalins

Lecithin

(b)

FIGURE 4-2 (Continued)

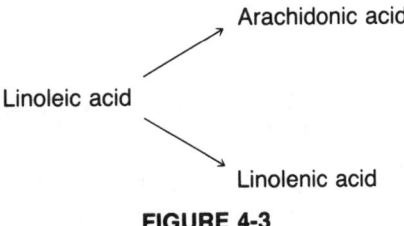

FIGURE 4-3

The top structure (Cephalins):

$$
\begin{array}{c}
\text{H} \quad\quad \text{O} \\
\text{H—C—O—C—R}_1 \\[4pt]
\quad\quad\quad\quad \text{O} \\
\text{H—C—O—C—R}_2 \\[4pt]
\quad\quad\quad\quad \text{O} \\
\text{H—C—O—P—CH}_2\text{—CH}_2\text{—NH}_2 \\
\text{H} \quad\quad \text{O}^-
\end{array}
$$

Cephalins

$$
\begin{array}{c}
\text{H} \quad\quad \text{O} \\
\text{H—C—O—C—R}_1 \\[4pt]
\quad\quad\quad\quad \text{O} \\
\text{H—C—O—C—R}_2 \\[4pt]
\quad\quad\quad\quad \text{O} \\
\text{H—C—O—P—O—CH}_2\text{—CH}_2\text{—N(CH}_3)_3 \\
\text{H} \quad\quad \text{O}^-
\end{array}
$$

Lecithin

(b)

FIGURE 4-2   (Continued)

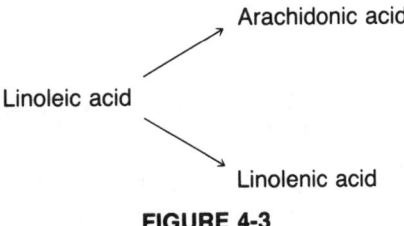

FIGURE 4-3

TABLE 4-1 COMMON FATTY ACIDS IN THE BODY

Common Name of Fatty Acid	Number of Carbons: Number of Double Bonds	Food Sources
Linoleic acid	18:2	Safflower oil, sunflower oil, and corn oil
Linolenic acid	18:3	Soybean oil
Arachidonic acid	20:4	Animal fat

Iodine number Number of grams of iodine absorbed by 100 g of fat.

greater the number of double bonds, the higher the **iodine number** and the greater the degree of unsaturation. Some iodine numbers of vegetable and animal sources of fats are:

- Vegetable fats: iodine numbers range from 90 to 200+
    Examples: corn oil: 115–124
              soybean oil: 130–138
- Animal fats: iodine numbers range from 25 to 65
    Examples: butter: 25–40
              lard: 50–65[3]

Coconut oil is a vegetable oil that has a low iodine number (8–10). It is actually more saturated than some animal fats. Coconut oil is often used in nondairy creamers and nondairy whipped toppings.

FUNCTIONS OF SATURATED AND UNSATURATED FATS

Saturated Fats	Unsaturated Fats
Source of energy (9 kcal/g)	Source of energy (9 kcal/g)
Raise the serum cholesterol level and increase the risk of developing atherosclerosis	Aid the liver in converting cholesterol to bile acids
	Enhance the liver's ability to decrease excess fatty acids (see Fig. 4-4)

Essential fatty acid A fatty acid (e.g., linoleic acid) that cannot be manufactured by the body in adequate quantities and, therefore, must be obtained from the diet. Its absence results in a specific deficiency disease.

ESSENTIAL AND NONESSENTIAL FATTY ACIDS

A fatty acid may be described as being either **essential** or **nonessential.** Linoleic acid, a polyunsaturated fatty acid, is the essential fatty acid required by the body for healthy cell membranes.

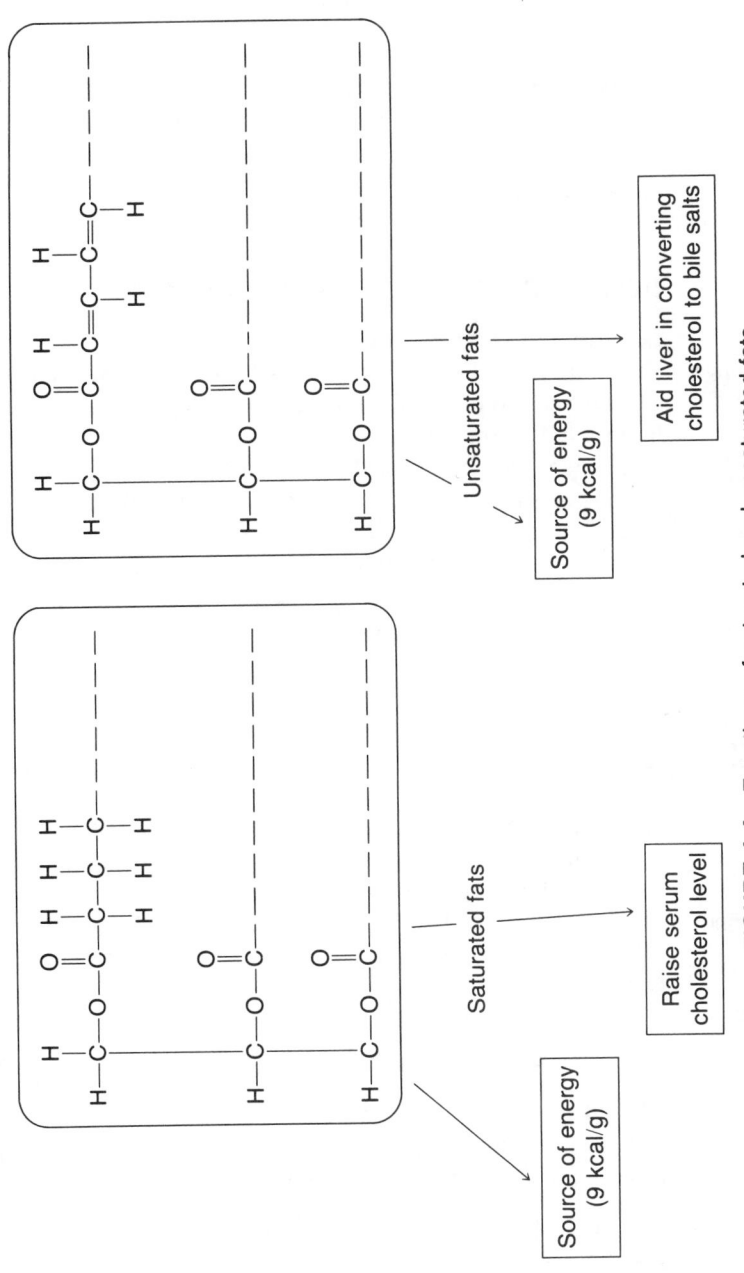

FIGURE 4-4 Functions of saturated and unsaturated fats.

TABLE 4-2 FOODS RICH IN LINOLEIC ACID

Plant Foods	% Linoleic Acid	Animal Foods	% Linoleic Acid
Safflower oil	74.1	Poultry	19.5
Sunflower oil	65.7	Fish, salmon	4
Corn oil	58.0	Pork	10.2
Wheat germ oil	54.8	Shortening	6
Cottonseed oil	51.5		

DEFICIENCY OF ESSENTIAL FATTY ACIDS

Dermatitis Inflammation of the skin, evidenced by itching and redness.

Diets that are deficient in linoleic acid are rare, but when they occur the skin may become irritated and reddened (**dermatitis**). Deficiencies are usually seen in hospital patients receiving liquid diets intravenously and infants fed formulas that are lacking in linoleic acid. Foods that are rich in linoleic acid are presented in Table 4-2.

The prevention or relief of dermatitis is actually not the result of linoleic acid; rather, it is due to the presence of arachidonic and linolenic acids. Since linoleic acid is widely available in foods compared to arachidonic and linolenic acids, linoleic acid is important as a precursor for the synthesis of the other two.[2]

PHOSPHOLIPIDS

Lecithin A phospholipid found in the body.

Cephalin A phospholipid found in the body.

A phospholipid molecule is very similar to a triglyceride. It is composed of glycerol and two fatty acids, but in place of the third fatty acid there is a phosphate and nitrogenous compound (see Fig. 4-5). Two important phospholipids in the body are **lecithin** and **cephalin**. Phospholipids differ from each other according to the nitrogenous compound they contain.

LOCATION AND FUNCTIONS

All cell membranes are composed of proteins and phospholipids. The cells in the brain, nervous tissue, and liver are especially rich in phospholipids. The functions of phospholipids are (see Fig. 4-5):

Emulsifying agents Substances that increase the surface area of fats for ease of absorption.

- Structural components of cell membranes
- Powerful **emulsifying agents**
- Transport agents of other lipids in the body

Phospholipids are nonessential nutrients. Liver, brains, heart, and egg yolk are good food sources.

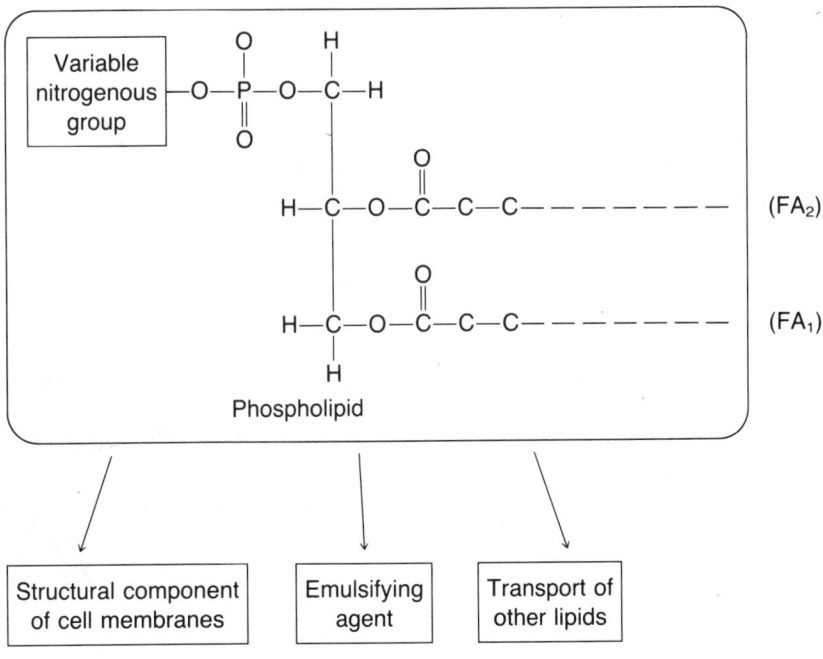

FIGURE 4-5   Functions of phospholipids.

STEROLS

Sterols, a subclass of lipids, have a completely different chemical structure from the triglycerides and phospholipids. Their chemical structure consists of four fused rings (see Fig. 4-6). Cholesterol is the most important nutritional sterol.

Steroid hormones
Hormones secreted by the adrenal cortex and other endocrine glands that have a typical steroid shape.

LOCATION AND FUNCTION

Cholesterol is located in cell membranes. It is a precursor of both **steroid hormones** such as estrogen, testosterone, aldosterone, and cortisone and

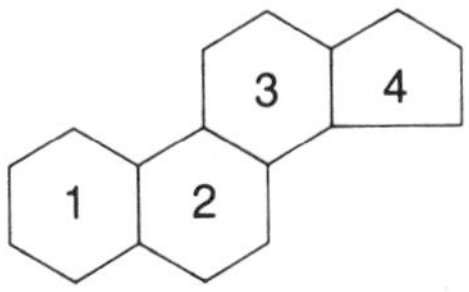

FIGURE 4-6   A cholesterol molecule as well as other steroids are composed of four fused rings. (From T. Randall Lankford, *Integrated Science for Health Students,* 3rd ed., 1984. Reprinted by permission of Reston Publishing Company, a Prentice-Hall Company, 11480 Sunset Hills Road, Reston, Va. 22090.)

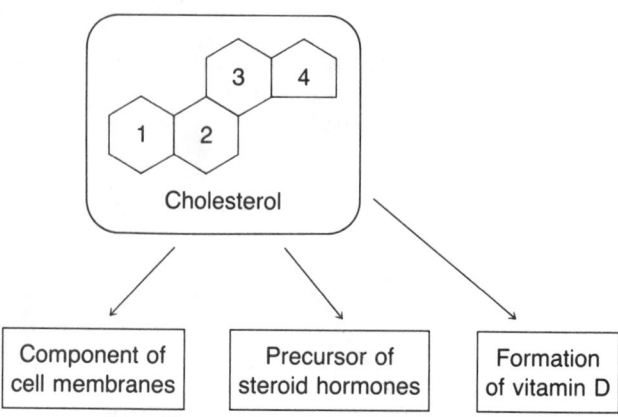

FIGURE 4-7 Functions of cholesterol.

of bile acids. Cholesterol can by synthesized by the body, and about 60% of it in the body is synthesized by the liver and intestine.

The functions of cholesterol are (see Fig. 4-7):

- A component of cell membranes
- A precursor of steroid hormones

Plaques Mounds of lipid material, smooth muscle cells, and calcium.

Cardiovascular disease Disease of the blood vessels and the heart.

Cholesterol has many beneficial functions in the body; however, high levels in the blood have been associated with the development of fatty **plaques** in arteries and ultimately with atherosclerosis. The normal concentration of cholesterol in the blood ranges from 150 to 300 mg/100 ml (150 to 300 mg%) of blood. When the concentration is persistently well above 300 mg%, the chances of developing **cardiovascular disease** are higher than if the cholesterol level is within the normal range.

FOOD SOURCES OF CHOLESTEROL

Since approximately 40% of cholesterol comes from food, we need to be aware of which foods are rich in it. They include egg yolks, butter, cream, cheese, sweetbreads, liver, and other organ meats, and shellfish (lobster, shrimp, and oysters).[4]

LIPOPROTEINS

Lipoprotein lipid with a protein coat around it.

A **lipoprotein** is a lipid with a protein coat around it. The body combines the two together so that the lipids are soluble in blood and **lymph** (remember, lipids are insoluble in water and blood in primarily water).

Lipoproteins are synthesized in intestinal cells and the liver. The lipids transported are primarily triglyceride, cholesterol, and phospholipids.

Blood lipid profile A measurement of the amounts of different classes of lipoproteins.

The level of lipoproteins in the blood can be determined by a **blood lipid profile,** and if low-density lipoproteins (LDL) are abnormally high, a person has a greater risk of developing cardiovascular disease. The classes of lipoproteins and their composition are discussed next.

CLASSIFICATION AND COMPOSITION OF LIPOPROTEINS

Lipoproteins are classified into five types on the basis of their lipid composition and density of the protein coat:

Chylomicrons. Made in the intestinal cells and transport just-eaten triglycerides to the liver, where they are dismantled and new lipids synthesized. Chylomicrons have a thin protein coat and therefore a low density. They can be seen floating at the top of a blood sample, where they form a creamy layer.

VLDL (very-low-density lipoproteins). Made primarily by liver cells and transport triglycerides and some cholesterol to the tissues. They circulate in the blood for a few hours and are then converted to IDL.

IDL (intermediate-density lipoproteins). Formed in the liver after triglycerides are removed from VLDL and then converted to LDL.

LDL (low-density lipoproteins). Made in the liver, they are composed of about 50% cholesterol, which they transport to the tissues (see Fig. 4-8). LDL can combine with blood calcium to form **plaques** in arteries.

HDL (high-density lipoproteins). Very dense due to the amount of protein coat they contain. HDL contain about 20% cholesterol, which they transport from tissues and plaques to the liver (see Fig. 4-8), where the cholesterol is degraded and secreted in bile.

CARDIOVASCULAR DISEASE AND LIPOPROTEINS

Research has shown that there is a correlation between the levels of LDL and HDL and the risk of developing cardiovascular disease. The risk of plaque formation and cardiovascular disease increases with a high level of blood cholesterol. Cholesterol is transported through the blood by lipoproteins, especially LDL; therefore, a high level of LDLs correlates closely with an increased risk of cardiovascular disease. LDL have a tendency to accumulate in the inner lining of arteries, possibly as a result of their protein coat.

Since HDL transport cholesterol as well as LDL, why is there a reduced risk of cardiovascular disease with an increase in the level of HDL? The

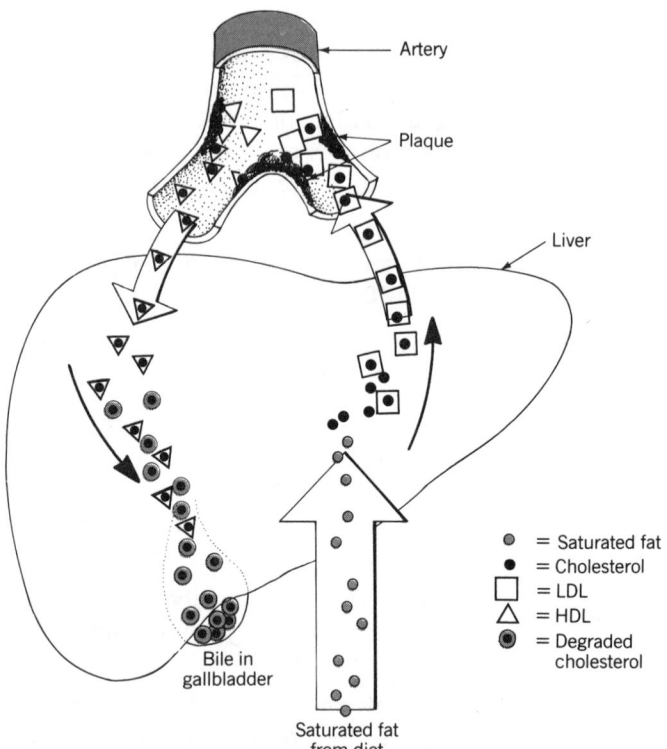

FIGURE 4-8 Formation and function of LDL and HDL are shown. Saturated fat in the diet is converted to cholesterol by the liver. LDL carries cholesterol from the liver through the blood, possibly resulting in the formation of plaques. HDL transports cholesterol from plaques to the liver, where it is degraded and secreted in bile. Plaques tend to form at points where arteries branch, since mechanical stresses are greater at these points.

reason is that as described above, HDL transport cholesterol from the tissues and plaques to the liver, where it is decomposed. Since HDL tend to reduce the risk of cardiovascular disease, they are sometimes called "good cholesterol." Research on raising HDL shows that consumption of fish rather than meat is helpful. However, the best way to raise HDL is by exercise—prolonged, intense, and frequent.

$$\uparrow \text{LDL level} = \uparrow \text{cholesterol level} = \uparrow \text{risk of heart attack}$$

$$\uparrow \text{HDL level} = \downarrow \text{cholestrol level} = \downarrow \text{risk of heart attack}$$

FUNCTIONS OF LIPIDS

Much information has been published in recent years on the harmful effects of cholesterol and saturated fats in the body. Logically, then, many people may conclude that fats should be eliminated from the diet as much as possible. This belief is incorrect. Lipids have some very important functions in the body, such as (see Fig. 4-9):

Concentrated source of energy. Fat provides more than twice as much as energy as carbohydrates and proteins: 9 kcal/g for fat as opposed to 4 kcal/g for carbohydrates and proteins.

Important component of cell membranes. Phospholipids and cholesterol are important structural components of cell membranes. One reason why swallowing kerosene, gasoline, or paint thinner is often fatal is that these compounds dissolve the phospholipids and cholesterol in the cells composing the digestive tract.

Aid absorption of fat-soluble vitamins. Fat-soluble vitamins cannot be absorbed into the blood and lymph unless fat is present.

Padding for the body's organs. All of the vital organs that maintain homeostasis are surrounded by a layer of fat. The kidneys, eyeballs, and heart are three examples.

Help maintain body temperature. Fat located below the skin helps to insulate the body against rapid loss of heat during the winter. This function results from the fact that fat does not conduct heat.

Component of various important chemical reactions. Bile salts help emulsify fats for fat digestion. All of the steroid hormones and vitamin D are synthesized from cholesterol.[1]

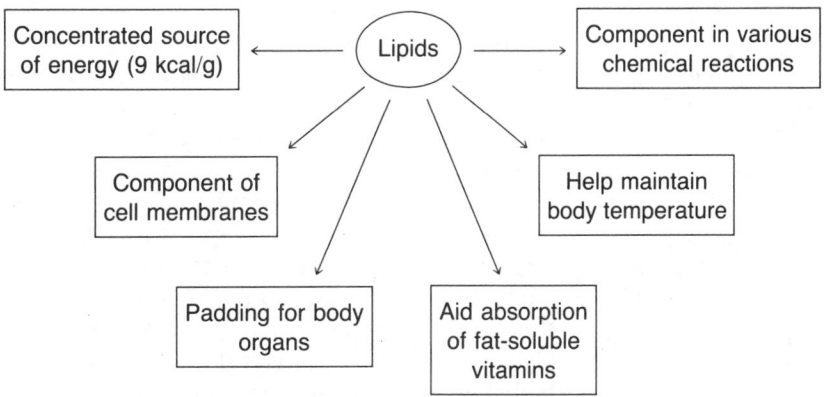

FIGURE 4-9 Functions of lipids.

DIGESTION AND ABSORPTION OF LIPIDS

Triglycerides, phospholipids, cholesterol, and sterols all are composed of large molecules. They cannot be absorbed into the blood and lymph from the digestive tract until they have been digested to smaller molecules. In this section, we will discuss how triglycerides are prepared by digestion for absorption and then used by the body.

EMULSIFICATION AND DIGESTION

Globules Small masses of material. Fat globules are small masses of fat.

Bile salts Clear yellow or orange fluid secreted by the liver.

Water soluble Refers to substances that dissolve in water. Fats become water soluble when a protein coat is secreted around them (see the discussion of water-soluble vitamins in Chapter 6).

Chylomicrons Lipoproteins synthesized in the intestines that transport triglycerides through the lymph and blood to the liver.

Lacteals Lymph vessels.

Leftsubclavianvein Vein that receives the majority of lymph and chylomicrons.

Portal vein Vein that brings blood rich in nutrients into the liver. Blood from the intestines, stomach, and spleen drain into the portal vein.

Monoglycerides Glycerides that contain one fatty acid chain.

No chemical digestion of triglycerides occurs until they reach the duodenum of the small intestine. When fats reach the duodenum, they are in the form of **globules,** which cannot be effectively broken down. The entrance of fats into the duodenum stimulates the release of **bile salts** from the gallbladder into this organ. Bile acts as an emulsifier and breaks up globules into small droplets (see Fig. 4-10). Emulsification increases the surface area of fat molecules, enabling pancreatic lipase enzymes to break down the triglyceride molecules more rapidly. The pancreatic enzymes are emptied into the duodenum by the pancreatic duct at the same point at which bile enters through the common bile duct.

Lipase enzymes break down about 25% of the triglycerides into fatty acids and glycerol. The other 75% are broken down into **monoglycerides.** Enzymes split off two of the fatty acids (usually the ones on the ends) in a triglyceride molecule, resulting in the formation of a monoglyceride.

ABSORPTION

After triglyceride molecules have been digested, they are absorbed through the intestinal lining into either blood vessels or lymph vessels.

In order for these digested materials (three triglycerides and one glycerol) to be absorbed, they must become **water soluble** (remember, lipids are insoluble in water), since blood and lymph are composed primarily of water. This process is accomplished by two methods—by combining with bile salts and by forming lipoproteins (**chylomicrons**). Bile salts combine with fatty acids and monoglycerides, which then pass into intestinal wall cells. The intestinal cells synthesize new triglyceride molecules, which are then wrapped in a thin membrane of phospholipid and lipoprotein. This water-soluble package is a chylomicron, and the larger ones are absorbed into the **lacteals** (see Figs. 4-11 and 4-12), whereas the smaller ones and short chain fatty acids are absorbed into the blood. The lymph vessels transport the larger chylomicrons into the blood (**left subclavian vein**) near the heart (see Fig. 4-12). Blood carries the smaller chylomicrons and short chain fatty acids initially into the liver through the **portal vein** (see Fig. 4-12).

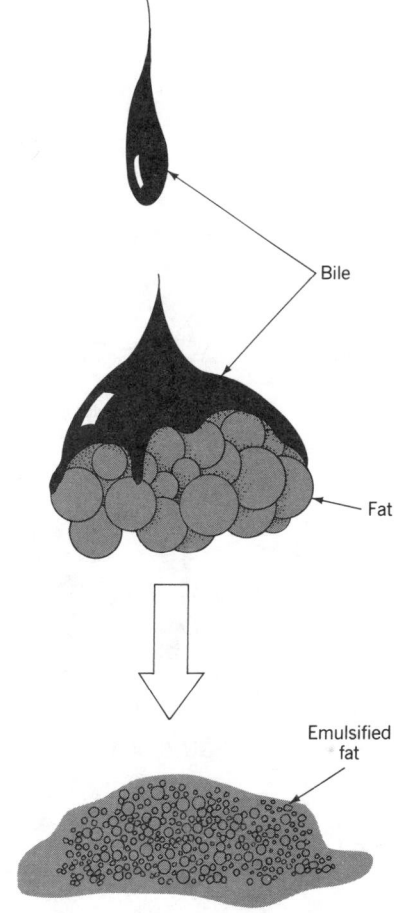

FIGURE 4-10   Emulsification of fat by bile.

METABOLISM

The liver, cardiac, and skeletal muscle cells metabolize triglycerides for energy. The majority of triglycerides, however, are removed by fat depots and stored as energy.[4]

In addition to metabolizing triglycerides for energy, the liver cells carry out the following fat metabolism functions:

- Synthesis of triglycerides from carbohydrates
- Synthesis of phospholipids and lipoproteins from proteins
- Synthesis of cholesterol from triglycerides
- Clearance or degradation of phospholipids, cholesterol, and lipoproteins from the blood

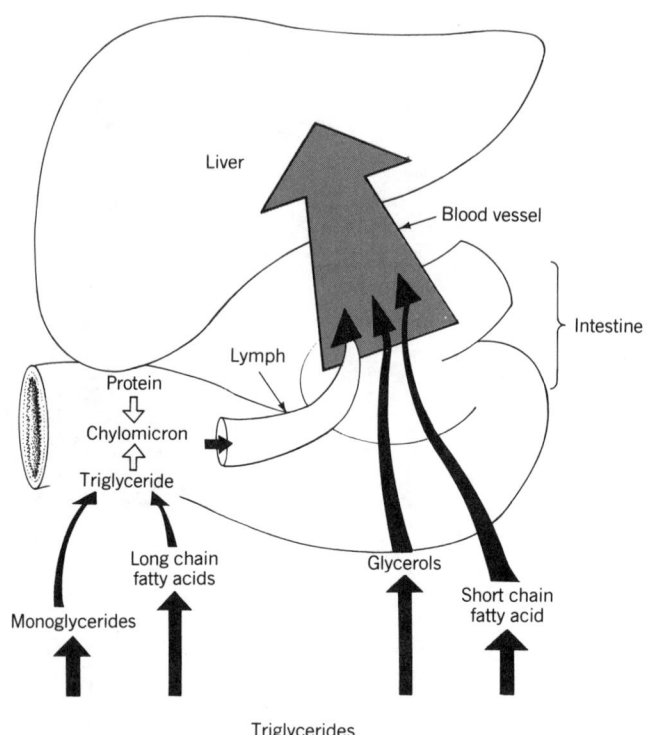

FIGURE 4-11 Absorption, synthesis, and transport of lipids.

STORAGE OF FAT

Adipose tissue Fat tissue.

The majority of triglycerides in the body are stored in fat cells composing **adipose tissue.** The number of fat cells probably reaches its maximum at adulthood or during pregnancy. Therefore, increased deposition of fat in an adult occurs primarily by increasing the amount of fat in each cell. Research shows that fat cells in an obese person may be 100 times larger than in a thin person. The size of fat cells also depends on their location in the body. In children, the cells of **subcutaneous** adipose tissue are larger than those in deeper tissues. In an adult, regions where fat is stored and percentages for each are:

Subcutaneous Under the skin.

Subcutaneous tissue—50%

Around kidneys—12%

Omenta A serous membrane attached to the visceral organs.

Omenta—10–15%

Genital areas—20%

Between muscles—5–8%[5]

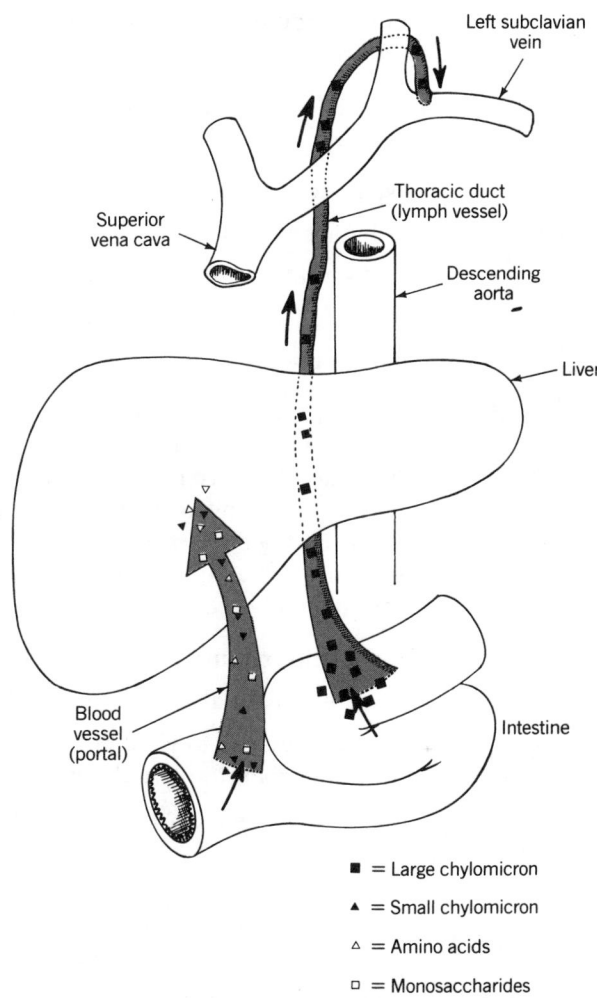

FIGURE 4-12 Large chylomicrons are absorbed into lacteals and transported by lymph into the left subclavian veins. Small chylomicrons, together with amino acids and monosaccharides, are transported by blood from the intestines to the liver.

PROBLEMS ASSOCIATED WITH DIGESTION AND ABSORPTION OF FATS

Steatorrhea Abnormally large amounts of fats in the feces.

Dehydration Excessive water loss from the tissues (see Chapter 9).

There are several conditions that can result in an inability to digest and absorb fats normally. The basic symptom that indicates the existence of this malabsorption problem is **steatorrhea.** The stools are light, mushy, greasy, and foul-smelling. This malabsorption problem may also result in severe diarrhea, **dehydration,** and **electrolyte depletion.**

Pancreatic enzyme deficiency A deficiency in the amount of enzymes secreted by the pancreas. This deficiency is especially a problem with pancreatic lipase, which breaks down triglycerides.

Cystic fibrosis A hereditary disease characterized by secretion and accumulation of excessively thick mucus that blocks the secretion of pancreatic enzymes (see Chapters 20 and 22).

Short bowel Surgical shortening of the length of the small intestine. Normally done as a therapeutic procedure to aid person in losing weight.

Gluten intolerance A disorder in which gluten (protein) causes the destruction of intestinal villi, thereby preventing the absorption of fats and other nutrients (see Chapter 19).

Some conditions that can result in steatorrhea and other previously described problems are:

Pancreatic enzyme deficiency

Cystic fibrosis

Bile salts deficiency

Lymphatic obstruction

Liver disease

Short bowel

Gluten intolerance

In each of the above conditions, *long chain triglycerides (LCT)* are not absorbed and are lost in feces. The reason is that they must go through the complex digestive processes in order to be absorbed, and due to the above problems, this does not effectively occur. In order to compensate for these problems, *medium chain triglycerides (MCT)* were developed synthetically several years ago. These MCT can provide compensation for the following reasons:

• They do not require bile salts for digestion or absorption.

• They are rapidly absorbed, even with a short bowel.

• They are digested to yield fatty acids that are absorbed into the portal vein rather than the lymphatic vessels.

• They can be mixed with LCT, which improves LCT digestion and absorption.[6]

FAT AND THE EXCHANGE GROUPS

Two food exchange groups that contain considerable amounts of fat are meat and fat. Some foods on the bread and milk exchange lists also contain fat (see below). The meat and fat exchange lists whose foods contain considerable amounts of fat will be discussed below.

MEAT

This group is subdivided into three categories according to fat content:

Low-fat meats. These meats contain 3 g of fat per exchange and a total of 55 kcal. Examples of low-fat meats are given in the meat exchange list in Appendix A.

Medium-fat meats. This category contains 5.5 g of fat per exchange and a total of 75 kcal or add one-half of a fat exchange (see the meat list in Appendix A).

High-fat meats. Meats in this category contain 8 g of fat per exchange and 100 kcal or add one fat exchange (see the meat list in Appendix A).

Many people believe that meats in the high-fat category are better quality than meats in the medium- and low-fat categories. There are 7 g of protein per exchange in each of the three meat categories. The quantity of fat does increase from 3 to 8 g per exchange in moving from the low- to high-fat meats categories. Therefore, high-fat meats are certainly not better in terms of protein but, rather, contain more fat and are more tender than the low- and medium-fat meats.

One should be aware that a meat exchange is 1 oz of meat, which is not a normal serving size. For meal planning, 4 oz of meat or four meat exchanges is considered normal. A small fast-food hamburger is about 2 oz when cooked.

FAT

A fat exchange is a serving of food that contains about 5 g of fat and about 45 kcal. The protein and carbohydrate contents are negligible.

Most people think of meat as being primarily protein. However, an analysis of a quarter-pound hamburger (not including the bun and other ingredients) reveals some interesting facts.

Protein	Fat
27 g	32 g
× 4 kcal/g	× 9 kcal/g
108 kcal	288 kcal
Total kcal = 396	

Notice that the meat contains 5 g more fat than protein. Since fat contribute 9 kcal/g compared to 4 kcal/g of protein, fat contributes 180 more calories to the total than does protein. Fat contributes about 72% and protein 28% of the total kilocalories in the meat. The fat is also saturated rather than unsaturated.

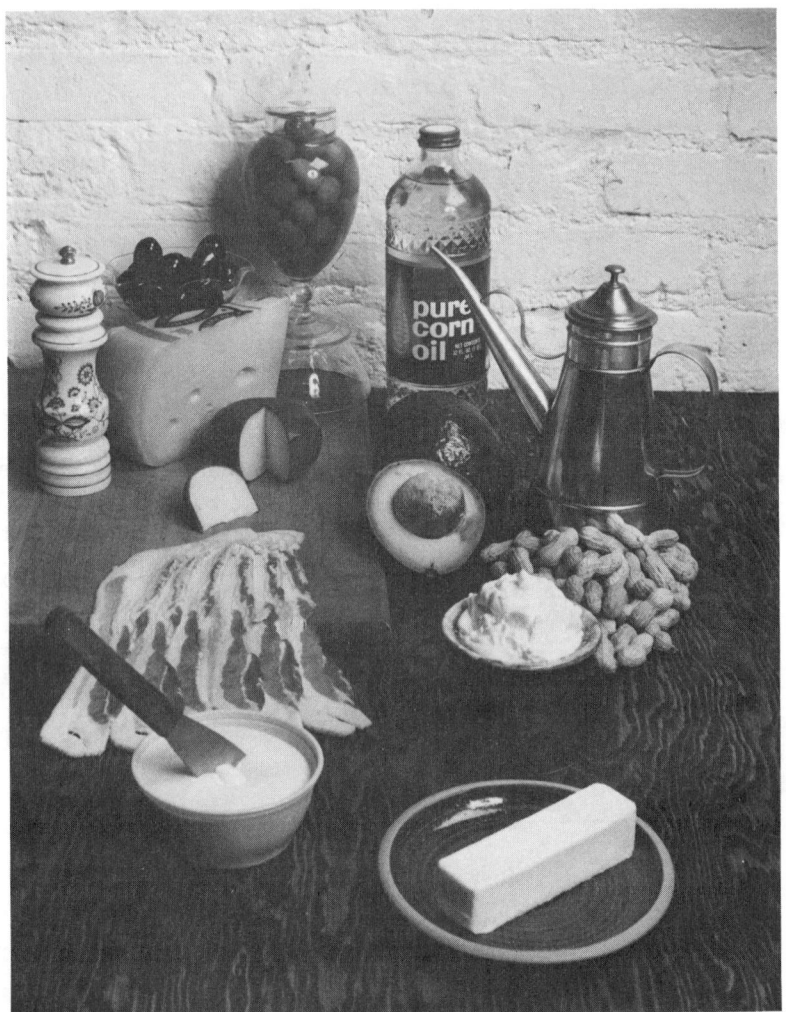

FIGURE 4-13 Foods in the fat exchange group. (Courtesy of Nickola M. Sargent.)

Some examples of foods that contain 1 fat exchange are (see Fig. 4-13):

- 1 tsp of butter or margarine
- $\frac{1}{8}$ of an avocado
- 5 small olives
- 2 large pecans
- 1 tsp french dressing
- 2 tbsp sour cream
- 1 tbsp heavy cream
- 1 strip of bacon

The milk exchange group list is based on 1 cup of skim milk. Therefore, if a person drinks 1 cup of whole milk, he or she is actually getting 10 g of invisible fat. In other words, "invisible" fat is not obvious when one looks at foods. Visible fat is that which can be seen, such as the strip of fat around beef cuts.

Some bread exchanges contain fat. Examples are:

1 biscuit—2-in. diameter (add 1 fat exchange)

1 piece of cornbread—2 × 2 × 1 in. (add 1 fat exchange)

8 french fried potatoes—(add 1 fat exchange)

15 potato chips—(add 2 fat exchanges)

1 pancake—5 × $\frac{1}{2}$ in. (add 1 fat exchange)

1 waffle—5 × $\frac{1}{2}$ in. (add 1 fat exchange)

In order for a diet to be balanced, it must contain the following in regard to fat:

• Thirty percent of the total calories should come from fat.

• The fat ingested should be one-third saturated fats, one-third mono-unsaturated fats, and one-third polyunsaturated fats.[7]

	Higher-Fat Menu	*Restricted-Fat Menu*
Breakfast	2 fried eggs, $\frac{1}{2}$ cup hashed brown potatoes, 2 slices toast, 2 tsp butter or margarine, coffee, cream, sugar	1 cup ready-to-eat cereal, 1 cup low-fat milk, 4 oz orange juice, coffee, milk
Lunch	cheeseburger, roll, french fries, tomato slices, lettuce, iced tea	sliced chicken sandwich with 2 slices bread, tomato slices, lettuce, 1 tsp mayonnaise, 1 cup skim milk
Dinner	6 oz steak, 1 large baked potato with 2 tbsp sour cream, $\frac{1}{2}$ cup peas, $3\frac{1}{2}$ oz red wine, coffee, cream, sugar, slice of apple pie, 1 scoop ice cream. This menu derives about 42–45% percent of its kilocalories from fat; cholesterol: approximately 900 mg.	4 oz roast veal, $\frac{1}{2}$ cup rice, salad (spinach, lettuce plus 1 tbsp french dressing, $\frac{1}{2}$ cup broccoli with lemon juice), coffee, milk, sugar, 1 medium apple. This menu derives about 30–35% of its kilocalories from fat; cholesterol: approximately 250 mg.

It is difficult for the average person to know whether a diet meets all of these criteria. However, the two menus on the previous page are examples of higher- and lower-fat meals plus kilocalories and cholesterol.

These menus are not nutritionally adequate, but rather represent typical meal selections commonly available in restaurants and fast-food establishments.[8]

The milk and bread exchange lists contain certain foods that contain fat (see Appendix A).

OUTLINE

INTRODUCTION

Lipid: Any biological substance that is insoluble in water and is greasy or oily to the touch.

Four Subclasses: glycerides, phospholipids, sterols, and lipoproteins.

CHEMISTRY OF LIPIDS
Glycerides

1. Compose 95–98% of fats eaten and in the body.
2. Triglyceride is the most common example; composed of glycerol and three fatty acids.
3. Long chain fatty acids are 18–20 carbon atoms in length; medium chain fatty acids are 14–16 carbon atoms in length; short chain fatty acids are 8–12 carbon atoms in length.

Saturated and Unsaturated Fatty Acids

1. Saturated: contains no double bonds and a maximum number of hydrogen atoms.
2. Unsaturated: contains double bonds and fewer hydrogen atoms.
3. Dietary sources of saturated fatty acids: animal foods (beef, butter, eggs, and whole milk).
4. Dietary sources of unsaturated fatty acids: vegetable oils (corn, olive, and safflower).

Polyunsaturated Fatty Acids (PUFA)

1. Contain two or more double bonds.
2. Can reduce serum cholesterol levels.
3. Linoleic, arachidonic, and linolenic acids are three important PUFA in the body.
4. Iodine number of fatty acids measures the degree of unsaturation; higher numbers indicate a greater number of double bonds.

Functions of Saturated and Unsaturated Fats

1. Saturated: Act as a source of energy and raise the serum cholesterol level.
2. Unsaturated: Act as a source of energy; aid the liver in converting cholesterol to bile acids; help the liver decrease excess fatty acids.

Essential and Nonessential Fatty Acids

1. Essential: The body cannot manufacture them, and their absence can result in deficiency disease.
2. Nonessential: The body can synthesize them if proper quantities of carbon, hydrogen, and oxygen atoms are present.

3. Deficiency: Can result in skin irritation; usually seen in hospitalized patients receiving formulas and intravenous fluids.

PHOSPHOLIPIDS
Composition
Glycerol, two fatty acids, and a nitrogenous group.

Location
All cell membranes, with brain, nerve, and liver tissues especially rich.

Functions
Structural components of the cell membrane; powerful emulsifying agents; transport other lipids.

STEROLS
Composition
Composed of four fused rings; cholesterol is the most common example.

Location
Cell membranes.

Functions
Component of cell membranes; precursor of steroid hormones

Food Sources of Cholesterol
40% comes from food and 60% is synthesized by the body; primary sources are egg yolks, butter, cream, cheese, and shellfish.

LIPOPROTEINS
Structure
Protein is wrapped around lipid molecules in order to make them water soluble.

Classification
Low-density lipoproteins (LDL) and high-density lipoproteins (HDL).

Functions: LDL transport cholesterol from liver through blood to tissues; HDL transport cholesterol from blood to liver, where it is degraded.

FUNCTIONS OF LIPIDS

1. Concentrated source of energy.
2. Important component of the cell membrane.
3. Aid absorption of fat-soluble vitamins.
4. Padding for body's organs.
5. Help maintain body temperature.
6. Component of various important chemical reactions.

DIGESTION, ABSORPTION, AND USE OF LIPIDS

Triglycerides, phospholipids, cholesterol, and sterols cannot be absorbed until they have been digested to their chemical building blocks.

Emulsification and Digestion

Bile breaks down large globules into smaller particles, which enables lipase enzymes to digest particles to glycerol, fatty acids, and monoglycerides.

Absorption

Glycerol, fatty acids, and monoglycerides pass into intestinal cells, where new triglycerides (chylomicrons) are synthesized; large chylomicrons are absorbed into lymph vessels (lacteals); small ones are absorbed into blood.

Use

Liver, cardiac, and skeletal muscle cells metabolize triglycerides for energy; the majority are stored in cells as energy reserves. The liver also carries out the following metabolic functions: synthesis of triglycerides from carbohydrates; synthesis of phospholipids and lipoproteins from proteins; synthesis of cholesterol from triglycerides; clearance or degradation of phospholipids, cholesterol, and lipoproteins from the blood.

STORAGE

The majority of triglycerides are stored in adipose tissues.

The number of fat cells reaches a maximum at adulthood; obesity increases the deposition of fat in cells rather than increasing the number of cells.

PROBLEMS ASSOCIATED WITH DIGESTION AND ABSORPTION OF FATS

The basic symptom of fat malabsorption is steatorrhea.

LCT cannot be absorbed with fat malabsorption problems.

MCT can be absorbed rapidly into blood without being digested and without the need of bile.

FAT AND THE EXCHANGE GROUPS

Meat and fat groups are the only two that all foods on the exchange lists contain fat.

Meat

Subdivided into three categories—low, medium, and high—based on the amount of fat present.

Fat

One exchange contains 5 g of fat; some foods contain invisible fat (e.g., milk, biscuits, pancakes, waffles, and cornbread).

REVIEW QUESTIONS

TRUE (A) OR (B) FALSE

Questions 1–18

1. A triglyceride molecule is composed of a glycerol atom and three fatty acid atoms.
2. A saturated fat differs from an unsaturated fat in that saturated fats contain hydrogen atoms at every possible carbon bond.
3. Polyunsaturated fatty acids (PUFA) are valuable nutritionally because they are low in kilocalories compared to saturated fatty acids.
4. Three essential PUFA are glycerol, cholesterol, and arachidonic acid.
5. An iodine number is a measure of the degree of unsaturation of a fatty acid.
6. Animal fats typically have higher iodine numbers than vegetable fats because they tend to be more unsaturated than vegetable fats.
7. An essential fatty acid is one that the body has to make for physiological activities.
8. Three functions of phospholipids are: precursor of steroid hormones, component of fatty plaques, and powerful emulsifying agents.
9. The majority of cholesterol in the body is synthesized by liver and intestine cells.
10. Foods rich in cholesterol are egg yolks, butter, cream, cheese, sweetbreads, and shellfish.
11. Emulsification of globules increases their surface area, which enables lipase enzymes to break down the molecules.
12. Most glycerol and fatty acids are not changed as they pass through intestinal cells into the blood or lymph.
13. High-density lipoproteins (HDL) tend to lower blood cholesterol levels by transporting cholesterol from tissues to the liver, where it is broken down.
14. Steatorrhea is a basic symptom of abnormal fat digestion and absorption.
15. Some examples of fat digestion and absorption disorders are atherosclerosis, eczema dermatitis, and steatorrhea.
16. High-fat meats not only contain more fat but also more protein than low-fat meats.
17. People should be aware that some foods, such as biscuits, cornbread, and waffles, contain invisible fat.
18. A balanced diet should derive no more than about 30% of the total kilocalories from fat.

MULTIPLE CHOICE

19. Functions of unsaturated fats are:
    A. a source of energy (9 kcal/g).
    B. to raise the serum cholesterol level.
    C. to aid the liver in converting cholesterol to bile acids.
    D. A, C.
    E. B, C.

20. A phospholipid is composed of:
    1. glycerol
    2. three fatty acids
    3. phosphate and nitrogenous compound
    4. fused rings
    A. 1, 2, 3.   B. 2, 4.   C. 1, 3.   D. 4.
    E. all of these.

21. The formation of lipoproteins is important because they:
    A. contain essential fatty acids.
    B. enable insoluble fats to be transported in blood and lymph.
    C. are precursors of steroid hormones.
    D. are stored in fat cells.
    E. none of these.

22. Lipase enzymes break down triglycerides to:
    A. fatty acids.
    B. glycerol.
    C. monoglycerides.
    D. A, C.
    E. A, B, C.

23. Short chain fatty acids are absorbed and transported by:
    A. lymph.
    B. blood.
    C. protoplasm.
    D. cellular fluid.
    E. none of these.

24. Medium chain triglycerides (MCT) can compensate for fat malabsorption problems by:
    A. not requiring bile salts to be absorbed.
    B. being absorbed slowly.
    C. being absorbed into blood.
    D. A, B.
    E. A, C.

25. Which of the following in regard to meat categories and fat plus kilocalories is (are) incorrect?
    A. low fat—3 g and 55 kcal.
    B. medium fat—5.5 g and 80 kcal.
    C. high fat—8 g and 100 kcal.
    D. all of these.
    E. none of these.

Questions 26–31 apply to the meals below. The information necessary to answer these questions is found in Table 2-5.

	Exchanges	Fat (g)	Saturated (S), Unsaturated (U)	kcal
Breakfast				
1 egg	1 meat + ½ fat	—	S	—
1 slice toast	—	0		70
1 tsp margarine	1 fat	—	U	45
Lunch				
1 cup skim milk	1 milk	0		—
2 slices bread	2 bread	0		140
1 oz cottage cheese	—	—	S	55
1 banana	2 fruit	0		—
Dinner				
6 oz fish	6 oz low-fat or lean meat	—	S	330
½ cup green beans	1 vegetable	0		—
½ cup carrots	—	0		25
1 plain roll	1 bread	0		70
1 tsp margarine	—	—	U	45
1 cup skim milk	1 milk	0		80

26. The breakfast meal contains _____ g fat and _____ kcal.
    A. 10—225
    B. 5—190
    C. 0—115
    D. 10—190

27. The lunch meal contains _____ g of fat and _____ kcal.
    A. 3—355
    B. 10—215
    C. 6—160
    D. 0—245

28. The dinner meal contains _____ g of fat and _____ kcal.
    A. 3—675
    B. 9—525
    C. 23—575
    D. 14—425

29. The three meals contain a total of _____ g of fat and _____ kcal.
    A. 13—1365
    B. 36—1120
    C. 25—1575
    D. 23—925

30. For all three meals, the number of kilocalories contributed by fats is _____ kcal, which is _____ % of the total kilocalories for all three meals.
    A. 324—29
    B. 258—39
    C. 456—47
    D. 189—25

31. In reference to adequacy, the total kilocalories contributed by fats is _____ .
    A. higher than the 30% of total kilocalories/day.

B. within the recommended 30% or less of total kilocalories/day.

DISCUSSION QUESTIONS

1. Give six functions of lipids.
2. Differentiate between low-density lipoproteins (LDL) and high-density lipoproteins (HDL) in terms of functions and correlation with increased heart attack.
3. Name the basic symptom indicative of an inability to digest and absorb fats and give three conditions that can cause this symptom.
4. Give three reasons why medium chain triglycerides (MCT) can compensate for fat malabsorption problems.

REFERENCES

1. S.J. Wickham. *Human Nutrition: A Self-Instructional Text.* Bowie, Md.: Robert J. Brady Co., 1982, pp. 61–62.
2. J.J.B. Anderson. *Applied Nutrition for Health Professions: Basic Nutrition.* Chapel Hill, N.C.: School of Public Health, University of North Carolina, 1983, pp. 95–96.
3. E.N. Whitney and E.M. Hamilton. *Understanding Nutrition,* 2nd ed. St. Paul, Minn.: West Publishing Co., 1981, p. 68.
4. T.R. Lankford. *Integrated Science for Health Students,* 3rd ed. Reston, Va.: Reston Publishing Co., 1984, p. 416.
5. G.J. Tortora and N. P. Anagnostakos. *Principles of Anatomy and Physiology,* 3rd ed. New York: Harper & Row, 1981, p. 651.
6. L. Aftergood and R.B. Slater. "Dietary fat—An ongoing controversy," *Nutrition and the M.D.,* 8, 1–2 (1982).
7. E.M. Hamilton and E.N. Whitney. *Nutrition: Concepts and Controversies,* 2nd ed. St. Paul, Minn.: West Publishing Co., 1982, pp. 120–121.
8. D.H. Calloway and K.O. Carpenter. *Nutrition and Health.* Philadelphia: W.B. Saunders Co., 1981, p. 41.

5 PROTEINS

OBJECTIVES

INTRODUCTION

Protein The most fundamental constituent of living matter. Proteins are
essential for the growth
and repair of animal tis-
sue.

The term **protein** comes from the Greek word *proteios,* meaning of prime
importance or primary. This is a most appropriate name for this group,
since proteins are the most fundamental constituents of living matter.
Proteins function as major structural and functional components of every
living cell.

CHEMISTRY OF PROTEINS

Proteins are organic compounds that are composed of carbon, hydrogen,
oxygen, and nitrogen atoms. They differ from carbohydrates and lipids
in that they contain nitrogen atoms in addition to carbon, oxygen, and
hydrogen; some proteins also contain sulfur.

Amino acid The fundamental building block of
proteins.

The fundamental chemical building block of proteins is the **amino
acid.** Figure 5-1 shows the amino and carboxyl acid groups that compose
amino acids. These two groups form the core of each of the 20 different
amino acids. What distinguishes one amino acid from another is the
R-group (see Fig. 5-2). The R-group can be thought of as being "the rest
of the molecule"; it varies from one hydrogen atom to a complicated
group of carbons and hydrogens. The R-groups also vary in their elec-
trical charge.[1]

R-group The rest of the
amino acid that is at-
tached to the amine and
acid portions of the molecule.

ESSENTIAL AND NONESSENTIAL
AMINO ACIDS

Nonessential amino acids
Amino acids that can be
synthesized by the adult
body from carbohydrates,
lipids, and other amino
acids.

Ten of the approximately 20 amino acids that are widely distributed,
can be synthesized by the adult body from carbohydrates, lipids and
other amino acids. These 10 are designated **nonessential amino acids.**

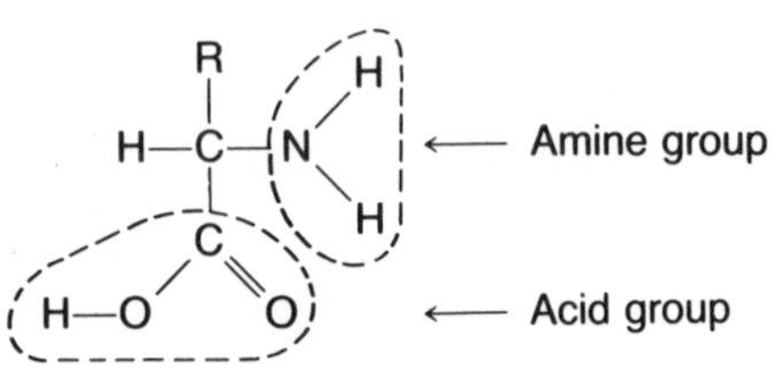

FIGURE 5-1   The core of an amino acid consists of amine and acid groups. (From
T. Randall Lankford, *Integrated Science for Health Students,* 3rd ed., 1984. Reprinted by permission of Reston Publishing Company, a Prentice-Hall Company,
11480 Sunset Hills Road, Reston, Va. 22090.)

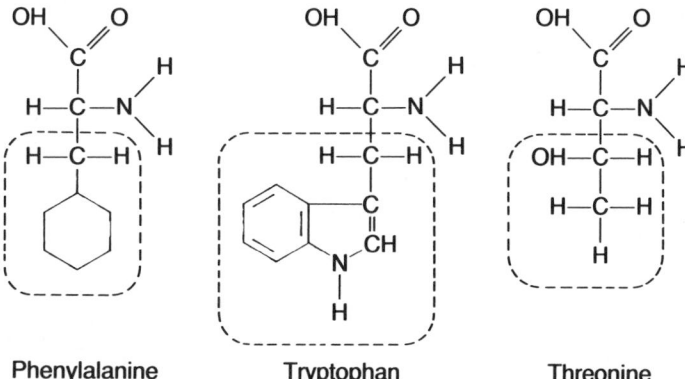

Phenylalanine   Tryptophan   Threonine

FIGURE 5-2 Three amino acids with their R-groups shown within the dashed lines. (From T. Randall Lankford, *Integrated Science for Health Students,* 3rd ed., 1984. Reprinted by permission of Reston Publishing Company, a Prentice-Hall Company, 11480 Sunset Hills Road, Reston, Va. 22090.)

TABLE 5-1 ESSENTIAL AND NONESSENTIAL AMINO ACIDS

Glycine

Alanine

Valine[a]

Leucine[a]

Isoleucine[a]

Serine

Threonine[a]

Aspartic acid

Glutamic acid

Lysine[a]

Arginine[b]

Cystine (composed of two cysteine)

Methionine[a]

Tyrosine

Phenylalanine[a]

Tryptophan[a]

Proline

Histidine[c]

Glutamine

Asparagine

[a]Essential amino acids.
[b]Synthesized in the body too slowly for metabolic needs.
[c]Essential in diets of children only.

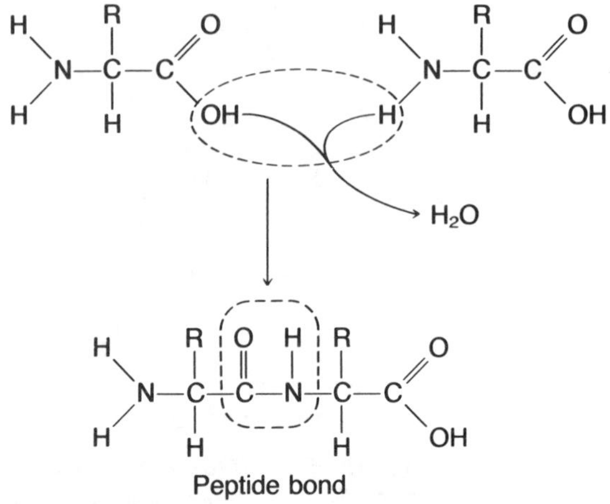

$$H-\underset{\underset{H}{|}}{N}-\underset{\underset{H}{|}}{\overset{\overset{R}{|}}{C}}-\overset{\overset{O}{\|}}{C}-(OH) \qquad (H)-\underset{\underset{H}{|}}{N}-\underset{\underset{H}{|}}{\overset{\overset{R}{|}}{C}}-\overset{\overset{O}{\|}}{C}-OH$$

$$\longrightarrow H_2O$$

$$H-\underset{\underset{H}{|}}{N}-\underset{\underset{H}{|}}{\overset{\overset{R}{|}}{C}}-\overset{\overset{O}{\|}}{C}-\underset{\underset{H}{|}}{N}-\underset{\underset{H}{|}}{\overset{\overset{R}{|}}{C}}-\overset{\overset{O}{\|}}{C}-OH$$

Peptide bond

FIGURE 5-3 A peptide bond joins two amino acids together. (From T. Randall Lankford, *Integrated Science for Health Students,* 3rd ed., 1984. Reprinted by permission of Reston Publishing Company, a Prentice-Hall Company, 11480 Sunset Hills Road, Reston, Va. 22090.)

Essential amino acids Amino acids that must be present in the diet, since they cannot be synthesized by the body.

The other 10 are known as **essential amino acids** and must be present in the diet (see Table 5-1). Eight of the 10 essential amino acids are essential throughout life. Histidine is essential during childhood only, and arginine is synthesized in the body too slowly for metabolic purposes. It should be emphasized that "essential" and "nonessential" refer only to whether or not an amino acid needs to be present in the diet and is not related to its importance in body functions.

PROTEIN STRUCTURE

Peptide bonds Chemical bonds that connect amino acids.

Proteins are very large molecules and frequently are composed of several hundred amino acids bonded together into long chains. **Peptide bonds** (see Fig. 5-3) join amino acids. Many proteins are composed of two or more connected chains that are twisted and folded into definite shapes (see Fig. 5-4).

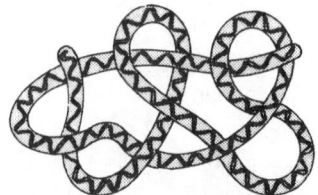

FIGURE 5-4 A twisted coiled shape of a protein is shown. (From T. Randall Lankford, *Integrated Science for Health Students,* 3rd ed., 1984. Reprinted by permission of Reston Publishing Company, a Prentice-Hall Company, 11480 Sunset Hills Road, Reston, Va. 22090.)

COMPLETE AND INCOMPLETE PROTEINS

Complete proteins Proteins that contain all of the essential amino acids in amounts needed by the body.

Complete proteins are found in animal products: meat, milk, cheese, and eggs. **Incomplete proteins** are found in plant products: grains, kidney beans, garden peas, lima beans, seeds, and nuts (see Fig. 5-5).

Incomplete proteins Proteins lacking one or more of the essential amino acids.

SEQUENCE OF AMINO ACIDS IN PROTEINS

The sequence in which amino acids are arranged in a protein is precise and important. The body can synthesize so many different proteins because of the almost infinite number of ways the 20 amino acids can be arranged. The function of each protein is directly related to its amino acid sequence and to the shape of the molecule. To illustrate the importance of amino acid sequence to function, see the Clinical Application "Sickle Cell Disease."

Sickle cell disease A disease characterized by abnormal hemoglobin that results in sickle-shaped red blood cells.

DENATURATION OF PROTEINS

Denaturation A change in the chemical structure of a molecule; often occurs with protein molecules when certain conditions exist.

As stated previously, all proteins have a characteristic structure that determines their functions. If the structure of a protein is **denatured** (see

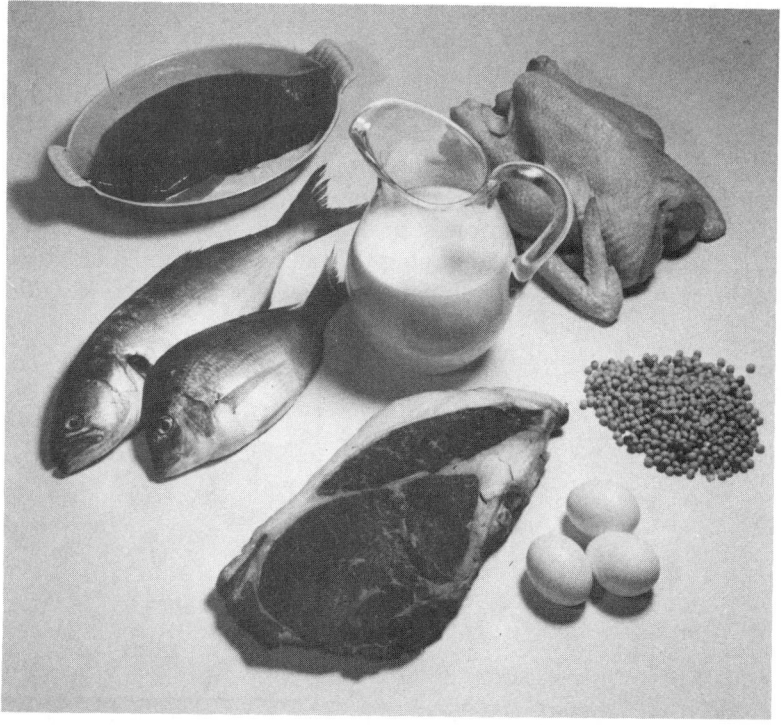

FIGURE 5-5 These foods contain complete and incomplete proteins.

CLINICAL APPLICATION: SICKLE CELL DISEASE

Hemoglobin A protein molecule composed of four amino acid chains with one iron atom in each.

Sickle cell disease is characterized by abnormal **hemoglobin** in red blood cells (RBCs). Normal hemoglobin is composed of two kinds of amino acid chains. One chain in sickle cell hemoglobin is normal. In the other chain, the sixth amino acid should be *glutamine* but has been replaced by *valine*. This one alteration in the sequence of amino acids results in a hemoglobin molecule that cannot transport oxygen efficiently to the tissues. This condition is called *sickle cell disease* because the abnormal RBCs take on a stiff sickle shape (see Fig. 5-6 and Table 5-2). Due to their shape, the RBCs tend to become clogged in small capillaries, resulting in great pain and destruction of the cells. This problem is an inherited recessive trait and is seen almost exclusively in blacks. Initial signs and symptoms are frequently seen in children under 2 years of age.[2]

Acidosis A condition in which the pH of blood is below 7.35; can result in the denaturation of proteins.

Alkalosis A condition in which the pH of blood is above 7.45; can result in the denaturation of proteins.

Keratin A protein substance in hair and nails.

Fig. 5-7), the functions of the protein are lost or altered. There are several factors that can cause proteins to be denatured in the body, such as high temperature and pH changes (**acidosis** or **alkalosis** conditions) in the blood. When these factors change, it is generally for a short period of time. As a result, the proteins are only temporarily denatured, resuming their normal shape once the condition is corrected. If the above changes persist, the proteins may be permanently denatured. An example of purposefully denaturing proteins is cooking an egg. Eggs are rich in complete proteins, but they are cooked or denatured before eating. Shampooing the hair is an example of temporary protein denaturation. The shampoo and water cause the **keratin** protein in hair to change

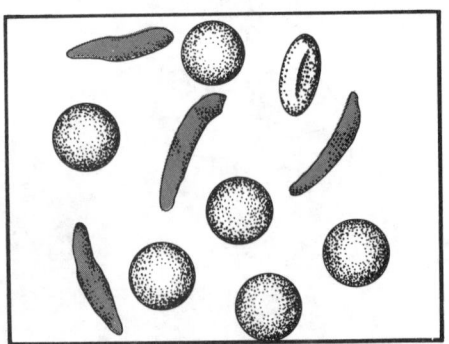

Normal RBCs and sickle cells

FIGURE 5-6   Normal red blood cells versus sickle cells.

**TABLE 5-2 NORMAL
VERSUS SICKLE CELL
SEQUENCE OF AMINO
ACIDS IN ONE CHAIN
OF HEMOGLOBIN**

Normal		Sickle Cell Disease
Valine	1	Valine
Histidine	2	Histidine
Leucine	3	Leucine
Threonine	4	Threonine
Proline	5	Proline
Glutamine	6	Valine
Glutamine	7	Glutamine
Lysine	8	Lysine

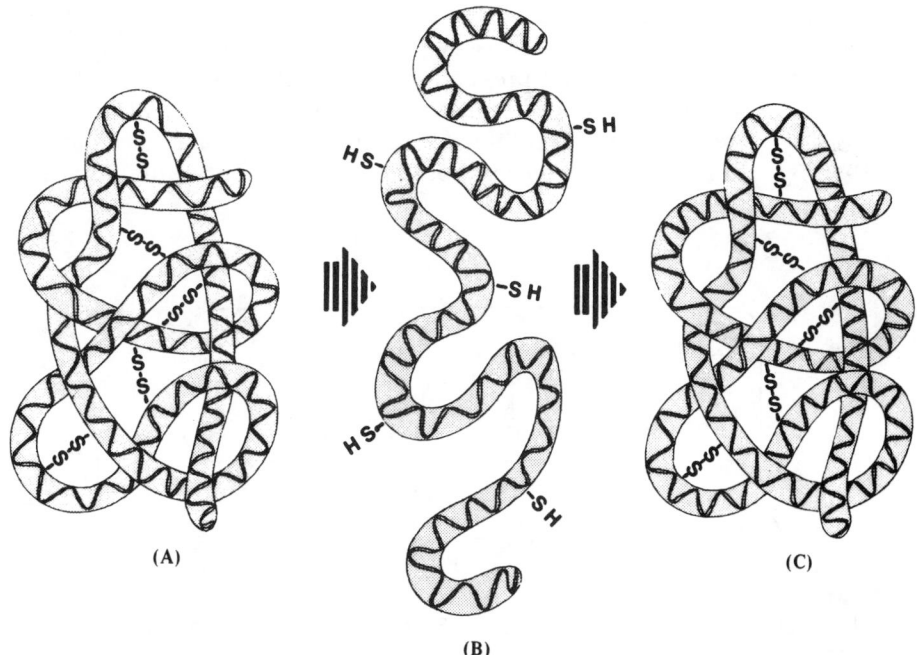

(A)

(B)

(C)

FIGURE 5-7 (*a*) Normal shape of a protein molecule. (*b*) Protein denatured or uncoiled. (*c*) Normal shape of protein restored. (From T. Randall Lankford, *Integrated Science for Health Students,* 2nd ed., 1979. Reprinted by permission of Reston Publishing Company, a Prentice-Hall Company, 11480 Sunset Hills Road, Reston, Va. 22090.)

shape temporarily, as indicated by the straightening of the hair. Once the hair is dried, the keratin protein molecules resume their normal shape, as evidenced by the appearance of the hair.

FUNCTIONS OF PROTEINS

Proteins have the greatest diversity of functions of the three energy nutrients. Several of the more important functions are discussed below.

GROWTH AND REPLACEMENT
(See Fig. 5-8)

Collagen Fibrous, insoluble protein found in connective tissue.

Epithelial Cells that form the outer layer of the skin.

As stated previously, proteins are the most fundamental constituent of living tissues; therefore, the growth and production of new tissues as well as replacement of old, worn-out cells require a constant input of essential and nonessential amino acids to the tissues. The cells then synthesize structural proteins such as **collagen** in connective tissue and *keratin* in hair. New tissue production occurs, for example, in a growing child and during pregnancy in both fetal and maternal tissues.

Examples of cell replacement include replacement of worn-out RBCs; replacement of **epithelial** cells that line intestinal tract and last for about a month; and constant loss and replacement of the outer layer of skin cells.

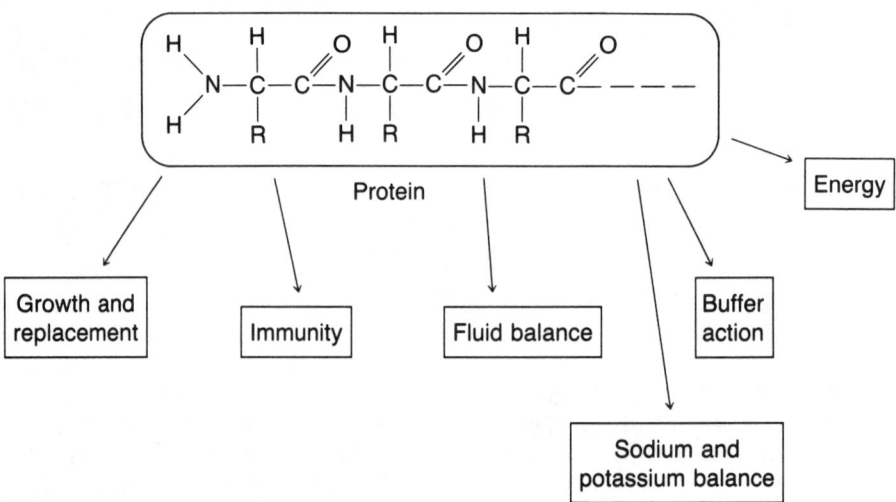

FIGURE 5-8 Functions of proteins.

IMMUNITY

Antibodies Proteins formed by the body to combat antigens.

Antigens Foreign substances (usually proteins) that invade the body; can cause infections and allergic reactions.

One of the most important functions of proteins is to protect the body against infection from bacteria. **Antibodies** are the proteins that provide this protection. Specifically shaped antibodies are produced by white blood cells (WBCs) to inactivate **antigens.** Most of the time, the antibodies protect a person by destroying or inactivating a harmful antigen.

FLUID BALANCE

Osmotic pressure Pressure on the cell membrane due to the inability of solutes to pass through it.

Proteins help to maintain levels of fluids in cells as well as in blood vessels. Proteins inside cells cannot diffuse across cell membranes and thereby create **osmotic pressure.** Osmotic pressure is very important in helping to maintain a balance of fluid between cells and tissues (see Fig. 5-9). Proteins in blood plasma, **albumin** for example, cannot move across blood vessel walls and thereby help to maintain fluid volumes in blood.

Albumin A protein found in blood plasma that is important in maintaining fluid volumes in the blood.

SODIUM AND POTASSIUM BALANCE

Extracellular Fluid outside cells, such as plasma and interstitial fluid.

Intracellular Fluid within cells.

Sodium (Na^+) and potassium (K^+) ions are very important to the normal functioning of many cells. Sodium is concentrated outside cells (**extracellular**) and potassium is concentrated inside cells (**intracellular**). Cells

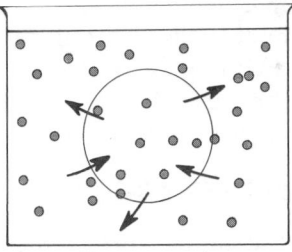

Free movement

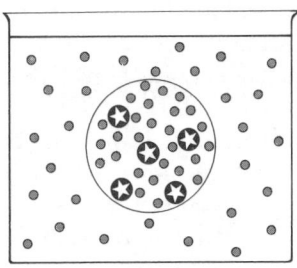

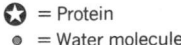
= Protein
= Water molecule

FIGURE 5-9 Proteins inside cells help create intracellular osmotic pressure, which maintains the correct amount of water inside the cell.

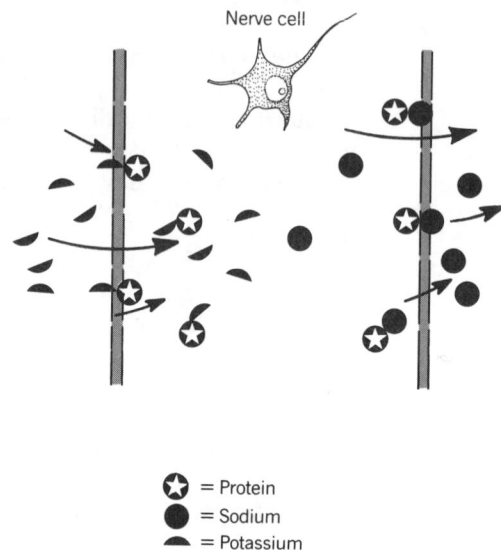

= Protein
= Sodium
= Potassium

FIGURE 5-10   Proteins transport sodium out of and potassium into cells.

Sodium-potassium pump
Protein carriers in cell
membranes that transport
sodium and potassium
ions back to their original
positions.

maintain the position of these two ions by means of protein carriers in
their membranes. Sodium and potassium ions tend to diffuse into and
out of cells, respectively. The protein carriers transport the ions back to
their original positions (see Fig. 5-10), a process often referred to as the
sodium-potassium pump. The normal functioning of nerve and muscle
cells requires the sodium-potassium pump.

BUFFER ACTION

Buffers   Compounds in
the blood that resist
changes in pH with the
addition of acids and
bases.

The normal pH of the blood, 7.35–7.45, is maintained by means of
buffers, with blood proteins being one of the most important. Body
processes constantly produce acids and bases that are transported by
the blood to excretory organs. Negatively charged side chains of amino
acids attract hydrogen (H^+) ions, thereby preventing the blood condition
acidosis (pH below 7.35). If a large number of hydroxyl (OH^-) ions enter
the blood, the condition alkalosis (pH above 7.45) exists. Protein buffers
correct this imbalance by causing their negative side chains to release
hydrogen ions, which combine with the hydroxyl ions to form water.
This action prevents the pH of the blood from becoming too alkaline or
increasing above 7.45. Ironically, proteins can be denatured by acids or
bases, but they can absorb hydrogen ions in small quantities without
causing their structure to change.

ENERGY

Proteins can be used as a source of energy (4 kcal/g), but at a high cost
to the body. This high cost results from the fact that the previous func-

tions of proteins are lost if they are used for energy. When the body does break down proteins for energy, the nitrogen atoms are not used, but rather are excreted. The nitrogen atoms are combined in the liver to form **urea,** which is excreted by the kidneys in urine.

As the body decomposes amino acids for energy, approximately half of them are converted to glucose and then oxidized to release energy. This action is important because the brain normally uses only glucose as a source of energy.[3]

Urea A nitrogen waste product that results from the metabolism or deamination of amino acids and is excreted in the urine (see Chapters 20 and 23).

DIGESTION AND ABSORPTION OF PROTEINS

In order for all of the protein functions to be possible, the digestive tract must break down proteins into amino acids and absorb them.

DIGESTION IN THE STOMACH

Pepsin A gastric enzyme that breaks down proteins into short chain polypeptides, proteoses, and peptides.

The stomach secretes hydrochloric acid (HCl) and the enzyme **pepsin,** which break down proteins into smaller fragments, **proteoses** and **peptones** (See Fig. 5-11).

Proteoses, Peptones Intermediate-sized protein segments.

DIGESTION IN THE SMALL INTESTINE
(see Fig. 5-11)

The proteoses and peptones move from the stomach into the duodenum region of the small intestine. Enzymes secreted by the pancreas break down proteoses and peptones into smaller fragments. This process is aided by secretion of sodium bicarbonate from the pancreas, which neutralizes the acidic fluid from the stomach.

A third group of enzymes secreted by the intestine function to break down the protein fragments into amino acids as well as **dipeptides, tripeptides,** and larger fragments.

Dipeptides Molecules composed of two amino acid molecules.

Tripeptides Molecules composed of three amino acid molecules.

ABSORPTION OF AMINO ACIDS,
DIPEPTIDES, AND TRIPEPTIDES

Ileum The terminal portion of the small intestine that is connected to the large intestine.

Amino acids, dipeptides, and tripeptides are absorbed by the jejunum and **ileum** regions of the small intestine. Once inside the intestinal cells, the dipeptides and tripeptides are broken down into amino acids, which are absorbed into the blood capillary vessels (see Fig. 4-12 for absorption of amino acids).

Actual absorption of amino acids occurs at specific sites by means of protein carriers. There is great competition for the carriers by the amino

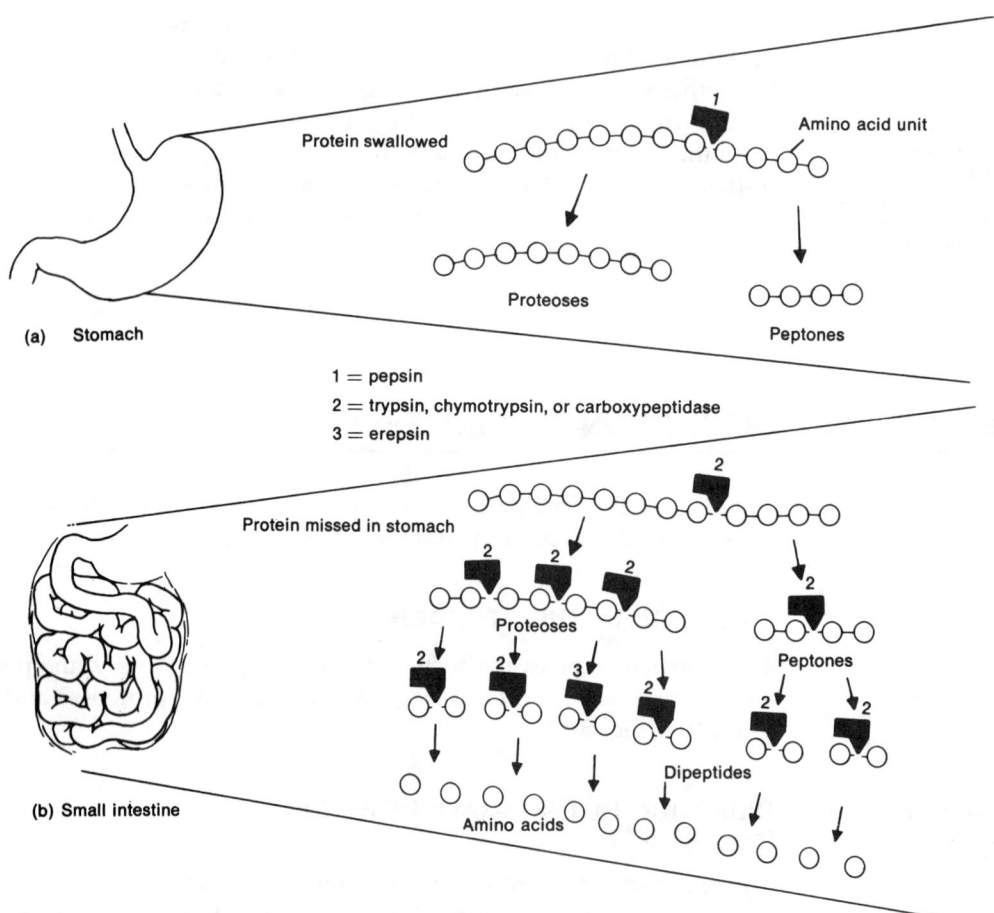

FIGURE 5-11 (a) Digestion of proteins in the stomach. (b) Digestion of proteins in the small intestine. (From *Principles of Anatomy and Physiology*, 2nd ed., by Gerard J. Tortora and Nicholas P. Anagnostakos. Copyright © 1975, 1978 by Gerard J. Tortora and Nicholas P. Anagnostakos. Reprinted by permission of Harper & Row, Publishers, Inc.)

acids. If too many amino acids are present in the intestines at one time, their absorption will be hindered and many of them will not be absorbed but rather excreted in the feces. This condition is possible if a person ingests one of the liquid protein preparations. These preparations contain predigested amino acids and, since the material already contains amino acids, no digestion is required in order for them to be absorbed. However, because so many amino acids are competing for the absorption sites, many of them cannot be absorbed.

Following absorption, amino acids are transported by the blood to the cells, where they are metabolized or synthesized into proteins.

METABOLISM OF PROTEINS

PROTEIN SYNTHESIS

Deoxyribonucleic acid (DNA) A nucleic acid found in the cell nucleus. It contains genetic information for the synthesis of specific proteins.

Amino acid pool A region in which large numbers of amino acids are maintained, such as in the liver. From the liver, the amino acids are distributed to the tissues.

Cells absorb amino acids from the blood and synthesize proteins, decompose them for energy, or convert them into other molecules. Each cell has a need for specific proteins, the synthesis of which is controlled by **deoxyribonucleic acid (DNA)** in the nucleus. For details of this complicated process, you may consult a biochemistry or physiology textbook.

If, during protein synthesis, a nonessential amino acid is unavailable, the cell will synthesize the amino acid and attach it to the growing protein chain. However, if an essential amino acid is not present, synthesis of the protein ceases. One might think that the incomplete amino acid chain is held by the cell until it obtains the essential amino acid, but it is not. Instead, the chain is decomposed and the amino acids are returned to the blood, which contains the **amino acid pool.** It is important, then, to eat the eight-essential amino acids within a 4-hour period. If they are not ingested during this period, many of the essential amino acids will be lost. People who eat foods such as meat, fish, poultry, cheese, eggs, or milk have no problems with this time frame, since these foods contain *complete proteins.* A strategy that vegetarians may wish to follow is one of *complementary protein* ingestion (mutual supplementation) (see Fig. 5-12). This strategy ensures that each food eaten supplies some amino acids that the others lack. By combining proper foods, one can get all of the essential amino acids. Some examples of complementary protein combinations are presented in Table 5-3.[4]

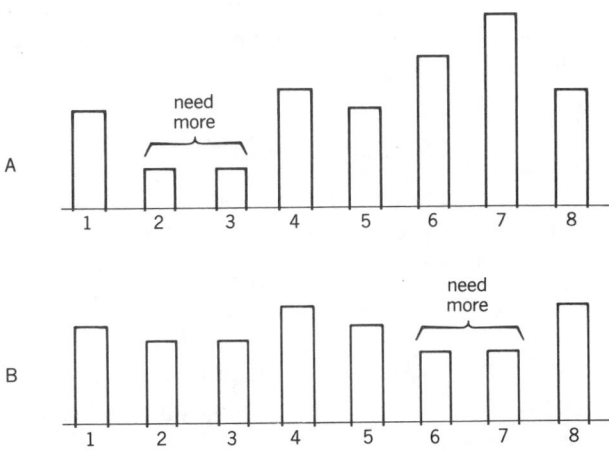

FIGURE 5-12 Example of protein mutual supplementation. Protein A lacks amino acids 2 and 3 but has sufficient quantities of amino acids 6 and 7. Protein B has sufficient quantities of amino acids 2 and 3 but lacks amino acids 6 and 7. Proteins A and B supplement each other.

TABLE 5-3 EXAMPLES OF COMPLEMENTARY PROTEIN COMBINATIONS

Complete protein: protein containing all of the essential amino acids.

Complementary protein combinations:
   Peanut protein goes with wheat, oats, corn, rice, coconut
   Soy protein goes with corn, wheat, rye, sesame
   Legumes go with cereals
   Leafy vegetables go with cereals

Traditional protein combinations:
   Soybeans go with rice (Indochina)
   Peas go with wheat (fertile Crescent)
   Beans go with corn (Central and South America)

CATABOLISM OF AMINO ACIDS

Catabolized Broken down.

Deamination The removal of an amine group (NH_2) from each amino acid.

Amino acids are **catabolized** primarily in the liver. The most important catabolic reaction of amino acids is **deamination** (see Fig. 5-13). After an amino group is removed, it is converted to ammonia and then to urea, all in the liver. The rest of the amino acid molecule may be oxidized to release energy (Fig. 5-14). If energy is not needed, the remains of the amino acids are converted to fat and stored in fat depots.

PROTEIN DIGESTIBILITY, QUALITY, AND RECOMMENDED DIETARY ALLOWANCE (RDA)

Digestibility Pertains to the ease of digestion.

The amount of protein that is recommended per day depends upon such factors as **digestibility**, the completeness of the protein, and the individual's state of health.

PROTEIN DIGESTIBILITY

The ability of the body to digest and absorb proteins from various sources varies, as can be seen below:

Protein	% Absorbed
Animal	90
Legumes	80
Cereals and other plants	60–90

As one can see from this list, if a person ate the same quantity of animal and cereal proteins, he or she would absorb considerably less cereal protein than animal protein.

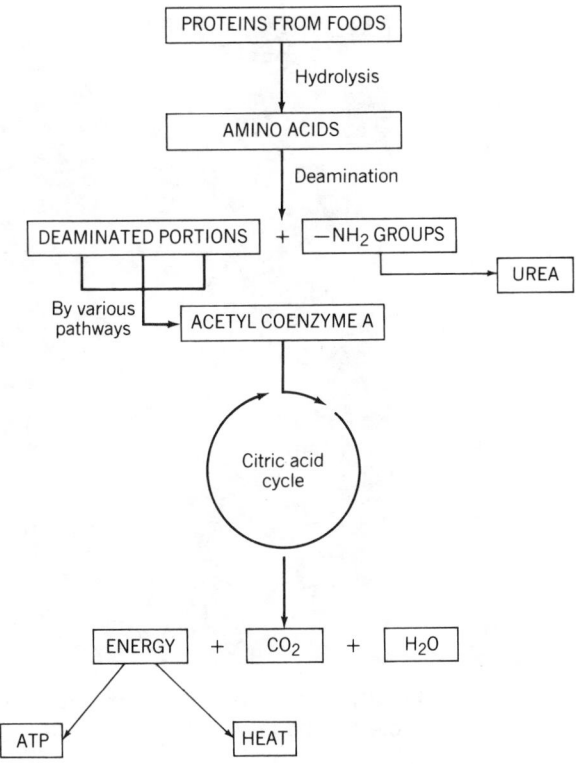

FIGURE 5-13 Deamination of a protein and metabolism of the remaining portion to release energy. (From Hole, John W., Jr., *Human Anatomy and Physiology,* 3d ed. © 1978, 1981, 1984 Wm. C. Brown Publishers, Dubuque, Iowa. All rights reserved. Reprinted by permission.)

PROTEIN QUALITY

Amino acid content The number of essential amino acids present.

The quality of each protein is determined by its **amino acid content, biological value (BV),** and **protein efficiency ratio (PER).**

Biological value (BV) Measures the absorbed nitrogen that is retained for growth or maintenance and not excreted through the feces, urine, or skin.

Amino Acid Content

A protein that contains all eight of the essential amino acids in exactly the right amounts is more completely used by the body than one that contains some of the essential amino acids in too small amounts.

Protein efficiency ratio (PER) Measures the growth of rats in relation to the amounts of protein eaten.

Biological Value (BV)

The BV of a protein is defined as follows:

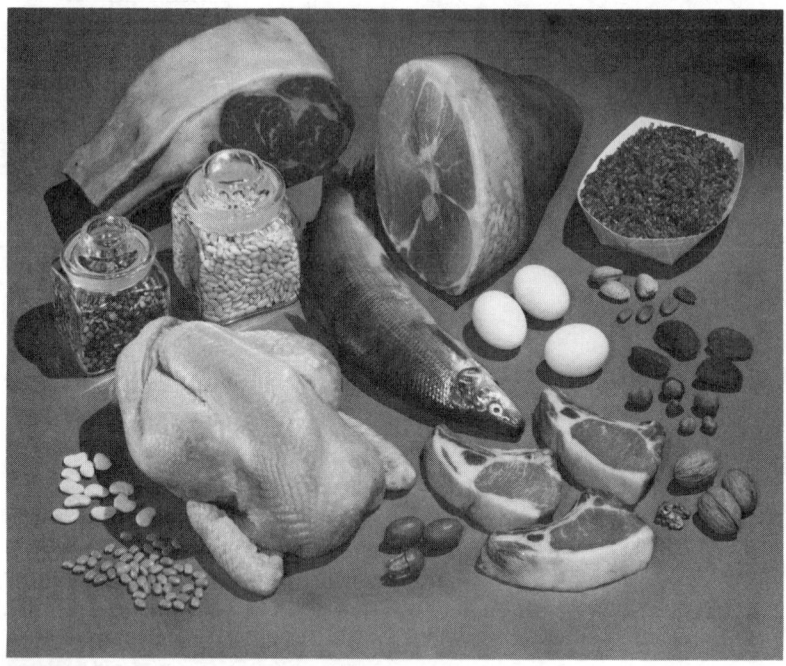

FIGURE 5-14 The milk and meat groups contribute large amounts of quality protein. (Courtesy of the National Dairy Council.)

$$BV = \frac{\text{quantity of nitrogen retained by the body}}{\text{quantity of nitrogen absorbed from dietary protein}} \times 100$$

A BV of 70 is the minimum for a protein that contributes to tissue growth, assuming that an adequate number of calories are also ingested.

PROTEIN EFFICIENCY RATIO (PER)

Another criterion for evaluating protein quality is the protein efficiency ratio (PER), which is defined as follows:

$$PER = \frac{\text{weight gain of the animal}}{\text{protein intake of the animal}}$$

There is a wide range of BV and PER values for proteins. Animal proteins, such as eggs, milk, meat, poultry, and egg protein, have the highest BV. Plant proteins tend to have lower BV than animal proteins. However, they can provide an adequate supply of essential amino acids, but only if consumed in quantities greater than those of animal proteins needed to meet the body's requirements. Some of the more common foods and their BV and PER values are:

Food	BV	PER
Hen's egg, whole	94	3.92
Cow's milk	84	3.09
Fish	83	3.55
Beef	74	3.20
Soybeans	73	2.32

By these criteria, the best-quality protein is egg protein. Therefore, egg protein is generally regarded as the reference protein, and all other proteins are measured against it. As stated previously, a BV of 70 can produce growth. Therefore, if a person eats protein of this quality, the U.S. RDA is 45 g/day. However, if the BV of protein is less than 70, then the U.S. RDA is 65 g/day.

RECOMMENDED DIETARY ALLOWANCE (RDA) FOR PROTEIN

Protein is the first nutrient discussed that has an RDA. There are no RDA values for carbohydrates and fats. Nitrogen balance studies provide the basis for RDA values. These studies show that nitrogen lost by excretion must be replaced by nitrogen consumed in food. In other words, nitrogen in must equal nitrogen out. Most healthy adults are in **nitrogen equilibrium.** Some people ingest more nitrogen than they excrete, and vice versa. The former are in **positive nitrogen balance** and the latter are in **negative nitrogen balance.**

Growing children, pregnant women, and people recovering from serious wounds should be in positive nitrogen balance. The reason is that they need to synthesize new tissues to replace the damaged ones.

Negative nitrogen balance occurs frequently in people who are bedridden or go on reducing diets. Their protein tissues degenerate more quickly than new protein tissue is produced. Astronauts who spend several inactive days in space tend to suffer from a negative nitrogen balance. They are unable to exercise their muscles adequately and therefore suffer from a decrease in muscle mass.

The optimal amount of dietary protein varies. In establishing the amounts in Table 5-4, the Food and Nutrition Board of the National Research Council considered that the protein in a diet would be mixed (complete and incomplete), that not all proteins are used with 100% efficiency, and that individual needs vary. Most individuals can consume two-thirds of

Nitrogen equilibrium Conditions in which the amount of nitrogen consumed is equal to the amount excreted.

Positive nitrogen balance A state that occurs when more nitrogen is ingested than excreted.

Negative nitrogen balance A state that occurs when more nitrogen is excreted than ingested.

TABLE 5-4 RDA
PROTEIN VALUES
FOR DIFFERENT
AGE GROUPS

Age (yr)	RDA (g/kg)
0–$\frac{1}{2}$	2.2
$\frac{1}{2}$–1	2.0
1–3	1.8
4–10	1.1
11–14	1.0
15–18	0.9
19 and up	0.8

the RDA for protein listed in Table 5-4, and be assured of meeting their bodies' needs.

Note that the criterion of 0.8 g/kg for adults in Table 5-4 is based on ideal weight rather than actual weight. The reason is that the amino acids are needed by lean body tissues rather than fat tissues. Infants need more protein per body weight than any other age group, since they are growing rapidly and producing new blood, bone, muscle, and other tissues daily. In order for infants, children, and adolescents to maintain a positive nitrogen balance, they need the amounts listed. Pregnant and lactating women also need a protein intake of 0.8 g/kg daily for their own body needs, as well as daily amounts of 30 and 20 g, respectively. During pregnancy, the increased protein provides for the needs of the developing fetus, as well as those of the mother.[5]

FOOD SOURCES OF PROTEIN

Nitrogen-fixing bacteria
Bacteria that can take in nitrogen from the air and soil and convert it into proteins.

Two groups in the exchange system contribute large amounts of quality proteins: milk and meat (see Table 5-5 and Fig. 5-14). Vegetables and bread groups contribute small amounts of complete proteins and significant amounts of incomplete proteins. One plant family contains a large amount of complete high-quality proteins: legumes. These plants are rich in protein because their roots have nodules that contain **nitrogen-fixing bacteria**. Legumes, often called "poor man's meat," are an inexpensive source of protein. They are also low in fat and high in B vitamins and iron. A cup of cooked legumes supplies 31% of the U.S. RDA for protein and 42% of the iron.

TABLE 5-5 PROTEIN CONTENT AND KILOCALORIES OF EXCHANGE GROUPS

Group	Serving Size	Carbohydrate (g)	Protein (g)	Fat (g)	Energy (kcal)
Milk (skim)	1 cup	12	8	0	80
Vegetable	½ cup	5	2	0	25
Fruit	1 serving	10	0	0	40
Bread	1 slice	15	2	0	70
Meat (lean)	1 oz	0	7	3	55
Fat	1 tsp	0	0	5	45

PROTEIN-CALORIE MALNUTRITION (PCM)

Protein-calorie malnutrition (PCM) Malnutrition that is caused by deficits of calories, proteins, or both.

Marasmus A type of protein-calorie malnutrition that results from a deficiency of proteins and calories.

Kwashiorkor A type of protein-calorie malnutrition that results from a decreased protein intake.

Hyperammonemia Excess ammonia in the blood.

Hypophosphatemia A deficiency of phosphates in the blood.

Protein-calorie malnutrition (PCM) may occur with deficits of calories, protein, or both. A calorie deficit results in a loss of body fat and, when either long-term or in the presence of depleted body fat stores, may result in decreased protein mass because the protein will be used as a source of calories. A protein deficit causes a loss of muscle or visceral protein mass regardless of the presence or absence of body fat. The deficit is due to the need for essential amino acids that the diet alone is not supplying. PCM is classified into two conditions: **marasmus** and **kwashiorkor.**

MARASMUS

Marasmus usually occurs in infants 6 to 18 months of age when the mother's breast milk provides insufficient proteins and calories due to malnourishment of the mother. The infant is characterized by being grossly underweight, with an aged appearance (see Fig. 5-15). The cheeks and eyes are sunken. The abdomen may be swollen but the child's extremities are very thin, which is evidence of the wasting of muscle mass. Edema is minimal or absent and diarrhea is common. Body height is retarded and the child is apathetic, listless, and unable to cry.

Diagnosis of marasmus is based on physical findings of severe fat and muscle wastage as a result of prolonged calorie deficiency. Marasmus patients have a starved appearance, and frequently their weight and height are less than 80% of the standard values. Since marasmus is a chronic rather than an acute illness, it should be corrected gradually. An overly aggressive approach should be avoided, since it may result in metabolic imbalances such as **hyperammonemia** or **hypophosphatemia.**

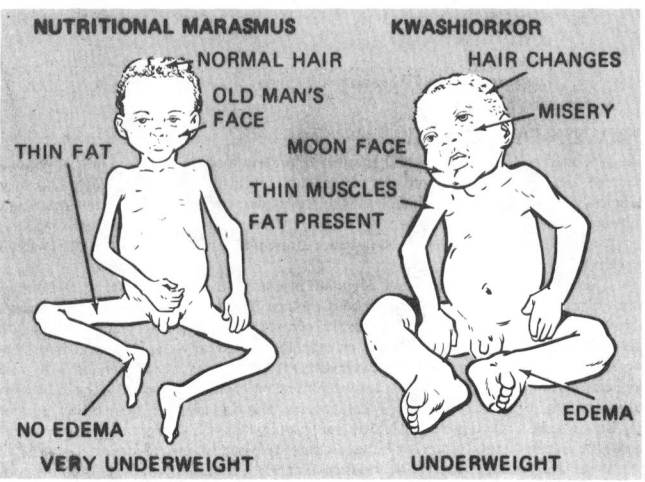

FIGURE 5-15 The appearance of children suffering from marasmus and kwashiorkor are shown. (From the U.S. Department of Health, Education and Welfare, Public Health Service Publication #1822, 1968.)

KWASHIORKOR

In contrast to marasmus, kwashiorkor results from decreased protein intake for a short period of time. In children, this condition often occurs in the second child after he or she has been weaned after 1 year of age from breast milk to a starchy, low-protein diet of gruel or sugar water. A kwashiorkor child develops the following symptoms, which result from protein deficiencies (see Fig. 5-15):

• Edema—results from decreased synthesis of the protein albumin.

• Muscular wasting.

• Diarrhea—deterioration of the intestinal lining as a result of protein deficiency.

• Susceptibility to infections—these children are very susceptible to common childhood infections, which are often fatal. This extreme susceptibility results from the inability to synthesize antibodies that provide immunity.

• Depigmentation of hair and skin.

Hypoalbuminemia A low level of albumin in the blood.

• **Hypoalbuminemia**

• Fatty infiltration of the liver.

• Decreased enzyme secretions of the pancreas.

• Severe vitamin A deficiency.

• Apathy—results from an inadequate amount of the protein hemoglobin, which carries oxygen to the cells, followed by release of energy.

In adults, kwashiorkor typically occurs in the hospitalized patient who is under acute stress from illness and surgery and is being supported with 5% dextrose solutions. Fat reserves and muscle mass tend to be normal or even above normal, which gives a deceptive appearance of adequate nutrition. Signs of kwashiorkor include easily pluckable hair, edema, and delayed wound healing. Characteristic laboratory values include severely depressed levels of proteins such as albumin, and the time of development may be as short as 2 weeks.

Parenteral feedings Feedings that bypass the intestine and are infused directly into the veins.

Unlike the treatment of marasmus, **parenteral feedings** are often used in an attempt to restore normal metabolic homeostasis rapidly. One of the first objectives is to correct the diarrhea and electrolyte inbalances.[6]

DISEASE AND PROTEIN REQUIREMENTS

In many disease states and with stress or trauma, protein requirements are increased because the body catabolizes large amounts of proteins for energy needs. As a result of the protein catabolism, the body is thrown into negative nitrogen balance and its weight declines.

In order to compensate for the protein losses, extra dietary protein together with calories must be provided. In severe cases, sometimes as much as 2–3 g of protein per kilogram of body weight may be necessary. However, in some disease states, particularly those involving the kidney or liver, protein intake must be decreased. The reason is that these two organs normally break down waste products of protein metabolism, but in a diseased state they cannot even handle normal amounts, much less increased amounts of waste products.

DISTRIBUTION OF PROTEIN KILOCALORIES IN BALANCED AND TYPICAL AMERICAN DIETS

As mentioned in Chapter 2, 10–15% of the total kilocalories in a balanced diet should come from proteins. This recommendation is for kilocalories only and is not specific for each individual. A much more formal recommendation for protein intake is the Recommended Dietary Allowance (RDA), which for an adult is 0.8 g of high-quality protein per kilogram of ideal body weight per day. If your ideal body weight is 55 kg, then $0.8 \times 55 = 44$ g of high-quality protein should be consumed each day. However, if you are consuming 1,500 kcal/day, then 10–15% is 150–225 kcal or 38–56 g. This example illustrates that the RDA for protein intake is based neither on the kilocalorie consumption nor on actual weight. Again, assume that your ideal body weight is 55 kg but that you actually weight 65 kg. Your RDA for protein is still 44 g, since the recommendation is based on ideal and not actual weight.

TABLE 5-6 SAMPLE MENU

	Exchange(s)	Quality	g (kcal)/Protein	kcal
Breakfast				
2 eggs	2 medium fat meat	high	14 (56)	150
1 cup skim milk	milk	high	8 (32)	80
1 slice toast	bread	low	2 (8)	70
1 tsp margarine	fat	—	—	45
Lunch				
1 quarter-pound cheeseburger				
2 buns	2 bread	low	4 (16)	140
3-oz patty	3 high fat meat	high	21 (84)	300
1-oz low-fat cheese	low fat meat	high	7 (28)	55
Dinner				
4-oz hamburger steak	4 meat	high	28 (112)	400
½ cup mashed potatoes	bread	low	2 (8)	70
2 rolls	2 bread	low	4 (16)	140
2 tsp margarine	2 fat	—		90
			Total 90 (360)	1540

PROTEIN CONTENT OF THE EXCHANGE GROUPS AND TYPICAL AMERICAN MEALS

Table 5-5 gives the protein quality and content of the exchange groups. Using this information, we will calculate the protein content of some typical American meals. Let us assume that a 150-lb (68-kg) college student is at his ideal weight, his RDA for protein is $0.8 \times 68 = 54$ g, and he eats the meals listed in Table 5-6.

The RDA for protein for this student is 54 g, and as the calculations show, he consumes a total of 90 g for the three meals. Also, remember that the U.S. RDA for high-quality protein is 45 g. He actually consumed almost all of his RDA for protein at breakfast and lunch. Were the three meals balanced in regard to the distribution of kilocalories from protein?

Kilocalories from protein = 360

Total kilocalories from all meals = 1,540

$$\text{Percent of kilocalories from protein} = \frac{360}{1540} \times 100 = 23\%$$

It is obvious that not only did the student consume (90 g) almost twice as much protein as is recommended (54 g), but the distribution of kilocalories (23%) from protein is almost twice as high as the recommended 10–15%. Unless the student's body is able to burn up the excess protein, it will be converted to fat and stored. In other words, in developed countries, people gain weight due to consumption not only of excess carbohydrates and fats but also of protein.[5]

OUTLINE

INTRODUCTION
Proteins are the most fundamental constituent and the major structural and functional component of living cells.

CHEMISTRY OF PROTEINS
Composition
Proteins consist of carbon, hydrogen, oxygen, and nitrogen atoms; some contain sulfur. Amino acid is the fundamental chemical building block. The R-group distinguishes the 20 different amino acids from each other.

Essential and Nonessential Amino Acids
Eight amino acids that cannot be synthesized by the body and have to be ingested in the diet are known as essential; 12 amino acids can be synthesized by the body and are known as nonessential.

Protein Structure
Proteins are very large and are sometimes composed of several hundred amino acids; peptide bonds join amino acids together.

Complete and Incomplete Proteins
Complete proteins contain all of the essential amino acids; incomplete proteins lack one or more of them.

Sequence of Amino Acids
The sequence of amino acids varies from protein to protein; sickle cell disease is an example of a protein (hemoglobin) that has one amino acid out of position.

Denaturation
If a protein loses shape, it is denatured. Factors that can cause denaturation include high temperature, acidosis, and alkalosis; permanent denaturation destroys the functions of proteins.

FUNCTIONS OF PROTEINS
Growth and Replacement
Synthesis and replacement of old tissues are important functions of proteins.

Immunity
Antibodies, specific proteins for antigens, protect the body against the invasion of bacteria.

Fluid Balance
Proteins create osmotic pressure inside and outside cells that helps maintain water equilibrium between cells and tissue fluids.

Sodium and Potassium Balance
Proteins help to maintain sodium (Na^+) and potassium (K^+) ions outside and inside cells, respectively.

Buffer Action
Proteins function as buffers to help maintain the normal pH of the blood (7.35–7.45) and prevent or correct acidosis and alkalosis.

Energy
Proteins can serve as a source of energy (4 kcal/g), but at the expense of the other functions of proteins.

DIGESTION AND ABSORPTION OF PROTEINS
Digestion in the Stomach
HCl and pepsin break down proteins to proteoses and peptones.

Digestion in the Small Intestine
Enzymes from the pancreas and small intestine break down proteoses and peptones to dipeptides, tripeptides, and larger peptides.

Absorption of Amino Acids, Dipeptides, and Tripeptides
These structures are absorbed into the cells of the jejunum and ileum regions of the small estestine. Dipeptides and tripeptides are digested to amino acids inside the cells. If too many amino acids are present and are attempting to be absorbed at one time, competition prevents many of them from being absorbed and they are excreted in feces.

METABOLISM
Protein Synthesis
DNA in the nucleus of each cell directs the specific synthesis of proteins in that cell. If a nonessential amino acid is unavailable, the cell synthesizes it and continues to synthesize protein. If an essential amino acid is unavailable, synthesis of protein ceases and it is decomposed.

Catabolism of Amino Acids
Deamination
The amino group is removed and converted to urea in the liver; the rest of the amino acid may be oxidized to release energy.

PROTEIN DIGESTIBILITY, QUALITY, AND RECOMMENDED DAILY ALLOWANCE
Protein Digestibility
Animal proteins are digested and absorbed better than are plant proteins.

Protein Quality

Protein quality is determined by its amino acid content, which is measured by its biological value (BV) and protein efficiency ratio (PER).

Amino Acid Content

The quality of a protein can be determined by the number of essential amino acids present.

Biological Value (BV)

The BV of a protein measures the amount of nitrogen that is retained for growth or maintenance; a BV of 70 is the minimum needed for a protein to contribute to growth; PER measures the weight gain of rats in relation to the amount of protein eaten.

Recommended Dietary Allowance (RDA) for Proteins

RDA values are based on nitrogen balance studies. With positive nitrogen balance, more protein is ingested than excreted; with negative nitrogen balance, more nitrogen is excreted than consumed; with nitrogen equilibrium, the amount of nitrogen consumed equals the amount excreted. The RDA for protein varies according to the age of the individual and the status (e.g., pregnant or lactating).

FOOD SOURCES OF PROTEIN

Milk and meat exchange groups contribute large amounts of high-quality proteins. Vegetables and bread groups contribute small amounts of complete proteins and large amounts of incomplete proteins. Legumes are vegetables that are an exception to this rule in that they contain large amounts of high-quality protein.

PROTEIN-CALORIE MALNUTRITION (PCM)

PCM occurs in the absence of calories, proteins, or both; a calorie deficit results in loss of body fat and in decreased protein mass; protein deficit causes loss of muscle or visceral protein mass.

Marasmus

Marasmus results from prolonged calorie deficiency and is a chronic rather than an acute problem. The adult patient exhibits a starved appearance. The condition usually occurs in children when the mother's breast milk provides insufficient proteins and calories due to malnourishment of the mother.

Kwashiorkor

Kwashiorkor is a chronic problem that can arise from decreased protein intake for a few weeks. In children it occurs in the second child after he or she is weaned from breast milk to a low-protein diet. Symptoms seen in children include edema, muscular wasting, diarrhea, susceptibility to infections, depigmentation of hair and skin, hypoalbuminemia, fatty infiltration of the liver, decreased enzyme secretions of the pancreas, vitamin A deficiency, and apathy. In adults it occurs in hospitalized patients who have been supported with 5% dextrose solutions for 2 weeks or longer; fat reserves and muscle mass tend to be normal, which is deceptive, but signs of the disease are easily pluckable hair, edema, and delayed wound healing.

Disease and Protein Requirements

Many diseases increase the catabolism of proteins for energy needs; extra protein (2–3 g/per kilogram of body weight) may be supplied to prevent this problem; however, diseases of the kidneys and liver frequently require protein intake to be decreased.

DISTRIBUTION OF PROTEIN KILOCALORIES IN BALANCED AND TYPICAL AMERICAN DIETS

From 10 to 15% of the total kilocalories in a balanced diet should come from proteins; protein RDA is 0.8 g per kilogram of ideal body weight for adults but is much higher in children.

Protein Content of the Exchange Groups and Typical American Meals

The protein content of typical American meals is much higher than the protein RDA.

REVIEW QUESTIONS

TRUE (A) OR FALSE (B)

Questions 1–21

1. The amino acid is the chemical building block of proteins, and the carboxyl group varies from one amino acid to another.
2. Nonessential amino acids can be synthesized by the body, whereas essential amino acids have to be ingested in the diet.
3. A complete protein is defined as one that contains peptide bonds in several chains that are twisted around each other.
4. To increase the intake of complete proteins, one would consume more meat, milk, cheese, and egg products.
5. Denaturation of proteins is a condition that results from a change in the amino acid sequence.

6. Normal body temperature and pH of the blood can denature proteins.
7. Protein functions include growth and replacement, storage form of glucose, immunity, fluid balance, source of vitamins, buffer action, and energy source.
8. In the stomach, proteins are digested to amino acids and absorbed into the blood.
9. Absorption of amino acids occurs in the jejunum and ileum regions of the small intestine at specific sites and by protein carriers.
10. During protein synthesis, if essential amino acids are absent from a cell, the unfinished chain is broken down.
11. A person can avoid the problem in question 10 by eating more complete proteins.
12. Deamination of proteins involves the removal of urea and the oxidation of the remainder of the molecule to release energy.
13. The BV of a protein is a measurement of the quantity of nitrogen that is retained for growth and maintenance and not excreted.
14. The PER of a protein is a measurement of how many essential complete amino acids are present.
15. A protein BV of 70 is the minimum for growth, and the U.S. RDA for protein of this value is 45 g.
16. A person who consumes protein with a BV of less than 70 must eat about twice as much, or the U.S. RDA of 90 g.
17. All nutrients, including protein, have an RDA value.
18. The protein RDA for adults is 0.8 g per kilogram of ideal weight; if a person's ideal weight is 160 lb (73 kg), then he should consume 58 g of protein a day.
19. A person who consumes 75 g of protein a day and excretes 35 g would be in positive nitrogen balance.
20. In a balanced diet, 10–15% of the total kilocalories consumed per day should be contributed by proteins.
21. In a diseased state, consumption of protein should always be decreased in order to lessen the work of the kidneys and liver.

MULTIPLE CHOICE

Questions 22–27

22. Amino acids that the body can synthesize are known as _____ , and proteins that contain all of the essential amino acids needed by the body are _____ .
    A. essential—complete proteins
    B. nonessential—incomplete

C. nonessential—complete
    D. essential—incomplete
23. Denaturation of proteins involves:
    1. loss of protein structure
    2. loss of protein functions
    3. acidosis and alkalosis
    4. high temperature
       A. 1, 2, and 3   B. 1, 3   C. 2, 4   D. 4
       E. all of these
24. Which of the following protein functions and descriptions is (are) incorrectly paired?
    A. growth and replacement—collagen and keratin proteins.
    B. sodium and potassium balance—proteins block the movement of these ions into and out of cells.
    C. buffer action—maintain blood pH of 7.35–7.45.
    D. energy—proteins provide 4 kcal per gram of energy.
25. Which of the following correctly describes digestion of proteins in the stomach?
    A. proteins $\xrightarrow[\text{pepsin}]{\text{HCl}}$ amino acids
    B. proteins $\xrightarrow[\text{pepsin}]{\text{HCl}}$ proteoses and peptones
26. Which of the following is correct in regard to digestion and absorption of proteins in the small intestine?
    A. Enzymes in the small intestine break down protein fragments into amino acids, dipeptides, and tripeptides.
    B. The pancreas secretes no protein digestive enzymes.
    C. Absorption of amino acids, dipeptides, and tripeptides occurs in the jejunum and ileum regions of the small intestine.
    D. A, C.
    E. B, C.
27. Synthesis of proteins is more efficient if _____ _____ proteins are present in the body, and before proteins can be catabolized for energy they must be _____ .
    A. complete—deaminated (removal of the NH₂ group)
    B. complementary—denatured
    C. incomplete—separated from urea
    D. essential—combined with DNA

MATCHING

Questions 28–39

___ 28. Biological value (BV)
___ 29. Protein efficiency ratio (PER)
___ 30. protein RDA for adult
___ 31. U.S. RDA for high-quality protein
___ 32. U.S. RDA for low-quality protein

A. 0.8 g per kilogram of ideal weight
B. amount of nitrogen retained for growth or maintenance
C. 45 g/day
D. 65 g/day
E. measures growth in relation to amount of protein eaten

Match the following descriptions and symptoms with marasmus and kwashiorkor.

___ 33. chronic protein deficiency   A. marasmus

___ 34. exhibit severe fat and muscle wastage   B. kwashiorkor

___ 35. edema and easily pluckable hair

___ 36. fat reserves and muscle mass tend to be normal

___ 37. child exhibits an aged appearance

___ 38. increased susceptibility to infections

___ 39. can occur in patients who have been supported on 5% dextrose solutions for 2 weeks or longer

Questions 40–45 apply to the meals below. The information necessary to answer these questions is found in Table 5-5.

	Exchange(s)	g protein (kcal)	kcal
Breakfast			
1 egg	1 meat + ½ fat or medium-fat meat	— (28)	75
1 slice toast	1 bread	— (8)	70
1 tsp margarine	1 fat	0	45
Lunch			
1 cup skim milk	1 milk	— (32)	80
2 slices bread	2 bread	— (16)	140
1 oz cottage cheese	1 lean meat	— (28)	55
1 banana	2 fruit	0	80
Dinner			
6 oz fish	6 lean meat	— (168)	330
½ cup green beans	1 vegetable	— (8)	25
½ cup carrots	1 vegetable	— (8)	25
1 plain roll	1 bread	— (8)	70
1 tsp. margarine	1 fat	0	45
1 cup skim milk	1 milk	(32)	80
		Total — (336)	Total 1120

40. The breakfast meal contains _____ g of protein and _____ total kcal contributed by carbohydrate, protein, and fat.
    A. 9—190   C. 28—195
    B. 16—32   D. 36—144
41. The lunch meal contains _____ g of protein and _____ kcal from all nutrients.

A. 29—116   C. 22—76
B. 19—355   D. 12—48

42. The dinner meal contributes _____ g of protein and _____ total kcal from all nutrients.
    A. 50—200   C. 56—575
    B. 42—725   D. 26—485
43. The three meals contribute a total of _____ g of protein and _____ total kcal from all nutrients.
    A. 84—1120   C. 336—1056
    B. 96—1678   D. 168—975
44. The number of kilocalories contributed by protein for all three meals is _____ , which is _____ % of the total kilocalories for all three meals.
    A. 336—30   C. 198—21
    B. 543—10   D. 336—26
45. Using the information from question 43, did these three meals provide this person with an adequate number of kilocalories from protein?
    A. No; 30% is much higher than the recommended 10–15%.
    B. Yes; 10% is within the recommended range.

DISCUSSION QUESTIONS

1. Discuss denaturation of proteins in terms of what happens to proteins and two causative factors.
2. Discuss digestion of proteins in the stomach and small intestine.
3. Calculate the protein RDA required for a person who weighs 172 lb. Give three examples of foods with high biological value (BV).
4. Discuss the protein-calorie malnutrition (PCM) problems, marasmus, and kwashiorkor in terms of causes and symptoms.

REFERENCES

1. T.R. Lankford. *Integrated Science for Health Students*, 3rd ed. Reston, Va.: Reston Publishing Co., 1984, pp. 36–37.
2. P.J. Long and B. Shannon. *Focus on Nutrition.* Englewood Cliffs, N.J.: Prentice-Hall Inc., 1983, pp. 117–118.
3. H.A. Guthrie. *Introductory Nutrition.* 5th ed. St. Louis: C.V. Mosby Co., 1983, pp. 73–75.
4. J.B. Anderson. *Applied Nutrition for Health Professions: Basic Nutrition.* Chapel Hill, N.C.: University of North Carolina Press, 1982, pp. 133–135.
5. N.W. Whitney and E.M.N. Hamilton. *Understanding Nutrition,* 2nd ed. St. Paul, Minn.: West Publishing Co., 1982, pp. 105–107, 137–151.
6. S.J. Wickham. *Human Nutrition: A Self-Instructional Text.* Bowie, Md.: Robert J. Brady Co., 1982, pp. 109–110.

6 VITAMINS

OBJECTIVES

Upon completion of this chapter you should be able to:

1. Define and give a general description of vitamins.

2. Recognize the functions of vitamins A, D, E, and K.

3. Give the animal and plant food sources for vitamins A, D, E, and K.

4. Describe the deficiency and toxicity problems associated with vitamins A, D, E, and K.

5. Describe how the general characteristics of water-soluble vitamins differ from fat-soluble ones.

6. Recognize the functions of the vitamins thiamin, riboflavin, niacin, pyridoxine, cobalamin, folacin, and ascorbic acid.

7. Give the animal and plant food sources for the vitamins thiamin, riboflavin, niacin, pyridoxine, cobalamin, folacin, and ascorbic acid.

8. Describe the deficiency and toxicity problems associated with the vitamins thiamin, riboflavin, niacin, pyridoxine, cobalamin, folacin, and ascorbic acid.

INTRODUCTION

Vitamins A group of organic substances that are essential for normal metabolism, growth, and development of the body. They do not generate energy.

In the previous chapters, much information was presented concerning the nutritional importance of carbohydrates, lipids, and proteins in the body. The functions of these substances will not be performed, however, unless **vitamins** are also present. Their importance is so great that the *vita* part of the word *vitamin* comes from the fact that they are vital to cellular functions of the body.

GENERAL DESCRIPTION

Noncaloric Non-energy-yielding.

Coenzymes A small nonprotein molecule that combines with an inactive protein to make it an active enzyme.

Fat soluble Able to be dissolved in fats.

Toxicity The quality of being poisonous; a condition that can result from consumption of excess amounts of some vitamins.

Hypervitaminosis A An excess amount of vitamin A that results in a toxicity condition.

Water soluble Able to be dissolved in water.

Vitamins differ from carbohydrates, lipids, and proteins in that they are **noncaloric** nutrients. The molecular size of vitamins is quite small compared to that of the energy nutrients. For example, a molecule of vitamin C is about the size of a glucose molecule. They are never combined to form large molecules, unlike amino acids, for example. Many vitamins serve as helpers or, more accurately, as **coenzymes** in the metabolism of carbohydrates, lipids, and proteins. In carrying out this coenzyme function, they are not normally used up by body processes. Practically speaking, this means that the amount of vitamins the body can use is limited.

Consuming excessive amounts of vitamins is expensive, unnecessary, and may lead to unpleasant side effects. **Fat-soluble vitamins** can be stored in the body. This means that we do not need to consume them every day. In fact, an excessive accumulation of some vitamins leads to **toxicity; hypervitaminosis A** is an example.

Vitamins are divided into two groups according to their solubility: fat and **water soluble**.

Table 6-1 presents a summary of the food sources, functions, and deficiency/toxicity problems of each vitamin.

FAT-SOLUBLE VITAMINS

Vitamins, A, D, E, and K are soluble only in fats and are therefore absorbed into the blood together with dietary fats. They are stored in the body in adipose and liver tissues. Since they are insoluble in water, they can be transported by the lymphatic vessels or the blood only after they have attached to a protein carrier.

TABLE 6-1 SUMMARY OF WATER- AND FAT-SOLUBLE VITAMINS

Name	Food Sources	Functions	Deficiency/Toxicity
Vitamin A (retinol)	Animal Liver Whole milk Butter Cream Cod liver oil Plants Dark green leafy vegetables Deep yellow or orange fruit Fortified margarine	Dim light vision Maintenance of mucous membranes Growth and development of bones	Deficiency Night blindness Xerophthalmia Respiratory infections Bone growth ceases Toxicity Cessation of menstruation Joint pain Stunted growth Enlargement of liver
Vitamin D (cholecalciferol)	Animal Eggs Liver Fortified milk Plants None	Bone growth	Deficiency Rickets Osteomalacia Poorly developed teeth Muscle spasms Toxicity Kidney stones Calcification of soft tissues
Vitamin E (alpha-tocopherol)	Animal None Plant Margarines Salad dressing	Antioxidant	Deficiency Destruction of RBCs Toxicity Hypertension
Vitamin K	Animal Egg yolk Liver Milk Plant Green leafy vegetables Cabbage	Blood clotting	Deficiency Prolonged blood clotting Toxicity Hemolytic anemia Jaundice

TABLE 6-1 (Continued)

Name	Food Sources	Functions	Deficiency/Toxicity
Thiamin (Vitamin B$_1$)	Animal: Pork, beef / Liver / Eggs / Fish / Pork / Beef. Plants: Whole and enriched grains / Legumes	Coenzyme in oxidation of glucose	Deficiency: Gastrointestinal tract, nervous, and cardiovascular system problems. Toxicity: None
Riboflavin (Vitamin B$_2$)	Animal: Milk. Plants: Green vegetables / Cereals / Enriched bread	Aids release of energy from food	Deficiency: Cheilosis / Glossitis / Photophobia. Toxicity: None
Pyridoxine (Vitamin B$_6$)	Animal: Pork / Milk / Eggs. Plants: Whole grain cereals / Legumes	Synthesis of nonessential amino acids / Conversion of tryptophan to niacin / Antibody production	Deficiency: Cheilosis / Glossitis. Toxicity: Liver disease
Vitamin B$_{12}$	Animal: Seafood / Meat / Eggs / Milk. Plants: None	Synthesis of RBCs / Maintenance of myelin sheaths	Deficiency: Degeneration of myelin sheaths / Pernicious anemia. Toxicity: None
Niacin (nicotinic acid)	Animal: Milk / Eggs / Fish / Poultry	Transfers hydrogen atoms for synthesis of ATP	Deficiency: Pellagra. Toxicity: Vasodilation of blood vessels

Vitamin	Sources	Functions	Deficiency/Toxicity
Folacin	Animal None Plants Spinach Asparagus Broccoli Kidney beans	Synthesis of RBCs	Deficiency Glossitis Macrocytic anemia Toxicity None
Biotin	Animal Milk Liver Plants Legumes Mushrooms	Coenzyme in carbohydrate and amino acid metabolism Niacin synthesis from tryptophan	Deficiency None Toxicity None
Pantothenic acid	Animal Eggs Liver Salmon Yeast Plants Mushrooms Cauliflower Peanuts	Metabolism of carbohydrates, lipids, and proteins Synthesis of acetylcholine	Deficiency None Toxicity None
Vitamin C (ascorbic acid)	Fruits All citrus Plants Broccoli Tomatoes Brussel sprouts Potatoes	Prevention of scurvy Formation of collagen Healing of wounds Release of stress hormones Absorption of iron	Deficiency Scurvy Muscle cramps Ulcerated gums Toxicity Raise uric acid level Hemolytic anemia Kidney stones Rebound scurvy

VITAMIN A (Retinol)

Nature and General Characteristics

Retinol A form of vitamin A that is found in
food.

Retinene A pigment
that is derived from vitamin A and results from
the breakdown of rho-
dopsin.

Most of the vitamin A we ingest (see Fig. 6-1) exists in a form called
retinol. Retinol is oxidized to **retinene,** which is the form that is functional in the response to vision in dim light (see Fig. 6-2).

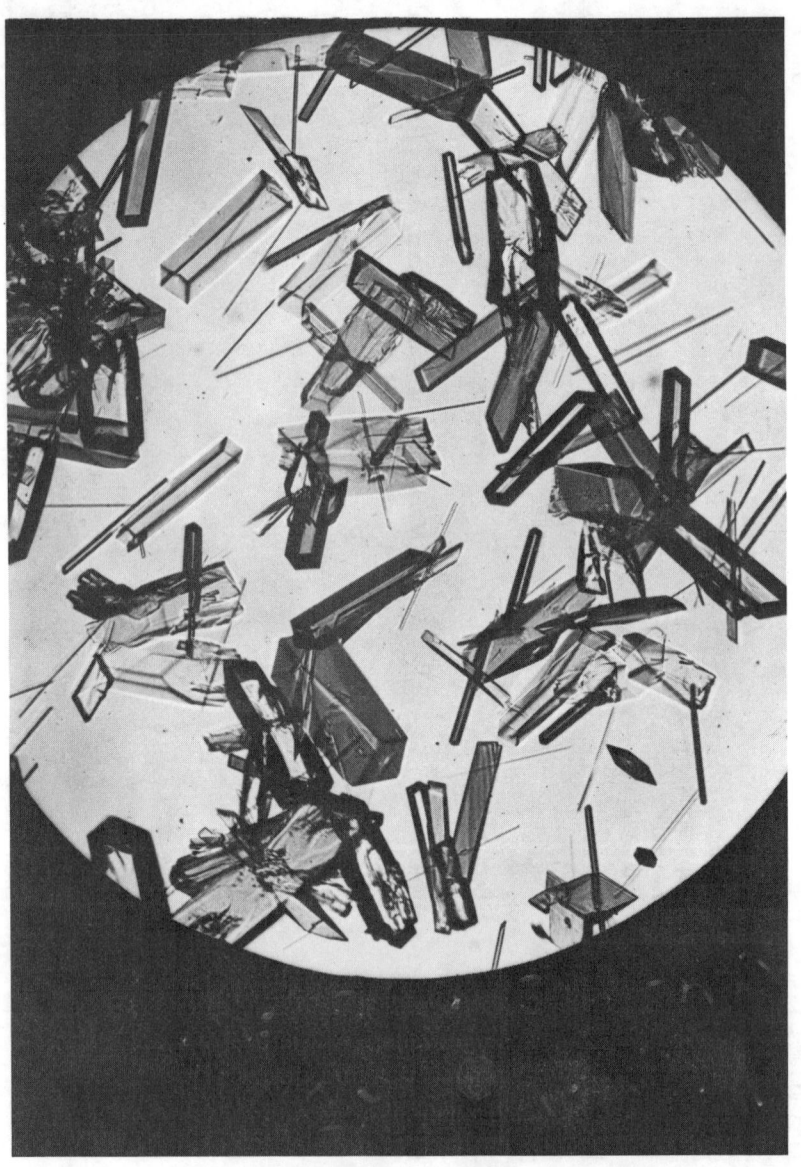

FIGURE 6-1   Vitamin A.

$$\text{Rhodopsin} \underset{\text{dark}}{\overset{\text{dim light}}{\rightleftharpoons}} \text{opsin} + \underset{\text{(vit. A)}}{\text{retinene}} \rightleftharpoons \underset{\text{(vit. A)}}{\text{retinol}}$$

FIGURE 6-2   Role of retinene (vitamin A) and retinol (vitamin A) in dim light vision.

Absorption, Storage, and Metabolism

Bile salts, along with fat, aid in the absorption of vitamin A through the intestinal mucosa into the blood. Vitamin A is transported to the liver, where 90% of it is stored and then distributed to the body tissues. Vitamin A is attached to a protein carrier in the liver before it is transported to the tissues to be metabolized. Therefore, if a person has a protein deficiency, transport of vitamin A and other fat-soluble vitamins is hindered.

Functions

Retina   The innermost layer of the eye that contains the visual receptors, rods, and cones.

Rods   Receptor cells in the retina of the eye that are sensitive to dim light.

Cones   Receptor cells in the retina of the eye, that are sensitive to bright light and colors.

Rhodopsin   The compound secreted by the rods in the retina.

Opsin   A protein pigment that combines with retinene in the rods to form rhodopsin.

Night blindness   The inability to see well in dim light.

Mucous membranes   Membranes that line the cavities that open to the outside of the body.

Keratinized   To become hard or horny.

Cornea   The outer covering of the eye.

Vitamin A has three primary functions: dim light vision, maintenance of skin and mucous membranes, and normal bone and teeth development.

1. **Dim light vision.** The **retina** of the eye contains two different receptor cells, **rods** and **cones**, that are sensitive to light and transform it into nerve impulses. Rods secrete a compound called **rhodopsin**, which is composed of the protein **opsin** and retinene (a form of vitamin A). The reaction of rhodopsin with light and its resynthesis in dark are shown in Figure 6-2.

   As indicated in Figure 6-2 when dim light strikes rhodopsin, it is decomposed to opsin and retinene, with much of the retinene being destroyed. The destroyed retinene is quickly replaced by the rods oxidizing retinol. If an adequate amount of retinol is present, there is no problem with the rods changing retinol to retinene and then the resynthesis of rhodopsin in darkness. Rods are very sensitive to dim light; thus, vitamin A and rhodopsin are important in dim light vision (see Fig. 6-2). However, if a deficiency of vitamin A exists, resynthesis of rhodopsin does not occur rapidly enough and the person experiences **night blindness.**

2. **Maintenance of mucous membranes. Mucous membranes** (see Fig. 6-3) are vitally important because they secrete mucus, which traps and removes invading bacteria, thereby protecting the body from infection. If the body is deficient in vitamin A, the mucous membranes lose their ability to secrete mucus and are transformed (**keratinized**) into a dry, hardened state. This condition reduces the ability of the membranes to resist infection. Two mucous membranes that often become keratinized are the respiratory mucosa and the **cornea** (see

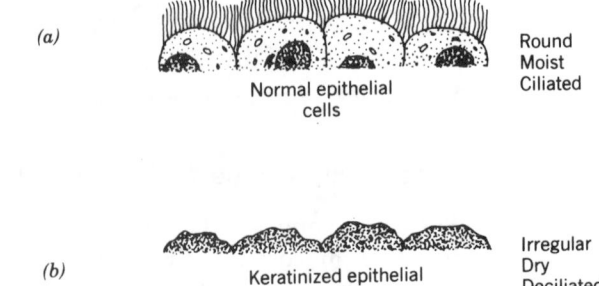

(a)   Normal epithelial   Round
                         cells   Moist
                                                    Ciliated

(b)   Keratinized epithelial   Irregular
                         cells   Dry
                                                     Deciliated

FIGURE 6-3   (*a*) Maintenance of the intestinal and respiratory linings by vitamin A. (*b*) Appearance of ciliated tissue with a vitamin A deficiency. (From Guthrie, Helen A.: *Introductory Nutrition*, ed. 5, St. Louis, 1983, The C.V. Mosby Co.)

Fig. 6-4). Keratinization of the cornea can result in blindness and increased eye infections. Respiratory infections are increased when the respiratory mucosa is keratinized.

3. **Growth and development of bones.** Vitamin A is important, in some unknown manner, to the growth of bones in length and diameter (see Fig. 6-5).

Body Requirements

The amount of vitamin A a person needs is proportional to body weight. The amount required by the body is stated in terms of daily quantities;

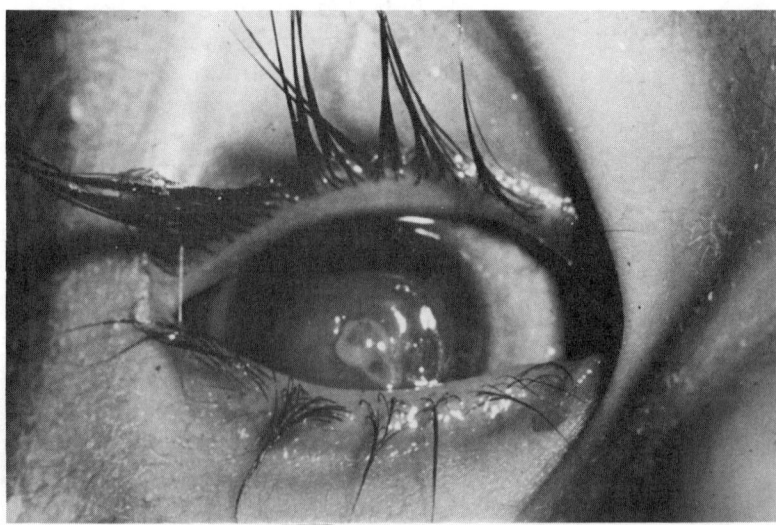

FIGURE 6-4   Keratinization of cornea due to vitamin A deficiency. (Courtesy of Dr. D.S. McLaren, American University, Beirut, Lebanon.)

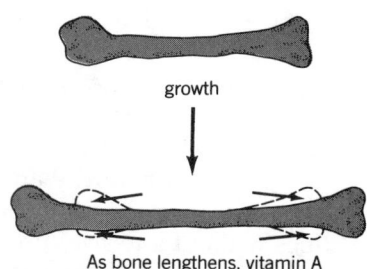

growth

As bone lengthens, vitamin A
helps remove old bone.

FIGURE 6-5 Role of vitamin A in the growth and development of bones.

however, since it is stored in the liver, it is not necessary to ingest it
daily. The Recommended Daily Allowances (RDA) for different people
is given inside the front cover.

Food Sources

Sources of vitamin A are as follows:

Animal	*Plant*
Liver	Dark green leafy vegetables
Whole milk	Deep yellow or orange fruit
Butter	Fortified margarine
Cream	
Egg yolk	
Cod liver oil	

Carotene A precursor of
vitamin A.

The vegetables and fruit mentioned above contain **carotene.** The body
is able to convert carotene to vitamin A in the intestinal mucosa cells.
Vitamin A in food is fairly stable in the presence of light and heat but
is easily destroyed by air (oxidized by reacting with oxygen) and sunlight
(ultraviolet rays). Vitamin E is very helpful in that it is oxidized, instead
of vitamin A, when they occur together. It is interesting that these two
vitamins frequently occur together in foods.

Toxicity and Clinical Deficiency

Since vitamin A is a fat-soluble vitamin, it is stored in the body; therefore,
the potential for toxicity problems exists. Some of the problems associated with vitamin A toxicity are joint pain, stunted growth, cessation
of menstruation, and enlargement of the liver.
Toxicity frequency occurs in children because of parental overconcern
about their getting the proper amounts of vitamins. These parents may

inadvertently give their children too much vitamin A when they feed them breakfast cereals, milk, and chewable, candylike vitamins, all fortified with vitamin A. A daily dose of vitamin A in the amount of 5,000 retinol equivalents (RE) for a month has been reported as having toxic effects in infants. The ingestion of toxic levels of vitamin A may be a greater health hazard than a deficiency if one is consuming vitamin A in capsule form. Foods containing vitamin A can be eaten in large quantities without a toxicity problem, with the possible exception of liver.

A deficiency of vitamin A probably does not become clinically evident until after about a year of dietary deficiency. The reason is that the body can store about a year's supply of vitamin A in the liver. Clinical evidence of vitamin A deficiency is first seen in the eyes. Some examples of deficiency are summarized in Table 6-1 and below.

1. **Night blindness.** Since vitamin A is essential for the resynthesis of rhodopsin in the retina, this symptom is very common. It is difficult to detect in young children, and the doctor has to rely on the mother's noticing whether the child's vision at night is impaired.

Xerophthalmia A condition in which the cornea becomes thickened and opaque.

2. **Xerophthalmia.** The cornea becomes thickened and opaque, resulting in blindness due to the decreased ability of light rays to enter the eye.

3. **Respiratory infections.** The mucosa of the respiratory tract also becomes keratinized (see Fig. 6-3) and therefore is not able to protect the individual from invading microorganisms.

4. Cessation of bone growth. Since vitamin A is important for normal bone growth and development, a deficiency can result in the failure of bones to grow and develop.

Vitamin A deficiency is widespread in India, South and East Asia, Africa, and Latin America. In the United States, it is most pronounced in Spanish-American and black children under 6 years of age.[1,2]

VITAMIN D (Cholecalciferol)

Nature and General Characteristics

Vitamin D is a steroid compound that has hormonelike functions (see Fig. 6-6). Some people believe that it should be classified as a hormone, since it is synthesized in the skin. It is unique in another way: It occurs naturally in only a few common foods, but it can be formed in the body by the interaction of the skin and ultraviolet rays from the sun.

Absorption, Storage, and Metabolism

Vitamin D is absorbed through the small intestine with the aid of bile and is then carried into the general circulation by lymph. Vitamin D is

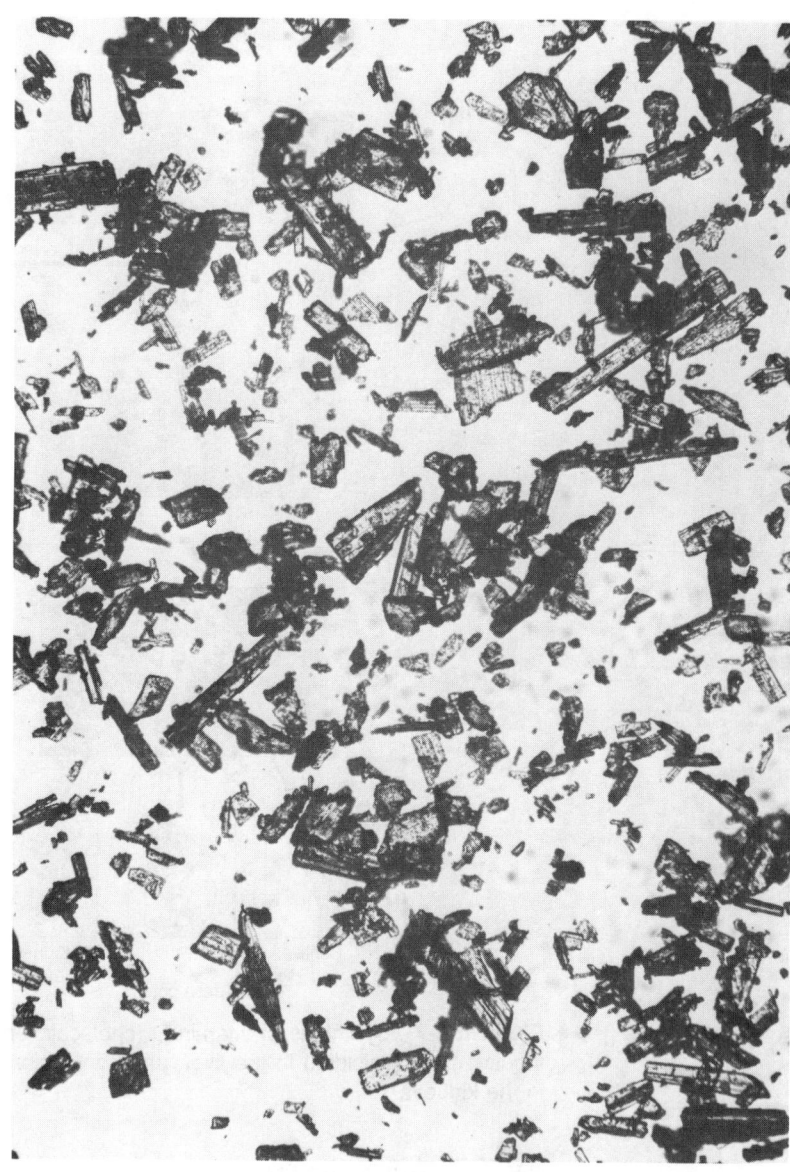

FIGURE 6-6 Vitamin D.

Calcidiol The inactive form of vitamin D that is stored in the liver.

Cholecalciferol Chemical name for vitamin D.

Target organs Organs that are stimulated by hormones.

Calcitriol The active form of vitamin D.

removed from the blood and stored in the liver as **calcidiol.** It is also synthesized in the skin. Ultraviolet light rays from the sun convert cholesterol in the skin to **cholecalciferol,** or vitamin D_3 (see Fig. 6-7), which is transported from the skin and stored as calcidiol in the liver. Calcidiol is the most common form of vitamin D circulating in the blood but is an inactive form; therefore, it has little or no activity in **target organs. Calcitriol** is formed by the conversion of calcidiol in the kidneys (see

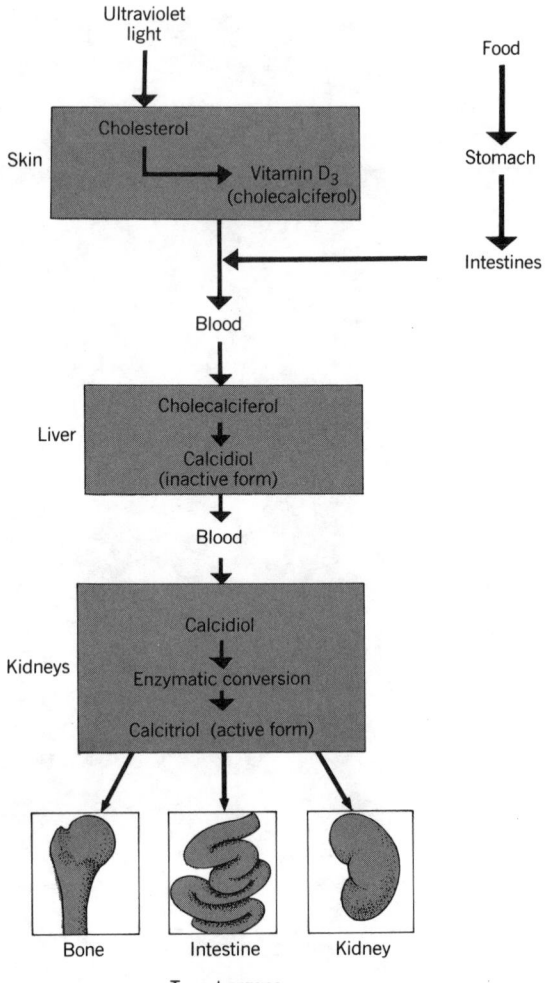

FIGURE 6-7 Synthesis of vitamin D (cholecalciferol) in skin, conversion to the inactive form (calcidiol) in the liver, and conversion to the active form (calcitriol) in the kidneys.

Fig. 6-7), where the necessary enzyme is found. Calcitriol then travels through the blood to three primary target organs: the intestines, kidneys, and bones. Since calcitriol is secreted into the blood and travels to target organs, it is often described as a hormone.

Functions

The primary function of vitamin D is to aid the growth of bones (see Fig. 6-8). It does this in two ways. First, it increases the absorption of calcium and phosphorus from the small intestine. Second, it influences

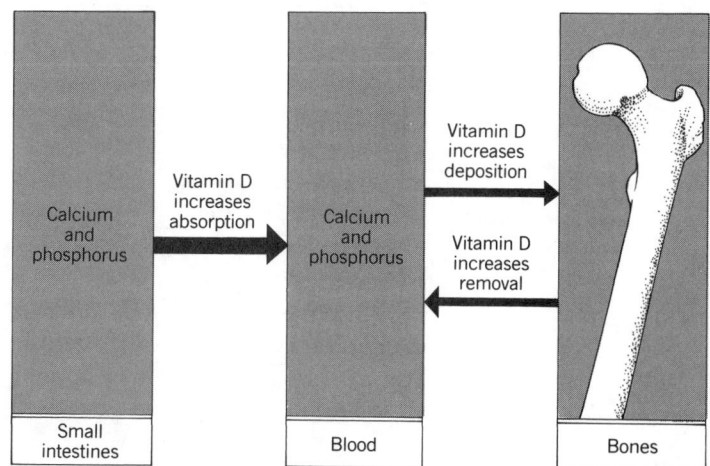

FIGURE 6-8 Role of vitamin D in the growth and development of bones.

the deposition into and removal of calcium and phosphorus from bone tissue (see Fig. 6-8).

Body Requirements

The amount of vitamin D needed in the diet is difficult to establish, since the skin synthesizes some of it. However, the Food and Nutrition Board's recommended daily intakes are listed inside the front cover.

Food Sources

Fortified The addition of nutrients to a food to make it richer than the unprocessed food.

As stated earlier, vitamin D is found naturally in only a few common foods: eggs, liver, butter, and cream. Therefore, we rely on **fortified** foods to make sure that we get our daily RDA. Milk is the best example of a food that is fortified with vitamin D. An adult who drinks two glasses of fortified milk daily can be assured of meeting the RDA even if he or she is not exposed to sunlight.[3]

Toxicity and Clinical Deficiency

Hypercalcemia A condition in which the blood calcium level is elevated.

Anorexia A loss of appetite.

Calcification The hardening of soft tissues due to an accumulation of calcium.

Some of the problems associated with a toxic level of vitamin D are **hypercalcemia**, **anorexia**, **calcification** of soft tissues, head pain, and reduction in the growth rate of children (see Fig. 6-9). These toxic effects are summarized in Table 6-1, and hypercalcemia and calcification of soft tissues is discussed below.

1. **Hypercalcemia** (see Fig. 6-9). This condition results from an excessive amount of calcium being withdrawn from bones and absorbed into

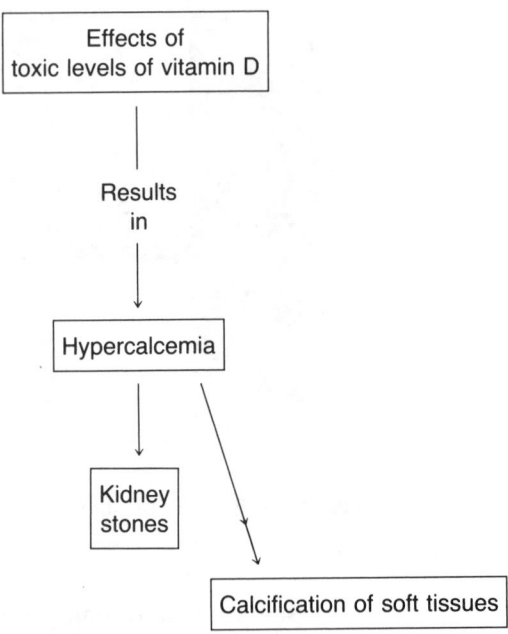

FIGURE 6-9   Effects of toxic levels of vitamin D.

the blood from the intestines as a result of high levels of vitamin D. This condition can lead to other problems as follows:

A. **Kidney stones** *and renal damage.* An excessive amount of calcium in the blood that circulates through the kidneys can result in the formation of kidney stones. Irreversible kidney damage can also result from excessive amounts of calcium being filtered by the kidneys.

B. **Calcification of soft tissues.** Certain soft tissues (blood vessels, kidneys, and lungs) may calcify due to the accumulation of calcium in them (see Fig. 6-9). Kidney tissue is very prone to calcification, leading to kidney failure. Recent evidence indicates that exceedingly large doses of vitamin D may contribute to the development of atherosclerosis.

A deficiency of vitamin D can cause rickets in children, **osteomalacia** in adults, poorly developed teeth, muscle spasms, and involuntary twitching (see Fig. 6-10). These problems are summarized in Table 6-1 and below.

1. **Rickets in children.** This problem has almost disappeared in the United States, primarily due to the fortification of milk. Cases are still seen in both Canada and Great Britain. Rickets is characterized by inadequate calcification of bones; as a result, the body weight causes

Kidney stones The stones formed in the kidneys as a result of certain dietary and chemical changes (see Chapter 23).

Osteomalacia The softening of the bones due to the loss of calcium or demineralization.

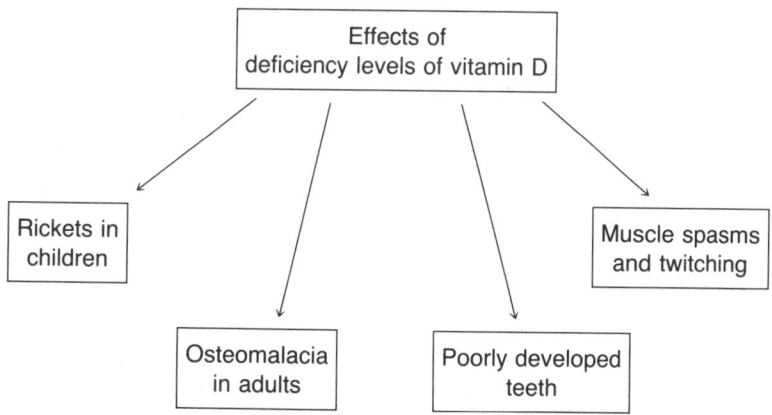

FIGURE 6-10   Effects of vitamin D deficiency.

the legs to bow (see Fig. 6-11). More serious bone deformities are bowed ribs and delayed closing of fontanels, which results in rapid enlargement of the head.

2. **Osteomalacia in adults.** This problem is also rare in adults unless the individuals have diseases that interfere with vitamin D absorption, such as **nontropical sprue**, obstruction of bile ducts, and pancreatic insufficiency. Osteomalacia is characterized by softening of bones due to the loss of calcium or demineralization. The limbs are deformed as well as the thorax, vertebral column, and pelvis. Bone fractures are also quite common.

Nontropical sprue An alternative term for adult celiac disease (malabsorption disorder) (see Chapter 19).

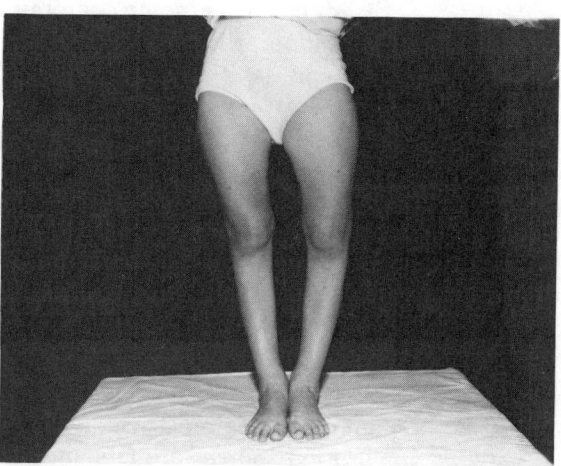

FIGURE 6-11   Rickets is characterized by inadequate calcification of the bones. As a result, the body weight causes the legs to bow.

3. **Poorly developed teeth.** Calcium is important for proper development of teeth. A deficiency causes slow eruption, improper development, and a greater tendency for tooth decay.

4. **Muscle spasms and twitching.** The blood calcium level is low in vitamin D deficiency, resulting in muscle twitches and spasms.[4]

VITAMIN E (Alpha-Tocopherol)

Nature and General Characteristics

Vitamin E is chemically known as alpha-tocopherol (Greek: to bear offspring) (see Fig. 6-12). This name is derived from its function as an antisterility compound in rats. However, this function, as well as other nutritional roles of vitamin E (increasing male sexual potency and reducing heart problems) in humans, has not been substantiated after many years of research. There are four forms of the vitamin, but alpha-tocopherol is the most active form.

Absorption and Metabolism

Vitamin E is absorbed into the blood, as are other fat-soluble vitamins, with bile salts and fat being required.

Functions

Antioxidant A compound that prevents oxidation.

The only documented nutritional role of vitamin E in humans is that of an **antioxidant.** Compounds such as vitamin A or polyunsaturated fatty acids (PUFA) cannot be used as well by the body after they have been oxidized. However, some compounds react more readily than others in the oxidation process. When such a compound is present in a mixture of compounds, it probably will be oxidized rather than the others. Vitamin E acts as an antioxidant for vitamin A and PUFA because it is more readily oxidized, thereby protecting them.

Body Requirements

The RDA for different people for vitamin E is given in the RDA table (inside front cover).

Food Sources

Vitamin E is the most widely available vitamin in common foods. The major food sources are fats and oils, particularly unsaturated fat products. This is a very fortunate coincidence, since the vitamin requirement apparently increases with the PUFA intake. Approximately 60% of the vitamin E we ingest comes from margarines, salad dressings, and short-

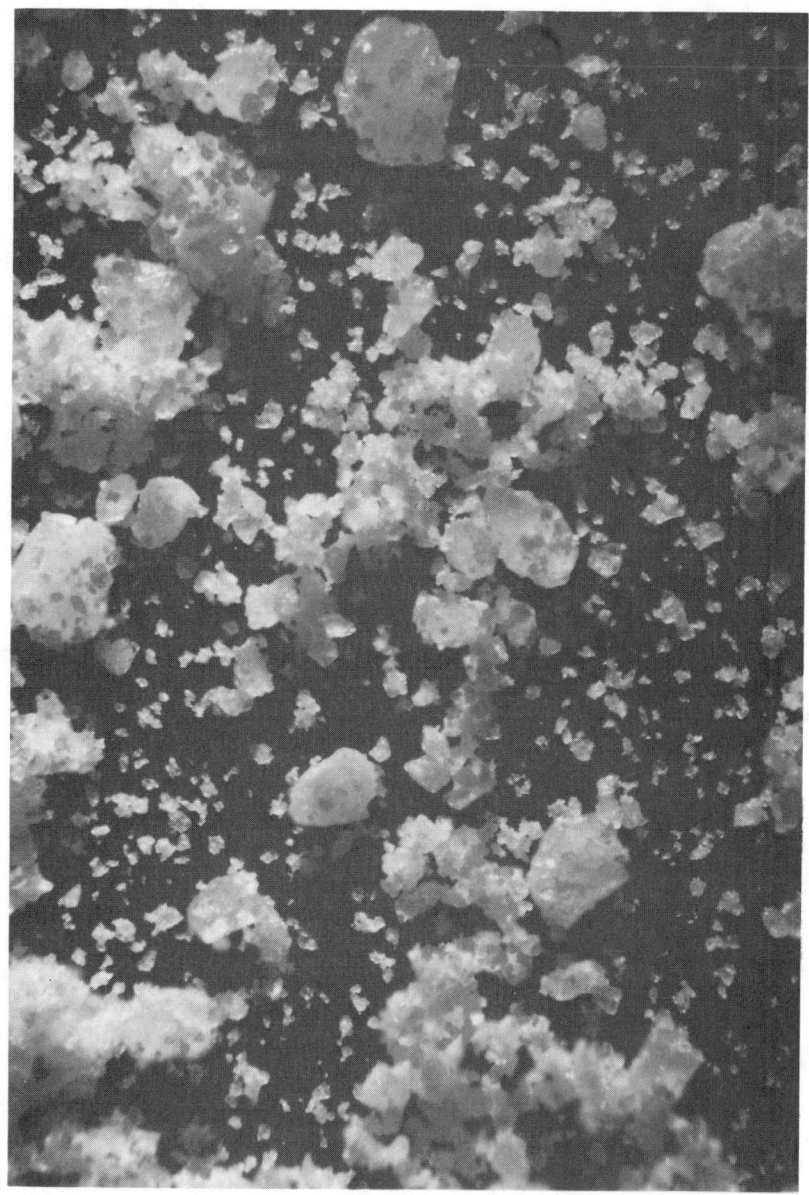

FIGURE 6-12 Vitamin E.

enings. Ten percent comes from fruits and vegetables, and a small percentage comes from grains such as soybeans and wheat. Soybean oil and wheat germ oil contain very high concentrations of vitamin E. Green leafy vegetables are moderate sources, as are liver and eggs. Animal foods other than the two just mentioned are generally poor sources of the vitamin.

Toxicity and Clinical Deficiency

Hypertension Elevated
blood pressure.

Prolonged excessive intake of vitamin E apparently can produce **hyper-tension**. In addition, some studies have shown that large doses increase the time required for blood to clot.

Erythrocytes Red blood
cells.

Hemolyzed Broken
down.

A deficiency of vitamin E in humans has been shown to be detrimental to **erythrocytes** when blood levels of vitamin E drop below 100 mg/dl. The red blood cells (RBCs) are **hemolyzed** and spill out hemoglobin. This serious problem is thought to result from the oxidation of PUFA in the RBC membranes. One way that oxidation occurs is by the addition of oxygen to a compound. PUFA in RBCs are very susceptible to this condition when the RBCs pass through capillaries in the lungs, where they exchange CO_2 for O_2. As described previously, normal amounts of vitamin E act as an antioxidant to protect PUFA and thereby prevent RBC hemolysis.

VITAMIN K

Nature and General Characteristics

Quinones A group of
chemical compounds that
includes vitamin K.

There are several forms of vitamin K, all of which belong to a chemical group called **quinones**. Bacteria in the large intestine produce vitamin K in quantities that are usually adequate for the body's needs. However, the intestine of a new born infant is sterile. Therefore, no vitamin K production occurs until about the third or fourth day of life, when the bacteria have colonized the intestine.

Absorption and Metabolism

Vitamin K is absorbed with the aid of bile. Then chylomicrons transport the molecule to the liver, where most of it is stored and used. Any disorders that interfere with secretion of bile (such as cholecystitis) or absorption of fat (such as celiac sprue or cystic fibrosis) will interfere with absorption and transport of vitamin K. Water-soluble or water-miscible forms of vitamin K are available in these cases.

Functions

Prothrombin A blood
protein that contributes to
blood clotting.

Vitamin K plays a role in blood clotting when a person is hemorrhaging by aiding in the synthesis of the protein **prothrombin** (see Fig. 6-13). Vitamin K aids in the synthesis of other blood-clotting factors as well.

Body Requirements

The recommended amount of vitamin K is presented in the inside back cover which gives the estimated safe and adequate daily dietary intakes

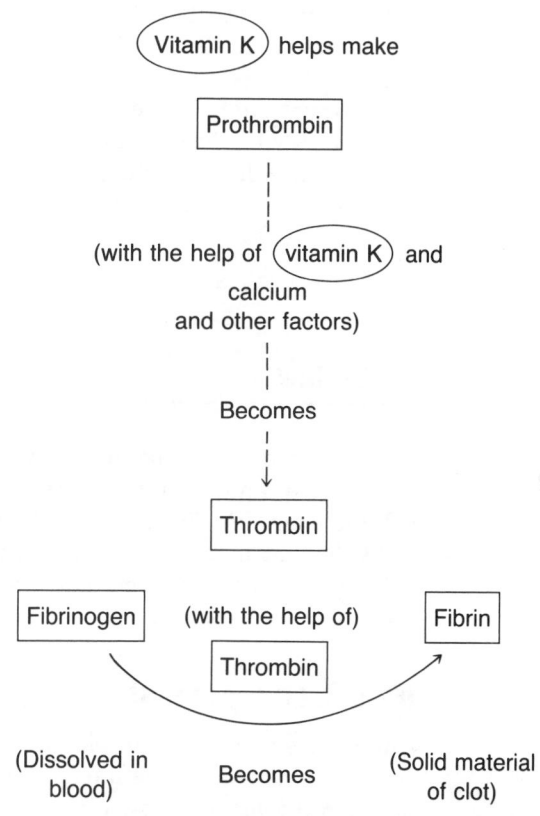

FIGURE 6-13 Role of vitamin K in blood clotting.

(ESADDI). The amounts for adults are small, since intestinal bacteria generally synthesize enough for daily needs. Newborn infants and especially premature infants, however, are a special case, since only a limited amount of the vitamin is transported across the **placenta** into the infant's body during pregnancy. Also, as previously mentioned, the intestinal bacteria are not established for a few days after birth. Therefore, many authorities suggest that a newborn term or premature infant receive 1 mg of vitamin K in order to prevent hemorrhage problems.

Placenta A structure present within the uterus of a pregnant woman that is connected to the developing fetus and exchanges wastes and nutrients.

Food Sources

Green leafy vegetables, cabbage, and milk are good sources of vitamin K. Egg yolk and some types of liver (pork) contain moderate amounts.

Hemolytic anemia A condition that results in the destruction of red blood cells (RBCs) at a faster than normal rate.

Jaundice Yellow discoloration of the whites of the eyes and the skin.

Toxicity and Clinical Deficiency

Large amounts of vitamin K given to an infant over a prolonged period of time may produce **hemolytic anemia** and **jaundice**.

A deficiency of vitamin K normally is rare unless a person has difficulty in absorbing it, such as in a deficiency of bile. Another example is a person who has been taking large amounts of antibiotics (sulfonamides and tetracycline). These compounds either kill the intestinal bacteria or depress vitamin K synthesis. As a result, if an artery or vein is cut, the person will hemorrhage, since the blood-clotting process has been hindered.[5]

WATER-SOLUBLE VITAMINS

Certain vitamins are soluble in water and easily absorbed into blood. Excessive quantities of them are excreted rather than stored, unlike fat-soluble vitamins. Since water-soluble vitamins are readily excreted, it is unlikely that a person would store them to the point of developing toxicity problems. Water-soluble vitamins include B complex vitamins and ascorbic acid.

B COMPLEX VITAMINS

There are six major B complex vitamins and six minor ones. RDAs have been established for thiamin (B_1), riboflavin (B_2), B_6, B_{12}, niacin (nicotinic acid), and folacin (folic acid).

Several of the B vitamins function as coenzymes. The coenzymes have several specific functions, but they all have one thing in common: They are necessary for enzyme function.

THIAMIN (Vitamin B_1)

General Characteristics, Absorption, and Metabolism

Vitamin B_1 is called *thiamin* because it contains a sulfur molecule and an amine group (see Fig. 6-14). It is absorbed from the duodenum into the general circulation, which carries it to the tissues. Alcohol and barbiturates hinder its absorption.

Functions

The principal function of thiamin is that of a coenzyme in the process of oxidizing glucose to form adenosine triphosphate (ATP), which is the basic energy molecule of the body. Thiamin prepares compounds (see

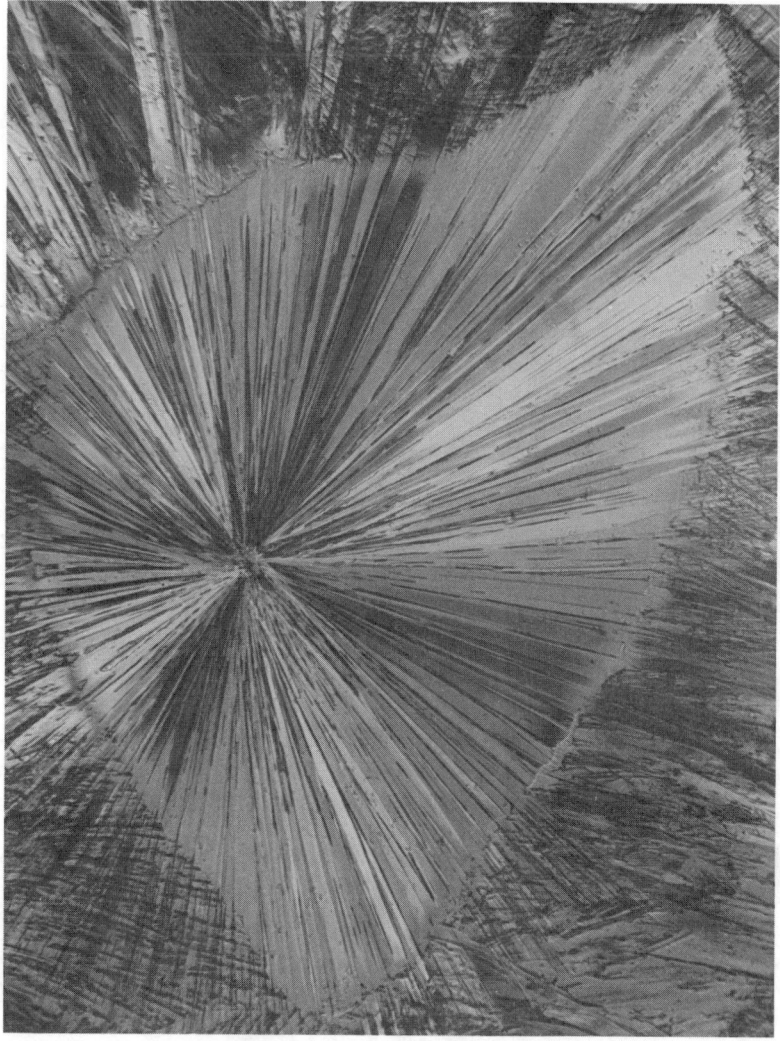

FIGURE 6-14 Thiamin (vitamin B₁).

Fig. 6-15) to enter the Krebs (citric acid) cycle, which is very important in the synthesis of ATP molecules.

Body Requirements

The need for thiamin increases with the need for calories. Thus, increased thiamin is quite important during growth periods, pregnancy and lactation, infections, and chronic illness.

The basic RDA is 0.5 mg/1,000 kcal/day. For example, if a 1-year-old

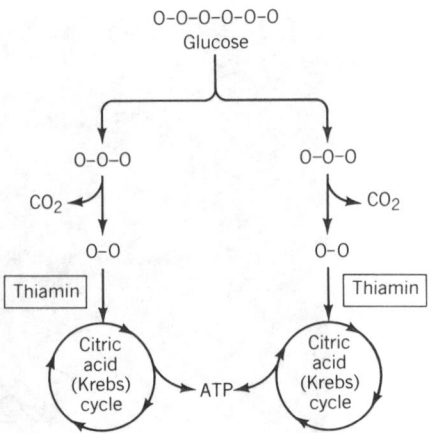

FIGURE 6-15 Role of vitamin in the synthesis of ATP.

child ingested 1,300 kcal/day, the RDA would be about 0.7 mg. A 19-year-old boy who ingested 3,000 kcal/day would need about 1.5 mg.

Food Sources

Good sources of thiamin are lean pork, beef, liver, whole or enriched grains, and legumes. Eggs, fish, and a few vegetables are fair sources. Thiamin is not as widely found in foods as are some of the other vitamins, such as A and C. Therefore, a person on an average diet, especially one low in calories, may have a thiamin deficiency.

Toxicity and Clinical Deficiency

It is almost impossible to develop a toxicity problem with any of the B complex vitamins, since they are not stored in large quantities in the body. Deficiencies of thiamin produce clinical disorders in the gastrointestinal, nervous, and cardiovascular systems. *Beriberi* is the term often used to describe this condition. The underlying cause of the symptoms is a decrease in the amount of energy released. Thiamin deficiency is most often seen in chronic alcoholics, since their diets are often inadequate in the proper amounts and types of foods. The nervous system is most dramatically affected. The earliest symptom indicating deterioration of the nervous system is heaviness of the legs. A burning sensation in the feet is often followed by progressive weakness of the toes, feet, legs, and thighs. In the cardiovascular system, the heart may weaken, followed by heart failure. The peripheral blood vessels are often weakened, resulting in **peripheral edema**. If the thiamin deficiency is persistent, an alcoholic can ultimately develop a mental disorder called **Wernicke-Korsakoff disease** (see Chapter 26 for more details).

Peripheral edema Excess accumulation of interstitial fluids within the extremities.

Wernicke-Korsakoff disease A mental disorder caused by a thiamin deficiency.

RIBOFLAVIN (Vitamin B$_2$)

General Characteristics

Flavins A group of chemicals that are fluorescent.

Vitamin B$_2$ is a member of a group of chemicals called **flavins**, which are fluorescent (see Fig. 6-16). Attached to the flavin part of the molecule is the five-carbon sugar, ribose, hence the name *riboflavin*.

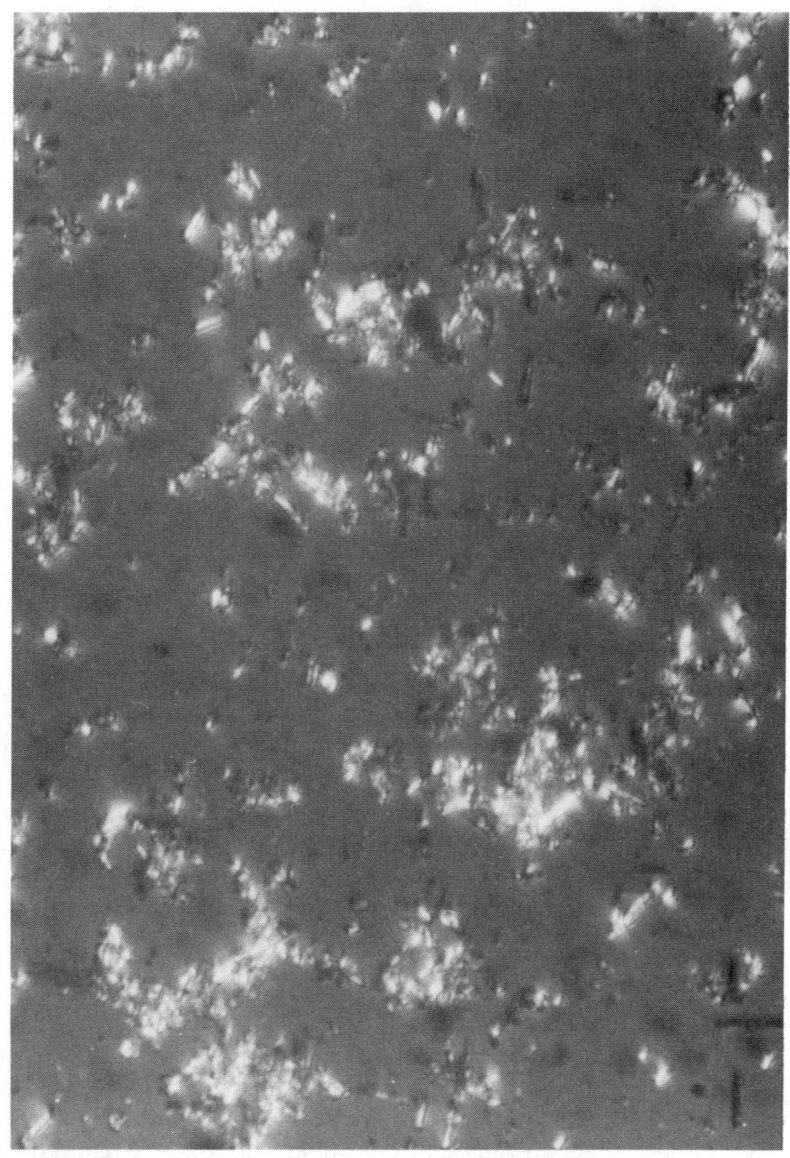

FIGURE 6-16 Riboflavin (vitamin B$_2$).

Absorption of riboflavin occurs in the upper portion of the gastrointestinal tract by a specific transport system. The amount absorbed is higher in older compared to younger people. More riboflavin is absorbed when eaten with food than when taken separately.

Several drugs affect the metabolism of riboflavin, with tetracycline antibiotics and the thiazide diuretics increasing urinary excretion.

Functions

Flavin adenine dinucleotide (FAD) An electron transfer compound that transfers electrons and hydrogen atoms from the Krebs cycle through the cytochrome system to oxygen.

Cytochrome A molecule in the electron transport system.

Similar to thiamin, riboflavin functions in the release of energy from food (see Fig. 6-14). Riboflavin is a component of the electron transfer compound called **flavin adenine dinucleotide (FAD)**. FAD transfers electrons and hydrogen atoms from the Krebs cycle through the **cytochrome** system to oxygen. It is this transfer process that produces the majority of ATP or energy molecules for the body. Riboflavin also participates in the first step of the decomposition of fatty acids for the production of energy.

Body Requirements

The RDA for riboflavin are based on energy intake and are given on the inside front cover. As with thiamin, increased riboflavin intake is important during pregnancy and lactation, growth periods, infections, and chronic illness.

Food Sources

It is ironic that riboflavin is widely distributed in food, but only in small amounts in foods that we commonly eat. Examples of foods that are rich in riboflavin are milk, green leafy vegetables, cereals, and enriched bread.

Cheilosis Cracks at the corner of the mouth due to a deficiency of vitamin B$_2$.

Glossitis Smooth, purplish appearance of the tongue due to a deficiency of vitamin B$_2$.

Photophobia Sensitivity of the eyes to light and strain.

Riboflavin is destroyed by ultraviolet rays (sunlight). This is one of the reasons why milk is no longer sold in transparent glass bottles. Transparent plastic bottles filter out more light and help to reduce the destruction of riboflavin.

Toxicity and Clinical Deficiency

There is no known toxicity from vitamin B$_2$. A deficiency of this vitamin can cause the following problems and is summarized in Table 6-1: **cheilosis, glossitis**, and **photophobia**. A riboflavin deficiency rarely occurs in isolation, but rather with other vitamin deficiencies.[5]

PYRIDOXINE (Vitamin B$_6$)

General Characteristics, Absorption, and Metabolism

Vitamin B$_6$ actually refers to several related compounds that are interconvertible and biologically active. Like the other water-soluble vitamins, vitamin B$_6$ is readily absorbed into the blood together with water from the small intestine. A small amount is stored in muscle tissue.

Functions

Pyridoxine is primarily involved with reactions involving the synthesis and catabolism of amino acids and, therefore, is important for protein synthesis.

1. **Synthesis of nonessential amino acids.** Vitamin B$_6$ aids in changing amino acids that occur in abundance to forms that the cells need at a given time. In other words, it aids in the synthesis of nonessential amino acids (see Fig. 6-17).

Tryptophan An amino acid.

2. **Conversion of amino acid tryptophan to the vitamin niacin.** Vitamin B$_6$ converts **tryptophan** into the vitamin niacin (see Fig. 6-17) (discussed shortly).

3. **Antibody production.** Vitamin B$_6$ aids in the production of antibodies (see Fig. 6-17) that protect the body against the invasion of foreign antigens.

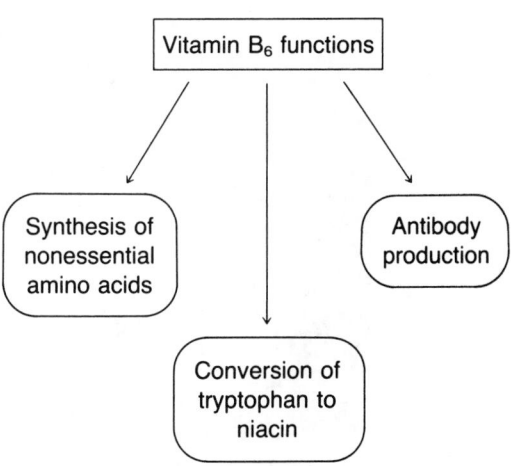

FIGURE 6-17 Functions of vitamin B$_6$.

Food Sources

The best food sources of vitamin B_6 are pork, wheat germ, whole-grain cereals, legumes, and bananas. Milk and eggs provide small amounts.

Toxicity and Clinical Deficiency

Convulsions Involuntary spasms or contractions of groups of muscles.

Deficiencies can result in cheilosis (see Fig. 6-18) and glossitis (see Fig. 6-19). The nervous system shows the deficiency by conducting an abnormal number of nerve impulses, which can result in **convulsions** and abnormal brain wave patterns.[6]

In addition to dietary deficiencies of vitamin B_6, several drugs interfere with its metabolism. Some examples are isoniazid (INH), levodopa (L-dopa), chloramphenicol, and particularly oral contraceptives.

COBALAMIN (Vitamin B_{12})

General Characteristics, Absorption, and Metabolism

Vitamin B_{12} is a complicated molecule that contains the mineral cobalt, hence the name *cobalamin*.

Absorption of vitamin B_{12} is difficult due to its large size. To facilitate

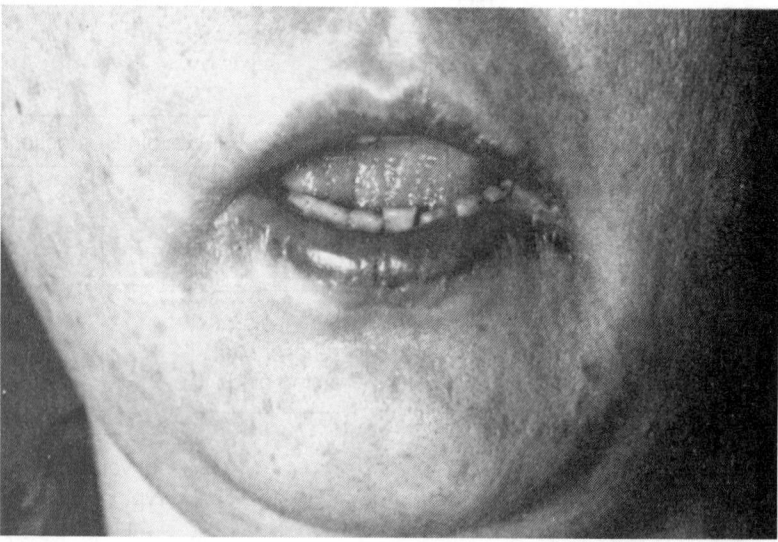

FIGURE 6-18 Cracking of skin at the corners of the mouth (cheilosis) due to deficiency of pyridoxine. (Courtesy of R.H. Kampmeier, M.D., Vanderbilt University.)

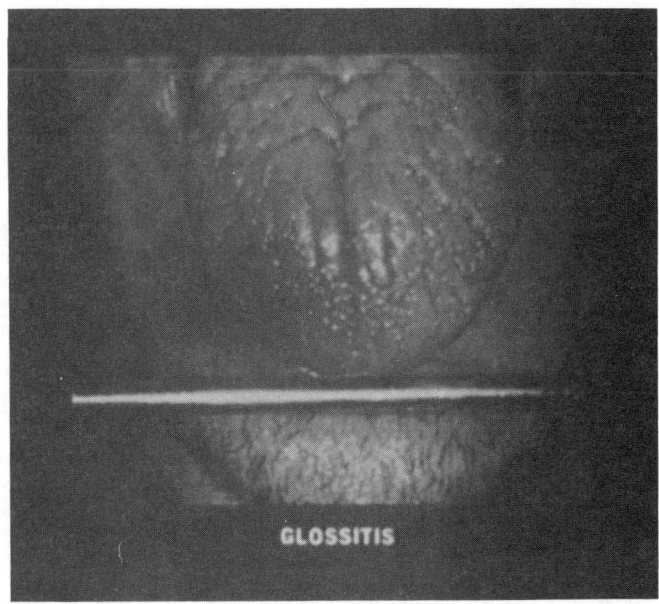

FIGURE 6-19 A deficiency of vitamin B_6 (pyridoxine) may cause the tongue to become smooth (glossitis). (From Sandstead, H.H., Carter, J.P., and Darby, W.J. "How to diagnose nutritional disorders in daily practice," *Nutrition Today*, *4*, 2 (Summer 1969.)

Intrinsic factor A protein that is secreted by the gastric mucosa and combines with vitamin B_{12}, thereby making its absorption possible.

Extrinsic factor A compound that refers to vitamin B_{12} and is formed outside the body.

Gastritis Inflammation of the stomach lining.

Myelin sheath A sheath, composed of fatty material, that surrounds and insulates some nerve fibers.

absorption, it combines with an **intrinsic factor** synthetized by the stomach mucosa. Vitamin B_{12} is called the **extrinsic factor**, since its source is outside the body. The intrinsic and extrinsic factors combine in the stomach to form a complex (see Fig. 6-20) that enables vitamin B_{12} to be absorbed from the small intestine.

The rate of vitamin B_{12} absorption tends to decrease with age, with pyridoxine deficiency, with **gastritis**, and in people who have congenital intrinsic factor deficiency. Interestingly, pregnancy enhances its absorption.

Functions

Vitamin B_{12} interacts with the cardiovascular and nervous systems to help maintain homeostasis. It also interacts with the red bone marrow in the synthesis of RBCs (see Fig. 6-21). The importance of this function cannot be overemphasized, since RBCs carry oxygen gas molecules to the cells, resulting in the release of energy. Vitamin B_{12} is important to the nervous system, since it helps to maintain the **myelin sheath** that surrounds and insulates some nerve fibers.

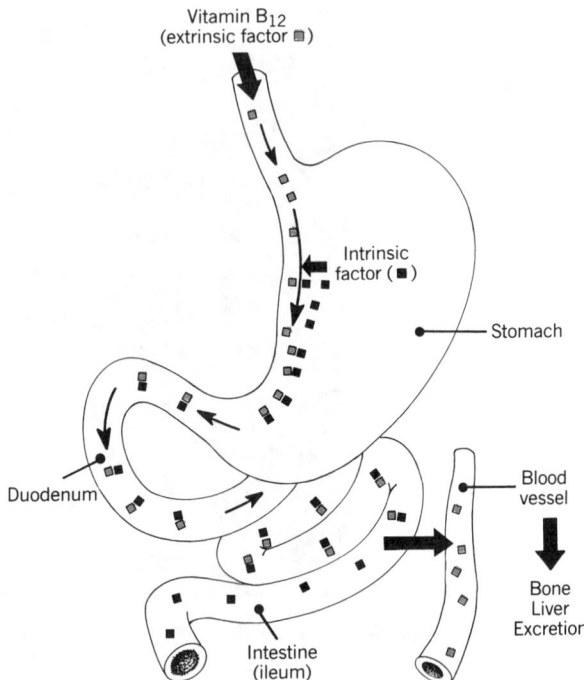

FIGURE 6-20   Combination of vitamin B_{12} (extrinsic factor) and intrinsic factor to aid the absorption of vitamin B_{12}.

Body Requirements

The body needs very little vitamin B_{12} to be effective, as indicated in the RDA table (inside front cover).

Food Sources

Vitamin B_{12} occurs in animal products only; none is found in plants. Seafood, meat, eggs, and milk are good sources. Strict vegetarians may become deficient in this vitamin and should consider vitamin supplements.

Toxicity and Clinical Deficiency

Toxicity problems are rare, since vitamins B_{12} is stored in the liver and muscle tissues in small amounts. The amount stored, however, is often adequate to last for 3 to 5 years. This is evidenced by the fact that when a subtotal gastrectomy (partial removal of the stomach) is performed (see Chapter 19), it takes 3 to 5 years before a vitamin B deficiency occurs.

A vitamin B_{12} deficiency may cause degeneration of myelin sheaths,

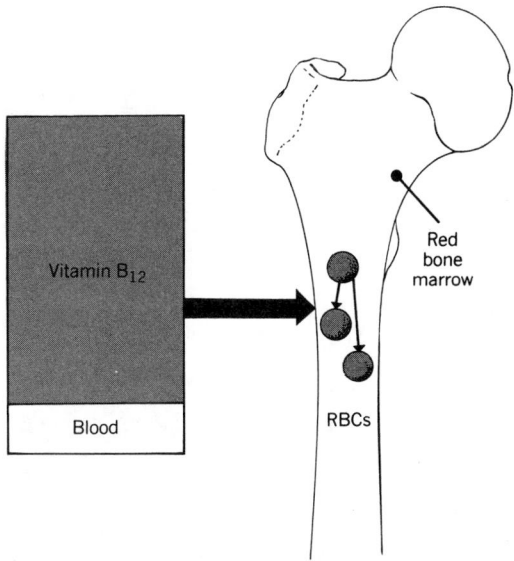

FIGURE 6-21 Role of vitamin B_{12} in the synthesis of red blood cells (erythropoiesis) in red bone marrow.

Pernicious anemia Anemia that results from a deficiency of vitamin B_{12} because of a lack of the intrinsic factor.

Gastrectomy Surgical removal of the stomach.

Macrocytic anemia A type of anemia in which red blood cells are larger than normal.

Intramuscular injections Injections of substances into muscles.

resulting in numbness in the limbs, difficulty and poor coordination in walking, and coldness of the extremities. In severe deficiencies, the person may suffer from mental deterioration.

People who inherit the inability to synthesize the intrinsic factor cannot absorb adequate amounts of vitamin B_{12} and therefore suffer from **pernicious anemia.** In addition, people who have undergone **gastrectomies** face potential pernicious anemia. The reduced number of RBCs is frequently much larger than normal (**macrocytic anemia**) (see Fig. 6-22). Early detection of pernicious anemia is important to avoid the nervous system problems mentioned above.

Pernicious anemia, in relation to the two problems discussed above, cannot be prevented by increasing the intake of foods high in vitamin B_{12} or by taking supplements. The person must receive vitamin B_{12} by **intramuscular injections** or by parenteral infusion (see Chapter 17 for details of parenteral infusion of nutrients).

NIACIN (Nicotinic Acid)

General Characteristics, Absorption, and Metabolism

Two forms of niacin exist: niacin and nicotinamide (NAD) (see Fig. 6-23). The body converts niacin to nicotinamide, which is the active func-

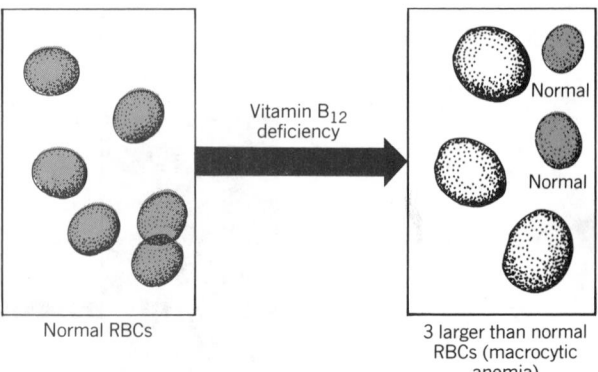

FIGURE 6-22 Normal red blood cells and larger than normal red blood cells (macrocytic anemia) due to vitamin B_{12} deficiency.

tional form of the vitamin. Niacin is absorbed in the upper part of the small intestine and is stored in very small quantities. The metabolism of niacin also includes its synthesis from the amino acid tryptophan. Research has shown that approximately 60 mg of tryptophan is converted to 1 mg of niacin.

Functions

Niacin is part of a coenzyme (NAD) that is vital in obtaining energy from glucose. NAD transfers hydrogen atoms and their energy to the electron transport system in cells for the purpose of synthesizing high-energy ATP molecules. Each NAD molecule receives two hydrogen atoms from a glucose ($C_6H_{12}O_6$) molecule (see Fig. 6-24).

Body Requirements

The RDA for niacin, given on the inside front cover, is based on kilocalorie intake due to its role in obtaining energy from glucose.

Food Sources

Good sources of tryptophan are milk and eggs. Good sources of niacin are meat, poultry, and fish.

Toxicity and Clinical Deficiency

Large amounts of niacin may result in **vasodilation** of blood vessels in the skin. **Pellagra** is a disease that may result from a niacin deficiency. It is characterized by the three Ds—diarrhea, **dementia**, and dermatitis. Diarrhea occurs when the intestinal mucosa becomes inflamed, excreting large amounts of watery feces.

Vasodilation Increased diameter or size of blood vessels.

Pellagra A condition that is caused by a niacin deficiency.

Dementia A severe mental disorder involving impairment of mental ability.

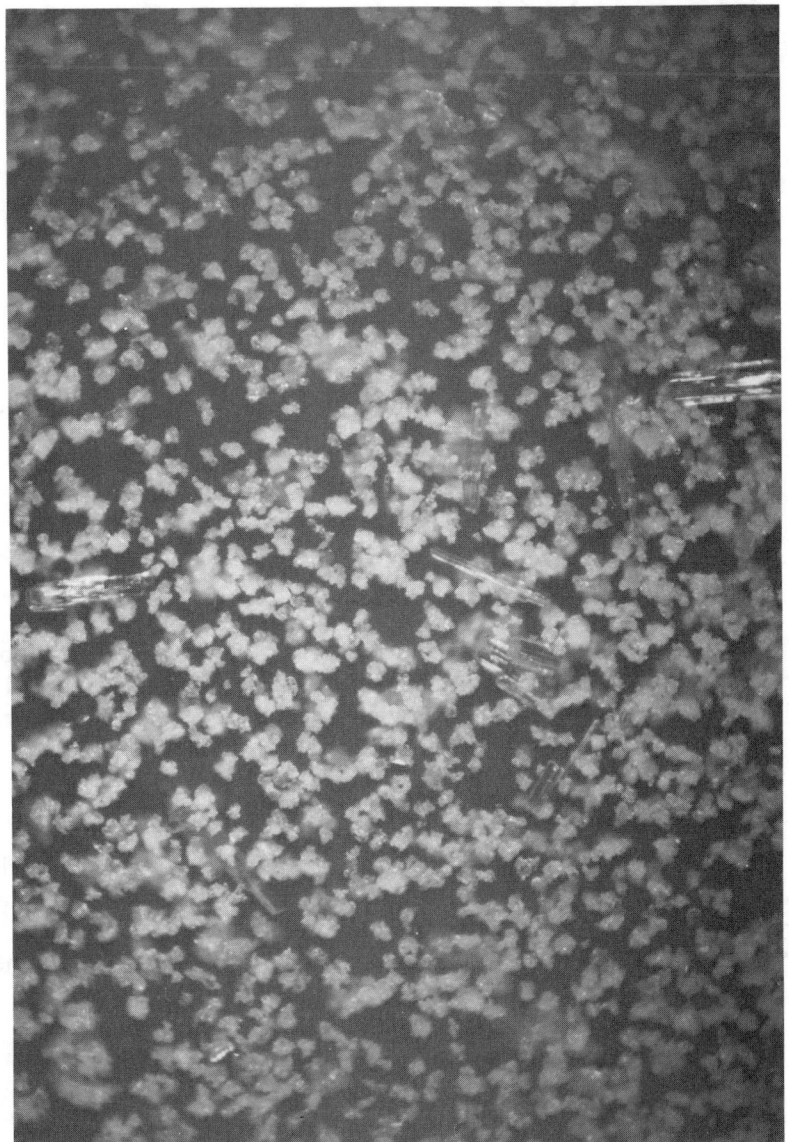

FIGURE 6-23 Niacin.

A person suffering from dementia, may exhibit mental confusion, anxiety, and depression. These problems occur when the nervous system does not get enough energy.

Dermatitis occurs on parts of the skin exposed to the sun, with the neck being a common location.

Most pellegra has been eliminated in the United States. It is still found,

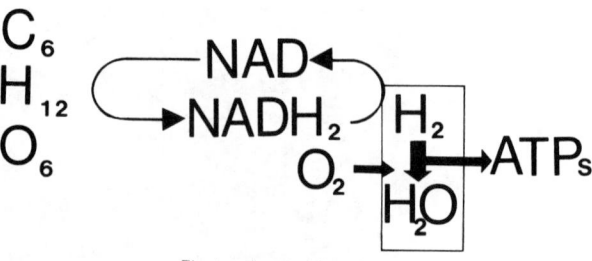

Electron transport system

FIGURE 6-24 The role of niacin (as a component of NAD) in transferring hydrogen (H_2) atoms in the electron transport system and synthesis of ATP.

however, in some Third World countries where protein malnutrition is rampant.[1,3,7]

FOLACIN

General Characteristics, Absorption, and Metabolism

Folacin is actually a group of related compounds that have the same basic functions. It is absorbed into the blood from the upper intestine. Alcoholics have a decreased ability to absorb folic acid, since alcohol interferes with its absorption.

Functions

Erythropoiesis The synthesis of red blood cells.

The most important function of folacin is the synthesis of the heme portion of hemoglobin molecules that are located in RBCs. Since hemoglobin molecules are the main constituent of RBCs, **erythropoiesis** (see Fig. 6-25) is dependent upon an adequate amount of folacin in addition to vitamin B_{12}.

Body Requirements

The RDAs for folacin are given on the inside front cover. Notice the increased amount recommended during pregnancy. The reason is that a pregnant woman produces more RBCs in order to furnish oxygen gas and other nutrients not only for herself but also for the fetus.

Food Sources

Vegetables are an excellent source of folacin. In fact, the terms *folacin* and *foliage* are derived from the same root word. A strict vegetarian will obtain more than an adequate amount of folacin but may be deficient in vitamin B_{12}. Vegetables that are high in folacin are kidney beans, spinach, asparagus, and broccoli.

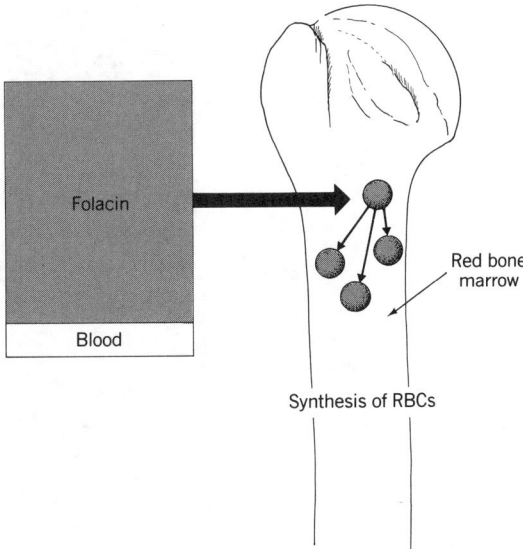

FIGURE 6-25 Role of folacin in the synthesis of red blood cells in red bone marrow.

Toxicity and Clinical Deficiency

Toxicity from folacin is very rare, since it is water soluble and therefore not stored in great quantities in the body.

Clinical deficiencies of folacin primarily affect the gastrointestinal tract and blood. The surface of the tongue may become smooth (glossitis), and the person may experience diarrhea.

A deficiency of folacin may result in a deficiency of RBCs or macrocytic anemia. Since these conditions are identical to a deficiency of vitamin B_{12}, what may appear to be a folacin deficiency may actually be a vitamin B_{12} deficiency. Also, a strict vegetarian may consume more than an adequate amount of folacin but not enough vitamin B_{12}. The deficiency of vitamin B_{12} may be masked because the folacin allows the RBCs to develop to their proper size and number, but this deficiency can lead to degeneration of myelin sheaths and thus to nerve damage.

BIOTIN

General Characteristics, Absorption, and Metabolism

Biotin is a sulfur-containing molecule and is absorbed in the upper part of the small intestine. Most of the biotin used by humans is synthesized by bacteria in the large intestine (see Fig. 6-26). Little is known about the metabolism and storage of biotin.

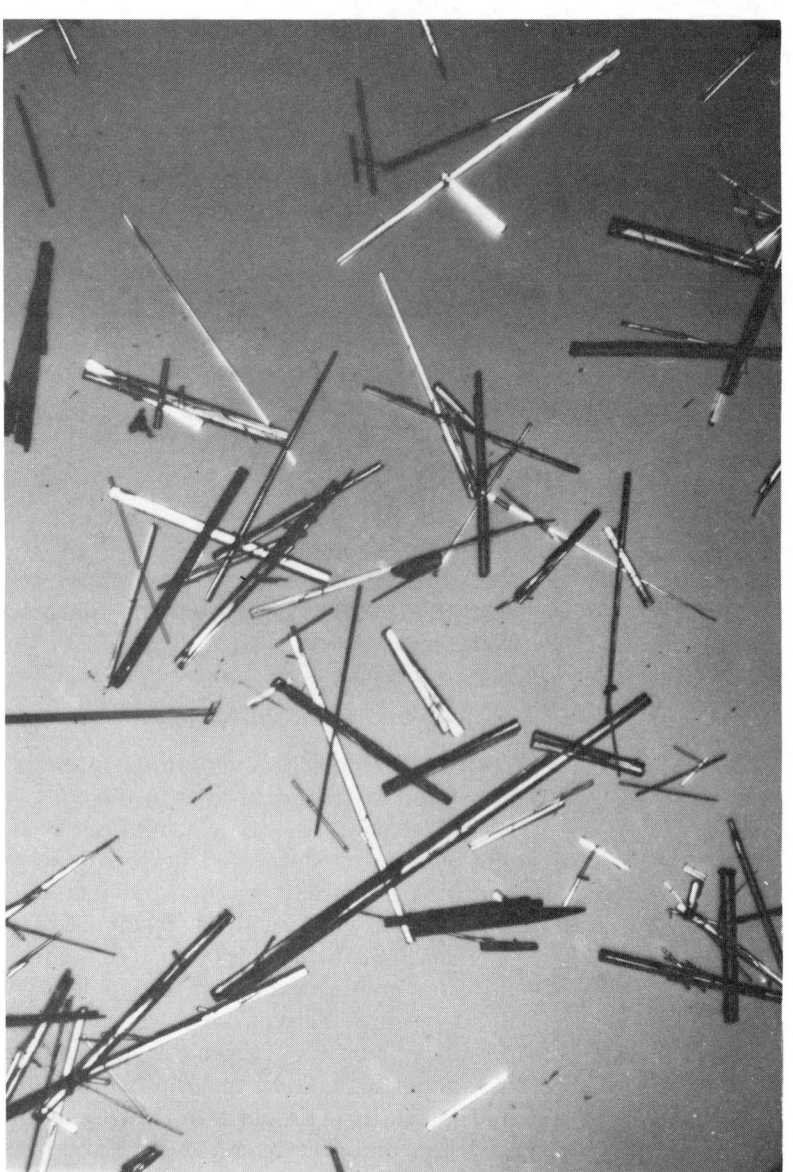

FIGURE 6-26 Biotin.

Functions

Biotin functions as a coenzyme in several biochemical reactions; carbohydrate and amino acid metabolism are examples. Other possible functions are niacin synthesis from tryptophan, formation of antibodies, and
synthesis of pancreatic amylase. Research shows that the functions of
biotin appear to be closely related to those of vitamin B_{12} and folic acid.

Body Requirements

The estimated safe and adequate daily dietary intake for biotin is given on the inside back cover. A normal American diet contains at least this much, and intestinal bacteria secrete a substantial amount of biotin.

Food Sources

Milk, liver, egg yolks, mushrooms, and legumes all contain biotin. Many foods have not been analyzed for their biotin content.

Toxicity and Clinical Deficiency

No toxicity or clinical deficiency problems in humans have been documented. Some deficiencies have been produced in experimental animals by dietary means.

PANTOTHENIC ACID

General Characteristics, Absorption, and Metabolism

The name *pantothenic acid* is derived from the Greek word *pantos*, meaning everywhere. It is found extensively in all plants and animals. Little is known about where and how it is absorbed. It is stored in the liver, brain, kidney, and heart.

Functions

Acetylcholine A neuro-transmitter substance that is secreted at the axion ends of many neurons.

Pantothenic acid has two basic functions: metabolism of carbohydrates, lipids, and proteins and synthesis of **acetylcholine**.

Body Requirements

The estimated safe and adequate daily dietary intake is given on the inside back cover.

Food Sources

The best sources of pantothenic acid are eggs, liver, yeast, and salmon. Good sources are mushrooms, cauliflower, molasses, and peanuts. Fruits and milk are poor sources. Grains are a good source of pantothenic acid, but approximately 50% is lost in the milling process.

Toxicity and Clinical Deficiency

Research has yet to find any problems in humans with excessive quantities or deficiencies of pantothenic acid. Problems with the nervous system and eyes, as well as a decrease in growth, have been observed with deficiencies of pantothenic acid in experimental animals.[2,7]

SUMMARY OF IMPORTANT POINTS ABOUT B VITAMINS

When one reviews the functions and deficiencies of the B vitamins, some general facts stand out:

1. **Nervous system malfunctions.** The nervous system depends heavily on glucose metabolism and therefore on thiamin. A deficiency of thiamin often causes nervous system disorders.

2. **Deficiency in RBC synthesis.** Erythropoiesis is especially important upon vitamins such as folic acid and cobalamin (vitamin B_{12}). Anemia is one of the first symptoms of a deficiency of these two vitamins.

3. **Abnormal appearance of the tongue.** The tongue frequently shows signs of vitamin deficiencies and is readily observable. Since the tongue is part of the gastrointestinal tract, its abnormal appearance may be an indication of other gastrointestinal problems.

VITAMIN C (Ascorbic Acid)

General Characteristics, Absorption, and Metabolism

The term *ascorbic acid* is a derivative of the word *antiscorbutic*, meaning without scurvy. This term indicates that ascorbic acid is important in preventing scurvy. Vitamin C has a structure similar to that of monosaccharides. It is water soluble, absorbed from the small intestine into blood, and transported to the liver and **spleen.** Even larger amounts are stored in the **adrenal gland.**

Spleen A large glandular organ composed of lymphatic tissue.

Adrenal gland A gland located on top of the kidneys that secretes several different hormones.

Scurvy A disease that is characterized by weakness, skin degeneration, ulcerated gums, loss of teeth, and hemorrhages in the skin.

Collagen A protein that is important in the structure of skin, teeth, bones, and muscle.

Functions

1. *Prevention of* **scurvy** (see Fig. 6-27). This disease is characterized by weakness, skin degeneration, ulcerated gums, (see Fig. 6-28), loss of teeth, and skin hemorrhages. The symptoms of scurvy are related to breakdown of collagen.

2. *Formation of collagen.* Ascorbic acid aids in the synthesis of **collagen,** which is important in the structure of the skin, teeth, bones, and muscle.

3. *Healing of wounds.* Vitamin C aids in the healing of wounds. It does this by moving to the site of injury, where it promotes the formation

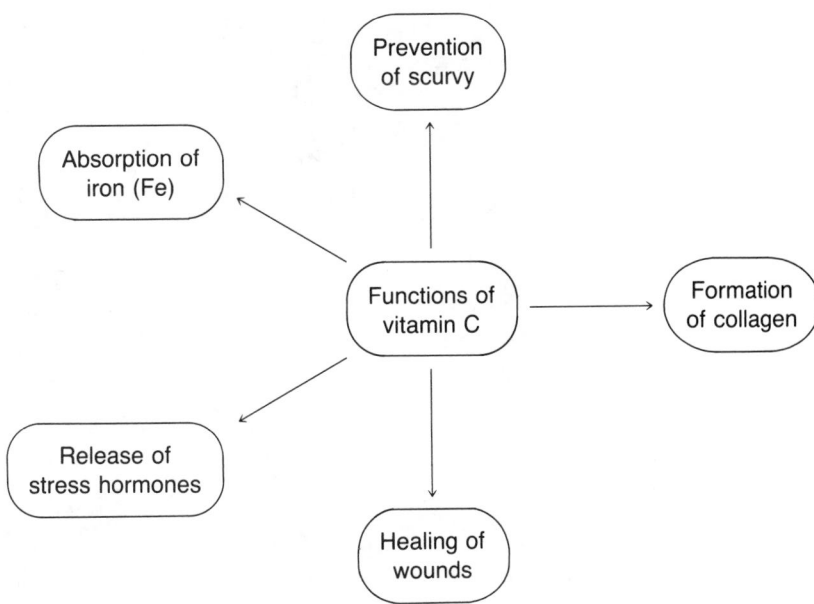

FIGURE 6-27 Functions of vitamin C.

of collagen in scar tissue. Vitamin C is often prescribed in large quantities for burn patients and patients who have had surgery to enhance the healing process.

4. *Release of stress hormones.* Vitamin C levels decrease in times of stress because it aids in the release of epinephrine and **norepinephrine** from the adrenal gland. These hormones prepare the body to overcome stress conditions.

5. *Absorption of iron.* Iron (Fe) exists in two states in the body: **ferric** (Fe^{3+}) and **ferrous** (Fe^{2+}), with the ferrous form being more readily absorbed. Vitamin C and hydrochloric acid (HCl) function to keep iron in the more absorbable form.

Since iron is the mineral that is present in RBCs, vitamin C is indirectly involved in the synthesis of RBCs.

Body Requirements

The RDA for ascorbic acid is given on the inside front cover. These normal amounts must be increased for people who are under stress or heavy cigarette smokers, or who are ill and have a fever. The amount of vitamin C needed for wound healing and formation of scar tissue following major operations or extensive burns may be as high as 1,000 mg/day or even more.

Norepinephrine A neurotransmitter secreted by the sympathetic nerves and as a hormone secreted from the adrenal gland.

Ferric Chemical form of iron, Fe^{3+}; a less absorbable form than ferrous iron.

Ferrous Chemical form of iron, Fe^{2+}; more absorbable form than ferric iron.

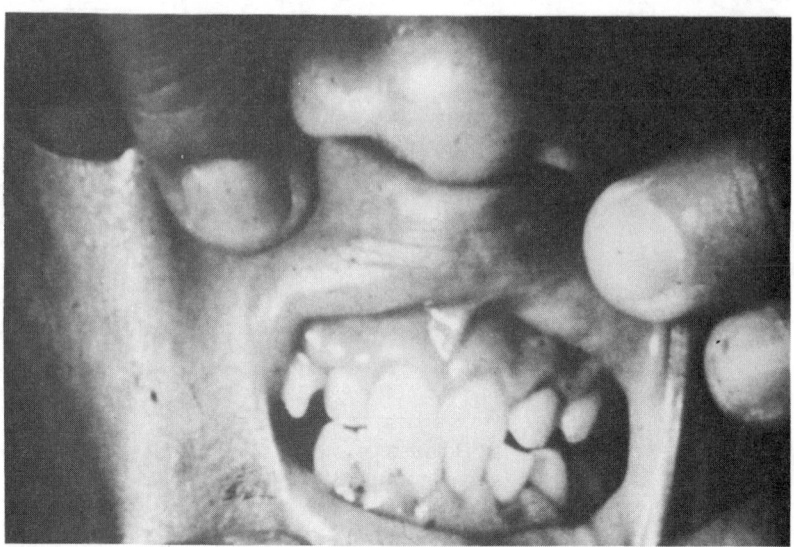

FIGURE 6-28 A deficiency of vitamin C can result in deteriorated or ulcerated gums. (Courtesy of the Centers for Disease Control, Atlanta, Ga.)

Food Sources

Ascorbic acid is found in all citrus fruits, canteloupe, and strawberries. Vegetable sources include broccoli, tomatoes, brussel sprouts, greens, and potatoes (each potato contains only a small amount of vitamin C, but people eat potatoes so often).

Ascorbic acid is one of the vitamins most easily destroyed by heat, air, light, prolonged storage, copper and iron cookware, and the use of baking soda to preserve food color. Some suggestions for obtaining the maximum amount of ascorbic acid from preparation of foods are:

- Use the water that vegetables are cooked in. Since vitamin C is water soluble, some of it will be lost from vegetables when they are cooked.
- Quick-freeze foods that are being preserved.
- Fresh foods containing the vitamin should be refrigerated.
- Boil cooking water for at least 1 minute before adding food. Boiling rids the water of dissolved oxygen, which oxidizes vitamin C.
- Frozen foods should be placed directly in boiling water (not thawed in advance).

Toxicity and Clinical Deficiency

In recent years, many people have advocated the ingestion of large doses of vitamin C to prevent the common cold. As a result, there have been

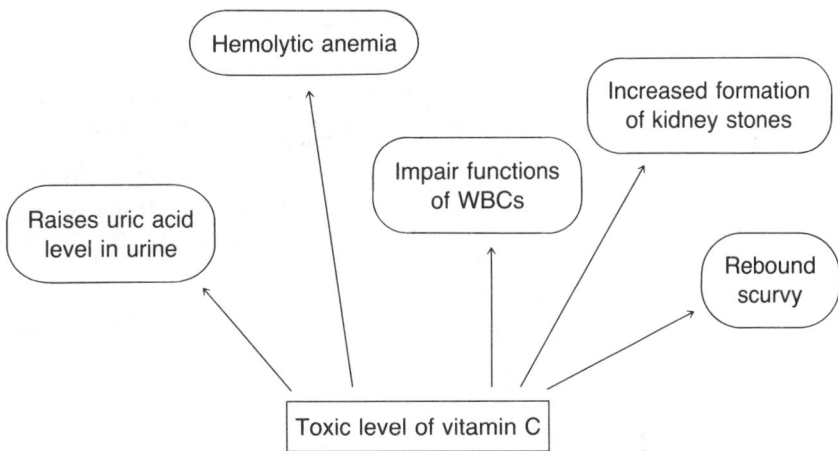

FIGURE 6-29 Effects of toxic levels of vitamin C.

Gout A metabolic disease characterized by an inability to metabolize purines and an elevated uric acid level in the blood.

many cases of toxicity, which have allowed scientists to study vitamin C toxicity. Some of the problems with vitamin C toxicity include raising the uric acid level in urine (see Fig. 6-29) and thereby increasing the chances of **gout** development in people who are already so predisposed. The toxic level of vitamin C may also cause hemolytic anemia in some ethnic groups such as blacks, Jews, and Orientals. High vitamin C levels have also been found to impair the ability of white blood cells to give immunity to the body. An increase in kidney stones has been found to occur in some people. One of the most interesting problems with vitamin C toxicity is rebound scurvy. This condition also occurs in adults who stop taking megadoses of vitamin C abruptly as opposed to decreasing their intake gradually.

Deficiencies can result in scurvy, muscle cramps, aching bones, dry, rough skin, and ulcerated gums (see Fig. 6-27)[1,5,7]

CAN VITAMIN C REALLY PREVENT COMMON COLDS?

There has been much controversy regarding vitamin C since Linus Pauling's book *Vitamin C and the Common Cold* was published in 1970. Pauling advocated the use of massive doses (1,000–2,000 mg/day) of vitamin C in order to prevent colds. Numerous studies have been conducted to determine whether vitamin C does have these effects. A summary of some of the results from these studies is as follows:

1. The decrease in the number of colds averaged 0.1 per year in one study, which is not statistically significant.

2. The massive doses possibly decrease the duration of colds very slightly.
3. Whatever beneficial effects the massive doses of vitamin C have on colds, there is a danger of toxic side effects (described above).

The results of the studies do not support the claims made by Pauling and others that massive doses of vitamin C can prevent colds. However, this is a controversial subject, and research will continue.

SUGGESTIONS FOR OBTAINING THE MAXIMUM AMOUNT OF VITAMINS WHEN HARVESTING, STORING, AND COOKING FOODS

Harvest vegetables immediately before they are to be cooked or stored

Vitamin C especially and other vitamins are lost the longer vegetables are held before they are eaten or properly stored (see below for proper storage).

Store vegetables and fruits properly

While the best source of vitamins is fresh vegetables and fruits, the vitamin content can be decreased significantly by not storing them properly. The best ways to store foods, in decreasing order, are:

Frozen
This method preserves the vitamin content best because it stops the enzyme activity that destroys the vitamins.

Fresh
If a person harvests vegetables or fruits from a home garden and allows them to remain at room temperature before eating, the enzyme activity that destroys the vitamins continues with great losses.

If a person cannot eat fruits and vegetables immediately after harvesting them, but plans to do so within a few days, they should be kept in the refrigerator.

To reduce evaporation of water, fresh vegetables and fruits should be stored in covered containers or plastic bags.

Canned

This method causes the greater nutrient loss of the three because of the high temperatures required. In addition, water-soluble vitamins are lost in the water in which they are prepared.

Reduce preparation and cooking of vegetables

The more preparation and cooking of vegetables is required before eating, the greater the nutrient loss. To reduce the losses:

- Avoid soaking vegetables in water.
- When possible, cook vegetables in their skins.
- Cook in as little water as possible.
- Bake, steam, or broil vegetables.
- When boiling, uses tight-fitting lids to diminish evaporation of water.
- Cook vegetables in as short a time as possible. Long cooking times destroy more vitamin C, folacin, and vitamin B_6 than short ones.

Cook frozen vegetables in the frozen state

This practice reduces the loss of vitamins compared to thawing the vegetables before cooking.

Avoid cutting vegetables and fruits before cooking

The more vegetables and fruits are cut up before cooking, the more exposure to air they receive and the greater the loss of vitamins, especially vitamin C.

Avoid adding soda to vegetables

If soda is added to green vegetables to preserve their color, an alkaline medium is created that will destroy more vitamin C than an acid medium.

OUTLINE

INTRODUCTION

Functions of carbohydrates, lipids, and proteins are dependent upon vitamins; they are vital to the cellular functions of the body.

GENERAL DESCRIPTION

Vitamins differ from the other nutrients (carbohydrates, lipids, and proteins) in that they do not yield energy; they are very small molecules and are not normally used up by the body processes. Consuming large amounts of vitamins is expensive and unnecessary, and in some cases can lead to undesirable side effects.

FAT-SOLUBLE VITAMINS

Included are vitamins A, D, E, and K; they have to attach to a carrier in order to be transported through the blood or lymph.

Vitamin A (Retinol)
Nature and General Characteristics
Most vitamin A is absorbed in the retinol form, which is oxidized to a form called *retinene*.

Absorption, Storage, and Metabolism
Absorption is aided by bile salts; 90% is stored in the liver and is transported from the liver by a protein carrier to tissues, where it is metabolized.

Functions
- Dim light vision
- Maintenance of mucous membranes
- Growth and development of bones

Body Requirements
The amount required is proportional to the body weight. The RDA for vitamin A is given on the inside front cover.

Food Sources
Animal sources: liver, whole milk, butter, egg yolk, cream.
Plant sources: dark green vegetables, deep yellow or orange fruit.

Toxicity and Clinical Deficiency
Vitamin A is stored and therefore creates a potential for toxicity; problems associated with toxicity are joint pain, stunted growth, cessation of menstruation and enlargement of the liver. Deficiency of vitamin A can cause night blindness, xerophthalmia, respiratory infections, and cessation of bone growth.

Vitamin D (Cholecalciferol)
Nature and General Characteristics
Vitamin D is a steroid compound; it can be formed in the body by the interaction of skin and ultraviolet rays from the sun.

Absorption, Storage, and Metabolism
Vitamin D is absorbed with the aid of bile; it is stored in the liver in an inactive form called *calcidiol*; the kidneys activate calcidiol to the active form *calcitriol*, which then travels to three primary target organs—intestines, kidneys, and bones.

Functions
- Vitamin D aids the growth of bones, firstly by increasing the absorption of calcium and phosphorus and secondly by influencing the deposition and removal of calcium and phosphorus from bone tissue.

Body Requirements
The RDA for vitamin D is given on the inside front cover.

Food Sources
Eggs, liver, butter, and cream are good sources; in addition, fortified foods such as milk provide vitamin D.

Toxicity and Clinical Deficiency
Toxicity problems include hypercalcemia, anorexia, kidney stones and renal damage, and calcification of soft tissues. Deficiency problems include rickets in children, osteomalacia in adults, poorly developed teeth, muscle spasms, and involuntary twitching.

Vitamin E (Alpha-Tocopherol)
Nature and General Characteristics
The name *alpha-tocopherol* is derived from its antisterility role in rats; this role in humans and others has not been substantiated.

Absorption and Metabolism
These processes are dependent upon the amount of bile acids; normally, 10–30% is absorbed, and vitamin A can interefere with its absorption; it is stored in liver, muscle, and adipose tissue.

Functions
- The only documented function of vitamin E is that of an antioxidant for vitamin A and poly-

unsaturated fatty acids (PUFA); since vitamin E is oxidized rather than vitamin A and PUFA, the latter two compounds and the tissues they are contained in are protected.

Food Sources
Major sources: fats and oils with margarines, salad dressings and shortenings.
Moderate sources: green leafy vegetables, liver, and eggs.

Toxicity and Clinical Deficiency
Toxicity causes hypertension and increased blood-clotting time. Deficiency causes destruction of RBCs as a result of decreased protection of PUFA.

Vitamin K
Nature and General Characteristics
There are several forms of the vitamin, all of which belong to the quinone group; it is produced by bacteria in the large intestine in amounts that are usually adequate for the body's needs; the intestines of a newborn are sterile and do not synthesize vitamin K for several days until they are colonized by bacteria.

Absorption and Metabolism
Absorption is affected by the amount of bile; vitamin K is transported by chylomicrons to the liver, where it is primarily used and a small amount is stored.

Toxicity and Clinical Deficiency
Toxicity: hemolytic anemia and jaundice in infants. Deficiency: Rare in adults unless they have bile deficiency and fat malabsorption problems; a person who has been taking large amounts of antibiotics (such as sulfonamides and tetracycline) may be deficient due to destruction of bacteria.

WATER-SOLUBLE VITAMINS

B Complex Vitamins
Six major vitamins that have RDA values are thiamin (vitamin B_1), riboflavin (vitamin B_2), niacin (nicotinic acid), pyridoxine (vitamin B_6), cobalamin (vitamin B_{12}), and folic acid; several B vitamins function as coenzymes, which are small nonprotein molecules that combine with inactive proteins to make them active.

Thiamin (Vitamin B_1)
General Characteristics, Absorption, and Metabolism
It is called *thiamin* because it contains a sulfur molecule attached to an amine group.

Function
- It acts as a coenzyme in the process of oxidizing glucose to form ATP; thiamin prepares compounds to enter the Krebs (citric acid) cycle.

Body Requirements
The body's need increases with the kilocalorie intake; the RDA is 0.5 mg/1,000 kcal/day.

Food Sources
Good sources: lean pork, beef, liver, whole or enriched grains, and legumes.
Fair sources: eggs, fish, and a few vegetables.

Toxicity and Clinical Deficiency
Toxicity: very rare
Deficiency: results in disorders in the gastrointestinal, nervous, and cardiovascular systems, with the deficiency often referred to as *beriberi*.
 Deficiency is most often seen in alcoholics, with the nervous system being most seriously affected; symptoms include heaviness of the legs, burning sensation of the feet, and progressive weakness of the toes, feet legs and thighs; the heart and peripheral blood vessels may weaken, with resultant edema.

Riboflavin (Vitamin B_2)
General Characteristics, Absorption, and Metabolism
Vitamin B_{12} is a member of a group called *flavins*, which are fluorescent; ribose, a five-carbon sugar, is attached to the flavin part of the molecule. Absorption is increased with age; several drugs affect its metabolism with tetracycline and thiazide diuretics, increasing its urinary excretion.

Functions
- Release of energy from food. Riboflavin is a component of the electron transfer compound flavin adenine dinucleotide (FAD), which is important in the transfer of hydrogen atoms and the release of energy from glucose.
- Decomposition of fatty acids for release of energy.

Body Requirements
This is based on energy intake and is given in the RDA table on the inside front cover.

Food Sources
Rich sources: milk, green leafy vegetables, cereals, and enriched bread. Ultraviolet rays in sunlight destroy the vitamin in milk; this is part of the reason why milk is rarely found in clear glass bottles.

Toxicity and Clinical Deficiency
Toxicity: no problems
Deficiency: cracks at the corners of the mouth (cheilosis); the tongue becomes smooth and purplish (glossitis); the eyes become sensitive to light and susceptible to strain (photophobia).

Pyridoxine (Vitamin B₆)
General Characteristics, Absorption, and Metabolism
Vitamin B₆ refers to several related compounds that are interconvertible and active.

Functions
- Synthesis of nonessential amino acids
- Conversion of the amino acid tryptophan to the vitamin niacin
- Antibody production

Food Sources
Rich sources: pork, wheat germ, whole grain cereals, legumes, bananas
Poor sources: milk, eggs

Toxicity and Clinical Deficiency
Deficiency: cheilosis, glossitis, and abnormal brain wave patterns.

Cobalamin (Vitamin B₁₂)
General Characteristics, Absorption, and Metabolism
Vitamin B₁₂ is a large vitamin with a cobalt molecule in the center. Absorption is possible only when cobalamin combines with an intrinsic factor secreted by the gastric mucosa or the lining of the stomach. The rate of absorption decreases with age, with gastritis (inflammation of the stomach), and in people who have congenital intrinsic factor deficiency.

Functions
- Synthesis of RBCs or erythrocytes
- Maintenance of myelin sheath on the nerves

Body Requirements
Very little B₁₂ is required, as indicated by the values in the RDA table on the inside front cover.

Food Sources
Vitamin B₁₂ occurs almost exclusively in animal (as opposed to plant) products; seafood, meat, eggs, and milk are examples; vegetarians or vegans may become deficient in vitamin B₁₂ if they do not consume supplements.

Toxicity and Clinical Deficiency
Toxicity problems are rare.
Deficiency: may cause degeneration of myelin sheaths on nerves, with person experiencing numbness in limbs, difficulty in walking, and coldness of extremities. Severe deficiencies may result in mental deterioration. Pernicious anemia results when a person cannot synthesize the intrinsic factor. The RBCs are larger than normal; therefore, the condition is often called *macrocytic anemia.*

Niacin (Nicotinic Acid)
General Characteristics, Absorption, and Metabolism
Two forms exist: niacin and nicotinamide (NAD); the body converts niacin to NAD, which is the active functional form of the vitamin. Niacin can be synthesized from the amino acid tryptophan.

Functions
- Synthesis of ATP molecules. Niacin is part of the coenzyme NAD, which is important for transferring hydrogen atoms and their energy to the electron transport in cells for the purpose of synthesizing ATP molecules.

Body Requirements
The RDA for niacin is based on the kilocalorie intake, since it is important in obtaining energy from glucose.

Food Sources
Tryptophan: milk eggs
Niacin: meat, poultry, fish

Toxicity and Clinical Deficiency
Pellagra is the disease that may result from a deficiency of niacin; it is characterized by diarrhea, dementia, and dermatitis.

Folacin
General Characteristics, Absorption, and Metabolism
Folacin is absorbed into the blood from the upper intestine; alcoholics frequently do not absorb folic acid well.

Functions
Synthesis of RBCs

Body Requirements
Increased amounts are required during pregnancy, since the woman produces more RBCs for herself and the fetus.

Food Sources
Folacin is found almost exclusively in plants, as the term *folic*, from foliage, indicates. Vegetables high in folacin are kidney beans, spinach, asparagus, and broccoli.

Toxicity and Clinical Deficiency
Toxicity: rare
Deficiency: deficiencies primarily affect the gastrointestinal tract and blood, with glossitis and anemia resulting; the anemia is characterized by very large RBCs or by macrocytic anemia, which is identical to vitamin B_{12} deficiency.

Biotin
General Characteristics, Absorption, and Metabolism
Biotin is a sulfur-containing molecule; it is synthesized by bacteria in the large intestine.

Functions

- Coenzyme in several biochemical reactions; carbohydrate and amino acid metabolism are examples.
- Other possible functions are niacin synthesis from tryptophan, formation of antibodies, and synthesis of pancreatic amylase.

Body Requirements
The body's requirement for biotin is given on the inside back cover for the estimated safe and adequate daily dietary intake compounds; the body does not require much biotin to be consumed in the diet, since it is synthesized by intestinal bacteria.

Food Sources
Milk, liver, egg yolks, mushrooms, and legumes are good sources of biotin.

Toxicity and Clinical Deficiency
Toxicity: rare
Deficiency: has not been documented in humans.

Pantothenic Acid
General Characteristics, Absorption, and Metabolism
Pantothenic acid is found extensively in all plant and animal foods; little is known about how it is absorbed; some is stored in the liver, brain, kidney, and heart.

Functions
- Metabolism of carbohydrates, lipids, and proteins
- Synthesis of acetylcholine

Body Requirements
The estimated safe and adequate daily dietary intake for pantothenic acid is given on the inside back cover.

Food Sources
Rich sources: eggs, liver, yeast, salmon
Moderate sources: mushrooms, cauliflower, molasses, peanuts
Poor sources: fruits, milk

Toxicity and Clinical Deficiency
There are no documented toxicity or deficiency problems with pantothenic acid.

Ascorbic Acid (Vitamin C)
General Characteristics, Absorption, and Metabolism
Ascorbic acid is a derivative of the term *antiscorbutic*, meaning without scurvy; the structure of vitamin C is similar to that of glucose; it is transported to liver, spleen, and adrenal gland after being absorbed.

Functions
- Prevention of scurvy
- Formation of collagen
- Healing of wounds
- Release of stress hormones
- Absorption of iron

Body Requirements
The RDA for vitamin C is given on the inside front cover; these amounts must be increased in people who are under stress, are heavy cigarette smokers, or who are ill and have fever; the amount of vitamin C needed for wound healing and formation of scar tissue may be as high as 1,000 mg/day or more.

Food sources
Fruits: all citrus, cantaloupe
Vegetables: tomatoes; broccoli, potatoes, greens

Toxicity and Clinical Deficiency
Toxicity: raises the uric acid level, causes hemolytic anemia, impairs the ability of white blood cells to provide immunity, causes an increased tendency to form kidney stones, and causes rebound scurvy.

Deficiency: scurvy, muscle cramps, aching bones, dry, rough skin, and ulcerated gums.

REVIEW QUESTIONS

TRUE (A) OR FALSE (B)

Questions 1–25

1. Vitamins are caloric compounds needed in large quantities.
2. Vitamin A functions in dim light vision, maintenance of mucous membranes, and synthesis of collagen.
3. Dark green vegetables or orange fruit are good sources of vitamin A.
4. Vitamin D is important for bone development by increasing the synthesis of protein molecules.
5. A deficiency of vitamin E can result in hemolysis of RBCs due to the destruction of polyunsaturated fatty acids (PUFA).
6. Since bacteria in the large intestine can synthesize vitamin K, a newborn infant has immediate protection against hemorrhaging.
7. Good food sources of thiamin are pork, beef, liver, and enriched grains.
8. Riboflavin is important in the development of bones.
9. A deficiency of pyridoxine may result in macrocytic anemia.
10. Vitamin B_{12} is important for the development of collagen and immunity.
11. Ascorbic acid is important for prevention of scurvy, formation of collagen, healing of wounds, and absorption of iron.
12. Vitamin E and A are often found together in foods, since vitamin E helps to protect vitamin A from being oxidized.
13. Carrots are an excellent source of carotene, which can be converted to vitamin D by the body.
14. Vitamin D aids the growth of bones by stimulating division of new bone cells.
15. A toxic level of vitamin D can result in osteomalacia, poorly developed teeth, and muscle spasms.
16. A deficiency of vitamin K is rare, since bacteria in the large intestine synthesize it.
17. The principal function of thiamin is to oxidize glucose for the formation of high-energy ATP molecules.
18. The best food sources of pyridoxine are milk and eggs.
19. A person who cannot synthesize the intrinsic factor is vitamin B_6 deficient and may exhibit megaloblastic anemia.
20. Niacin is an example of a vitamin that the body can make from the amino acid tryptophan.
21. Pellagra is a niacin deficiency disease and is characterized by diarrhea, dementia, and dermatitis.
22. A strict vegetarian is likely to have an adequate intake of folacin but may be deficient in cobalamin.
23. A deficiency of vitamin B_{12} may mask a folacin deficiency and, over a long period, lead to nerve damage.
24. Deficiencies of the B vitamins frequently result in nervous system malfunctions, RBC deficiency, and an abnormal appearance of the tongue.
25. Megadose levels of ascorbic acid increase its ability to form collagen, heal wounds, and absorb iron.

MULTIPLE CHOICE

Questions 26–34

26. Toxicity problems with vitamin A include:
    1. joint pain.
    2. xerophthalmia.
    3. enlargement of the liver.
    4. night blindness.
       A. 1, 2, 3.   B. 1, 3.   C. 2, 4.   D. 4.
       E. all of these.
27. The RDA for vitamin D can easily be satisfied by consuming:
    A. 6 oz of beef.
    B. green vegetables.
    C. two glasses of fortified milk.
    D. legumes.
    E. potatoes.
28. The major food sources of vitamin E are:
    A. fats.
    B. carbohydrates
    C. proteins.
    D. oils.
    E. A, D.
29. Vitamin K aids the blood-clotting process by:
    A. the synthesis of collagen.
    B. the conversion of fibrinogen to prothrombin.
    C. the synthesis of prothrombin.
    D. the breakdown of platelets.
    E. none of these.
30. The principal function of thiamin is to:
    A. act as a coenzyme in the oxidation of glucose to form ATP.
    B. aid the conversion of amino acids.

C. convert iron into a more absorbable form.
D. act as an antioxidant.

31. _____ is a good food source of riboflavin, but this vitamin can be easily destroyed by _____.
    A. Meat—oxygen.
    B. Corn—cold temperatures.
    C. Fruit—sunlight.
    D. Liver—cooking.
    E. none of these.

32. Which of the following is (are) functions of pyridoxine?
    A. synthesis of nonessential amino acids.
    B. conversion of tryptophan to niacin.
    C. antibody production.
    D. A, C.
    E. A, B, C.

33. Which of the following is (are) *not correct functions* of cobalamin?
    A. synthesis of collagen.
    B. conversion of tryptophan to niacin.
    C. release of stress hormones.
    D. aid in blood clotting.
    E. all of these.

34. Which of the following foods is (are) good sources of vitamin C?
    A. citrus fruit, beef, eggs, milk.
    B. citrus fruit, broccoli, tomatoes, potatoes.
    C. strawberries, bread, meat, legumes.
    D. cantaloupe, corn, bananas, liver, milk.

MATCHING

Questions 35–41. Answers to Questions 35–41 may be used more than once.

___ 35. osteomalacia   A. vitamin D toxicity
___ 36. hypercalcemia   B. vitamin A deficiency
___ 37. xerophthalmia   C. vitamin K deficiency
___ 38. respiratory   D. vitamin E deficiency
___   infections   E. vitamin D deficiency
___ 39. RBC hemolysis
___ 40. prolonged blood-clotting time
___ 41. kidney stones

Questions 42–46. Answers may be used only once.

___ 42. folic acid   A. pernicious anemia
___ 43. thiamin   B. aids oxidation of glucose
___ 44. riboflavin   C. pellagra
___ 45. niacin   D. megaloblastic anemia
___ 46. cobalamin   E. cheilosis

DISCUSSION QUESTIONS

1. Discuss why a person suffering from chronic bronchitis, chronic obstructive pulmonary disease (COPD), or cystic fibrosis should consume large amounts of vitamins A and C.
2. Explain why a kidney disease may cause a person to experience vitamin D deficiency problems such as osteomalacia.
3. Explain why the amounts of riboflavin, niacin, and thiamin should be increased during growth periods, pregnancy and lactation, infections, and chronic illness.
4. Discuss pernicious anemia in terms of basic causes and effects. Give two examples of individuals who are most likely to develop this condition and the appropriate treatment for it.
5. Discuss four functions of ascorbic acid. Name the food sources of this vitamin. State four possible problems that may result from vitamin C toxicity.

REFERENCES

1. J.B. Anderson. *Applied Nutrition for Health Professionals: Basic Nutrition.* Chapel Hill, N.C.: University of North Carolina, 1982, pp. 183–203.
2. L.H. Bodinski. *The Nurse's Guide to Diet Therapy.* New York: John Wiley & Sons, Inc., 1982, pp. 13–20.
3. L. Anderson et al. *Nutrition in Health and Disease,* 17th ed. Philadelphia: J.B. Lippincott, 1982, pp. 131–158.
4. "Marginal vitamin deficiency." *Nutrition and the M.D.,* 9 2–3 (1983).
5. S.J. Wickham. *Human Nutrition: A Self-Instructional Text.* Bowie, Md.: Robert J. Brady Co., 1982, pp. 165–183.
6. "Clinical aspects of vitamin B_6 (pyridoxine) metabolism." *Nutrition and the M.D., 9,* 1–2 (1983).
7. H.A. Guthrie. *Introductory Nutrition,* 5th ed. St. Louis: C.V. Mosby Co., 1983, pp. 223–328.
8. P.J. Long and B. Shannon. *Focus on Nutrition.* Englewood Cliffs, N.J.: Prentice-Hall, Inc., 1983, p. 187.

7 MAJOR MINERALS

OBJECTIVES

Upon completion of this chapter, you should be able to:

1. Distinguish between major and trace minerals.

2. Give the functions and food sources and describe the deficiency diseases of calcium.

3. Discuss the dietary factors that affect calcium absorption.

4. List the functions and food sources of phosphorus.

5. Describe the functions and food sources of potassium.

6. Discuss elevated blood potassium (hyperkalemia) and decreased blood potassium (hypokalemia).

7. List the functions and food sources of sodium

8. Discuss hypertension and sodium intake.

9. Give the functions, food sources, and imbalances of chloride ions.

10. Describe the functions and food sources of magnesium.

11. List the functions and food sources of sulfur.

INTRODUCTION

Minerals Small, inorganic elements that yield no energy.

Acid-base balance A balance of the amount of acid and base ions so that blood pH is within the normal range, 7.35–7.45.

Cations Minerals that are positively charged.

Anions Minerals that are negatively charged.

Major minerals Minerals that are present in the body in quantities greater than 5 g and are required at levels of 100 mg/day.

Trace minerals Minerals that are present in the body in quantities of less than 5 g.

Minerals are small inorganic elements that yield no energy. They constitute only about 4% of the body weight but are essential as structural components and in many vital processes, such as regulation of the **acid-base balance** of body fluids and osmotic pressure. Even though minerals are inorganic, they are often combined with organic molecules as iron in hemoglobin and as iodine in thyroxin. Some minerals are found in the body as salts, such as calcium salts in bone. **Cations** include calcium, magnesium, potassium, and sodium ions. **Anions** include chlorine, fluorine, and iodine.

Minerals are divided into two groups:

Major minerals. Minerals present in the body in quantities greater than 5 g (1 tsp) and are required at levels of 100 mg/day or more. Examples are calcium (Ca), phosphorus (P), potassium (K), sulfur (S), sodium (Na), chlorine (Cl), and magnesium (Mg).

Trace minerals. Minerals present in quantities of less than 5 g. Examples are iron (Fe), iodine (I), fluoride (F), zinc (Zn), manganese (Mn), copper (Cu), selenium (Se), molybdenum (Mo), and chromium (Cr).

Major minerals will be discussed in this chapter; trace minerals will be covered in Chapter 8.

RDA values have been established for calcium, phosphorus, iodine, iron, magnesium, and zinc (for RDA values, see inside front cover).

Table 7-1 presents a summary of the food sources, functions, and deficiency/toxicity problems of each major mineral.

MAJOR MINERALS

CALCIUM (Ca^{2+})

General Characteristics

Calcium (Ca) is the most abundant mineral in the body, and 99% is stored in the bones and teeth. The remaining 1%, present in the blood and other tissue fluids, has several important functions, which will be discussed shortly.

Absorption

The amount of calcium absorbed into the blood depends upon the needs of the body. Normally, in adults, 10–30% of dietary calcium is absorbed;

TABLE 7-1 SUMMARY OF MAJOR MINERALS

Name	Food Sources	Functions	Deficiency/Toxicity
Calcium (Ca)	Milk exchanges Milk, cheese Meat exchanges Sardines Salmon Vegetable exchanges Green vegetables	Development of bones and teeth Permeability of cell membranes Transmission of nerve impulses Blood clotting	Deficiency Osteoporosis Osteomalacia Rickets
Phosphorus (P)	Milk exchanges Milk, cheese Meat exchanges Lean meat	Development of bones and teeth Transfer of energy Component of phospholipids Buffer system	(Same as calcium)
Potassium (K)	Fruit exchanges Oranges, bananas Dried fruits	Contraction of muscles Maintaining water balance Transmission of nerve impulses Carbohydrate and protein metabolism	Deficiency Hypokalemia Toxicity Hyperkalemia
Sodium (Na)	Table salt Meat exchanges Beef, eggs Milk exchanges Milk, cheese	Maintaining fluid balance in blood Transmission of nerve impulses	Toxicity Increase in blood pressure
Chlorine (Cl)	Table salt Meat exchanges	Gastric acidity Regulation of osmotic pressure Activation of salivary amylase	Deficiency Imbalance in gastric acidity Imbalance in blood pH
Magnesium (Mg)	Vegetable exchanges Green vegetables Bread exchanges Whole grains	Synthesis of ATP Transmission of nerve impulses Activator of metabolic enzymes Relaxation of skeletal muscles	
Sulfur (S)	Meat exchanges Eggs, poultry, fish	Maintaining protein structure Formation of high-energy compounds	

however, growing children and pregnant women absorb 50–60%. Dietary factors that influence calcium absorption are (see Figure 7-1):

Presence of an acid environment. Foods that increase the acidity of the gastrointestinal tract increases the absorption of calcium. Cereals and protein foods are examples of acid-forming foods.

Intake of calcium and phosphorus in a ratio of 1:1 to 2:1. Absorption of calcium is increased when the diet contains a calcium: phosphorus ratio of 1:1 to 2:1. The average ratio of calcium to phosphorus in American diets is 1:1.6, which obviously is the reverse of what it should be for maximum calcium absorption. Apparently, part of the reason for the high level of phosphorus is the large number of soft drinks, rich in phosphorus, consumed by Americans. The end result of consuming this much phosphorus is less calcium absorption.

Increased intake of vitamin D. Vitamin D increases the absorption of calcium. Since milk contains large amounts of calcium, one can understand why milk is vitamin D fortified.

Presence of lactose. The lactose (sugar) in milk increases the absorption of calcium, as does vitamin D.

Functions

The reason 99% of the calcium is stored in the bones is that calcium is essential for the proper development and maintenance of bones and teeth (see Fig. 7-2).

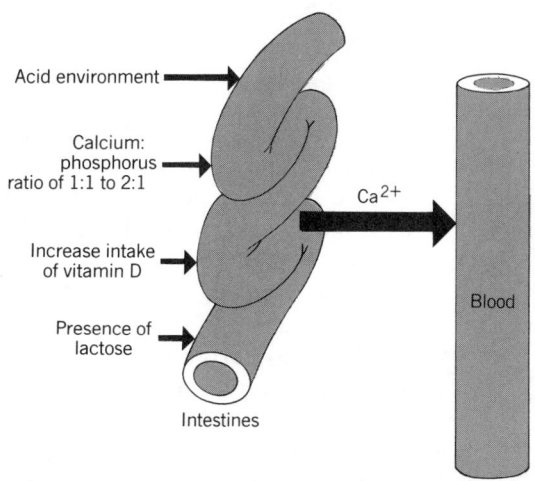

FIGURE 7-1 Factors that influence calcium (Ca^{2+}).

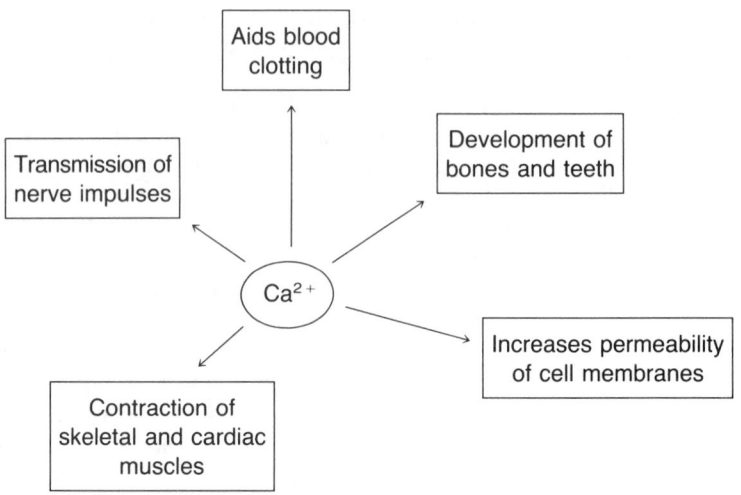

FIGURE 7-2 The functions of calcium.

Permeability A state of being permeable, or allowing the passage of materials.

Ions Atoms or molecules that have either a positive or a negative charge.

Synapse The junction between two neurons where an impulse is transmitted.

Binder compounds Substances that inhibit absorption of calcium.

Oxalic acid An acid found in some foods such as cocoa, rhubarb, and spinach. It inhibits the absorption of calcium, iron, and magnesium.

Phytic acid A binder compound that forms an insoluble calcium complex.

Calcium is important to the **permeability** of cell membranes. Apparently it functions in the transport of certain **ions** into and out of cells through their membranes.

The contraction of skeletal and cardiac muscle tissues is dependent upon a certain level of calcium ions.

Transmission of nerve impulses at **synapses** between nerves and between nerve and muscle tissue depends upon calcium.

Blood clotting depends upon several cofactors, one of which is calcium. There are approximately 14 cofactors in blood clotting; calcium, vitamin K, and plasma proteins are examples.[2]

Food Sources

The best food sources of calcium are found on the milk exchange list, 1. Lactose and vitamin D in milk increase its absorption. The meat exchange list, 5L, contains an excellent source of calcium—canned fish with bones; canned sardines and salmon are examples. The vegetable exchange list, 2, includes foods that contain calcium, such as dark green vegetables, but they also contain **binder compounds**. The binder compound in dark green vegetables is **oxalic acid**, which combines with calcium to form complexes that are insoluble (see Fig. 7-3). Cereal grains also contain **phytic acid**, which forms an insoluble calcium complex (see Fig. 7-3).[1] Children who have milk allergy or lactose intolerance can obtain calcium from sources such as fortified soy milk and from calcium salt supplements such as calcium gluconate, lactate, sulfate, and carbonate.

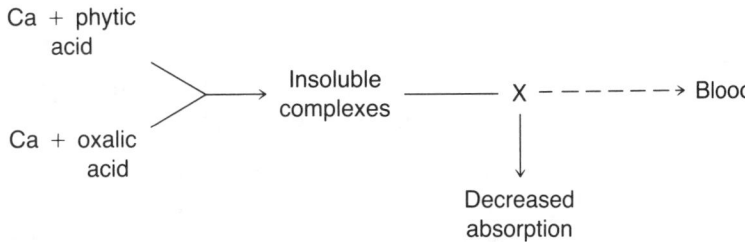

FIGURE 7-3 Binder compounds, oxalic and phytic acids, form insoluble complexes with calcium.

It is recommended that men consume 800 mg/day (one glass of milk contains 300 mg of calcium) and women 1000 mg/day. Pregnant women are advised to consume 1,500 mg/day in order to protect the skeleton from loss of calcium to the developing fetus. It is recommended that postmenopausal women consume 1,500 mg/day in order to reduce **osteoporosis**, which will be discussed in more detail next.

Osteoporosis A progressive demineralization of bones that results in the reduction of bone tissue.

Calcium Deficiency Diseases: Rickets and Osteoporosis

Osteoporosis. The ultimate result of osteoporosis is that bones become so fragile that they fracture quite easily. This condition is very prevalent in women between 40 and 60 years of age. The reasons why osteoporosis is more common in women and the possible causes are (see Table 7-2):

Menopause A permanent cessation of menstruation when ovaries, fallopian tubes, uterus, vagina, and breasts atrophy.

Hormonal changes following menopause. Osteoporosis occurs more frequently in women after they have undergone a decrease in sex hormones (primarily estrogen). The exact mechanism by which a decrease in estrogen results in loss of calcium from bones is unknown. However, research shows that the loss of total body calcium increases from an average of 0.22% per year for premenopausal women to an average of 1.5% per year after menopause.

Low calcium intake over many years. Apparently osteoporosis is not

TABLE 7-2 CAUSES OF OSTEOPOROSIS AND OSTEOMALACIA

Osteoporosis	Osteomalacia
Decreased hormone (estrogen) levels after pregnancy	Prolonged malabsorption
Impaired calcium absorption	Renal failure
Low calcium intake over many years	Inadequate intake of calcium during pregnancy

caused by a low calcium intake only as an adult, but rather by a low intake starting in childhood and continuing into the adult years.

Impaired calcium absorption. Prolonged impairment of calcium absorption possibly can result in osteoporosis.[3]

The pelvic bone and vertebrae exhibit the fragility characteristics of osteoporosis more than any other bones. It is very common for elderly people to fall and fracture their hip into so many small fragments that it cannot be repaired and must be replaced with an artificial hip.

It is very important for postmenopausal women to be informed about the need to consume large amounts of calcium, approximately 1,500 mg/day (1.5 g/day).[4] Consumption of 5 glasses of milk per day will satisfy these amount or consumption of **calcium supplements.** This increased intake is needed not only to offset the losses from bone but also to offset the decreased amount of calcium that is absorbed by the intestines. The efficiency of calcium absorption decreases after age 45 in women and age 60 in men.[5]

Rickets. The clinical signs of rickets include stunted growth, bowing of the legs, enlargement of the wrists and ankles, and a hollow chest.

Osteomalacia. Factors that commonly cause osteomalacia in the United States (see Table 7-2) are as follows:

Prolonged malabsorption. Long periods of malabsorption and decreased calcium intake will result in removal of calcium stored in bones for use in various physiological functions (clotting of blood, transmission of nerve impulses) (see Fig. 7-2). **Sprue** and **steatorrhea** (see Chapter 19) for details of these two diseases) are two malabsorption problems that may result in osteomalacia.

Renal failure. The kidneys are important for calcium absorption because vitamin D is activated by the kidneys; therefore, kidney failure will result in a decreased amount of vitamin D, decreasing the absorption of calcium.

Inadequate intake of calcium during pregnancy. Women are susceptible to osteomalacia due to an increased need for calcium. Women who have undergone several pregnancies and had a diet inadequate in vitamin D and calcium are especially susceptible.[6]

PHOSPHORUS (P)

General Characteristics

Phosphorus is the second most important mineral in the body. Approximately 85% of phosphorus is combined with calcium in bones to

---

Calcium supplements
Calcium supplements vary as to the amount of calcium that is present. Calcium carbonate tablets are 40% calcium, or a 600 mg tablet contains 240 mg of calcium. Calcium lactate contains 13% and calcium gluconate 9% calcium.

form calcium phosphate, $Ca(PO_4)_2$. The rest of the phosphorus is located in body cells as the phosphate ion (PO_4).

Absorption

The absorption of phosphorus is closely related to that of calcium, and the factors (see page 170) that influence its absorption also affect phosphorus. However, approximately 70% of dietary phosphorus is absorbed compared to 10–30% of dietary calcium.

Functions

The functions of phosphorus (see Fig. 7-4) are as follows:

Development of bones and teeth. Phosphorus combined with calcium is very important in the proper development of teeth and bones.

Transfer of energy in cells. Phosphorus is an important component of adenosine triphosphate (ATP) molecules, which store and transfer energy in cells. Phosphorus must also combine with B vitamins before they can play major roles in energy metabolism.

Component of phospholipids. Phospholipids are a major component of cell membranes, in which they help regulate what enters the cells. Phospholipids also help to transport other lipids in the blood, since they are normally insoluble in water.

Buffer system. One of the buffer systems in the blood that helps to maintain its acid-base balance contains phosphorus.[2]

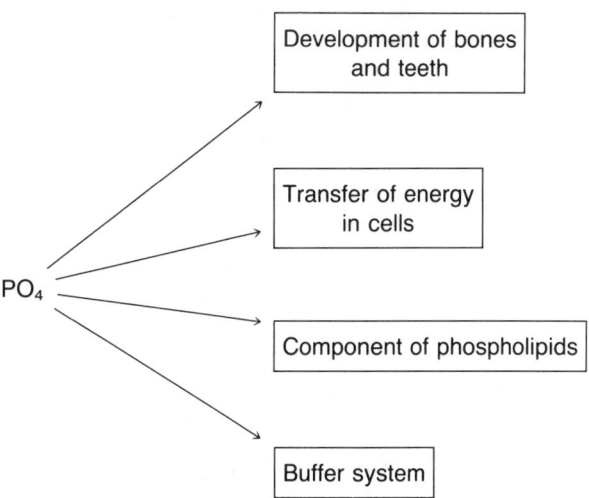

FIGURE 7-4 The functions of phosphorus.

Food Sources

As with calcium, the milk exchange list 1 is the best source of phosphorus. Since muscle tissue contains a high level of ATP for metabolism, lean meat on the meat exchange list 5 is a good source of phosphorus. Some foods are high in phosphorus as a result of the addition of phosphorus-containing compounds in their processing. Some examples are carbonated beverages, cheeses, and processed meats.

Phosphorus Imbalance Diseases

A deficiency of phosphorus (hypophosphatemia) can result from various problems. End-stage renal disease can result in a phosphorus deficiency due to a decreased level of activated vitamin D, thereby reducing its absorption. Malabsorption diseases such as sprue can cause phosphate deficiency due to a decreased ability to absorb vitamin D and phosphate. In addition, people who chronically take large amounts of antacids may have a low phosphate level and may experience weakness, anorexia, bone pain, and bone demineralization.

An excess of phosphorus (hyperphosphatemia) often results from renal disorders where decreased urination occurs. Since the level of phosphorus is inversely related to that of calcium, a hyperphosphatemic condition also results in a low blood calcium level. The end result can be muscle tetany.

POTASSIUM (K$^+$)

General Characteristics

Potassium is the most abundant cation in the intracellular fluid of cells (see Fig. 7-5). Approximately 98% of the potassium in the body is located in the cells. However, the small amount in the blood has some very important functions, as described below. The level of potassium in the blood is regulated by the hormone aldosterone.

Contraction of muscles. Potassium is very important in the contraction of skeletal and especially cardiac muscle tissue.

Maintenance of water balance. The osmotic pressure inside cells is due to the concentration of potassium ions; therefore, the shifting of water into cells is due to the pressure created primarily by potassium ions. Imbalances in the amount of potassium and the resultant shifting of fluids will be discussed later in this section.

Transmission of nerve impulses. Transmission of nerve impulses through muscles and along nerves is strongly dependent upon the concentration of potassium as well as sodium ions.

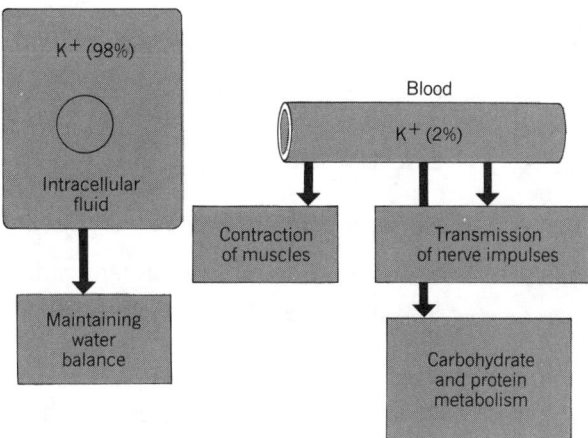

FIGURE 7-5 The roles of potassium in the blood.

Carbohydrate and protein metabolism. Potassium is important in glycogenesis. It functions as a catalyst in the synthesis of proteins.[7]

Food Sources

The best sources of potassium are foods on the fruit exchange list 4.
Fruits that are high in potassium are oranges, bananas and dried fruits.
Foods from the meat exchange list 5 and the vegetable exchange list 2
contain smaller amounts. Specific amounts of potassium in various foods
are given in Appendix I.

Diseases Related to Potassium Deficiencies
and Excesses

Hyperkalemia Elevated
blood potassium levels.

Hypokalemia Decreased
blood potassium levels.

Most problems related to potassium are grouped under **hyperkalemia**
and **hypokalemia.**

Hyperkalemia. Potassium excess frequently results from oral or intravenous overdosages when potassium is given for the correction of electrolyte imbalances. Other common causes of potassium excess are renal
failure and severe dehydration.

The previously mentioned functions of potassium that are affected by
hyperkalemia are weakness of heart contractions and of respiratory muscles. The nervous system is also affected, with the patient displaying
mental confusion.

Diuretics Agents that
promote urine excretion
and are used to alleviate
edema (see Chapters 20
and 23).

Hypokalemia. Potassium deficiency may result from the chronic use of
diuretics, surgery, diarrhea, and vomiting. A major problem of low

Tachycardia Rapid and irregular heartbeat.

blood potassium is that it produces **tachycardia.** With prolonged use of diuretics in certain medical situations, foods high in potassium or supplements should be given to help eliminate hypokalemia.[8]

SODIUM (Na⁺)

General Characteristics

Sodium is the most abundant cation in extracellular fluid, with about two-thirds being located in the blood. The other one-third is located in bones.

Absorption and Excretion

Aldosterone A hormone secreted from the adrenal gland that regulates the levels of sodium and potassium.

Sodium is easily absorbed into blood from the intestines. The blood level of sodium is controlled by the kidneys; they excrete excess quantities in urine, and when the blood level is low they conserve it. The hormone **aldosterone** controls the activities of the kidneys; an increase in the aldosterone level results in greater sodium absorption, and a decrease results in reduced absorption. A person can also lose sodium via perspiration, from gastric secretions lost as a result of vomiting, and from the repeated use of diuretics.

Functions

The functions of sodium are similar to those of potassium. They include (see Fig. 7-6) the following:

Maintenance of fluid balance in the blood. Sodium is the major ion in the blood and therefore plays a major role in maintaining the osmotic pressure and fluid level of the blood. Whenever the level of sodium in the blood is normal, so is the level of water. Likewise, whenever the level of sodium is high or low, the level of water will be adversely affected. More details about this condition will be presented at the end of this section.

Transmission of nerve impulses. The transmission of impulses along nerves and muscles is dependent upon a normal concentration of sodium ions.

Maintenance of acid-base balance. Two of the buffer systems that help maintain the normal pH of the blood are sodium monohydrogen phosphate ($Na_2HPO-[4]$) and sodium dihydrogen phosphate (NaH_2PO_4).

Food Sources

The most predominant source of sodium in the daily diet is table salt (NaCl), 40% of which is sodium. Generally speaking, animal foods con-

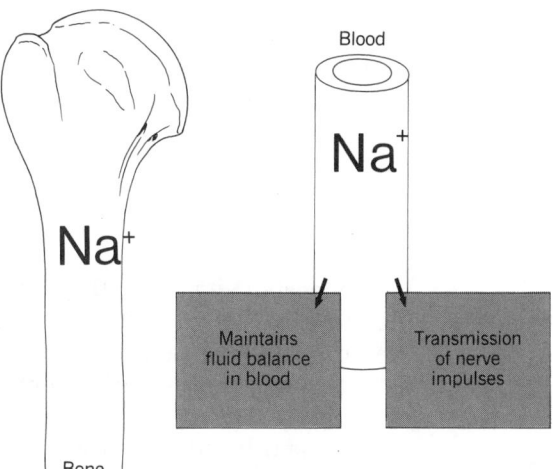

FIGURE 7-6 Sodium and its roles in the body.

tain more sodium than plant foods. Good sources of sodium include cheese, milk, processed meat, poultry, shellfish, fish, and eggs. Cereals, fruits, and vegetables are lower in sodium unless it is added during processing. Other foods high in salt are those that have been preserved with salt, such as cured ham and bacon. Specific amounts of sodium in various foods are given in Appendix I. Processed foods generally have salt added to them for taste; however, food companies have recently started marketing some processed foods with no added salt.

An often overlooked source of sodium is the public water supply. The sodium standard for public water is 20 mg/liter, but the water may contain more or less depending on the geographic location. Water containing over 100 mg per liter of sodium could have an effect on hypertensive persons, who should probably consider using bottled, distilled water for drinking and cooking.

There is no RDA value for sodium, since it is so readily abundant in our diet and drinking water. Also, since the kidneys regulate the level of sodium in the blood very effectively, a person could consume large amounts but have a normal concentration in the blood. The average American diet contains 10 g table salt and 4 g sodium (40% of 10), which is about twice as much sodium as the body requires for normal maintenance. For adults with no hypertension, an intake of about 5 g salt or 2 g sodium has been recommended. Hypertension and its relationship to sodium is discussed next.

Hypertension and Sodium Intake

Hypertension is related to many factors—obesity, genetic predisposition, smoking, personality type, and stress. It may be helped or hindered

$$\uparrow \begin{array}{c} \text{High level} \\ \text{of Na}^+ \text{ in} \\ \text{blood} \end{array} = \uparrow \begin{array}{c} \text{High blood} \\ \text{osmotic} \\ \text{pressure} \end{array} = \uparrow \begin{array}{c} \text{Increased} \\ \text{movement of} \\ \text{H}_2\text{O into} \\ \text{blood} \end{array} = \uparrow \begin{array}{c} \text{Increased} \\ \text{blood volume} \end{array} = \uparrow \begin{array}{c} \text{Increased} \\ \text{blood pressure} \end{array}$$

FIGURE 7-7 The relationship between the level of blood sodium, blood volume, and blood pressure.

by the level of sodium in the diet. If a person with hypertension has a high level of blood sodium, this condition will result in a high osmotic pressure, pulling a large volume of water into the blood. This increased blood volume causes the person's already high blood pressure to rise even higher. The relationship between the level of blood sodium, blood volume, and blood pressure is shown in Figure 7-7. Likewise, if a hypertensive person decreases the intake of sodium, this will generally help to decrease the blood pressure. It is recommended that people with hypertension consume no more than 1–2 g salt (0.4 and 0.8 g sodium, respectively). Low-sodium diets and specific foods will be discussed in Chapter 21.[9] Sodium deficiency in the blood is uncommon but can be caused by severe vomiting, very heavy perspiring, and certain diseases such as cystic fibrosis and **Addison's disease.** Deficiency symptoms include nausea, vomiting, acid-base imbalance, and diarrhea.

Addison's disease A disease caused by insufficient secretion of adrenal hormones.

CHLORINE (Cl⁻)

General Characteristics

Chloride (Cl^-) is the form in which chlorine is present in the body. This anion is found primarily in the extracellular fluid, with gastric secretions and cerebrospinal fluid being the two most common examples. Chloride ions in gastric secretions are combined with hydrogen ions to form hydrochloric acid.

Absorption

Chloride ions are absorbed readily into the blood from the intestines, and the kidneys control this level by either excreting the excess or conserving chloride ions. The body can also lose chloride ions by excessive perspiration, diarrhea, and vomiting.

Functions

The functions of chlorine in the extracellular fluid are the following (see Fig. 7-8):

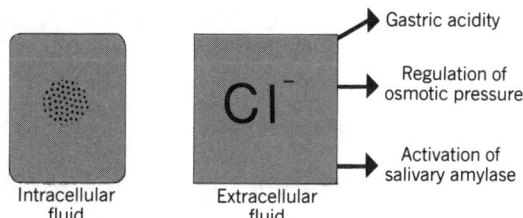

FIGURE 7-8 Chloride ions in extracellular fluid and its roles.

Gastric acidity. Chloride ions combine with hydrogen in the stomach to form hydrochloric acid, which is essential for digestion of protein and for conversion of iron into a more absorbable form.

Regulation of osmotic pressure. Chloride ions combine with sodium ions in the blood to help maintain the osmotic pressure, thereby helping to maintain a normal blood volume.

Activation of salivary amylase. Chloride ions in the saliva function to activate salivary amylase, which is an enzyme that begins the breakdown of starch.

Food Sources

The most common dietary source of chlorine is table salt, or sodium chloride (NaC1). Foods that are high in sodium typically are high in chlorine; meats, seafood, milk, and eggs are examples.

Chlorine Deficiency Diseases

Prolonged vomiting results in the loss of chlorine that is in the hydrochloric acid of gastric secretions. These losses can cause the pH of the stomach to shift from the acid to the alkaline range, interfering with protein digestion and iron absorption. Diarrhea can cause losses of chlorine from the intestinal tract, resulting in an acid-base imbalance in the blood.

High levels of chlorine in the body are rare, since the kidneys will remove any excess and excrete it in the urine.

MAGNESIUM (Mg^{2+})

General Characteristics

Magnesium is the second most important cation in the cells or intracellular fluid. However, approximately 70% of it is located in the bones, where it is combined with calcium and phosphorus salts. The other 30%

is in the cells of the soft tissues and in body fluids, where its functions are described next.

Functions

The most important roles of magnesium (see Fig. 7-9) are as follows:

Synthesis of ATP. Magnesium activates the enzymes necessary to add the third phosphate group to ADP to form ATP.

Transmission of nerve impulses. Magnesium interacts with sodium and potassium to allow the transmission of impulses along nerves and muscles.

Activator of enzymes necessary for metabolism of carbohydrates, proteins, and fats. The metabolic pathway that results in the release of energy from carbohydrates, fats, and lipids involves many enzymes and magnesium helps to activate them.

Relaxation of skeletal muscles. The relaxation of muscles after contraction involves magnesium.

Food Sources

The exchange lists and examples of foods that are high in magnesium are:

Chlorophyll The green pigment found in most plant cells that is important for photosynthesis.

Vegetable list 2. Magnesium is a component of **chlorophyll**; therefore, most green vegetables are good sources.

Bread list 4. Whole grains are a good source of magnesium. Whole

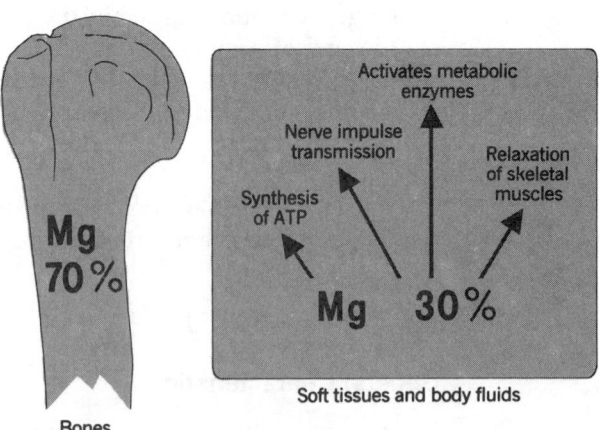

FIGURE 7-9 Magnesium in soft tissues and body fluids and its functions.

wheat bread, bakery products, and cereals rich in whole grains are excellent sources of magnesium.[10]

Magnesium Deficiency and Effects on the Body

Tetany Continuous, forceful muscle contraction.

Magnesium is widely available in the diet; therefore, a deficiency is rare. Some conditions that can result in magnesium deficiency are alcoholism, prolonged diarrhea, vomiting, and intestinal malabsorption. A prolonged deficiency can result in **tetany** and an increased startle response to sound and touch. Magnesium deficits in alcoholics are thought to be the cause of the hallucinations from which they often suffer.

SULFUR (S)

General Characteristics

Sulfur is present in all cells in the body, usually as a part of cell proteins. Keratin is the most common protein that contains sulfur. It is found predominantly in hair, skin, and nails.

Heparin An anticoagulant or substance that prevents blood clotting.

Three amino acids are composed of sulfur–cystine, cysteine, and methionine. Sulfur is also found in other organic compounds such as **heparin**, insulin, thiamin, and biotin.

Functions

The structure of protein molecules is maintained by disulfide (—S—S—) linkages that help to hold amino acid chains together in a distinct shape (see Fig. 7-10). The rigid structure of keratin protein in hair, skin, and nails is the result of its high sulfur content.

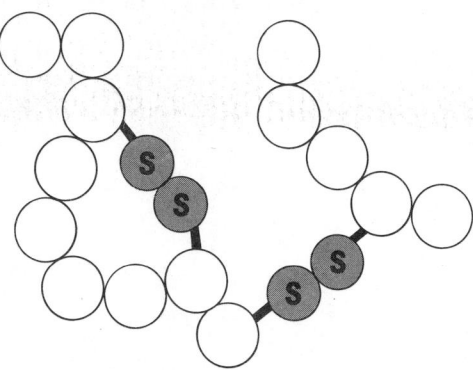

FIGURE 7-10 The role of sulfur in maintaining the structure of protein molecules.

Another important function of sulfur is the formation of some high-energy compounds in the energy metabolism pathways. Some enzymes in the energy pathway are activated by the presence of sulfur.

Food Sources

Proteins are the main source of sulfur in the diet, specifically proteins that contain cystine, cysteine, and methionine. Examples of foods that are rich in these amino acids are cheeses, eggs, poultry, and fish.[7]

OUTLINE

INTRODUCTION

Minerals are small, inorganic compounds that yield no energy; they are essential as structural components and in many vital processes, such as regulation of the acid-base balance and osmotic pressure of body fluids. Some minerals are combined with organic molecules; iron-hemoglobin and iodine-thyroxin are examples. Cations are positively charged ions such as calcium, magnesium, potassium, and sodium. Anions are negatively charged ions such as chlorine, fluorine, and iodine.

Major minerals are present in the body in quantities greater than 5 g and needed in the body at levels of 100 mg/day or more. Examples are calcium, phosphorus, potassium, sulfur, sodium, chlorine, and magnesium.

Trace minerals are present in quantities of less than 5 g. Examples are iron, iodine, fluorine, zinc, manganese, copper, selenium, molybdenum, and chromium.

MAJOR MINERALS

Calcium (Ca^{2+})
General Characteristics
Calcium is the most abundant mineral in the body; 99% stored in bones and teeth; the remaining 1% has several functions.

Absorption
From 10 to 30% of calcium is absorbed normally; growing children and pregnant women absorb 50 to 60%. Dietary factors that increase calcium absorption are:

- Acid environment in the gastrointestinal tract
- Calcium: phosphorus ratio of 1:1 to 2:1 in the diet
- Increased vitamin D intake
- Lactose in the diet

Functions

- Development of bones and teeth
- Permeability of cell membranes
- Contraction of skeletal and cardiac muscles
- Transmission of nerve impulses between nerves and from nerves to muscles
- Factor in blood clotting

Food Sources
Best sources: milk and foods on the milk list.
Other sources: sardines and salmon are good meat sources; dark green vegetables contain calcium but also contain binder compounds (oxalic acid) that reduce the absorption of calcium. Phytic acid is another binder compound found in cereal grains.

The recommendation for calcium is 800 mg/day for men and 1000 mg for women; 1,500 mg/day for pregnant women. A glass of milk supplies 300 mg of calcium.

Calcium Deficiency Diseases:
Rickets and Osteoporosis
Osteoporosis: Progressive demineralization of bones; the ultimate result is that bones become fragile and fracture easily. It is commonly seen in women between 40 and 60 years of age. The possible causes are:

- Hormonal changes following menopause
- Low calcium intake over many years
- Impaired calcium absorption

Postmenopausal women should consume 1,500 mg/day to reduce the risks and damage from osteoporosis; 5 glasses of milk will supply this amount.
Rickets: Bones of children are soft due to inadequate vitamin D and calcium absorption.
Osteomalacia: Bones are soft due to the reduction of calcium. The possible causes are:

- Prolonged malabsorption
- Renal failure
- Inadequate intake during pregnancy

Phosphorus (P)
General Characteristics
Phosphorus is the second most abundant mineral in the body; approximately 85% of phosphorus is combined with calcium in bones to form calcium phosphate.

Absorption
The same factors that affect the absorption of calcium also affect that of phosphorus; however, 70% of dietary phosphorus is absorbed, compared to 10–30% of calcium.

Functions

- Development of bones and teeth
- Transfer of energy in cells
- Component of phospholipids
- Buffer system

Food Sources
Best sources: milk and meat
Foods that have phosphorus added during their processing: carbonated beverages, cheeses, and processed meats

Phosphorus Imbalance Diseases

Deficiency Problems: End-stage renal disease can decrease the level of vitamin D, thereby resulting in a low level of phosphorus in the blood, or hypophosphatemia. Malabsorption diseases such as sprue also can result in hypophosphatemia. Excess consumption of antacids can result in hypophosphatemia, with person experiencing weakness, anorexia, bone pain, and bone demineralization.

Excess Phosphorus Problems: An excess of phosphorus can result from decreased urination, and thereby less phosphorus excretion. It results in a low calcium level and possibly tetany.

Potassium (K$^+$)

General Characteristics

Potassium is the most abundant cation in intracellular fluid. Approximately 98% of potassiusm in the body is located in its cells. It is readily absorbed into the blood, and excesses are excreted by the kidneys under the control of the hormone aldosterone.

Functions

- Contraction of muscles
- Maintenance of water balance
- Transmission of nerve impulses
- Carbohydrate and protein metabolism

Food Sources

Best sources: oranges, bananas, and dried fruits
Foods with smaller amounts: meats, vegetables

Diseases Related to Potassium Deficiencies and Excesses

Hyperkalemia (Elevated Blood Potassium Level): Hyperkalemia frequently results from oral or intravenous overdosages of potassium when it is administered to correct fluid-electrolyte imbalances. It can also result from renal failure and dehydration. Symptoms include weakness of heart contractions and respiratory muscles.

Hypokalemia (Decreased Blood Potassium Level): Hypokalemia may result from chronic use of diuretics, surgery, diarrhea, and vomiting; symptoms include tachycardia.

Sodium (Na$^+$)

General Characteristics

Sodium is the most abundant cation in extracellular fluid; about two-thirds is located in blood and one-third in bones.

Absorption and Excretion

Sodium is easily absorbed from blood. The kidneys control the excretion of excess amounts and increased absorption when there is a deficiency. The hormone aldosterone controls the activities of the kidneys. Sodium is also is lost through sweating, vomiting, and repeated use of diuretics.

Functions

- Maintenance of fluid balance in blood
- Transmission of nerve impulses

Food Sources

Predominant source: table salt, 40% of which is sodium.

Animal foods: generally contain more sodium than plant foods; cheese, milk, processed meat, poultry, shellfish, fish, and eggs are good sources.

Foods lower in sodium: cereals, fruits and vegetables are lower in sodium unless it is added during processing.

Processed foods: generally have salt added for taste; however, processors have started marketing foods with no salt added.

Public water supply: the standard amount of sodium is 20 mg/liter, but it may be more or less. Water containing over 100 mg/liter of sodium may have an effect on people with hypertension (high blood pressure).

No RDA value for sodium exists, since it is readily abundant in the diet and drinking water. The average American diet contains 10 g of table salt and 4 g of sodium, which is about twice as much as the body requires.

Hypertension and Sodium Intake

Hypertension is related to many factors—genetic predisposition, smoking, personality type, and stress. A high sodium intake with hypertension will only aggravate the problem. Hypertensive individuals are frequently advised to consume no more than 1–2 g salt per day.

Sodium deficiency is rare but can be caused by severe vomiting, very heavy perspiring, and certain diseases such as cystic fibrosis and Addison's disease. Deficiency symptoms include nausea, vomiting, acid-base imbalance, and diarrhea.

Chlorine (Cl$^-$)

General Characteristics

Chlorine is found primarily in gastric secretions and cerebrospinal fluid. Chloride ions in gastric secretions are combined with hydrogen ions to form hydrochloric acid. Chloride is absorbed readily, and the kidneys control its level by either excreting the excess or conserving chloride when the level is low. Chloride ions are lost by perspiration, diarrhea, and vomiting.

Functions

- Maintain gastric acidity for protein digestion
- Help regulate osmotic pressure of the blood
- Activate salivary amylase

Chlorine Deficiency Diseases

Prolonged vomiting results in a loss of chlorine. It causes the pH of the stomach to shift into the alkaline range, thereby interfering with protein digestion and iron absorption.

Food Sources

The most common source of chlorine is table salt, or sodium chloride (NaCl); foods high in sodium typically are high in chloride ions; processed meats, seafood, milk, and eggs are examples.

Magnesium (Mg^{2+})

General Characteristics

Seventy percent of magnesium is located in the bones, where it is combined with calcium and phosphorus; 30% is located inside cells.

Functions

- Synthesis of ATP
- Nerve impulse transmission
- Activation of enzymes for carbohydrate, fat, and protein metabolism
- Relaxation of skeletal muscles

Food Sources

Vegetable list: green vegetables
Bread list: whole grains

Magnesium Deficiency and Effects on the Body

Magnesium deficiency can result from alcoholism, prolonged diarrhea, vomiting, and intestinal malabsorption. The deficit in alcoholics is thought to be the cause of alcoholic hallucinations.

Sulfur (S)

General Characteristics

Sulfur is present in all cells, usually as a part of cell proteins. Keratin is a common example that is found predominantly in hair, skin, and nails; it is also found in other organic compounds such as heparin, insulin, thiamin, and biotin.

Functions

- Help maintain the structure of proteins
- Formation of high-energy compounds

Food Sources

Sources are proteins that contain cystine, cysteine, and methionine amino acids; examples are cheeses, eggs, poultry, and fish.

REVIEW QUESTIONS

TRUE (A) OR FALSE (B)

Questions 1–20

1. Major minerals differ from trade minerals in that major minerals are present in quantities greater than 5 g.
2. More calcium is absorbed when the calcium:phosphorus ratio in the diet is close to 2:1.
3. The greater the amount of lactose and vitamin D in the diet, the greater the amount of calcium that will be absorbed.
4. The functions of calcium include healing of wounds, maintaining osmotic pressure in blood, and maintaining the structure of protein molecules.
5. The best sources of calcium are foods that are on the milk exchange list.
6. Canned sardines and salmon are excellent sources of calcium, but absorption is hindered due to the presence of the binder compounds oxalic and phytic acids.
7. Osteoporosis is a calcium deficiency disease that is common in young women before menopause.
8. As the level of the sex hormone (estrogen) decreases, the absorption of calcium increases.
9. Women over 45 years of age need to consume 1,500 mg of calcium (5 glasses of milk per day) in order to offset the losses due to decreased estrogen and decreased calcium absorption by the intestines.
10. Two factors that can result in osteomalacia are renal failure and prolonged malabsorption.
11. Even though the same basic factors that affect calcium absorption affect phosphorus, approximately 70% of dietary phosphorus is absorbed compared to 10–30% of dietary calcium.
12. The majority of phosphorus is located in the blood, where it is a component of phospholipids and certain buffer systems.
13. Foods from the milk and meat exchange lists are the best sources of phosphorus.
14. Approximately 98% of potassium is found in extracellular fluids, where it functions in contractions of muscles, maintenance of water balance, and transmission of nerve impulses.
15. Foods from the meat and vegetable exchange lists are very high in potassium.
16. Sodium is an anion that is predominantly located inside cells, where it is quite important in the proper development of bones and teeth.

17. Forty percent of table salt (NaCl) is sodium, and the average American diet contains 10 g.
18. The average American diet contains about twice as much sodium (4 g) as is recommended.
19. A person with high blood pressure needs to increase the intake of sodium, since this will reduce the blood volume and thereby lower the blood pressure.
20. Sulfur is important in maintaining the structure of protein molecules.

MULTIPLE CHOICE

Questions 21–27

21. Which of the following dietary factors influence calcium absorption?
    1. presence of lactose
    2. increased intake of vitamin D
    3. intake of calcium and phosphorus in a 2:1 ratio
    4. alkaline environment in the gastrointestinal tract
    A. 1, 2, 3.   B. 1, 3.   C. 2, 4.   D. 4.
    E. all of these.
22. The _____ exchanges have some foods that are good sources of calcium, but they contain the 'binder compounds' _____ _____, which inhibit its absorption.
    A. meat—ascorbic and lactic acids.
    B. fruit—sulfate and phosphate.
    C. vegetable and bread—oxalic and phytic acids.
    D. milk and meat—carbonate and sulfate.
    E. none of these.
23. Osteoporosis is more common in postmenopausal than premenopausal women because of _____.
    A. low calcium intake.
    B. impaired calcium absorption.
    C. renal failure.
    D. reduced level of estrogen.
24. Which of the following are functions of phosphorus?
    1. development of bones and teeth
    2. contractions of muscles
    3. component of phospholipids
    4. maintaining water balance
    A. 1, 2, 3.   B. 1, 3.   C. 2, 4.   D. 4.
    E. all of these.
25. Which of the following foods are the best sources of potassium?
    A. meat, green vegetables, bread.
    B. oranges, bananas, dried fruits.
    C. oranges, milk, whole wheat bread.
    D. green vegetables, milk, cottage cheese.

26. Sodium is the most abundant _____ in _____ fluid.
    A. anion—intracellular.
    B. cation—extracellular.
    C. anion—extracellular.
    D. cation—intracellular.
27. The functions of sodium are _____ and _____.
    A. contractions of muscles—transmission of nerve impulses.
    B. blood clotting—development of bones and teeth.
    C. Component of phospholipids—maintain the structure of protein.
    D. maintenance of fluid balance—transmission of nerve impulses in blood.

Indicate in each of the following paired items whether the nutrient content of A is (a) appreciably higher, (b) appreciably lower, or (c) approximately the same as that of B.

		Column A	Column B
28.	__ calcium	milk	yogurt
29.	__ potassium	green beans	oranges
30.	__ magnesium	spinach	beef
31.	__ sodium	milk	eggs
32.	__ calcium	skim milk	whole milk
33.	__ phosphorus	meat	milk
34.	__ potassium	bananas	meat

DISCUSSION QUESTIONS

1. Discuss four dietary factors that influence calcium absorption.
2. Describe osteoporosis and discuss three reasons why this condition is more prevalent in women between 40 and 60 years of age.
3. Describe hyperkalemia and hypokalemia in terms of their basic causes and symptoms.
4. Discuss three functions of sodium. List the foods that are high in sodium and the average amount in the American diet compared to what is actually required for normal maintenance.
5. Explain the relationship between hypertension and sodium intake.

REFERENCES

1. B. Luke. *Principles of Nutrition and Diet Therapy.* Boston: Little, Brown, 1984, pp. 101–105.
2. R.S. Goodhart and M.E. Shils, Eds. *Modern Nutrition in Health and Disease.* Philadelphia: Lea & Febiger, 1980, pp. 294–309.

3. R.R. Recker. "Osteoporosis." *Contemporary Nutrition*, *8*(5), 1–2 (May 1983).
4. R. P. Heaney, J.C. Gallagher, C.C. Johnson, et al. "Calcium nutrition and bone health in the elderly." *American Journal of Clinic Nutrition, 36*, 986 (1982).
5. H. Spencer. "Osteoporosis: Goals of therapy." *Hospital Practice, 17,* 131 (1982).
6. S.R. Williams. *Nutrition and Diet Therapy*, 5th ed. St. Louis: C.V. Mosby Co., 1985, pp. 171–172.
7. E.N. Whitney and E. M. Hamilton. *Understanding Nutrition*. St. Paul: West Publishing Co., 1981, pp. 430–435.
8. T. Beaudette. "Fluid and electrolyte considerations in dietetic practice." *Nutrition in Practice, 2,* 15 (1983).
9. C.R. Kleeman. "Salt and Hypertension." *Nutrition and the M.D., 4,* 1–2 (April 1983).
10. P.J. Long and B. Shannon. *Focus on Nutrition*. Englewood Cliffs, N.J.: Prentice-Hall, Inc., 1983, pp. 218–219.

8 TRACE MINERALS

OBJECTIVES

Upon completion of this chapter, you should be able to:

1. Name the four forms of iron in the body and give their functions.

2. Discuss the four factors that increase the absorption of iron in the body.

3. Describe the four factors that decrease the absorption of iron in the body.

4. Give the food sources of heme and non-heme iron.

5. Describe iron deficiency anemia in terms of the appearance of RBCs, high-risk groups, and treatment.

6. Describe the functions of iodine and name good food sources.

7. Describe goiter and cretinism.

8. Give the functions and food sources of zinc.

9. Give the functions and food sources of copper, manganese, selenium, molybdenum, fluoride, and chromium.

INTRODUCTION

Basal metabolic rate
The rate at which the body uses energy for maintenance of homeostasis at rest.

As mentioned in Chapter 7 trace minerals are those present in the body in quantities of less than 5 g. Despite their small amounts, these minerals are involved in some very important functions—transport of oxygen and regulation of the **basal metabolic rate**. Three trace minerals—iron, iodine, and zinc—have been studied extensively enough so that recommended dietary allowances (RDAs) have been established for them. In 1980 the Committee on RDA published estimated safe and adequate daily dietary intakes (ESADDI) for six other trace minerals—manganese, fluoride, chromium, selenium, molybdenum, and copper. Only those trace minerals for which RDAs or ESADDI have been established will be discussed in this chapter. Less information concerning the effects of these six minerals on the body is known. Table 8-1 presents a summary of the food sources, functions, and deficiency/toxicity problems of trace minerals.

TABLE 8-1 SUMMARY OF TRACE MINERALS

Name	Food Sources	Functions	Deficiency/Toxicity
Iron (Fe)	Meat exchanges Meat, fish poultry	Transport oxygen and carbon dioxide	Iron deficiency anemia
Iodine (I)	Meat exchanges Seafood Iodized salt	Regulates basal metabolic rate	Deficiency: goiter, cretinism
Zinc (Zn)	Meat exchanges Eggs, oysters Milk exchange	Formation of collagen Component of insulin Component of many vital enzymes	
Copper (Cu)	Meat exchanges Oysters, liver	Oxidation of glucose	
Manganese (Mn)	Meat exchanges Nuts, peas, and beans	Component of metabolic enzymes	
Fluoride (F)	Drinking water, seafoods	Reduces dental caries	
Chromium (Cr)	Meat exchanges Eggs, meats	Binds insulin to cell membranes	
Selenium (Se)	Meat exchanges Liver, seafoods	Antioxidant	
Molybdenum (Mo)	Meat exchanges Liver, legumes Bread exchanges Whole grains	Metabolism of nucleic acids to uric acid	

IRON (Fe)

Iron is the best-known micromineral due to its important role in transporting oxygen to the cells. It is unusual in that there is no known mechanism that regulates its excretion. Iron balance is regulated at the intestinal site of absorption and will be discussed in detail later.

FORMS IN THE BODY

Iron is found in the body in five different forms with different functions.

Transport Iron

Transferrin (nonheme iron) A combination of iron and a globulin protein; important as the transport form of iron.

Most iron is combined with other molecules in the body, but one form, **transferrin (nonheme iron)**, is found circulating in the plasma (see Fig. 8-1). This form is important since it is the one that carries iron throughout the body to all cells.

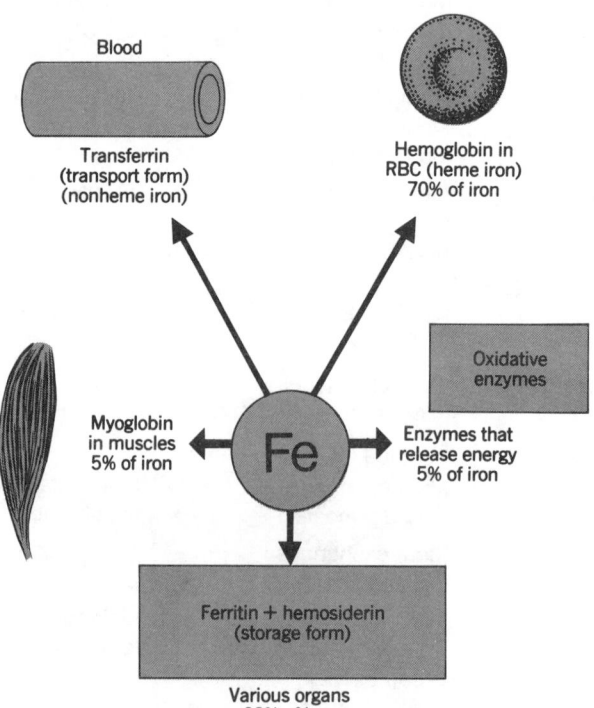

FIGURE 8-1 The five forms of iron and the percentage of each in the body.

Hemoglobin and Myoglobin

Myoglobin (heme iron)
A protein molecule composed of four amino acid chains, with one iron atom in each that is found in muscle tissue.

Approximately 70% of iron is found in red blood cells (RBCs) as hemoglobin (heme iron) (see Fig. 8-1). Another 5% of the iron is in the form of **myoglobin (heme iron)**. Hemoglobin is the most important form, since it transports oxygen to all of the cells, where it is used in the metabolism of glucose for energy. Myoglobin is important as a reservoir of oxygen in the muscles. It holds on to oxygen until the muscles need it during sustained muscle contractions.

Storage Iron

Ferritin A form of iron that is stored in the liver, spleen, and bone marrow.

Hemosiderin An insoluble form of iron that is stored in the liver.

About 20% of the total body iron is stored in various organs as **ferritin** and **hemosiderin** (see Figs. 8-1 and 8-2). Iron that is not taken up by RBCs and muscle tissue to form hemoglobin and myoglobin is stored as ferritin in the liver, spleen, and bone marrow. Hemosiderin is stored in the liver.

Enzymatic Iron

The remaining 5% of the iron in the body is found as a component of oxidative enzymes (see Fig. 8-1) that are vital to the release of energy from glucose.[1]

In summary, the majority of iron in the body exists in an active functioning form, hemoglobin. This form is vital in that it transports oxygen to the cells, where it is involved in the metabolism of glucose with the release of energy.

ABSORPTION, USE, AND EXCRETION

As mentioned earlier, there is no mechanism to control the excretion of iron; rather, it is controlled by the amount that is absorbed and stored. There are several factors that control the amount of iron absorbed. These factors are described and illustrated in some detail next.

Factors Affecting Absorption

Chemical form of iron. Iron usually enters the body in food as ferric iron (Fe^{3+}), which cannot be readily absorbed. The hydrochloric acid (HCl) in the stomach changes iron to the ferrous iron (Fe^{2+}) form, which can be easily absorbed (see Fig. 8-3). Ascorbic acid in the diet along with iron enchances its conversion to the ferrous state. This is one reason why the 1980 RDA for ascorbic acid for adults was raised from 45 to 60 mg.[2]

Physiological need for iron. When there is a greater need for iron in the body, as during growth periods and pregnancy, more iron is

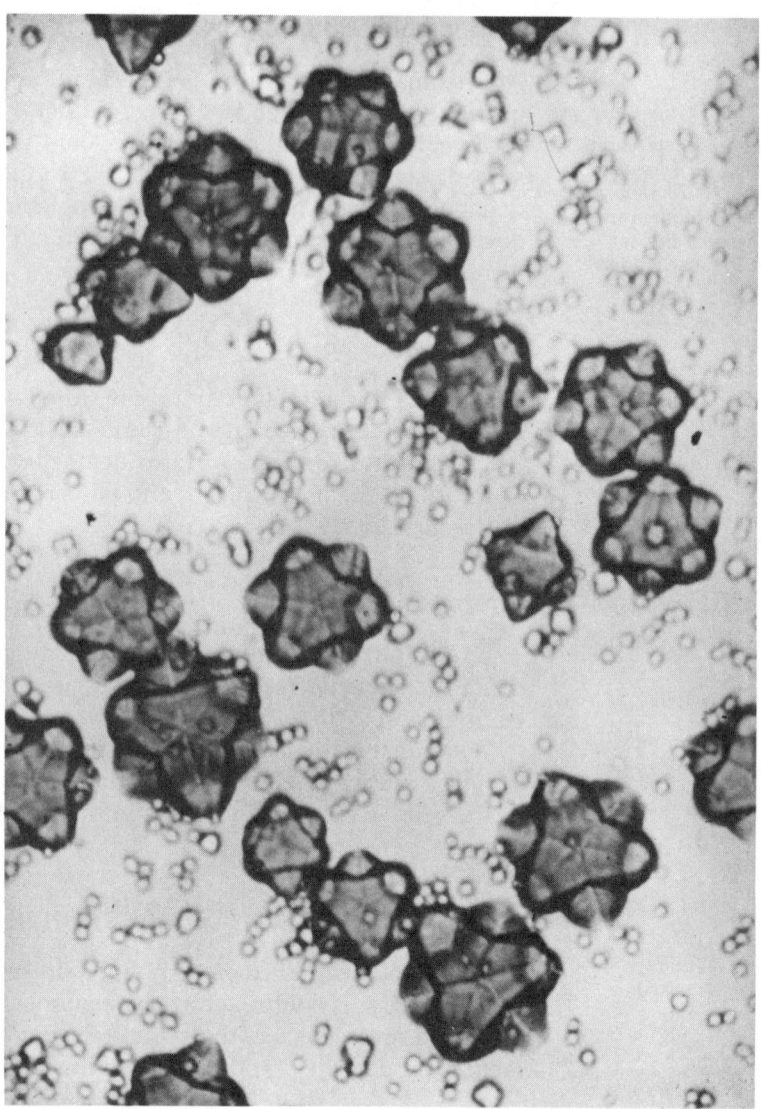

FIGURE 8-2 Crystals of human ferritin. (Courtesy of the Upjohn Company, Kalamazoo, Michigan.)

absorbed. Actually, what increases iron absorption during these periods is the amount of ferritin present in the cells of the mucosa lining the duodenum (see Fig. 8-3). The relationship between the amount of ferritin and absorption of iron is an inverse one, as shown below:

$$\frac{\text{Decreased}}{\text{ferritin}} = \frac{\text{increased}}{\text{absorption of iron}}$$

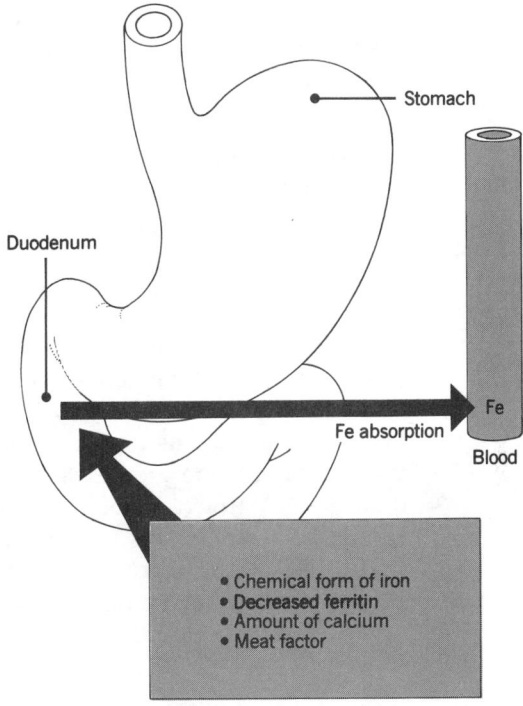

FIGURE 8-3

$$\frac{\text{Increased}}{\text{ferritin}} = \frac{\text{decreased}}{\text{absorption of iron}}$$

During periods of growth and pregnancy, mucosal ferritin levels decrease; during other periods they increase. Therefore, less iron is absorbed and excreted.

This relationship is important, since it increases the absorption of iron when the body actually needs it but prevents excess storage in tissues to the point of causing an iron toxicity problem.

Amount of calcium. Calcium binds to phosphate and phytate, which prevents them from inhibiting the absorption of iron (see Fig. 8-3).

Presence of "meat factor." Research results show that nonheme iron is absorbed better if meat, fish, or poultry (MFP) is present along with nonheme foods (See Fig. 8-3).

These factors increase the absorption of iron into the blood through the duodenum and jejunum regions of the small intestine, where the number of villi is greatest.

Factors that decrease the absorption of iron are:

High-fiber diet. A diet that is high in fiber tends to move food through the intestines so quickly that it reduces iron absorption.

Surgical removal of stomach. When the stomach or a portion if it is surgically removed, the amount of hydrochloric acid is decreased; therefore, the ability to convert iron from the ferric form to the ferrous form is reduced.

Diets high in cereals and grains. Phytic and oxalic acids tend to combine with iron and hinder its absorption.

Ulcerative colitis A disease of the large intestine that is characterized by inflammation of the intestinal mucosa and ulcers (see Chapter 19).

Malabsorption problems. Celiac sprue, **ulcerative colitis**, and diarrhea are examples of malabsorption problems that hinder iron absorption.

Generally, about 10% of iron in a mixed diet is absorbed, or about 1 mg out of 10 mg ingested. Absorption of iron from the heme iron pool (hemoglobin and myoglobin) is distinctly better than from the nonheme iron pool (ferritin and hemosiderin). Specifically, iron absorption from liver and other meats can be as high as 10–30%, whereas absorption of iron from nonheme sources such as grains and vegetables is usually less than 5%.[3] A true vegetarian who consumes no meat products at all should be aware of this very low absorption rate of iron.

The 1980 RDA for iron in adult men is 10 mg and for adult women 18 mg. Women have a higher value since they lose greater amounts of iron due to blood loss from menstruation.

Use

Cytochrome enzyme systems An iron-containing protein molecule that is important for the synthesis of adenosine triphosphate (ATP) molecules.

As mentioned earlier, most of the iron is removed from the blood and used by the bone marrow in the synthesis of hemoglobin to form RBCs (see Fig. 8-4). After about 120 days, RBCs are broken down, but approximately 90% of the iron is conserved and reused in their synthesis.

The other major way that the body actively uses iron is in the **cytochrome enzyme systems** that oxidize glucose with the release of energy (see Fig. 8-4).

Excretion

Very little iron is lost from the body. As mentioned earlier, when RBCs are destroyed in the liver and bone marrow, 90% is conserved and reused in the synthesis of new RBCs. A small amount of iron is lost daily in sweat, hair, shed skin cells, and urine (see Fig. 8-4).

FOOD SOURCES

The best food sources of iron (40% heme iron, 60% nonheme iron) are meat, fish, and poultry, (meat exchanges). Good sources (nonheme iron) are fortified breads and cereals (bread exchanges), dark green vegetables (vegetable exchanges), and raisins, prunes, and apricots (fruit exchanges).

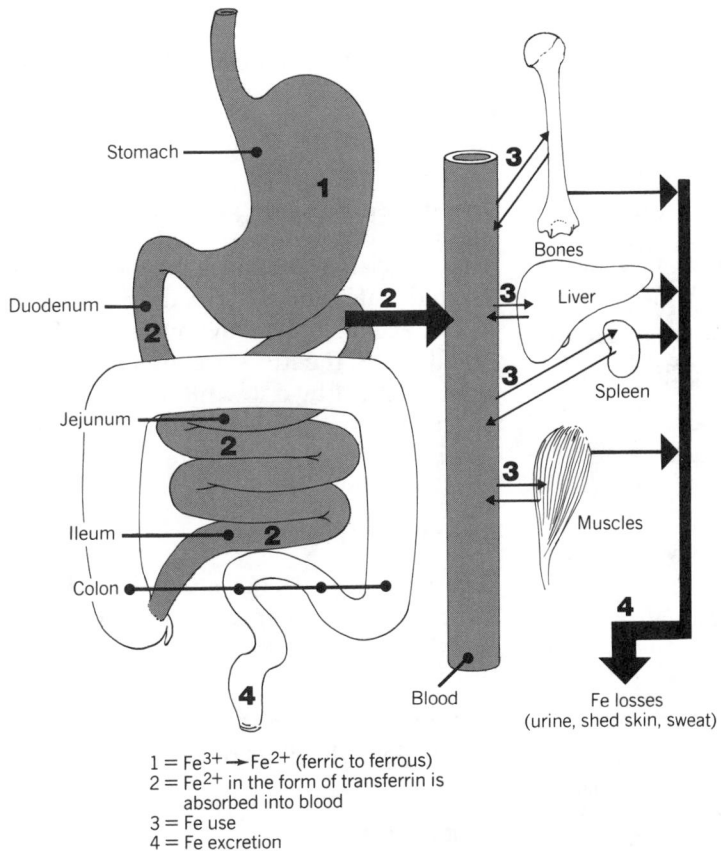

1 = Fe^{3+} → Fe^{2+} (ferric to ferrous)
2 = Fe^{2+} in the form of transferrin is
    absorbed into blood
3 = Fe use
4 = Fe excretion

FIGURE 8-4 Use of iron is shown. (1) The ferric form of iron (Fe^{3+}) is converted to the ferrous form (Fe^{2+}) by the stomach. (2) The ferrous form of iron is shown being absorbed into the blood, where 70% of iron will be in the hemoglobin molecules of red blood cells. Transferrin is the transport form in the blood. (3) Iron is shown moving into bones, where it is incorporated into red blood cells, stored in the liver and spleen, and functions as a component of mycoglobin within muscles.

Vegetables, bread, and fruit are not as good sources as meat because they contain only nonheme iron, which cannot be absorbed as well as heme iron in meat exchanges. Also, vegetables and fruit that are high in fiber tend to interfere with iron absorption. The absorption of non-heme foods can be improved by combining these foods with ascorbic acid or MFP. Apparently each 1 g of ascorbic acid or 1 g of MFP can enhance the absorption of nonheme iron. A meal containing nonheme iron could be iron enchanced if the following were incorporated:

(1) 4 fl oz orange juice (60 mg ascorbic acid)

(2) 2 oz sliced beef (60 mg MFP)

or

(3) 1 large sliced tomato (30 mg ascorbic acid)
plus

1 oz beef (30 mg MFP)[4]

IRON DEFICIENCY ANEMIA

Anemia A reduction in
the number of RBCs.

Iron deficiency anemia
A reduced number of
RBCs that are smaller
than normal.

Microcytic An RBC that
is smaller in size than
normal.

Hypochromic Pale in
color.

**Hypochromic microcytic
anemia** Anemic condi-
tion characterized by
RBCs that are smaller in
size and pale in color.

**Total iron-binding
capacity** A measurement
of the percentage of saturation of transferrin. It
evaluates the amount of
extra iron that can be carried.

Hematocrit A percentage of RBCs in a sample
of whole blood.

Iron deficiency **anemia** is the most common nutritional deficiency in the United States and is the leading cause of anemia. **Iron deficiency anemia** is characterized by a low number of RBCs, and the cells are **microcytic**. In addition, the RBCs are **hypochromic**. Since iron deficiency anemia is characterized by a low number of RBCs that are small in size and pale in color, this problem is often described as **hypochromic microcytic anemia**.

Laboratory Indicators

There are several biochemical laboratory determinations that can indicate iron deficiency anemia. Some determinations are:

Serum ferritin

Total iron-binding capacity

Hemoglobin/**hematocrit**

Symptoms

Iron deficiency anemia can result in a variety of abnormal changes in the body. Most of these changes are related to the fact that the anemic person's tissues must function with less oxygen and therefore have less energy. Fatigue followed by decreased work performance are two common symptoms. The risk of infection is also increased. Impairment of growth in infants can occur when their diets are iron deficient.

High-Risk Groups

There are four groups who are quite susceptible to the development of iron deficiency anemia.

Infants. Infants between the ages of 4 months and 3 years are vulnerable. During this period the child's iron stores are depleted, and the body size more than doubles; however, his or her diet is often composed almost exclusively of milk, which is a poor iron source.

Infants that are born to mothers who are iron deficient and low-birth-weight infants are very susceptible to iron deficiency anemia.

Adolescents. During adolescence, teenagers undergo rapid growth spurts and their blood volume expands tremendously. Their diets often do not contain enough iron for the body's increased needs.

Pregnant Women. During pregnancy the iron needs of the woman increase as her blood volume and tissues expand. In addition, iron is needed for the development of the fetus. It is common today for physicians to prescribe an iron supplement during pregnancy to prevent iron deficiency.

Intrauterine devices (IUDs) Objects inserted into the uterus for contraceptive purposes.

Menstruating Women. When women menstruate, their iron stores decrease due to the loss of blood. **Intrauterine devices (IUDs)** increase menstrual blood loss, whereas oral contraceptives decrease it.[5]

Iron Deficiency: Treatment

Ferrous sulfate An oral iron supplement that is often given to correct iron deficiency anemia.

Treatment of iron deficiency can take two forms—dietary management and iron supplementation. Dietary management involves increasing animal products—MFP. In addition, foods high in vitamin C should be increased, since they can double the absorption of iron from a meal. Likewise, milk and milk products should not be increased, since they can decrease the amount of iron absorbed from the same meal. Bottle-fed infants should receive iron-fortified formula. When solid foods are introduced, iron-fortified cereals and vitamin C–enriched apple juice are good choices. Iron supplementation involves the use of oral **ferrous sulfate**. The iron in the usual 300-mg tablets is absorbed best when taken between meals but is poorly tolerated. Iron is better tolerated if taken immediately after meals.[5]

IODINE (I)

Thyroid gland An endocrine gland located below the larynx and in front of the trachea. Secretes thyroxine and triiodothyronine hormones.

Iodine is a trace mineral that is present in the body in very small quantities—20–50 mg. Approximately 75% of it is concentrated in the **thyroid gland**.

FUNCTIONS

Thyroxine (T$_4$) A thyroid hormone that regulates the body's metabolism. Each thyroxin molecule contains four iodine atoms; therefore, it is designated as T$_4$.

Iodine functions as a component of two thyroid hormones, **thyroxine (T$_4$)** and **triiodothyronine (T$_3$)**. As Figure 8-5 shows, thyroxine contains four iodine molecules and triiodothyronine three. These hormones are secreted from the thyroid gland and regulate the basal metabolic rate, the rate at which the body uses energy for maintenance of homeostatis.

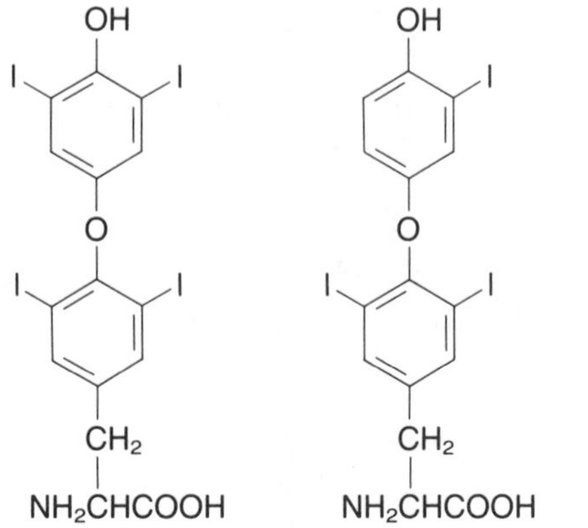

FIGURE 8-5   The two hormones, thyroxine (T_4) and triiodothyronine (T_3), in which iodine functions as a component are shown. (From Hole, John W., Jr., *Human Anatomy and Physiology*, 3d ed. (c) 1978, 1981, 1984 Wm. C. Brown Publishers, Dubuque, Iowa. All rights reserved. Reprinted by permission.)

As a result of this function, iodine is very important to the growth and development of the body tissues, especially the nervous system.

REQUIREMENT AND FOOD SOURCES

The adult RDA for iodine is only 150 μg/day. The RDA for pregnant and lactating women is 175 and 200 μg, respectively. The meat exchange list with seafood specifically is the best food source of iodine. However, the average diet does not provide an adequate amount of iodine unless it includes iodized table salt, which is the main dietary source of iodine. This situation is especially true in noncoastal geographic locations.

Goitrogens Substances that block the absorption or use of iodine.

Some foods contain a substance, **goitrogens**, which block the absorption or utilization of iodine. Foods of the cabbage family, such as rutabagas, turnips, and cabbage, contain goitrogens.

DISEASES RELATED TO DEFICIENCY AND EXCESS

Goiter An enlargement of the thyroid gland.

Cretinism A condition caused by an iodine deficiency in an infant.

People who are deficient in iodine may develop a **goiter** (see Fig. 8-6). The gland enlarges in order to capture the small amount of iodine present. These people exhibit a low metabolic rate, body temperature, and sluggishness. **Cretinism** (see Fig. 8-7) is a condition in which an infant is born with an iodine deficiency and is characterized by stunted growth, dwarfism, and varying degrees of mental retardation. These problems occur because the metabolic rate of the infant is inadequate for nervous system development and growth of tissues. Cretinism in the United

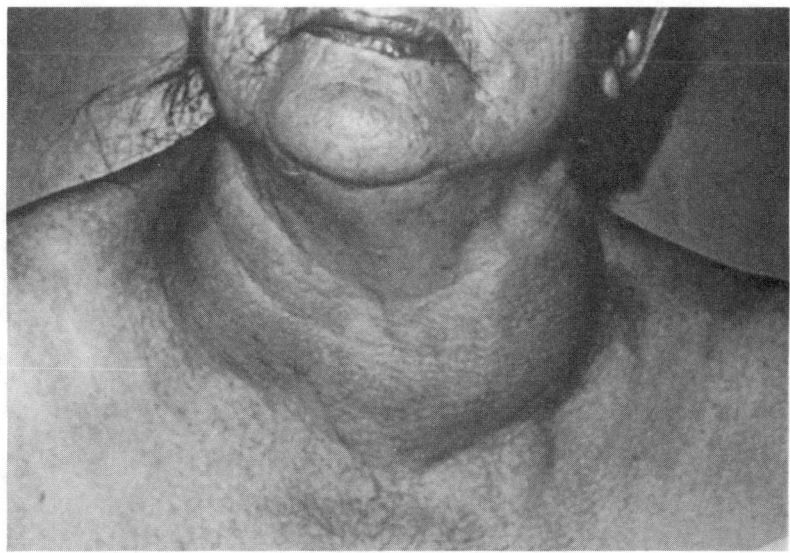

FIGURE 8-6 A goiter may develop as a result of an iodine deficiency.

States is rare but can occur in an infant whose mother was severely iodine deficient. Early detection and treatment with thyroid extracts can avoid much of the mental retardation and improve growth.

Excessive iodine intake may also result in the formation of a goiter. These people have high levels of thyroxin and triidothyronine, and exhibit a high metabolic rate, nervousness, and weight loss.

ZINC (Zn)

Zinc is second to iron in the amount present in the body. It is located in the eyes, reproductive organs, liver, muscle, and bones.

FUNCTIONS

Some important functions of zinc (see Fig. 8-8) are as follows:

Formation of collagen. The formation of collagen is dependent upon zinc. It is not surprising that a zinc deficiency can hinder wound healing and tissue repair.

Component of insulin. Insulin is a protein molecule with zinc as a component. It apparently increases the duration of insulin action after injection.

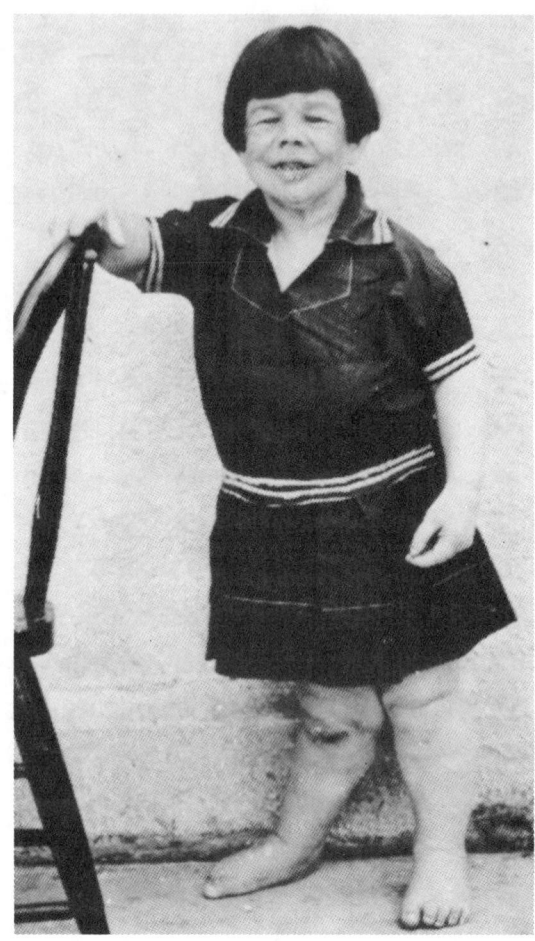

FIGURE 8-7   Cretinism is characterized by stunted growth, dwarfism, and varying degrees of mental retardation. (From Chaffee, E.E., and Lytle, I.M., *Basic Physiology and Anatomy*, 4th ed. Philadelphia, J.B. Lippincott Co., 1979. Reprinted with permission.)

Component of many vital enzymes. It is a component of many enzymes that are involved in metabolic activities such as the release of carbon dioxide from tissues to lungs; protein digestion and synthesis; and carbohydrate metabolism.

FOOD SOURCES

The best food sources of zinc are those on the milk list and, on the meat list, eggs and seafood, especially oysters. Poor food sources are those

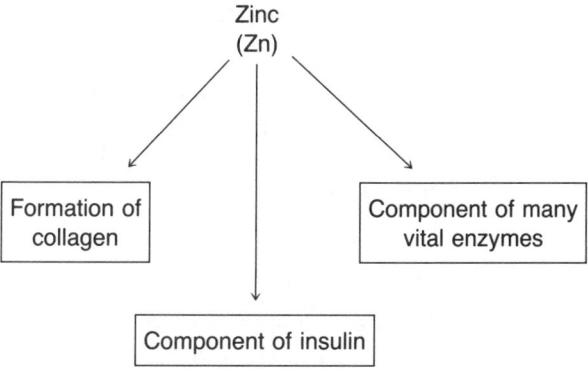

FIGURE 8-8 The functions of zinc.

on the vegetable list. Oxalic acids hinder the absorption of zinc in vegetables. Foods on the bread list are also poor in zinc. Phytic acid and fiber hinder absorption of zinc from grains.

TRACE MINERALS WITH ESTIMATED SAFE AND ADEQUATE DAILY DIETARY INTAKE

As mentioned at the beginning of the chapter, only three trace minerals have RDAs. Six trace minerals in 1980 were assigned ESADDI values (see inside back cover for the values for these minerals). Their essential nature has long been established, but is was not until 1980 that they were assigned values. The values for these six minerals appear as ranges of intake rather than as detailed, age-specific recommendations because of the uncertainty of the nutrient requirements.

COPPER (Cu)

Copper and iron are metabolized in much the same ways and, in addition, share some functions. Copper is involved with iron in the enzymatic reactions that oxidize glucose and release energy. Copper, along with iron, is involved in the synthesis of hemoglobin. It aids in the synthesis of collagen and the maintenance of the myelin sheath around nerve fibers.

The meat list is the best source of copper, with oysters, shellfish, liver, and legumes as examples. Fresh foods in general are better sources of copper than processed foods. Cow's milk is a poor source of copper, but human breast milk contains a large amount.

MANGANESE (Mn)

Manganese is a component of many enzymes that are involved in metabolic reactions. The site of most of the reactions include bones, reproductive organs, and liver.

Manganese is especially abundant in foods such as bran, coffee, tea, nuts, peas, and beans.

FLUORIDE (F)

Fluoride ions are found primarily in bone and the enamel of teeth. Research indicates that fluoride ions reduce the incidence of caries when fluoride ions are present in the drinking water, applied topically to teeth, or included in toothpaste. Fluoride acts by enhancing the ability of teeth to withstand the effects of acid formed by cavity-causing bacteria. Numerous studies have shown a reduction of dental caries by 50–70% when public water is fluoridated.[2]

The main dietary sources of fluoride are drinking water, tea, and seafoods.

Excess Intake

Tooth mottling Brown discoloration of the teeth.

Excessive intake of fluoride, such as in areas where fluoride is naturally high in the drinking water, can cause **tooth mottling**. Skeletal deformities can also occur with prolonged high fluoride intake. Fluoride toxicity is rare, since artificially fluoridated water levels are kept within a safe narrow range.

CHROMIUM (Cr)

Glucose tolerance factor A compound that helps to bind insulin to cell membranes.

Non-insulin-dependent diabetes Also known as *type II diabetes*; characterized by the inability of glucose to metabolize glucose.

Cirrhosis Inflammation and scarring of interstitial (between parts) tissue; commonly occurs in liver tissue. See Chapter 20.

Chromium is associated with a decrease in glucose tolerance. It is found in the body as a part of the **Glucose Tolerance Factor**.

Chromium levels tend to decrease with age, which leads some researchers to believe that chromium deficiency is related to maturity-onset diabetes (**non-insulin-dependent diabetes**.[9]

Dietary sources of chromium are egg yolks, meats, cheeses, beer, and whole grains.

SELENIUM (Se)

The best-known function of selenium in humans is an antioxidant one. Apparently, it works with vitamin E to prevent the oxidation of RBCs. Research also shows that selenium can help protect the liver against **cirrhosis**.

The best food source is the meat exchange list, with liver, seafoods, and other meats as examples.

MOLYBDENUM (Mo)

Molybdenum is a component of enzymes in the metabolism of nucleic acids to uric acid. It is an important enzyme in the uptake of nitrogen in legume plants. The highest amounts are found in the liver and kidneys.

A good food source is the meat list, with legumes and organ meats (liver and kidneys) being examples. The bread list with grains is another good source.

OUTLINE

INTRODUCTION

Trace minerals are compounds present in quantities of less than 5 g. RDA values have been established for only three trace minerals—iron, iodine, and zinc. In addition, six minerals have ESADDI values—manganese, fluoride, chromium, selenium, molybdenum, and copper.

IRON (Fe)

Iron is the best-known trace mineral, since it is important for the transport of oxygen to the cells. No known mechanism regulates its excretion; therefore, the iron level is regulated at the intestinal site of absorption.

Forms in the Body

- Transport iron: Transferrin (nonheme iron) is the form in which iron is transported through the blood.
- Hemoglobin and Myoglobin: Approximately 70% of iron is found in RBCs as hemoglobin (heme iron). Approximately 5% of iron is in myoglobin (heme iron), which is found in muscles.
- Storage iron: Approximately 20% of iron is stored in various organs as ferritin and hemosiderin.
- Enzymatic iron: The remaining 5% of iron in the body is found as a component of oxidative enzymes.

Absorption, Use, and Excretion
Factors Affecting Absorption

- Chemical form. Ferric iron (Fe^{3+}), consumed in food, is changed to ferrous iron (Fe^{2+}), which is the more absorbable form. Ascorbic acid enhances the conversion of ferric to ferrous iron.
- Physiological need. The greater the need for iron (as during increased growth and pregnancy), the more iron is absorbed. Actually, the absorption of iron is inversely related to the level of ferritin; decreased ferritin results in increased iron absorption.
- Amount of calcium. Calcium binds to phosphate and phytate, thereby preventing them from inhibiting the absorption of iron.
- Presence of meat factor. Nonheme iron is absorbed better if MFP are present along with nonheme foods.

Factors that decrease the absorption of iron are:

- High-fiber diet
- Surgical removal of stomach
- Diets high in cereals and grains
- Malabsorption problems

About 10% of iron in a mixed diet is absorbed. Absorption of iron from the heme iron pool (hemoglobin and myoglobin) is distinctly better (10–30%) than from the nonheme iron pool (ferritin and hemosiderin) (less than 5%).

Use
Most iron is used by red bone marrow in the synthesis of hemoglobin; approximately 90% of iron is conserved when RBCs are broken down and reused in the synthesis of hemoglobin. Iron is also used in the cytochrome enzyme system that oxidizes glucose and releases energy.

Excretion
Very little iron is lost from the body; a small amount is lost daily in sweat, hair shed skin cells, and urine; 90% is conserved and reused in synthesis of RBCs.

Food Sources
Best sources (40% heme iron, 60% nonheme iron): MFP
Good sources (nonheme iron): fortified breads, cereals, dark green vegetables, raisins, prunes, and apricots
  Vegetables are poorer sources than MFP because they contain nonheme iron, which is not as readily absorbed as heme iron.

Iron Deficiency Anemia
Iron deficiency anemia is the most common nutritional deficiency in the United States. It is characterized by RBCs that are quite small in size and pale in color. The condition is called *hypochromic microcytic anemia*.

Laboratory Indicators
Laboratory indicators are serum ferritin, total iron-binding capacity, hemoglobin, and hematocrit.

Symptoms
Symptoms include fatigue and decreased work performance.

High Risk Groups

- Infants. Between the ages of 4 months and 3 years, an infant's iron stores are depleted and milk is not high in iron.
- Adolescents. Adolescents need more iron but often do not eat enough in their diet.
- Pregnant women. More iron needed for the

mother's increased blood volume; extra iron is needed for development of the fetus.
- Menstruating women. Women lose iron when they lose menstrual blood.

Iron Deficiency: Treatment
There are two forms: dietary mangement and iron supplementation. Dietary management involves increases of MFP. In addition, vitamin C should be increased and milk should not be increased. Iron-fortified milk should be given to infants. Iron supplementation involves taking iron tablets, with 300 mg being a common size.

IODINE
Approximately 75% is concentrated in the thyroid gland.

Functions

- Iodine is a component of the thyroid hormones thyroxine and triiodothyronine, which regulate the basal metabolic rate.

Requirement and Food Sources
The iodine requirement for the average person is very low; increased amounts are needed for pregnant and lactating women.

Diseases Related to Deficiency and Excess
People deficient in iodine may develop a goiter or an enlarged thyroid gland. Cretinism is a condition in which an infant is born with an iodine deficiency. Excess iodine deficiency may also result in the formation of a goiter.

ZINC (Zn)
Zinc is second to iron in the amount present in the body.

Functions

- Formation of collagen
- Component of insulin
- Component of many vital enyzmes

Food Sources
Best sources: eggs, seafood, and milk
Poor sources: vegetables and bread

TRACE MINERALS WITH ESTIMATED SAFE AND ADEQUATE DAILY DIETARY INTAKE

Copper (Cu)
Functions

- Oxidation of glucose
- Synthesis of hemoglobin
- Synthesis of collagen and maintenance of the myelin sheath around nerves

Food Sources
Oysters, shellfish, liver, and legumes

Manganese (Mn)
Functions

- Component of many enzymes involved in metabolic reactions.

Food Sources
Bran, coffee, tea, nuts, peas, and beans.

Fluoride (F)
Function

- Reduces the incidence of caries (cavities).

Food Sources
Drinking water, tea, and seafoods.

Excess Intake
Can cause tooth mottling; skeletal deformities can also occur.

Chromium (Cr)
Function

- Component of Glucose Tolerance Factor, which helps to bind insulin to cell membranes.

Food Sources
Egg yolk, meats, cheeses, beer, and whole grains.

Selenium (Se)
Function

- Works with vitamin E as an antioxidant; helps protect the liver against cirrhosis.

Food Sources
Liver, seafoods, and other meats.

Molybdenum (Mo)
Functions

- Component of enzymes involved in the metabolism of nucleic acids to uric acid.

Food Sources
Liver, kidney, and breads.

TRUE (A) OR FALSE (B)

Questions 1–15

1. The transport form of iron is transferrin, which carries iron through the blood to all of the tissues.
2. Approximately 70% of iron is stored in RBCs as ferritin and hemosiderin.
3. The chemical form of iron that is most readily absorbed is ferric (Fe^{3+}) iron.
4. Iron absorption is constant despite the needs of the body.
5. Nonheme iron absorption is increased if meat, fish, or poultry (MFP) are included with nonheme foods.
6. Three factors that decrease the absorption of iron are a high-fiber diet, surgical removal of stomach, and diets high in cereals and grains.
7. In a mixed diet, about 50% of iron is absorbed, whereas a diet high in MFP increases iron absorption up to 70%.
8. The most important function of iron is that of transporting oxygen and carbon dioxide in RBCs.
9. Iron deficiency anemia is characterized by RBCs that are small in size, pale in color, and few in number.
10. Groups that are most likely to develop iron deficiency anemia are the elderly, postmenopausal women, and women taking oral contraceptives.
11. Iodine is important in regulating the body's metabolic rate.
12. Seafoods and vegetables in the cabbage family such as turnips, and cabbage are good sources of iodine.
13. An excess of iodine can cause cretinism and goiter.
14. Zinc is important in the formation of collagen, as a component of insulin, and as a component of many vital enzymes.
15. The vegetable and bread lists are good sources of zinc.

MULTIPLE CHOICE

Questions 16–24

16. Which of the following is correct?
    A. transport iron—transferrin
    B. hemoglobin—where 70% of the iron in the body is found
    C. ferritin—form of iron found in oxidative enzymes
    D. B, C
    E. A, B
17. Factors that increase the absorption of iron are:
    1. a change from ferric to ferrous iron
    2. a high-fiber diet
    3. presence of MFP in the diet
    4. a diet high in cereals and grains

    A. 1, 2, 3   B. 1, 3   C. 2, 4   D. 4
    E. none of these
18. The percentage of iron generally absorbed in a mixed diet is _____, and in a diet high in nonheme sources such as grains and vegetables, the percentage of iron absorbed is ____.
    A. 50—30
    B. 10—5
    C. 30—10
    D. 70—50
    E. none of these
19. Dietary management of iron deficiency anemia includes:
    A. increasing animal products
    B. taking more ferrous sulfate
    C. increasing the intake of foods high in vitamin C
    D. A, C
    E. B, C
20. The function(s) of iodine is (are) _____.
    A. formation of collagen
    B. a component of insulin
    C. as a component of hormones that regulate the basal metabolic rate
    D. a component of many metabolic enzymes
21. The average diet will be deficient in iodine unless _____ is (are) included.
    A. iodized salt
    B. green leafy vegetables
    C. cabbage
    D. vitamin C
22. Which of the following food lists are the best sources of zinc?
    1. vegetable   3. bread
    2. meat   4. milk
    A. 1, 2, 3   B. 1, 3   C. 2, 4   D. 4
    E. none of these
23. A diet that is low in iron and _____ can result in decreased synthesis of RBCs or anemia.
    A. manganese
    B. fluoride
    C. chromium
    D. selenium
    E. copper
24. Chromium is important in the body as a (an) _____.
    A. component of enzymes that metabolize nucleic acids to uric acid

B. component of the Glucose Tolerance Factor
C. compound that reduces the incidence of dental caries
D. none of these

MATCHING

Questions 25–29

___ 25. chromium   A. aids oxidation of glucose and release of energy

___ 26. fluoride   B. component of many enzymes involved in metabolic reactions

___ 27. selenium   C. reduces the incidence of dental caries

___ 28. manganese   D. helps bind insulin to cell membranes

___ 29. copper   E. functions as an antioxidant

DISCUSSION QUESTIONS

1. Discuss four factors that increase the absorption of iron in the body.
2. Name the food sources of heme and nonheme iron.
3. Discuss the four high-risk groups who are most susceptible to the development of iron deficiency anemia.
4. Discuss dietary management and iron supplementation as two forms of treatment for iron deficiency anemia.
5. Discuss the functions of iodine and state which foods can supply the RDA.

REFERENCES

1. B. Luke. *Principles of Nutrition and Diet Therapy.* Boston: Little, Brown, 1984, p. 125.
2. S. J. Wickham. *Human Nutrition: A Self-Instructional Text.* Bowie, Md. Robert J. Brady Co., 1982, pp. 231–249.
3. T. Beaudette. "Perspectives in iron nutrition." *Nutrition in Practice 2,* 4 (1982).
4. E. R. Monsen. "How to get more iron from the food you eat." *Nutrition and the M.D.,* 7,(6) 1–2 (1981).
5. "Iron Deficiency: Evaluation." *Nutrition and the M.D.,* 8,(6) 2–3 (1982).
6. S. R. Williams. *Nutrition and Diet Therapy,* 2nd ed. St. Louis: C.V. Mosby Co., 1985, pp. 193–195.

9 WATER

Upon completion of this chapter, you should be able to:

1. Give the percentage of total body weight composed of water and in the extracellular and intracellular compartments.

2. List and describe the five functions of water.

3. Define osmosis and describe its importance in the body.

4. Define osmolality and describe the two criteria that determine its level.

5. Define isotonic, hypertonic, and hypotonic fluids and their effects on the shift of fluids through membranes.

6. Determine in which direction water will shift, given specific osmolalities of fluids.

7. Describe how diarrhea results in a shift of fluids through membranes until dehydration occurs.

INTRODUCTION

Of all the nutrients in the body, water is one of the most important. This statement is evidenced by the fact that the body can survive a deficiency of all the other nutrients for long periods (months even years), but can survive for only a few days without water. This fact is a strong indicator of how important water is to the maintenance of homeostasis.

PERCENTAGE OF BODY WEIGHT AS WATER AND LOCATION

Water makes up 60% of the total body weight of an adult[1] and 75% of that of an infant. The reason for this difference is that an infant has a higher body surface area and metabolic rate than an adult. Another interesting point is that body water tends to decrease as body fat increases. Notice the following relationships:

	Percentage of Total Body Weight Composed of Water
Normal-weight person	60
Obese person	50
Lean person	70

One might think that an obese person has a greater percentage of body weight as water than a lean person, but this is not true. The reason is due to the fact that adipose tissue does not contain much water, but muscle tissue does. An interesting point in this regard is that 1 lb of protein tissue retains 4 lb of water. Therefore, if an obese person has struggled to lose 25 lb and then gains 1 lb of protein tissue, the result is the retention of 4 lb more of water.[1] It is easy to see why many obese people say that the smallest amount of food tends to make them gain weight and therefore that dieting is futile.

Water is located in fluid compartments throughout the body. These compartments, and the percentage of total body weight consisting of water in each, are (see Fig. 9-1):

Compartment	*Percentage of Body Weight*
Extracellular	20
Intracellular	<u>40</u>
	Total: 60

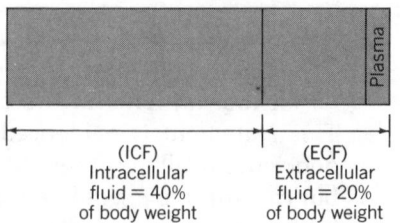

FIGURE 9-1 The fluid compartments and the percentage of water according to body weight. (From T. Randall Lankford, *Integrated Science for Health Students*, 3rd ed. 1984. Reprinted by permission of Reston Publishing Company, a Prentice-Hall Company, 11480 Sunset Hills Road, Reston, Va. 22090.)

Water shifts back and forth between these compartments as a result of changes in osmotic pressure, which will be discussed shortly.

FUNCTIONS OF WATER IN THE BODY

Water has several important functions in the body (see Fig. 9-2).

REACTANT

Reactant A substance that interacts with other substances to produce products.

Ionize Chemical process by which substances break apart into ions.

Water is a **reactant** in various chemical reactions. Ionic compounds **ionize** to electrolytes as a result of water molecules:

$$NaCl + H_2O \rightarrow Na^+ + Cl^- + H_2O$$

Several of the minerals discussed in Chapters 7 and 8 actually exist as electrolytes as a result of ionization in water. Carbohydrates, lipids, and proteins are broken down into their basic chemical components by water and enzymes, breaking chemical bonds.

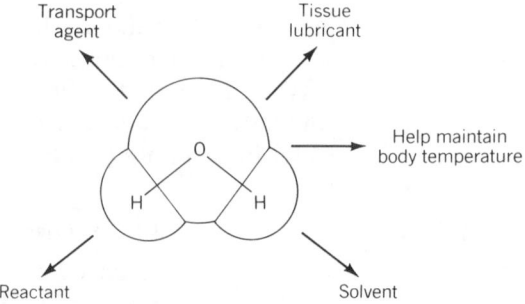

FIGURE 9-2 The functions of water in the body.

SOLVENT

Solvent A fluid that causes a solute to dissolve and form a solution.

A **solvent** is a fluid that causes a **solute** to dissolve, forming a solution. Water serves as the solvent for most chemical reactions in the body.

TRANSPORT AGENT

Solute A substance that dissolves in a solvent.

Blood, urine, and sweat are extracellular fluids composed primarily of water. They transport nutrients and wastes to and from cells.

HELPS MAINTAIN BODY TEMPERATURE

Celsius (C) A unit of temperature measurement on the Celsius scale.

Specific heat The amount of heat required to raise the temperature of 1 g of liquid 1°C (Celsius).

Synovial A fluid that lubricates bones articulating in joints.

Serous A fluid that lubricates body walls and organs that are coated with the fluid.

More heat is required for water than any other liquid to raise its temperature. The amount of heat required to raise the temperature of 1 g of liquid 1°C **(celsius)** is called **specific heat**. The high specific heat characteristic of water is the reason that it is slow to change from cold to hot or hot to cold. In other words, water does not change temperature very readily, which explains why it is used in hot water bottles and cold compresses. The high specific heat of water benefits the body by preventing rapid cooling or heating. As a result, body temperature is maintained at a fairly constant level.

TISSUE LUBRICANT

Water is the major constituent of **synovial** and **serous** fluids.[2]

MOVEMENT OF WATER BETWEEN FLUID COMPARTMENTS

Edema Accumulation of water in tissues.

Dehydration An excess loss of fluids from tissues.

As stated previously, water shifts back and forth between the fluid compartments. This shifting of fluids is a normal process and helps to maintain homeostasis. However, the shifting of the fluids between compartments is sometimes excessive, causing **edema** or **dehydration**. The mechanism responsible for the shifting of fluids between compartments and the conditions that can initiate the shift will be discussed next.

OSMOSIS

Osmosis The movement of water from a low-solute concentration to a high-solute concentration through a membrane permeable to water only.

The mechanism responsible for shifting of fluids back and forth between compartments is **osmosis**. Solutes are substances that dissolve in water. In order for osmosis to occur, a cellular membrane must be impermeable to the majority of solutes but permeable to water. Since solutes cannot pass across a membrane, they create a pressure called *osmotic pressure,* which varies directly with the concentration of solutes.[3] Osmotic pressure pulls water through the membrane from the low to the high-solute concentration. As water moves through the membrane, it lowers the solute concentration on the more concentrated side, since only water is in motion. Likewise, the solute concentration on the less concentrated side increases as water moves to the other side of the membrane. In other words, one side of the membrane becomes more concentrated as it loses water alone, and no solute, whereas the other side of the membrane is diluted as water alone moves to that side and the number of solute particles remains the same.

These changes occur until the concentrations of the solutions on both sides of the membrane are equal or an equilibrium is established. The underlying importance of osmosis is that it maintains or restores equal solute concentrations on both sides of a cell membrane, which is essential for maintenance of homeostasis.

OSMOLALITY

Osmolality The number of osmoles per kilogram of solvent.

Osmole The standard unit of measure of osmotic pressure.

Milliosmole (mOsm) Equals 1/1,000th of an osmole.

The concentration of a solute, and likewise of a solution, can be expressed in terms of **osmolality***. An **osmole** is the standard unit of measure for osmotic pressure. Generally, the osmole is too large a unit for satisfactory use in expressing the osmotic activity of a solution in the body. Therefore, the term **milliosmole** (mOsm) is commonly used.

Two criteria determine the osmolality of a solution. One criterion is the number of solute particles in a solution; the greater the concentration of a solution, the higher the osmolality or osmotic pressure. The second criterion is the size of the particles. The smaller the particles, the higher the osmolality or osmotic pressure. The reason is that more particles are hitting the membrane and therefore increasing the osmotic pressure.[3] The importance of the second criterion is illustrated by comparing two solutions with equal concentrations but different-sized particles, as shown below.

5% glucose	5% glycogen
5 g/dl	5 g/dl
Small particles	Large particles
High osmotic pressure	Low osmotic pressure

*The term *osmolarity* is commonly used by health professionals in expressing the osmotic activity of a solution. Osmolarity refers to the number of osmotically active particles per liter of solution (solvent plus solute). Clinical differences between the two terms are slight.

As shown above, the 5% glucose solution has a higher osmotic pressure than the 5% glycogen solution. The reason is that glucose particles are much smaller than glycogen particles.

Whole-protein molecules are very large and have little or no osmotic effect. However, individual amino acids are smaller particles that have an osmotic effect similar to that of low molecular weight carbohydrates.

Fats are not water soluble and thus have no osmotic effect.

Electrolytes such as sodium and potassium are comparatively small particles that have a great effect on the osmolality of a solution.

In summary, foods that contain high concentrations of simple sugars, electrolytes, and amino acids have the greatest effects on osmolality. See the Clinical Application "Osmotic Pressure."

OSMOLALITY OF BODY FLUIDS

The osmolality of normal body fluids is approximately 300 mOsm/kg. The body attempts to maintain the osmolality of its fluids by osmosis. Various problems can cause the osmolality of body fluids to become

---

CLINICAL APPLICATION: OSMOTIC PRESSURE

Tube Feeding

Elemental formulas
Liquid formulas that contain simple sugars and amino acids.

Some commercial tube formulas used in tube feeding are known as **elemental formulas** (see Chapter 17 for details on tube feeding and elemental formulas). These formulas create a very high osmotic pressure in the intestines; thus, if infused at full strength, they cause a large amount of water to shift into the intestines, resulting in diarrhea. To prevent this problem, the formulas are generally started at half strength, which reduces their osmotic pressure by half, and are gradually increased to full strength as the body adapts to the solution.

Cathartic Drugs

Cathartic Laxative drugs.

Many of the **cathartic** drugs used in treating constipation contain large amounts of salts that ionize into electrolytes when dissolved in intestinal fluids. This action creates a high osmotic pressure in the intestines, causing water to shift into and soften the feces. Some examples of these drugs are milk of magnesia (magnesium hydroxide), epsom salts (magnesium sulfate), and Fleet enema (sodium phosphate and sodium biphosphate).

higher or lower than the norm. Intravenous (IV) fluids as well as food and drink may be higher or lower than this value, which can result in a shift of fluids from one compartment to another.

The osmolality of foods and body fluids can be **isotonic, hypertonic,** or **hypotonic.** These osmolalities are discussed below.

Isotonic. Figure 9-3 shows that isotonic osmolality has no net effect on the amount of water in fluid compartments or cells. Water does shift

Isotonic A food or solution that has the approximate osmolality of body fluids: 300 mOsm.

Hypertonic A food or solution that has an osmolality of at least 340 mOsm or higher.

Hypotonic A food or solution that has an osmolality of 240 mOsm or lower.

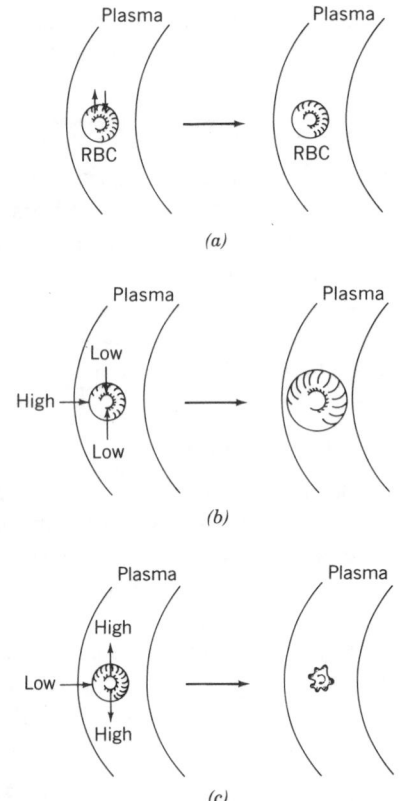

FIGURE 9-3 Isotonic, hypertonic, and hypotonic solutions and their effects on cells. (*a*) Isotonic: The osmolarities of the plasma and the RBC are equal. As a result, the movement of water into and out of the RBC is equal, and no net change occurs in the RBC. (*b*) Hypotonic: The osmolarity of the plasma is lower than that of the RBC. The result is a net movement of water into the RBC, as indicated by the arrows. (*c*) Hypertonic: The osmolarity of the plasma is higher than that of the RBC. The result is a net movement of water out of the RBC, causing the RBC to shrink or become crenated. (From T. Randall Lankford, *Integrated Science for Health Students*, 3rd ed., 1984. Reprinted by permission of Reston Publishing Company, a Prentice-Hall Company, 11480 Sunset Hills Road, Reston, Va. 22090.)

through membranes in this condition; however, the amount that shifts into a cell is equal to the amount that shifts out.

Two solutions that are isotonic to normal body fluids are 5% glucose and 0.9% sodium chloride (NaCl). Since the osmotic pressure exerted by these two solutions is equal to that of body fluids, they are known as **physiological solutions.** These two physiological solutions are frequently used in IV solutions, injections, and others.

Physiological solutions
Solutions in which the osmotic pressure exerted by the solutions is equal to that of body fluids.

Hypertonic. Figure 9-3 shows the effects of a hypertonic solution on compartments or tissue cells. Since this solution has a higher osmolality than adjacent fluid compartments or cells, it tends to pull fluids out of these regions. This action can result in shrinkage of cells and fluid compartments or dehydration.

Hypotonic. Figure 9-3 shows the effect of a hypotonic solution on fluid compartments or cells. Since the osmotic pressure of this solution is lower than that of adjacent cells or compartments, water tends to move from the solution into cells or fluid compartments.[3] See the Clinical Application: "Disorders That Can Cause Hypertonic, Hypotonic, and Fluid Imbalances."

OSMOLALITY OF CERTAIN FOODS

The approximate osmolality of common foods and beverages is as follows:

Food	mOsm/liter
Whole milk	275
Tomato juice	595
Coca cola	680
Apple juice	870
Ice cream	1150
Grape juice	1170[4]

Some of these foods and beverages such as ice cream and grape juice, are extremely hypertonic. They cause fluids to shift from the various compartments into the intestines, as shown in Figure 9-4. As a result of this shift, a person may experience the following:

Feeling of fullness

Increased peristaltic activity of the intestines

Nausea

Diarrhea

Dehydration

CLINICAL APPLICATION: DISORDERS THAT CAN CAUSE HYPERTONIC, HYPOTONIC, and FLUID IMBALANCES

Illnesses that result in prolonged vomiting or diarrhea can cause dehydration. This condition is due to a hypertonic imbalance that initially begins in the intestines (see p.220 and Figure 9-4 for details on diarrhea).

Edema is an abnormal accumulation of extracellular fluid within the interstitial spaces. One factor that can cause edema is a hypotonic condition in the blood due to a low protein concentration, such as protein-calorie malnutrition.

Examples of Intravenous Solutions That Are Isotonic, Hypertonic, and Hypotonic

Some examples of solutions that are administered intravenously are as follows:

Isotonic. D_5W, a 5% dextrose solution that is commonly administered intravenously.

Total parenteral nutrition (TPN) Solutions that are composed of dextrose for energy, amino acids for tissue synthesis, fats for energy, and essential fatty acids plus vitamins and minerals.

Hypertonic. $D_{10}W$ and $D_{20}W$ are 10 and 20% dextrose solutions, respectively. They are frequently used in **total parenteral nutrition (TPN)** (see Chapter 17 for details on these solutions and TPN). These solutions contribute more kilocalories than a 5% solution but are also hypertonic, thereby creating a potential for more fluid to be shifted into the vessels.

Hypotonic. 2.5% dextrose in 0.45% sodium chloride is an example of a hypotonic solution. This solution can be used to shift fluids into cells when the body is dehydrated.

The dehydration effect is the reason why one generally becomes thirsty after eating ice cream. Obviously, a food or beverage that has a lower osmolality will cause less water to be shifted into the intestines and should therefore be better tolerated than one of higher osmolality. Hospitalized patients who are receiving nutritional formulas, either orally or by tube, can tolerate a wide range of osmolalities if the formulas are administered slowly and additional fluids are given. However, certain patients are more likely to develop symptoms of intolerance when receiving formulas of high osmolality. These include:

Debilitated (very weak) patients

Gastrointestinal disorder patients

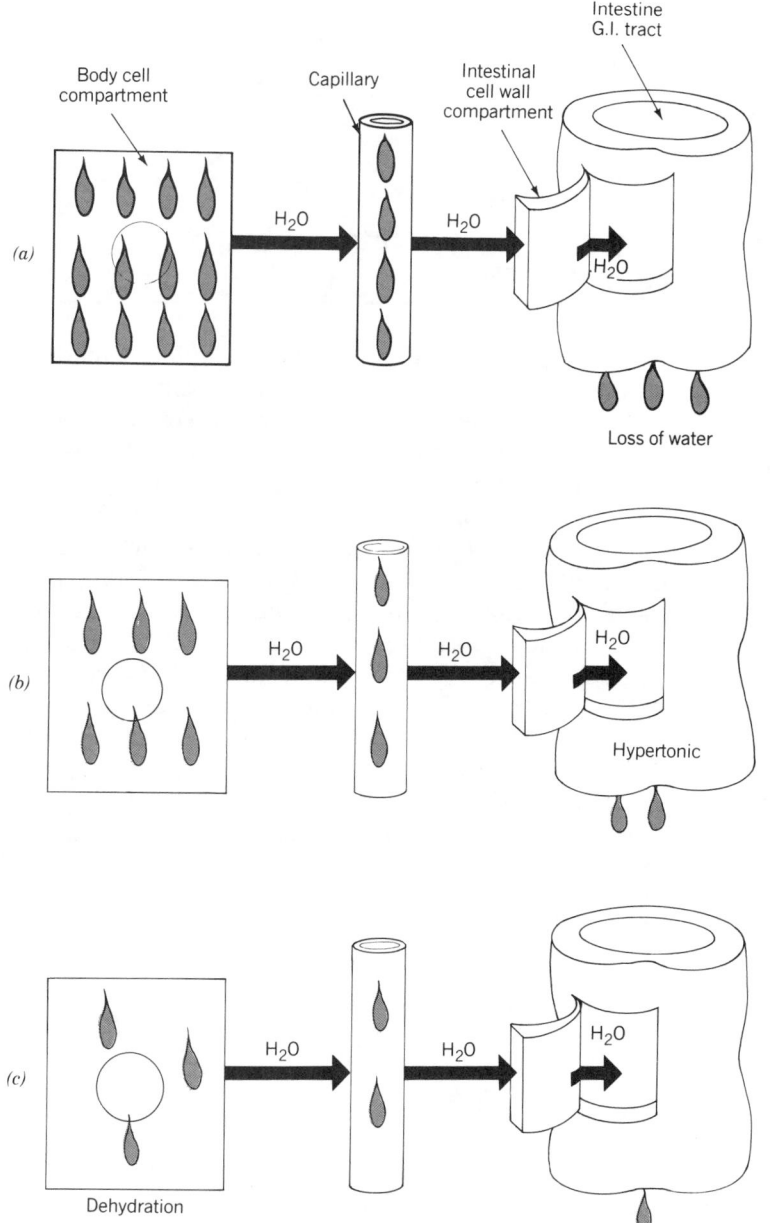

FIGURE 9-4 (*a*) The gastrointestinal tract and the adjacent compartments are shown, with H_2O loss from the gastrointestinal tract. (*b*) H_2O loss from the gastrointestinal tract causes it to become hypertonic, which results in a shift of water from each compartment toward the gastrointestinal tract. (*c*) The final result of this shift is that the body cell compartment becomes dehydrated.

Pre- and postoperative patients

Gastrostomy Feeding
directly into the stomach
through a specially cre-
ated opening.

Gastrostomy patients

Jejunostomy patients

DIARRHEA: EXAMPLE OF THE SHIFT OF WATER
OUT OF FLUID COMPARTMENTS

An example of how a change in one fluid compartment can result in
compensatory changes in all the compartments is diarrhea (see Fig. 9-
4). Prolonged diarrhea results in large losses of fluids from the intestines
or gastrointestinal tract fluid compartment. The large losses of fluids
compared to the loss of minerals causes the gastrointestinal tract to
become hypertonic (see Fig. 9-4). Water shifts from the intestinal wall
cell compartment into the gastrointestinal tract (water moving from the
low-solute concentration in the intestinal cell compartment to the high-
solute concentration in the gastrointestinal tract) in a compensatory move
to dilute the high-solute concentration in the gastrointestinal tract. This
original hypertonic condition and shift of fluids progresses until the body
cell compartment finally becomes dehydrated (see Fig. 9-4).

In summary, prolonged diarrhea initially results in a hypertonic condition in the gastrointestinal tract. The initial compensatory shift of fluids
causes each fluid compartment to be affected, in turn, by a change in
the concentration of fluids in adjacent compartments until dehydration
results.

OUTLINE

INTRODUCTION

PERCENTAGE OF BODY WEIGHT AS WATER AND LOCATION

Water makes up 60% of the total body weight in adults and 75% of that in infants; the obese body has less water than the lean body.

Water is located in two body compartments; the extracellular compartment has 20% of body weight and the intracellular compartment has 40% of body weight.

FUNCTION OF WATER IN THE BODY

Reactant
Water takes part in many reactions.

Solvent
Water acts to dissolve many solutes.

Transport agent
Water transports nutrients and wastes to and from cells.

Helps maintain body temperature
Specific heat of water aids in maintaining a fairly constant body temperature.

Tissue lubricant
Joints and surfaces of body organs are lubricated by fluids composed primarily of water.

MOVEMENT OF WATER BETWEEN FLUID COMPARTMENTS

Osmosis
Osmosis is the movement of water from a low-solute concentration to a high-solute concentration through a membrane permeable to water only. It is the mechanism responsible for shifting water between compartments. Osmotic pressure is responsible for pulling of water through membranes. The importance of osmosis is that it allows an equilibrium of concentration on each side of a membrane to be achieved.

Osmolality
Osmolality is the concentration of a solute and a solution. Two criteria determine the osmolality of a solution.

The number of particles in a solution: the greater the number of particles, the greater the osmolality.

The size of the particles: The smaller the particles, the greater the osmolality.

Osmolality of Body Fluids
The normal osmolality of body fluids is 300 mOsm per kilogram of solution. Three osmolalities of body fluids and IV fluids are:

- Isotonic: two fluids have equal osmolalities, normally 300 mOsm; 0.9% NaCl and 5% dextrose (glucose) are examples frequently used in IVs.
- Hypertonic: a food or solution that has an osmolality of at least 340 mOsm and usually much higher. A hypertonic solution will cause fluid to shift out of cells, resulting in dehydration.
- Hypotonic: food or solution that has an osmolality of less than 240 mOsm. Water moves out of this solution into adjacent cells or fluid compartments.

Osmolality of Certain Foods
Some foods have osmolalities that are isotonic, whereas those of many foods are hypertonic. It is important to know the osmolality of foods or solutions that are given to hospitalized patients in order to avoid problems such as fullness, nausea, diarrhea, and dehydration.

DIARRHEA: EXAMPLE OF THE SHIFT OF WATER OUT OF FLUID COMPARTMENTS

Diarrhea causes a hypertonic condition in the gastrointestinal tract that results in a shift of water until the cells finally become dehydrated.

REVIEW QUESTIONS

TRUE (A) OR FALSE (B)

Questions 1–11

1. Obese people have a greater percentage of their body weight as water than lean people.
2. The majority of water in the body is located in the extracellular fluid compartment.
3. Water is a solvent and causes solutes to dissolve, forming solutions.
4. The high specific heat characteristic of water is the reason why body temperature remains fairly constant.
5. Osmosis is the mechanism responsible for the shift of solutes through membranes.
6. Osmosis is defined as the movement of water from a low-solute concentration to a high-solute concentration through a membrane to water only.

7. If the concentration of a solution inside a cell is 2.0% NaCl and that outside the cell is 0.9%, water will tend to move into the cell.
8. Two criteria, the number of solute particles and the size of the particles, determine the osmolality of a solution.
9. A fluid such as grape juice that has an osmolality of 1,170 mOsm is hypotonic and causes fluids to shift out of the intestines into other body compartments.
10. A 0.9% NaCl solution and a 5% glucose solution are isotonic fluids and have osmolalities of about 300 mOsm.
11. The two fluids mentioned in question 10 will result in the net movement of water into the bloodstream when they are given in IVs.

MULTIPLE CHOICE

Questions 12–19

12. Which of the following is incorrect?

   1. Water composes 60–75% of the total body weight.
   2. Obese people have a smaller percentage of their body weight as water than lean people.
   3. Water composes about 75% of the total body weight of an infant.
   4. Less water is in the intracellular than in the extracellular compartment.

   A. 1, 2, 3,   B. 1, 3   C. 2, 4   D. 4
   E. all of these

13. Which of the following functions of water is (are) correct?

   1. reactant   2. solvent.
   3. transport agent   4. tissue lubricant
   A. 1, 2, 3   B. 1, 3   C. 2, 4   D. 4
   E. all of these

14. Osmosis is defined as the
   A. movement of water through a membrane from a low-water concentration to a high-water concentration.
   B. movement of water from a high-solute concentration to a low-solute concentration through a membrane permeable to water only.
   C. movement of water from a low-solute to a high-solute concentration through a membrane permeable to water only.
   D. none of these

15. Which of the following would cause a solution to have a high osmolality?
   A. very small particles
   B. very large particles
   C. large number of particles

D. B, C
E. A, C

16. Which of the following solutions has the highest osmolality?
   A. 5% glycogen
   B. 5% NaCl
   C. 5% protein
   D. 5% fat

17. If a person eats ice cream with an osmolality of 1,150 mOsm/liter, this food is _____ and will result in a shifting of fluids _____ the intestines.
   A. isotonic—equally into and out of
   B. hypotonic—out of
   C. hypertonic—out of
   D. hypotonic—into
   E. hypertonic—into

18. Hospitalized patients who might develop symptoms of intolerance when fed nutritional formulas of high osmolality, either orally or by tube, are _____ patients.
   A. debilitated (very weak)
   B. gastrointestinal disorder
   C. gastrostomy
   D. pre- and postoperative
   E. all of these

19. Diarrhea can result in dehydration because a (an) _____ condition is initially formed in the gastrointestinal tract that ultimately results in a shift of water _____ the intestines.
   A. hypotonic—out of
   B. hypertonic—into
   C. isotonic—out of
   D. hypotonic—into
   E. none of these

MATCHING

Questions 20–24. Each answer may be used more than once.

___ 20. fluid or food with an osmolality of less than 240 mOsm

A. hypotonic solution

___ 21. physiological solution

B. hypertonic solution

___ 22. solution that, in the gastrointestinal tract, can cause dehydration

C. isotonic solution

___ 23. 5% glucose, 0.9% NaCl

___ 24. solution that, in a cell, would cause a shift of fluids into it

DISCUSSION QUESTIONS

1. Describe five functions of water.
2. Define osmosis. Give two criteria that determine the osmolality of a solution.

3. Describe the basic osmotic balance problem that may occur with elemental tube formulas if they are not started at half strength.
4. Give the osmolalities of isotonic, hypertonic, and hypotonic IV fluids and an example of each that is used clinically.
5. Describe diarrhea in terms of the initial osmotic imbalance the starts the shift of water and which fluid compartment is ultimately affected.

REFERENCES

1. B. Luke, *Principles of Nutrition and Diet Therapy*. Boston: Little, Brown, 1984, p. 179.

2. P. Long and B. Shannon. *Focus on Nutrition*. Englewood Cliffs, N.J.: Prentice-Hall, Inc. 1983, p. 232.
3. T. R. Lankford. *Integrated Sciences for Health Students*, Reston, Va.: Reston Publishing Co., 1984, pp. 146, 147, 148–50.
4. "Osmolality." Monograph. Minneapolis: Doyle Pharmaceutical Co.

PART II

NUTRITION THROUGHOUT THE LIFE CYCLE

10. ENERGY, OBESITY, AND UNDERWEIGHT

11. NUTRITION DURING PREGNANCY AND LACTATION

12. NUTRITION DURING INFANCY, CHILDHOOD, AND ADOLESCENCE

13. NUTRITION AND THE ELDERLY

14. NUTRITION AND PHYSICAL FITNESS

10 ENERGY, OBESITY, AND UNDERWEIGHT

OBJECTIVES

Upon completion of this chapter, you should be able to:

1. Define and give the unit for measurement of energy in nutrition.

2. Distinguish between positive and negative energy balance and the results when there is a deficit or surplus of 3,500 kcal.

3. Estimate the total energy requirements of an individual using the three-step process.

4. Discuss why ideal weight is a misnomer and what it actually measures.

5. Give the percentage of body weight from fat that indicates obesity and the percentages above ideal weight that indicate overweight and obesity.

6. Discuss the four metabolic or internal causes of obesity.

7. Name the three critical periods when the number of fat cells can increase dramatically and therefore result in juvenile obesity.

8. Name and describe the three theories in terms of how the hypothalamus knows when the person is hungry or satiated.

9. Discuss the three external causes of obesity.

10. Describe the five nonrecommended methods for the treatment of obesity.

11. Describe the three recommended methods for the treatment of obesity.

12. Define underweight and describe anorexia nervosa as well as bulimia and bulimarexia.

INTRODUCTION

In Chapter 1, we mentioned that carbohydrates, fats, and proteins are designated as energy nutrients. They release energy when oxidized, which is used by the body to maintain homeostasis. The maintenance of homeostasis depends upon continual input of **energy.**

Energy The capacity to do work.

In this chapter, we will discuss energy in more detail, including energy balance and the results of imbalance: obesity and underweight.

MEASUREMENT OF ENERGY

Examples of how the body uses energy to accomplish work are contractions of the heart to move blood, movement of food along the digestive tract, and contraction of respiratory muscles in moving air into and out of the lungs. In other words, almost all body activities involve work and thereby require an expenditure of energy.

Energy is measured and expressed in nutrition in terms of heat units called *kilocalories (kcal)* (see Fig. 10-1). Chemists and physicists measure energy in terms of a **calorie (cal),** which is defined as the amount of heat required to raise the temperature of 1 g of water 1° Celsius (C) (see Fig. 10-1).

Calorie (cal) The amount of heat required to raise the temperature of 1 g of water 1°C.

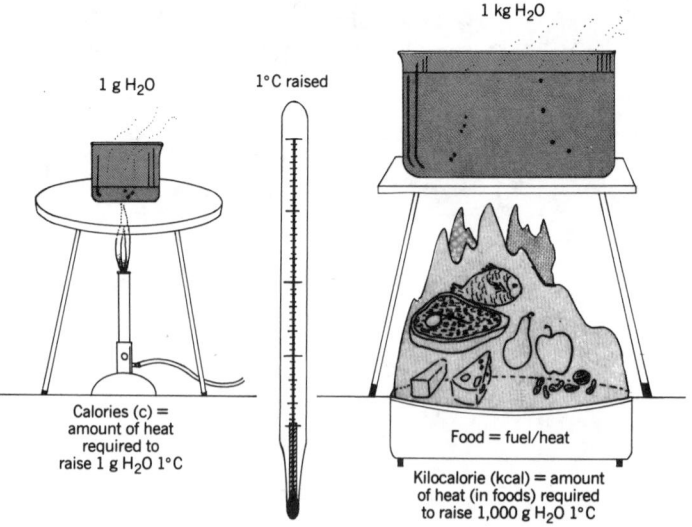

FIGURE 10-1   The two kinds of calories.

Recall that carbohydrates, proteins, lipids, and alcohol provide different amounts of energy; carbohydrates and proteins yield 4 kcal/g and triglycerides (fats) yield 9 kcal/g. Alcohol provides 7 kcal/g when oxidized.

ENERGY BALANCE

Energy balance The amount of energy remaining in the body when energy output is subtracted from energy input.

Energy balance refers to the amount of energy remaining in the body when energy output is subtracted from energy input:

Energy balance = energy input − energy output

A **positive energy balance** will result in weight gain. For example:

$$\text{Energy balance} = \underset{\text{input}}{2,500 \text{ kcal}} - \underset{\text{expenditure}}{2,000 \text{ kcal}}$$
$$= +500 \text{ kcal}$$

Positive energy balance A situation in which energy input is greater than energy expenditure.

If this positive 500-kcal energy balance continues every day for 1 week, the person will gain 1 lb, since a 3,500-kcal surplus equals 1 lb of weight gain. A positive energy balance results in weight gain and is the type of balance that can result in **overweight** and ultimately **obesity**.[1] Overweight and obesity will be discussed later in the chapter.

Overweight Body weight that is more than 10% above ideal weight.

A **negative energy balance** occurs when an adult has a greater energy expenditure than input:

Obesity Body weight that is 15–25% above ideal weight.

$$\text{Energy balance} = \underset{\text{input}}{2,000 \text{ kcal}} - \underset{\text{expenditure}}{2,500 \text{ kcal}}$$
$$= -500 \text{ kcal}$$

Negative energy balance A situation in which energy expenditure is greater than energy input.

If this negative 500-kcal energy balance continues every day for 1 week, the person will lose 1 lb, since a 3,500-kcal deficit equals 1 lb of weight loss. A negative energy balance is necessary for weight loss, which will be discussed later in the chapter.

If energy intake equals energy expenditure, the person's current weight will be maintained.

ENERGY INTAKE

Energy intake Energy supplied by the three energy nutrients: carbohydrates, fats, and proteins.

Foods from the three energy nutrients, carbohydrates, fats, and proteins, compose the **energy intake.** The Recommended Dietary Allowance (RDA) for energy for various age groups is given in Table 10-1. The man used as a reference figure is 5 feet 10 inches tall and weighs 154 lb (70 kg)

TABLE 10-1 MEAN HEIGHTS AND WEIGHTS AND RECOMMENDED ENERGY INTAKES

Age	Weight		Height		Energy Needs[a]	
(Years)	(kg)	(lb)	(cm)	(in.)	(kcal)	(MJ)[b]
Infants						
0.0–0.5	6	13	60	24	kg × 115 (95–145)	kg × 0.48
0.5–1.0	9	20	71	28	kg × 105 (80–135)	kg × 0.44
Children						
1–3	13	29	90	35	1,300 (900–1,800)	5.5
4–6	20	44	112	44	1,700 (1,300–2,300)	7.1
7–10	28	62	132	52	2,400 (1,650–3,300)	10.1
Males						
11–14	45	99	157	62	2,700 (2,000–3,700)	11.3
15–18	66	145	176	69	2,800 (2,100–3,900)	11.8
19–22	70	154	177	70	2,900 (2,500–3,300)	12.2
23–50	70	154	178	70	2,700 (2,300–3,100)	11.3
51–75	70	154	178	70	2,400 (2,000–2,800)	10.1
76+	70	154	178	70	2,050 (1,650–2,450)	8.6
Females						
11–14	46	101	157	62	2,200 (1,500–3,000)	9.2
15–18	55	120	163	64	2,100 (1,200–3,000)	8.8
19–22	55	120	163	64	2,100 (1,700–2,500)	8.8
23–50	55	120	163	64	2,000 (1,600–2,400)	8.4
51–75	55	120	163	64	1,800 (1,400–2,200)	7.6
76+	55	120	163	64	1,600 (1,200–2,000)	6.7
Pregnant					+300	
Lactating					+500	

[a]The energy allowances for the young adults are for men and women doing light work. The allowances for the two older age groups represent mean energy needs over these age spans, allowing for a 2% decrease in basal (resting) metabolic rate per decade and a reduction in activity of 200 cal/day for men and women between 51 and 75 years, 500 cal for men over 75 years, and 400 cal for women over 75. The customary range of daily energy output, shown in parentheses, is based on a variation in energy needs of ±400 cal at any one age, emphasizing the wide range of energy intakes appropriate for any group of people. Energy allowances for children through age 18 are based on median energy intakes of children these ages followed in longitudinal growth studies. The values in parentheses are 10th and 90th percentiles of energy intake, to indicate the range of energy consumption among children of these ages.

[b]MJ stands for megajoules (1 MJ = 1,000 kJ).

Source: Recommended Dietary Allowances, 9th rev. ed, National Academy of Science, Washington, D.C., 1980.

and needs about 2,700 kcal. The reference woman is 5 feet 4 inches tall and weighs 120 lb (55 kg) and needs about 2,000 kcal.[2] Obviously, most people do not exactly meet these average measurements; the reason for the 800-kcal range is to cover most individuals. A person can estimate what his or her energy needs quite accurately, as described on pages 234–236.

ENERGY EXPENDITURE

Energy is expended by the body to maintain the basal metabolic rate (BMR), physical activity, and specific dynamic action. Total energy expenditure is the sum of these three components.

BASAL METABOLIC RATE (BMR)

The expenditure of energy for the BMR is for the maintenance of homeostasis when the body is at rest. Body functions involved in maintaining homeostasis are heartbeat, breathing, nerve activity, kidney functions, and other basic functions.

Methods for estimating the BMR of an individual are given on pages 234 and 235, with examples.

Several factors influence the BMR (see Figure 10-2). They are discussed below.

Body Surface Area

Body surface area Total surface area of an individual, which can be determined from charts based on the person's height and weight.

The greater the **body surface area,** the higher the BMR. If a short, fat person and a tall, thin person both weighed 170 lb, the latter would have the higher BMR. The reason is that this individual has a greater skin surface area through which heat is lost; therefore, the BMR must be higher to replace the lost heat.

Sex

Men generally have a faster BMR than women. One reason is that men have a greater proportion of muscle tissue compared to fat tissue than women. Muscle (lean) tissue is more metabolically active than fat tissue. A lean man has a higher BMR than a man who is fatter and has a greater percentage of less active adipose tissue.

Fever

Fever Elevation of body temperature above normal.

Fever is an example of increased expenditure of energy by the cells to destroy the bacteria or viruses that are causing the infection. In order to provide this increased energy as well as the basal energy, the BMR will rise. Generally, the body needs approximately 7–10% more energy for each 1°F rise in temperature to maintain the BMR.[2] This increase can be accomplished only by increasing the amount of calories in the diet of the individual.

Hormones

Two hormones that influence the BMR are epinephrine and thyroxine (T_4). Epinephrine is released from the adrenal glands in times of stress. In order to overcome the stress, many body activities are activated, raising the BMR.

Thyroxine influences the BMR at all times by increasing the rate at which carbohydrates are catabolized or oxidized to produce energy. **Hyperthyroidism** usually results in elevated thyroxine levels (described in Chapter 8), which can increase the BMR by as much as 80% whereas **hypothyroidism** may reduce it by as much as 30%.

Hyperthyroidism Excessive activity of the thyroid gland, which results in increased secretion of thyroxine.

Hypothyroidism Decreased activity of the thyroid gland, which results in an underproduction of thyroxine.

Age

The BMR increases from birth to age 2 and then begins to drop slightly until puberty, when it increases again as the person goes through a growth spurt. After age 20 the BMR decreases by about 2% every 10 years. In many adults, this decrease in BMR may be greater than 2% because of decreased physical activity, decreased muscle tone, and increased body fat.

Pregnancy and Lactation

Pregnancy is a period when the mother's BMR increases because of the rapid growth and development of the fetus. Lactation also increases the BMR as the mother's body produces breast milk. The RDA for energy tables show 300 kcal more than the normal energy needs for a pregnant woman and 500 kcal more for a lactating woman (see Table 10-1).

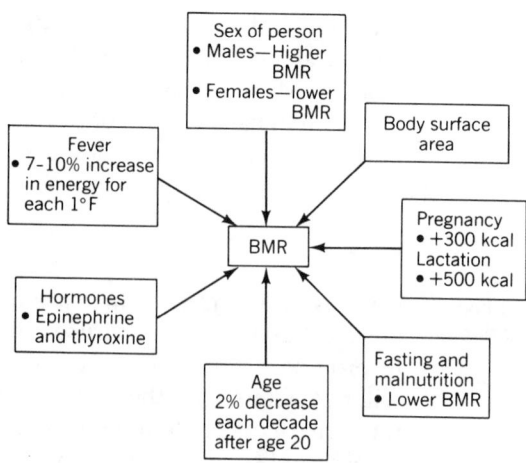

FIGURE 10-2   Factors that influence the BMR.

Fasting and Malnutrition

Fasting and malnutrition lower the BMR as a result of loss of muscle tissue and decrease in body functions. In reality, this BMR decrease is a homeostatic response to conserve energy, since the body is not receiving an adequate amount.

As stated previously, BMR is the minimum amount of energy the body needs to expend to maintain homeostasis when it is at rest. However, BMR accounts for about 50–70% of the total kilocalorie requirement for people who are sedentary or moderately active. Since this description fits most people in the United States, unless a person is very physically active, his or her energy requirements do not exceed the basal metabolism requirement. Physical activity and its influence on energy expenditure will be discussed next.

PHYSICAL ACTIVITY

Physical activity The amount of energy expended by the body to contract the skeletal muscles in voluntary activities.

A second component of energy expenditure is **physical activity.** The actual amount of energy expended for a physical activity depends on muscle involvement, on body weight, and on the length of the activity period. Table 10-2 gives some examples of the kilocalories expended per kilogram per hour.

TABLE 10-2 AMOUNT OF ENERGY EXPENDED FOR VARIOUS ACTIVITIES

Energy Level	Energy Cost (kcal/kg/hr)[a]
Sleeping	0.000
Lying still, relaxed	.12
Sitting or standing still (includes sewing, writing, eating, reading)	0.30
Very light activity (includes driving a car, walking at moderate speed on level ground)	0.90
Light exercise (includes light housework such as sweeping the floor, walking at moderate speed on level ground carrying books)	1.5
Moderate exercise (includes fast walking, dancing, bicycling at moderate speed)	2.4
Heavy exercise (includes fast dancing, walking almost at a run, or fast uphill walking)	3.9
Severe exercise (includes tennis, running)	6.3
Very severe exercise (includes wrestling, rowing, boxing, racing)	8.4

[a]Measured in kilocalories per kilogram of body weight per hour above basal energy.

Source: Adapted from R. Passmore and J.V.G.A. Purnin, "Human Energy Expenditure," *Physiological Reviews 35,* 801–840 (1955).

For any physical activity, the actual expenditure of energy depends upon the person's physical condition and the efficiency with which the exercise is carried out or its form. In other words, a person who is in good physical condition and is close to the ideal weight will actually expend less energy per hour for a particular physical activity than a person who is heavier and not in good physical condition.

A simple method of estimating the amount of energy expended on muscular activities is to classify the person's lifestyle and then add to the BMR a percentage for his or her particular classification, as shown below and discussed on pages 231 and 232.

Sedentary: BMR + 20%

Lightly active: BMR + 30%

Moderately active: BMR + 40%

Very active: BMR + 50%[3]

Typically, physical activity decreases as the person ages. On the average, the person's total energy needs (BMR + physical activity) decrease by about 5% per decade after the age of 20. Do not confuse this decrease with the 2% per decade for BMR only that was discussed earlier.

SPECIFIC DYNAMIC EFFECT

Specific dynamic effect
The expenditure of energy when food is consumed.

When a person consumes food, energy is expended. This energy is used in the digestion, absorption, and transport of nutrients in the body. This expenditure of energy is known as the **specific dynamic effect** or specific dynamic action of food. The amount of energy needed for specific dynamic action is calculated at 10% of the total kilocalories used for BMR and physical activity.[2]

CALCULATING TOTAL ENERGY REQUIREMENTS

The total energy needs of a person can be estimated or calculated by several short methods. Two methods will be discussed here and an example of each given. Method 1 involves three steps:

Step 1. Multiply the weight of a person in kilograms by a factor.
   Note: The factor used is 24 kcal/kg/day, which is arrived at by multiplying the basal energy requirement of 1 kcal/kg/hr × 24 hr/day.[4]

Step 2. Add a percentage to the BMR for the amount of physical activity.

The percentages for the different levels of physical activity are as follows:

Sedentary—BMR + 20%

Light activity—BMR + 30%

Moderate activity—BMR + 40%

Heavy activity—BMR + 50%

Step 3. Add a percentage for the specific dynamic effect of food.

In order to illustrate this method, we will estimate the energy needs of the reference man used for RDA energy values (see Table 10-1) who is in the age range 23–50. His weight is 70 kg (154 lb) and his energy range is 2,300–3,100 kcal, with a mean value of 2,700 kcal for doing light work. [Note: To convert weight in pounds (lb) to kilograms (kg), divide weight in pounds by 2.2 (lb/2.2 = kg).]

Step 1. $70 \dfrac{kg}{1} \times 24 \dfrac{kcal}{kg/day} = 1{,}680 \qquad BMR = 1{,}680 \dfrac{kcal}{day}$

Step 2. $1{,}680 \dfrac{kcal}{day} \times 0.30 = 504 \dfrac{kcal}{day}$

$1{,}680 \dfrac{kcal}{day} + 504 \dfrac{kcal}{day} = 2{,}184 \dfrac{kcal}{day}$

This calculation shows the amount of energy needed for BMR plus energy needed for physical activity.

Step 3. $2{,}184 \dfrac{kcal}{day} \times 0.10 = 218 \dfrac{kcal}{day}$

$2{,}184 \dfrac{kcal}{day} + 218 \dfrac{(kcal)}{day} = 2{,}402 \dfrac{kcal}{day}$

This 2,402 kcal/day is the estimated energy need for this man, which is within the RDA range but less than the mean value.

Method 2 involves only one step: multiplying the ideal body weight by a factor that takes into consideration BMR + energy for light activity + specific dynamic effect. It should be noted that these factors were determined from the RDA table for recommended energy intakes. As an example, Table 10-1 shows that a man in the age range 23–50 should weigh 70 kg and should need 2,700 kcal as a mean energy value. Therefore, to determine this group's energy factor, perform the following calculation:

$$2{,}700 \dfrac{kcal}{day} \times \dfrac{1}{70 \text{ kg}} = 39 \text{ kcal/kg/day}$$

This factor is rounded off to the nearest whole number.

The energy factors for men and women, according to the age range, are:

Men (age)	kcal/kg/day	kcal/lb/day
23–50	39	18
51–75	34	16
76+	29	13

These values allow for a 2% decrease in BMR per decade and a reduction in activity of 200 kcal/day for men and women between 51 and 75 years, 500 kcal for men over 75, and 400 kcal for women over 75. These factors also estimate the energy needs only for light activity.

Women (age)	kcal/kg/day	kcal/lb/day
23–50	36	17
51–75	33	15
76+	29	13

IDEAL OR DESIRABLE BODY WEIGHT AND BODY COMPOSITION

IDEAL OR DESIRABLE BODY WEIGHT

Ideal body weight The values that originated from the height and weight tables issued by the Metropolitan Life Insurance Company in 1942.

The term **ideal body weight** is actually a misnomer, since there is no scientific way to know what the ideal body weight for each individual should be. If this is the case, where did this term originate and how valid are the ideal body weight tables that are available in doctors' offices and other sources? The term *ideal body weight* originated from height and weight tables that were published in 1942 by the Metropolitan Life Insurance Company. The weights were ideal in the sense that they resulted in maximum longevity, which the insurance industry was interested in for establishing life insurance rates. In reality, they turned out to be the average weights for both sexes and given heights at age 30.

In 1959, Metropolitan Life published new height and weight recommendations but designated the recommended weights as *desirable weights*, since it was felt that no one really knew what the ideal weight was for any specific individual. Data for the 1959 tables also showed that the average body weights for persons 25 to 30 years of age are desirable weights for all older persons, and it is recommended that each individual maintain this desirable weight throughout life.

In 1983 Metropolitan Life published new height-weight tables (see Table 10-3). The recommended weights are not referred to as either ideal or desirable but simply as the 1983 Metropolitan Height and Weight Table. This new table indicates that the weights associated with the lowest mortality (longest longevity) have increased since 1959 but still remain below the average weight for all persons of a specific height.[5] The average weights for the whole U.S. population are given in Table 10-4. If one compares the new Metropolitan height and weight figures with the average weight for all persons, they are very close. Also, note at the bottom of Table 10-4 that this table permits weight to increase until middle age, whereas insurance tables assume that the weight that was ideal at age 25 is ideal throughout life.[3]

TABLE 10-3 1983 METROPOLITAN HEIGHT AND WEIGHT TABLE

Men					Women				
Height		Small Frame	Medium Frame	Large Frame	Height		Small Frame	Medium Frame	Large Frame
Ft	In.				Ft	In.			
5	2	128–134	131–141	138–150	4	10	102–111	109–121	118–131
5	3	130–136	133–143	140–153	4	11	103–113	111–123	120–134
5	4	132–138	135–145	142–156	5	0	104–115	113–126	122–137
5	5	134–140	137–148	144–160	5	1	106–118	115–129	125–140
5	6	136–142	139–151	146–164	5	2	108–121	118–132	128–143
5	7	138–145	142–154	149–168	5	3	111–124	121–135	131–147
5	8	140–148	145–157	152–172	5	4	114–127	124–138	134–151
5	9	142–151	148–160	155–176	5	5	117–130	127–141	137–155
5	10	144–154	151–163	158–180	5	6	120–133	130–144	140–159
5	11	146–157	154–166	161–184	5	7	123–136	133–147	143–163
6	0	149–160	157–170	164–188	5	8	126–139	136–150	146–167
6	1	152–164	160–174	168–192	5	9	129–142	139–153	149–170
6	2	155–168	164–178	172–197	5	10	132–145	142–156	152–173
6	3	158–172	167–182	176–202	5	11	135–148	145–159	155–176
6	4	162–176	171–187	181–207	6	0	138–151	148–162	158–179

Note: Weights at ages 25–59 based on lowest mortality. Weight in pounds according to frame in indoor clothing (5 lb for men and 3 lb for women), wearing shoes with a 1-in. heel.

Source: Courtesy of the Metropolitan Life Insurance Company.

TABLE 10-4 AVERAGE WEIGHTS OF U.S. CITIZENS: HANES SURVEY, 1980

Height (in.)	Weight (lb), Men Age 18–24	Age 25–34	Age 35–44	Age 45–54	Age 55–64	Age 65–74	Height (in.)	Weight (lb), Women Age 18–24	Age 25–34	Age 35–44	Age 45–54	Age 55–64	Age 65–74
62	130	141	143	147	143	143	57	114	118	125	129	132	130
63	135	145	148	152	147	147	58	117	121	129	133	136	134
64	140	150	153	156	153	151	59	120	125	133	136	140	137
65	145	156	158	160	158	156	60	123	128	137	140	143	140
66	150	160	163	164	163	160	61	126	132	141	143	147	144
67	154	165	169	169	168	164	62	129	136	144	147	150	147
68	159	170	174	173	173	169	63	132	139	148	150	153	151
69	164	174	179	177	178	173	64	135	142	152	154	157	154
70	168	179	184	182	183	177	65	138	146	156	158	160	158
71	173	184	190	187	189	182	66	141	150	159	161	164	161
72	178	189	194	191	193	186	67	144	153	163	165	167	165
73	183	194	200	196	197	190	68	147	157	167	168	171	169
74	188	199	205	200	203	194							

Note: Weights are given for older age groups. The insurance company tables assumed that the weight that was ideal at 25 would be ideal throughout life; this table permits weight gain to take place until middle age.

Source: U.S. Government Publication. Data from the National Health Examination Survey and the National Health and Nutrition Examination Survey. Weight by Height and Age for Adults 18–74 years, United States, 1971–1974, published in 1980.

RULE-OF-THUMB METHOD OF ESTIMATING IDEAL WEIGHT

A quick way to estimate the ideal weight for medium-frame men and women is:

Women	Men
1. Give the height of 5 feet (barefooted) an ideal weight of 100 lb.	1. Give the height of 5 feet (barefooted) an ideal weight of 110 lb.
2. For every inch above 5 ft, add 5 lb. The total should be expressed as plus or minus 10% to compensate for large and small frames.	2. For every inch above 5 feet, add 5 lb. The total should be expressed as plus or minus 10% to compensate for small and large frames.

Women	Men
3. For example, a women who is 5 ft 5 in. would add 25 lb to 100 for a total of 125 lb (plus or minus 10%).	3. For example, a man who is 5 ft 9 in. would add 45 lb to 110 for a total of 155 lb (plus or minus 10%).

In summary, as stated earlier, the term *ideal body weight* is a misnomer. There is no scientifically determined ideal or desirable body weight for each height. The height and weight tables give us the weights for a particular height that result in the longest longevity.

DETERMINING BODY FRAME SIZE

Body frame size The size of a person's body frame, with small, medium, and large being the three possibilities.

Another problem with ideal or desirable body weight is determining **body frame size.** Note in Table 10-3 that for each specific height there are weights for small, medium, and large frames. The problem, though, is, into which category does a person fit? Again, there is no scientific way to determine body frame size; therefore, when in doubt, assume a medium frame. When Metropolitan Life published its 1983 tables, it also described a method for determining body frame size based on the measurement of elbow breadth. The method is as follows:

1. Extend the arm with the fingers straight.

2. Bend the forearm upward at a 90-degree angle and turn the palm of the hand away from the body.

3. Place the thumb and index finger of the other hand on the two prominent bones on either side of the elbow.

4. Measure the space between the fingers against a ruler or use a caliper.

5. Compare the measurements with the figures in Table 10-5. The measurements given in the table are for medium-framed men and women. Measurements lower than those shown indicate a small frame and higher measurements indicate a large frame.[6]

BODY COMPOSITION AND DETERMINATION OF OVERWEIGHT AND OBESITY

Body composition is important in determining whether a person is overweight or obese, especially with the limitations of ideal or desirable body weight tables. A certain percentage of a person's body weight must be composed of fat due to its important functions (heat insulation, protection of vital organs, reserve energy source). Research has shown that

TABLE 10-5 ELBOW BREADTH FOR MEN AND WOMEN OF MEDIUM FRAME AND VARIOUS HEIGHTS

Men		Women	
Height (1" heels)	Elbow Breadth (inches)	Height (1" heels)	Elbow Breadth (inches)
5'2"–5'3"	$2\frac{1}{2}$–$2\frac{7}{8}$	4'10"–4'11"	$2\frac{1}{4}$–$2\frac{1}{2}$
5'4"–5'7"	$2\frac{5}{8}$–$2\frac{7}{8}$	5'0" –5'3"	$2\frac{1}{4}$–$2\frac{1}{2}$
5'8"–5'11"	$2\frac{3}{4}$–3	5'4" –5'7"	$2\frac{3}{8}$–$2\frac{5}{8}$
6'0"–6'3"	$2\frac{3}{4}$–$3\frac{1}{8}$	5'8" –5'11"	$2\frac{3}{8}$–$2\frac{5}{8}$
6'4"	$2\frac{7}{8}$–$3\frac{1}{4}$	6'0"	$2\frac{1}{2}$–$2\frac{3}{4}$

Note: Measurements lower than those listed indicate a small frame, and higher measurements indicate a large frame.

Source: Courtesy of the Metropolitan Life Insurance Company.

the following percentages are ideal in terms of fat as a percentage of body weight and the percentages that indicate obesity:

	Normal percentage of body weight	Percentage of body weight from fat that indicates obesity
Men	15–20	25
Women	20–25	30[7]

Densitometry A method of determining the body composition and body fatness of a person. The method involves measuring the body's specific gravity by immersing the individual in water.

Hydrometry A method of determining the body composition and body fatness of a person. It involves injection of deuterium oxide (heavy water) into the body.

Potassium-40 A radioactive isotope that is naturally present in the body, but in low quantities in fat tissue.

Anthropometric measurements Measurements of the size, weight, and proportions of the human body.

Four common methods used to determine body composition and body fatness are **densitometry, hydrometry, potassium-40,** and **anthropometric measurements.** Densitometry, hydrometry, and potassium-40 are less commonly used methods and will be briefly described. Anthropometric measurements constitute the most common method and will be described in more detail.

Densitometry. Fat has a specific gravity of 0.92, and bone and muscle tissue have a specific gravity of 1.1; therefore, the more fat tissue a person has, the closer to 0.92 the specific gravity will be. Likewise the more bone and muscle tissue a person has, the closer to 1.1 the specific gravity will be.

Hydrometry. After injection, a blood sample is taken to determine the amount of deuterium oxide that has been used in fat metabolism. Calculations can be made from the amount left to determine the amount of fat in the body.

Potassium-40. This method involves measuring the amount of radioactivity produced by potassium-40 and comparing this value to body

Calipers An instrument with two bent or curved legs. It is frequently used for measuring skinfold thickness.

Triceps A muscle located on the back of the upper arm.

size. A high potassium count in relation to body size is indicative of little fatty tissue, whereas a low count is indicative of a higher amount of fatty tissue.

Anthropometric Measurements

A trained individual can use **calipers** to measure the thickness of a fold of skin (see Fig. 10-3). This skinfold measurement is usually made on the **triceps** midway between the shoulder and elbow, with the arm

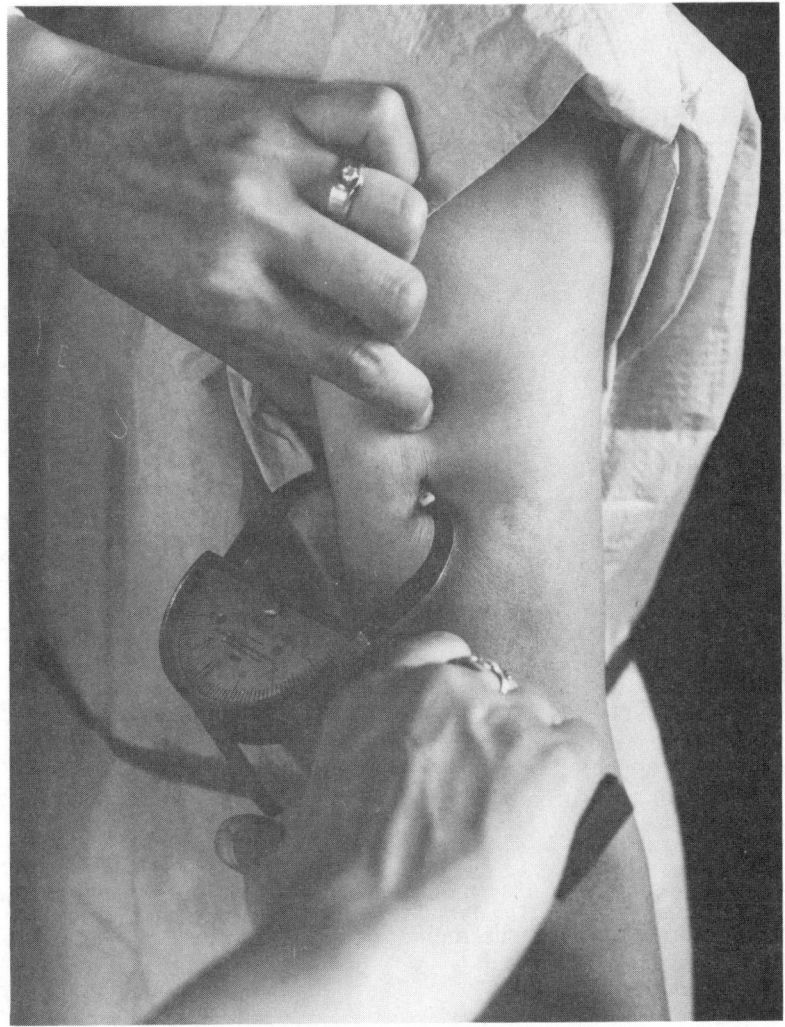

FIGURE 10-3 Measurement of a skinfold on the back of the upper arm with calipers. (Photo by Pilar A. Garcia.)

hanging freely. A skinfold measurement of 0.5 to 1 in. is normal, and measurements over 1 in. are indicative of obesity.

One major advantage of measuring obesity by body composition is that it allows one to distinguish overweight from **overfat.** For example, a muscular athlete who is active in strenuous sports may be overweight according to height-weight tables but not overfat. This overweight situation is not a nutritional problem, as is overfat, since the excess weight is due to a disproportionately high amount of muscle tissue.

Overfat Disproportionately high percentage of fat tissue.

OVERWEIGHT AND OBESITY

Despite the limitations of the ideal weight tables, they are still used as a guide to determine overweight and obesity. *Overweight* is defined as body weight that is more than 10% above the ideal weight. *Obesity* is defined as body weight that is 15–25% above the ideal weight, with 20% being the most common percentage. Likewise, a person who is more than 10% below the table weight is considered **underweight.**

Weights that are 30–100% above ideal weight are classified as **severe obesity; massive or morbid obesity** refers to weights that are more than 100% above normal.[8]

In summary, obesity can be determined by three different methods—measuring body composition, anthropometric measurements, and comparing a person's body weight with ideal weight tables. The specific measurements that indicate overweight or obesity for each method are given below:

Underweight Body weight that is more than 10% below the ideal weight.

Severe obesity Body weight that is 30–100% above the ideal weight.

Massive (morbid) obesity Body weight that is more than 100% above the ideal weight.

	Overweight	Obesity
Body composition Various measurements		Man: 25% of body weight is due to fat Woman: 30% of body weight is due to fat
Anthropometric measurements		Skinfold measurement greater than 1 in.
Ideal weight tables	10% above ideal weight	15–25% above ideal weight, with 20% being most common

Overweight and obesity are examples of a positive energy balance, in which more kilocalories are being consumed than used.

INCIDENCE OF OBESITY

Various studies have been conducted to determine the incidence of obesity in the United States. These studies estimate that 25–30% of adults and at least 10% of children are either overweight or obese. They also show that obesity is more common among women than men. It is greatest among black women between the ages of 45 and 74 and those below the poverty level.[7]

CAUSES OF OBESITY

Some experts consider obesity to be America's number one malnutrition problem and believe that the problem has been expanding to epidemic proportions rather than diminishing in recent years. Obesity, as stated earlier, is a problem of positive energy balance, in which more kilocalories are consumed than expended, resulting in the storage of fat and weight gain. The question, then, is, why do so many people overeat and create a positive energy balance? Research has found that the factors that lead to obesity can be placed into two major categories—**metabolic** (internal) and **regulatory** (external).

Metabolic factor (internal) An internal factor that can lead to obesity.

Regulatory factor (external) An external factor that can lead to obesity.

Metabolic (internal). Some of the metabolic factors that will be discussed in more detail are genetic, physiological, and hormonal.

Regulatory (external). Psychological, social, and cultural factors and lack of exercise are regulatory factors that will be discussed in more detail.

Metabolic (Internal) Factors

Genetic Congenital or inherited.

Genetic Factors. A considerable body of data suggests that a predisposing factor in obesity is **genetic** background. Figure 10-4 shows that if both parents are lean, the incidence of obesity in their children is about 9–14%. If one parent is obese, the incidence rises to 41–50%. If both parents are obese, it rises to 66–80%. The research done on obesity as an inherited trait shows that if a person inherits genes from obese parents, he or she has simply inherited the potential for being obese; however, the environment actually determines whether or not this potential is expressed. In studies done with identical twins in which both inherited genes from obese parents, but were raised by different families, in some cases one twin became obese because of the poor eating habits learned from his parents. The other twin remained lean because of positive eating behaviors learned from his parents. In summary, the evidence that peo-

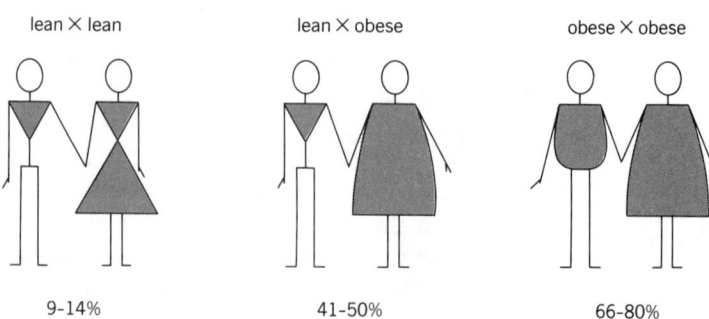

FIGURE 10-4   Genetic chances of a child's developing obesity. (Reprinted with permission from Weinsier, Roland L., and Butterworth, C.R., Jr.: *Handbook of Clinical Nutrition*, St. Louis, 1981, The C.V. Mosby Co.)

Fat cell hypothesis The theory that the body has the potential to accumulate an excess number of fat cells during three periods of life: the last 3 months of fetal development, the first 3 years of life, and adolescence.

Hyperplasia A dramatic increase in the number of fat cells.

Hypertrophy An increase in the size of fat cells.

Juvenile-onset obesity Obesity beginning during the last 3 months of fetal life, the first 3 years of life, and adolescence.

Adult-onset obesity Obesity beginning in adulthood.

ple can be genetically predisposed to obesity is strong; however, the environment can inhibit or enhance this predisposition.

Related to the genetic factor is the controversial **fat cell hypothesis** concerning a possible cause of obesity in juveniles and adults. The number of fat cells in an infant is genetically determined; however, research shows that during three critical phases of growth, the body has the potential to accumulate an excess number of fat cells. The three periods when the potential for **hyperplasia** occurs are during the last 3 months of fetal development, the first 3 years of life, and adolescence. After 18 months of age, fat cells increase not only in number but also in size (**hypertrophy**) until approximately adulthood, when the number is fixed; however, they can continue to grow in size indefinitely.[10] **Juvenile-onset obesity** can result from both hyperplasia and hypertrophy. **Adult-onset obesity** results from hypertrophy of fat cells alone. In some cases of morbid obesity (greater than 170% of ideal body weight), hyperplasia of fat cells may start again.[11]

Evidence shows that those who became obese during childhood generally have a harder time losing weight than those who became obese as adults. The fat cell hypothesis states that this is because the greater the number of fat cells, the more hungry the person will be; therefore, juvenile-obese people will always feel hungry more often than lean or even adult-obese individuals. Also, the juvenile-obese individual will always have an excess number of fat cells, making long-term weight loss very difficult.

The fat cell hypothesis has been heavily criticized. Many experts feel that there is no convincing proof that obesity develops as a result of having a large number of fat cells. However, these critics do agree on the three critical phases of growth. If obesity occurs during these times, it may be very hard, if not impossible, to lose this weight.

Hunger An inborn instinct that causes a physiological response to the body's need for food.

Appetite A learned psychological response to food that is initiated for reasons other than the need for food.

Satiety A sensation of fullness that follows a meal.

Hypothalamus An area at the base of the brain that contains centers of hunger and satiety and secretes the antidiuretic hormone.

Glucostatic theory The theory that when the blood glucose level is high, a person will feel full, and when it is low, the person will feel hungry.

Lipostatic theory The theory that the tissues, especially the fat tissues, signal the brain when the level of fat is increased above or decreased below a certain level.

Set point theory The theory that the body is programmed to maintain a certain amount of fat.

Physiological Factors. Obesity is often the result of an inability to respond adequately to **hunger** and **appetite** as well as satiety sensations. For example, the smell of frying bacon can make a person want to eat even though he or she may already be full. **Satiety** is the sensation of fullness that follows a meal, and is thought to be a combination of physiological and psychological responses.

The **hypothalamus** (see Fig. 10-5) region of the brain receives nerve impulses from various regions of the body concerning the body's energy needs. It can interpret these impulses as either hunger or satiety sensations.

How does the hypothalamus know when the body needs food or is full? This has long been an intriguing question for nutritionists, especially since the answer might help to explain why people become obese. Three widely accepted theories that attempt to answer this question are the **glucostatic, lipostatic,** and **set point theories.**

Glucostatic theory. Figure 10-6 shows that the brain (the hypothalamus apparently being the primary site) is able to monitor the blood glucose level; when it is low (below 70 mg/dl), the hunger sensation is the result. Figure 10-6 also shows that when the blood glucose level is high (above 120 mg/dl), a satiety sensation is produced.

In other words, this theory states that there is an inverse relationship between blood glucose level and hunger; that is, as the blood glucose

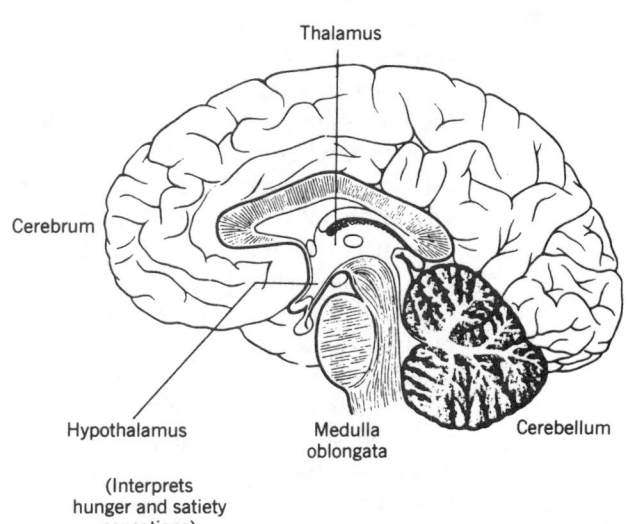

FIGURE 10-5 The hypothalamus region of the brain, where interpretation of hunger and satiety signals occurs. (From T. Randall Lankford, *Integrated Science for Health Students,* 3rd ed., 1984. Reprinted by persmission of Reston Publishing Company, a Prentice-Hall Company, 11480 Sunset Hills Road, Reston, Va. 22090.)

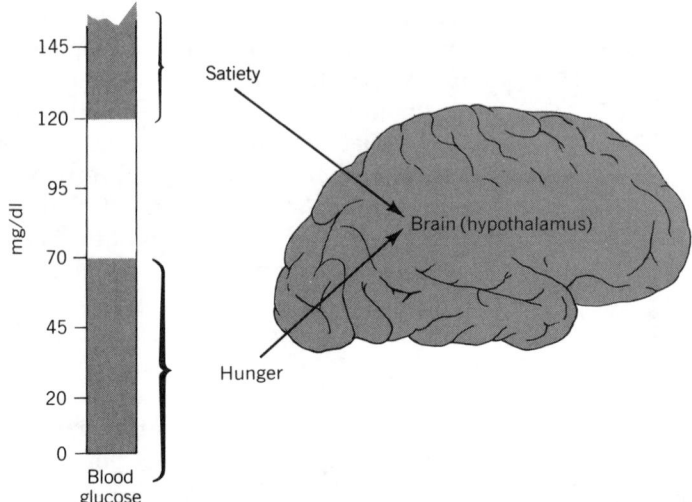

FIGURE 10-6 Glucostatic theory. The hunger sensation results from a drop in
the blood glucose level below 70 mg/dl, and a satiety sensation results from a
blood glucose level above 120 mg/dl.

level decreases, the sensation of hunger increases. The relationship between blood glucose and satiety is direct; as the blood glucose level
increases, so does the sensation of satiety. This mechanism monitors
short-term needs as the blood glucose level varies from hour to hour.

Lipostatic theory. The lipostatic theory states that the tissues, especially
the fat tissues, signal the brain when they are satiated (see Fig. 10-7).
Likewise, when fat decreases below a certain level, the brain interprets
this action as a need for food and a hunger sensation is created. People
with more fat cells have to eat more food before they experience satiety.
This mechanism involves long-term regulation, since the content of fat
cells changes slowly.

Set point theory. Since the number of fat cells is theorized to be fixed
by adulthood, an obese person has a greater number of fat cells and
thus a greater amount of fat to maintain. According to this theory, each
person has a body weight that functions as a "set point" (which may
be an obese weight in some people) (see Fig. 10-8); when this weight is
exceeded, the hypothalamus recognizes the need to lose weight. Likewise, when the body weight is below the set point, the hypothalamus
recognizes the need to gain weight. People who try to lose weight below
their set point may actually lose lean tissue rather than fat tissue, as
shown in rat studies.[12]

Whether the hypothalamus recognizes hunger and satiety according
to the glucostatic, lipostatic, or set point theories or combinations of
them, obesity results from their malfunctions. The obese person may

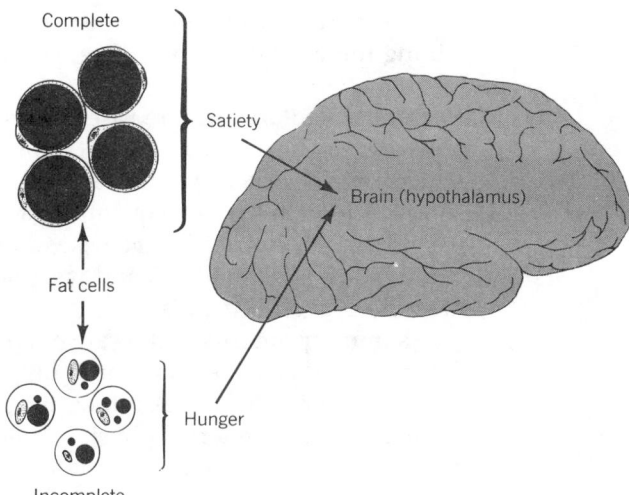

FIGURE 10-7 Lipostatic theory. Satiety sensations result from the fat tissues being "full" of fat. Hunger sensations result from emptiness of the fat tissues.

have a defective monitoring system, so that the hypothalamus does not recognize when the blood glucose level is back to normal; therefore, food may be consumed beyond the satiety level. Likewise, since an obese person has to consume more food to fill the fat cells than a lean person, the hypothalamus may not recognize when the obese person has reached a satiety level. Finally, it may be that some people are destined to be

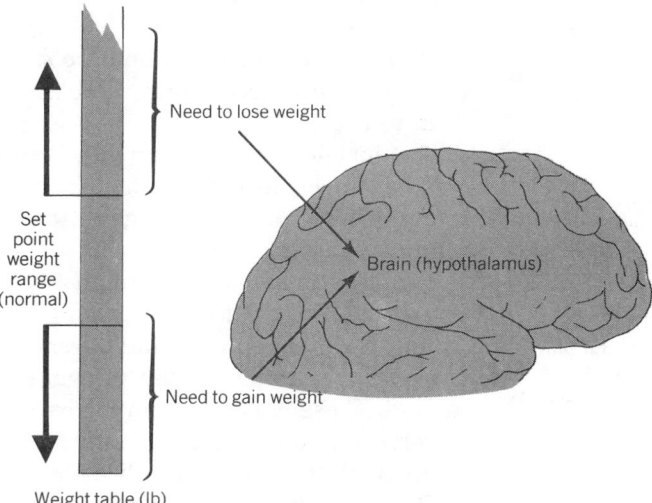

FIGURE 10-8 Set point theory. When the set point weight is exceeded, the hypothalamus interprets this condition as a need to lose weight. When body weight drops below the set point, the hypothalamus recognizes a need to gain weight.

overweight and obese due to their set point; therefore, losing and maintaining the weight loss may be impossible for them.

Hormonal Factors. In rare cases, obesity may be caused by hormonal imbalances. The most common example is a decreased level of thyroxine, which results in a lowering of the BMR. If the person continues to consume food in the same quantities as before the lowering of the BMR, weight gain is inevitable. Likewise, an increased level of thyroxine will result in an increased BMR and weight loss if there is no change in the quantity of food consumed.

In summary, internal factors are not related to the environment (except for the role that the environment plays in hindering or enhancing the predisposition to be obese); rather, the problems originate internally and are influenced by internal physiological changes. A very small percentage of obese cases are due to these internal physiological factors. The majority are due to regulatory or external factors, which are discussed next.

Regulatory (External) Factors

Regulatory factors that can result in obesity are independent of physiological factors and instead are related to the environment. People who become obese due to external factors are not very sensitive to internal cues such as hunger and satiety sensations. Instead, they are very susceptible to external cues such as the time of day and the availability, sight, and taste of food.

Psychological Factors. Some people eat to satisfy needs other than hunger. These needs form the basis of psychological factors that can lead to obesity.

The inability of some individuals to recognize and express emotions such as anger, fear, frustration, rejection, and anxiety may lead to abnormal eating patterns. **Binge eating** is an example of an eating pattern that may result in obesity.

People who are under emotional or physical stress often find relief by overeating. In addition to overeating, stress results in the release of large amounts of epinephrine and **adrenocorticotrophic (ACTH)** hormones, which increase the amount of energy used to overcome the stress situation. These hormones can increase energy by stimulating the release of large amounts of glucose, fatty acids, and amino acids. If the stressed individual does not metabolize all of these energy nutrients, the body will convert them to fat. In addition, if stress results in the lowering of the blood glucose level, a hunger sensation is created and the person may overeat soon after the situation is over. Lean and overly thin people

Binge eating Consumption of large amounts of food in a short period of time.

Adrenocorticotrophic hormone (ACTH) A hormone that is secreted by the anterior pituitary gland.

respond in an opposite manner; they tend to reject food and metabolize their energy nutrients more efficiently.

Psychotherapy has been found, in some cases, to be a successful treatment for obesity that results from basic psychological disorders.

Social Factors. Social and cultural habits are external factors that can result in obesity in children and adults. Some cultures view a fat baby as healthy and obese adults as wealthy and powerful individuals.

Cultural norms (see Chapter 1 for more details on cultural influences on food habits) determine acceptable foods, attitudes toward eating, and obesity. It is very important for medical personnel to have knowledge of or access to the food patterns of major cultures in the United States in order to assess responses to diets more efficiently and to teach nutrition concepts to patients.

Socioeconomic factors also influence attitudes toward obesity, as evidenced by data that show that poor black women have higher rates of obesity than white women. However, black men have lower rates than white men.

Lack of Exercise. Probably the single most important causative factor in obesity is inactivity. This conclusion is partially validated by recent food consumption data showing that people are consuming fewer kilocalories today than they did a few years ago. This inconsistency is partially explained by people's reduced physical activity due to the availability of convenience appliances in the home, machines at work, and modern transportation to carry them back and forth. Little exercise is required in today's society to carry out daily activities. Therefore, to increase energy expenditure today, a person has to make a constant effort to exercise.

Two other points about lack of exercise and obesity concern the consumption of fewer kilocalories by obese compared to normal-weight people and the role of exercise in regulating the physiological appetite. Studies show that obese people often consume fewer kilocalories than lean ones; however, these obese people were so inactive that they still managed to have a positive energy balance. Other studies have shown that active people are better able to regulate their physiological appetite mechanism and are less influenced by external cues. Apparently, the more sedentary a person is, the greater the chance of failure of the hunger-satiey mechanism and the greater the chance the person will be influenced by the environment.[13]

NONRECOMMENDED TREATMENTS OF OBESITY

Many methods have been used to treat obesity; some are recommended by nutritional experts and others are not. Table 10-6 presents a summary of the nonrecommended methods.

One writer has estimated that there are about 2,000 weight reduction diets, and more than 50% of them are unsafe.[14] A logical question to ask is, "How can I distinguish a fad diet from a recommended weight loss diet?" Below are some of the typical claims made by fad diets; these diets should be avoided:

The diet promises ease and comfort in weight loss. Successful weight loss takes a great deal of work and sometimes involves discomfort in regard to exercise.

The diet promises extremely rapid weight loss. Claims such as a loss of 5–8 lb/week are impossible except on starvation or very-low-carbohydrate diets. The early weight loss is almost totally water, not fat, and the rate of loss decreases the longer one remains on such a diet.

The diet restricts or includes only a few foods. Examples are the grapefruit or egg diet. The results are inadequate nutrient intake, boredom, and quick abandonment of the diet.

The diet requires you to purchase a "secret formula" or "magic pill." Most of the claims made for these aids have not been scientifically verified and are frequently quite expensive.

The diet is published in a book or magazine. In a free society, anyone can publish anything, true or not, if he or she can find someone who will publish it.

RECOMMENDED TREATMENTS OF OBESITY

The recommended and proven treatments of obesity are:

- A nutritionally balanced caloric diet
- A reasonable increase in physical activity
- An understanding of behavior modification

NUTRITIONALLY BALANCED DIET

As stated earlier, weight loss cannot occur unless a person has a negative energy balance, that is, expending more energy than he or she is con-

TABLE 10-6 NONRECOMMENDED METHODS FOR TREATING OBESITY

Method	Comments
A) Drugs	
Diet pills	Diminish appetite
	Can cause serious side effects (nervousness and insomnia)
	Danger of addiction if used over a long period
Hormones	Hormone injected along with a 400- to 500-kcal diet.
HCG (human chorionic gonadotropin)	Claim that HCG suppresses appetite has not been substantiated; side effects are unknown and possibly dangerous
Thyroid	Increases BMR but may result in loss of lean tissue
	May cause adverse effects on heart if not medically controlled
Diuretics	Causes water loss, not loss of fat tissue
	Long-time use can lead to dehydration and potassium deficiency
B) Fasting	May be used in hospital settings for morbid obesity when the patient is allowed noncaloric fluids, vitamins, and mineral supplements
	Rapid weight loss at first, but declines as BMR decreases
	Does not teach new food behavior patterns
	Loss of lean tissue and ketosis may occur
C) Fad diets	
The Beverly Hills Diet	No scientific justification for the premise that food combining causes weight loss.
	No scientific evidence to support the claim that enzymes in fresh fruit can burn up or oxidize fat
	The narrow variety of foods does not provide an adequate range and quantity of nutrients to maintain health
	Diet does not teach good eating habits that meet the body's need for all essential nutrients
The Complete Scarsdale Medical Diet	High-protein, low-carbohydrate diets can result in mineral deficiencies
	Unsound guidelines are given for vegetarian diets; the sample meals do not include milk, eggs, legumes, or other foods that could improve the protein quality of a vegetarian diet
	Dietary concepts for disease states are unsound and outdated
The Cambridge Diet Plan	Provides only 330 kcal/day; 44 g carbohydrate, 33 g high-grade protein, 3 g fat
	Protein intake is less than 75% of the RDA for adult women and less than 60% of that for adult men
	Low level of kilocalories is potentially dangerous to people with cardiovascular disease, stroke, kidney disease, and diabetes

TABLE 10-6 *(Continued)*

Method	Comments
D) Surgery Intestinal bypass surgery	Surgical removal or tying off of a large portion of the small intestine to decrease the absorption of food Generally used only on patients who are 100 lb or more overweight in whom the risks to health from obesity are greater than those from surgery Can result in severe side effects: liver failure, kidney stones, and malnutrition; mortality reports range from 2 to 10%

suming. The starting point, then, is to estimate the person's specific energy needs (the methods for doing so were presented on pages 234 and 235 in this chapter). This estimate should be based on the person's ideal weight, not on the actual caloric intake.

Once the person's energy needs have been determined, one can calculate how many kilocalories must be cut in order to achieve a negative energy balance. Let us assume that Jane is overweight and needs 2,500 kcal to maintain her recommended ideal weight. She wants to lose weight only at the recommended rate, which is 1–2 lb/week. In order to reach this goal, Jane has to reduce her daily intake by 500–1,000 kcal. Remember that to lose 1 lb, a person has to have a 3,500-kcal deficit. Let us assume that Jane wants to lose 2 lb/week:

2,500	Kilocalories needed to maintain her recommended ideal weight
− 1,000	Daily kilocalorie deficit needed to lose 2 lb/week
1,500	Jane cannot consume more than 1,500 kcal/day in order to lose up to 2 lb/week. Table 10-7 presents an example of a 1,500-kcal diet.

It is important to emphasize that nutritional adequacy cannot be maintained on fewer than about 1,200 kcal/day—1,000 at the very least. After the total kilocalories that can be consumed per day is determined, the specifics of the diet need to be planned. They should include the following factors:

Adequacy. As pointed out in regard to the fad diets in Table 10-6, most of them are not adequate in nutrients. It is important that the diet have the proper amounts of servings from the four food groups but stay within kilocalorie limits.

Emphasis on nutrient density. To achieve an adequate diet, foods that are high in nutrients but low in kilocalories have to be emphasized.

TABLE 10-7 SAMPLE MEAL PLAN FOR A 1,500-KCAL DIET

	Exchange	kcal/ Exchange	Total kcal
Breakfast			
Skim milk, 1 cup	1 milk	80	80
Eggs, 2	2 meat + 1 fat	110, 45	155
Orange juice, $\frac{1}{2}$ cup	1 fruit	40	40
Bagel, 1	2 bread	70	140
Margarine, 1 teaspoon	1 fat	45	45
Coffee/tea	free	0	0
Lunch			
Tuna, $\frac{1}{2}$ cup	2 meat	55	110
Onions, celery, $\frac{1}{2}$ cup	1 vegetable	25	25
Mayonnaise, 1 teaspoon	1 fat	45	45
Rye bread, 2 slices	2 bread	70	140
Lettuce, pickle	free	0	0
Peach, medium	1 fruit	40	40
Tea	free	0	0
Snack			
Yogurt, 2% milk, 1 cup	1 milk + 1 fat	80 + 45	125
Banana, small, $\frac{1}{2}$	1 fruit	40	40
Dinner			
Chicken, baked, no skin, 4 ounces	4 meat	55	220
Green beans, 1 cup	1 vegetable	25	25
Salad: tomatoes, onions, celery, radishes, $\frac{1}{2}$ cup total	1 vegetable	25	25
Lettuce, wine vinegar	free	0	0
Corn, $\frac{1}{3}$ cup	1 vegetable	25	25
Potato, small	1 bread	70	70
Wine, dry white, 3 ounces	1 bread	70	70
Total kilocalories for day:			1490

Source: Patricia J. Long and Barbara Shannon, *Focus on Nutrition,* © 1983, p. 177. Reprinted by permission of Prentice-Hall, Inc., Englewood Cliffs, N.J.

Refer to Chapter 1 for examples of skim milk as opposed to whole milk or lean meat as opposed to medium- or high-fat meat. This will require familiarizing the person with the six exchange lists (discussed in Chapter 1 and presented in Appendix A). Refer to Table 10-7 for specific examples in a 1,500-kcal diet.

Emphasis on balance. Remember from Chapter 1 that a nutritious diet needs to be balanced—55–60% of kilocalories from carbohydrates, 30% from fat, and 10–15% from protein. Fad diets are frequently negligent in that they are often extremely low in carbohydrates and sometimes in protein. It is important to include some fat in each meal, since fat will increase satiety and prolong the onset of hunger pains.

Readily adaptable to family meals or public eating places. It is very important that the diet be practical or include foods that are readily available and exclude foods that are exotic or that the person does not like. Fad diets frequently consist of foods that are not readily available or are exotic.

Plateaus Periods during weight reduction in which the person is not losing weight.

In addition to planning the diet, it should be emphasized that dieter will reach **plateaus** in the weight loss period. It might help the dieter get through these periods if he or she understands why they occur in the first place. Essentially, plateaus result from the temporary increase and retention of water in the tissues. The increase in water results from the oxidation, or burning up, of fat tissue. Retention results because it takes water a long time to move from the tissues into the lymph and blood before it can be excreted by the kidneys.

INCREASE IN PHYSICAL ACTIVITY

An important accompaniment to a nutritional diet in losing weight is increasing physical activity. It is much easier to achieve a negative energy balance if one exercises rather than remaining sedentary. It is important to dispel the common myth that increasing exercise stimulates the appetite, making it more difficult to create a negative energy balance. Studies show that people who engage in moderate exercise such as running, swimming, or calisthenics for 1 hour/day do not experience an increase in appetite.[15] In fact, as mentioned earlier, the active individual is more sensitive to the appetite mechanism than the more sedentary person.

What kind of exercise is the most productive of weight loss? The answer is, many kinds. However, in deciding what exercise to engage in, the person should choose one that can be incorporated into the daily routine. Preferably, the exercise should employ large muscle groups and should be rhythmic. Walking, riding a bicycle, swimming, and running are ideal. Table 10-8 gives the amount of time required, when performing these activities, to burn up 3,500 kcal or to lose 1 lb. The minimum length of time that exercise should be engaged in is 20–30 minutes at least three times per week.[7]

BEHAVIOR MODIFICATION

The third and final component of a successful weight loss program is to identify unhealthy eating habits and then help the obese person to learn constructive behaviors. This component is critical to the long-term success of the weight loss program. Almost any person can diet for a period of time and lose a few pounds, but it is much more difficult to maintain the weight loss for an extended period of time.

TABLE 10-8 TIME REQUIRED TO BURN UP 3,500 KCAL WHEN PERFORMING CERTAIN ACTIVITIES

Activity	Time (hr)
Walking (3.5 mph)	11.2[a]
Riding bicycle	7.1[b]
Swimming	5.2[c]
Running	3.0[d]
Reclining	78.0[e]

[a]Energy cost of walking for a 70-kg person = 312 kcal/hr.
[b]Energy cost of riding a bicycle = 492 kcal/hr.
[c]Energy cost of swimming = 672 kcal/hr.
[d]Energy cost of running = 1,164 kcal/hr.
[e]Energy cost of reclining = 78 kcal/hr.

Source: F. Konishi, "Food and energy equivalents of various activities," Copyright The American Dietetic Association. Reprinted by permission from *Journal of the American Dietetic Association, 46,* 18 (1965).

Behavior modification An approach to the correction of undesirable eating habits. This procedure involves the manipulation of environmental and behavioral variables.

Food diary A record of what a person eats, the mood he or she is in while eating, and the circumstances in which eating occurs.

Stimuli Changes in an environmental condition that cause a response.

Three steps are often involved in **behavior modification** for weight control:

Keeping a food diary. Many obese people do not realize that have a tendency to eat foods at certain times when they are in various moods. Also, they do not realize that they frequently eat too fast and are not sensitive to satiety signals. In order to identify these factors, a person needs to keep a **food diary** (see Fig. 10-9). It enables the dieter to judge whether eating occurs because of hunger or in response to cues from the environment. Ultimately, the diary provides clues concerning what prompts the person to overeat.

Controlling the stimuli aassociated with eating. The second step involves designing the environment so that there is a decrease in the **stimuli** that prompt the person to eat. Examples are restricting meals to certain rooms at certain times and requiring the person to eat slowly and consume bulky foods first.

Reinforcement for appropriate behavior. This step involves a formal reward to appropriate behavior and should be something the individual prizes or enjoys doing.

The dieter may find that peer support is very helpful in behavior modification. Groups like Weight Watchers and Take Off Pounds Sensibly (TOPS) offer weekly meetings at which the person can receive support, evaluate the progress and become educated.

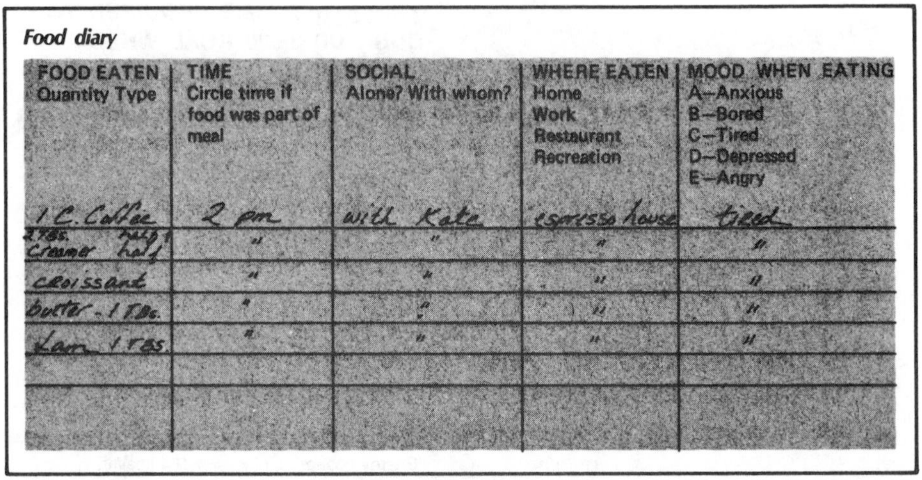

Food diary

FOOD EATEN Quantity Type	TIME Circle time if food was part of meal	SOCIAL Alone? With whom?	WHERE EATEN Home Work Restaurant Recreation	MOOD WHEN EATING A—Anxious B—Bored C—Tired D—Depressed E—Angry
1 C. Coffee 2 Tbs. milk creamer half	2 pm	with Kate	espresso house	tired
croissant	"	"	"	"
butter - 1 Tbs.	"	"	"	"
jam 1 tsp	"	"	"	"

FIGURE 10-9 An example of a food diary, which is important in behavior modification. (From Patricia J. Long, Barbara Shannon, *Focus on Nutrition,* © 1983, p. 173. Reprinted by permission of Prentice-Hall, Inc., Englewood Cliffs, N.J.)

UNDERWEIGHT, ANOREXIA NERVOSA, BULIMIA, AND BULIMAREXIA

UNDERWEIGHT

Underweight is defined as a body weight that is 15–20% below the ideal weight tables. People generally do not consider underweight to be a problem in the United States. Despite the view that underweight is not a problem and may even be healthy, research shows that underweight persons have decreased resistance to infection, tend to become easily fatigued, and are often sensitive to a cold environment.[7]

ANOREXIA NERVOSA

Anorexia nervosa A self-starvation disease that is characterized by severe disruption of the person's eating behavior.

Anorexia nervosa is actually a misnomer, since the person actually does not have a loss of appetite. Most anorexics are girls in their mid-teens and typically exhibit these characteristics:

- They are well educated.
- They have been raised in a middle- to upper-class family.
- They are preoccupied with thinness and exercise.
- They are highly competitive and perfectionistic.

Why would a girl with all these characteristics go on a starvation diet to the point where she might weigh only 65–70 lb and be on the verge of death? The answer is that this is a complicated psychological disorder. Psychologically, anorexics have a distorted perception of their body image and view themselves as fat even though they may have reached the lower end of their recommended weight range. This disorder is not a problem because of the mortality but rather because of the size of the population at risk. According to the American Psychiatric Association, as many as 1 out of every 250 girls between the ages of 12 and 18 may become anorectic every year.[16]

BULIMIA AND BULIMAREXIA

Bulimia An enormous appetite that is satisfied by eating binges.

Bulimarexia Purging of food.

Two complications of anorexia are **bulimia** and **bulimarexia.** An anorexic may eat several pounds of sweet, fattening foods. These binges are followed by bulimarexia, in which an attempt is made to remove the food from the body by inducing vomiting, taking large doses of laxatives, or using enemas. Bulimia is not as life-threatening as anorexia, but it can cause disturbances in electrolyte balance and dehydration.[3]

The treatment of an anorexic is a three-stage process. The first stage is restoration of normal nutrition. This step is often a problem, since the anorexic is not very receptive to voluntary eating. Hospitalization may be required, with either IV feeding by **hyperalimentation** or nasogatric tubes into the stomach. The advantage of these methods is that the patient cannot get rid of the nourishment by vomiting.[16]

Hyperalimentation Injection of hyperosmolar fluids directly into the superior vena cava vein.

Psychotherapy Any of a number of related techniques for treating mental illness by psychological methods. It is often used in the second stage of treating anorexia nervosa.

The second stage begins when the person's weight starts to return to normal and involves **psychotherapy.** This stage is critical to the long-term success of reversing anorexia nervosa. The individual and her family must be cooperative, must acknowledge the problem, and must motivate themselves to overcome it. Behavior modification and group therapy have been shown to be effective.

The third stage involves teaching the anorectic and her family proper nutritional concepts, as well as helping them eliminate misconceptions about nutrition.

OUTLINE

MEASUREMENT OF ENERGY

The kilocalorie (kcal) is the unit used to measure energy in nutrition; it is defined as the amount of heat required to raise the temperature of 1 kg of water 1°C.

ENERGY BALANCE

Energy balance is energy input minus energy expenditure.

Positive energy balance: energy input is greater than energy expenditure; if it continues, the person will gain weight. A 3,500-kcal surplus equals a gain of 1 lb.

Negative energy balance: energy expenditure is greater than energy input; if it continues, the person will lose weight. A 3,500-kcal deficit equals loss of 1 lb.

ENERGY EXPENDITURE

Basal Metabolic Rate (BMR)
Expenditure of energy for maintenance of homeostasis when the body is at rest. Factors that influence BMR are body surface area, sex, fever, hormones, age, pregnancy and lactation, fasting, and malnutrition. It decreases about 2% per decade.

Physical Activity
The actual amount of energy expended depends upon the involvement of the muscles, the weight of the person, and the length of time the activity is engaged in. BMR plus physical activity decreases by about 5% per decade.

Specific Dynamic Effect
This is energy expended in the digestion, absorption, and transport of nutrients. The amount of energy needed is 10% of the total kilocalories used for BMR plus physical activity.

CALCULATING TOTAL ENERGY REQUIREMENTS

Step 1. Multiply the weight of the person in kilograms by a factor (24 kcal/kg/day).
Step 2. Add a percentage to the BMR for the amount of physical activity (see text for specific percentages).
Step 3. Add a percentage for the specific dynamic effect of food.

A second method involves only one step, in which the ideal body weight is multiplied by a factor (see text for factors).

IDEAL OR DESIRABLE BODY WEIGHT AND BODY COMPOSITION

Ideal or Desirable Body Weight
This term is a misnomer, since there is no scientific evidence to determine the ideal or desirable body weight; medical personnel use weight tables published by Metropolitan Life Insurance Company as the guide to what is considered ideal or desirable body weight. See text for the rule-of-thumb method for estimating ideal weight.

Body Composition and Determination of Overweight
Body composition. A certain percentage of body weight should be fat for important functions; the normal percentages of body weight that should be fat and those that indicate obesity are as follows:

	Normal percentage of body weight that should be fat	Percentage of body weight from fat that indicates obesity
Men	15–20	25
Women	20–25	30

Four common methods are used to determine body composition and body fatness: densitometry, hydrometry, potassium-40 measurements, and anthropometric measurements. Anthropometric measurements, whereby calipers are used to measure the thickness of the skin on the back of the upper arm, are the most common method.

OVERWEIGHT AND OBESITY

Overweight is body weight that is more than 10% above ideal weight; obesity is body weight that is 15–25% above ideal weight, with 20% being the most common figure. Weights that are 30–100% above ideal weight are classified as severe obesity. Morbid obesity is more than 100% above normal.

Incidence of Obesity
From 25 to 30% of adults and at least 10% of children are overweight or obese. The incidence is higher in certain groups; for example, as black women have a higher percentage of obesity than white women.

Causes of Obesity
Metabolic (Internal) or Regulatory (External)
Metabolic Factors
Genetic: Evidence suggests that a person can be genetically predisposed to obesity, but the envi-

ronment ultimately determines whether or not the person becomes obese.

Fat Cell Theory: The number of fat cells in an infant is genetically determined. However, there are three periods when the number of fat cells can dramatically increase (hyperplasia)—the last 3 months of fetal life, the first 3 years of life, and adolescence. After 18 months of age, fat cells increase not only in number but also in size (hypertrophy). Obesity occurring during any of the three periods is called juvenile-onset obesity and can result in both hyperplasia and hypertrophy.

Physiological Factors: Obesity frequently results from an inadequate response to hunger and satiety signals. The hypothalamus region of the brain is where satiety and hunger signals are interpreted. Three theories on how the hypothalamus knows when the person is hungry or full are as follows:

1. Glucostatic Theory: The person feels full when the blood glucose level is high and hungry when it is low.
2. Lipostatic Theory: When the level of fat in fat cells is low, the brain interprets this condition as hunger; When the level of fat is high, the brain interprets this condition as satiety.
3. Set Point Theory: Each person has a set point weight. When he or she exceeds it, the hypothalamus recognizes the need to lose weight; likewise when body weight drops below the set point, the hypothalamus recognizes the need to gain weight.

Hormonal Theory
A low level of thyroxine can result in a lowered BMR and thereby in weight gain.

External Factors
Psychological Factors
Some people eat to satisfy needs other than hunger; this practice can lead to overconsumption and obesity.
Social Factors
Social and cultural habits consider overweight and obesity differently. Some cultures view obesity in a different manner than others. It is important for nutritionists to have access to the food patterns of major cultural groups in the United States in order to assess responses to diets and teach nutrition to patients.
Lack of Exercise
Probably the single most important factor in causing obesity is lack of activity. Many obese people consume less food than lean people, but they are so inactive that they still have a positive energy balance. Active people regulate their physiological appetite mechanism better than inactive ones.

NONRECOMMENDED TREATMENTS OF OBESITY

Claims made by fad diets that are nonrecommended methods for treatment of obesity are as follows:

- They promise ease and comfort in weight loss.
- They promise extremely rapid weight loss.
- They restrict or include only a few foods.
- They require the purchase of a secrete formula or magic pill.
- The diet is published in a book or magazine.

RECOMMENDED TREATMENT OF OBESITY

Nutritionally Balanced Diet
The diet should include all four food groups. The caloric level of the diet, to be adequate, should be no lower than 1,200 kcal a day, or 1,000 kcal at the very least.

Increase in Physical Activity
It is much easier to create a negative energy balance by increasing one's physical activity than by remaining less active. The physical activity the person decides to engage in should be one that can be easily built into the daily routine. The minimum length of time that exercise should be engaged in is 20–30 minutes at least three times per week.

Behavior Modification
This component involves identifying unhealthy eating habits and helping the obese person to learn constructive behaviors. Three steps are involved:

- Keeping a food diary. This record shows what a person eats, the mood at the time, and the circumstances.
- Controlling the stimuli associated with eating. The environment is modified to remove the stimuli that prompt the person to overeat.
- Reinforcement for appropriate behavior. The individual is rewarded for positive behavior in losing weight.

UNDERWEIGHT, ANOREXIA NERVOSA, BULIMIA, AND BULIMAREXIA

Underweight
This is body weight that is 15–20% below the ideal weight. Research shows that underweight persons have decreased resistance to infection, tend to become easily fatigued, and are often sensitive to a cold environment.

Anorexia Nervosa
This is a serious self-starvation disease. Most victims are girls who are well educated, raised in a

middle- to upper-class family, preoccupied with being thin and exercise, and highly competitive and perfectionistic. The cause is thought to be a psychological disorder; psychotherapy is very important in ultimately overcoming it.

Bulimia and Bulimarexia

These are two complications of anorexia, characterized by eating several pounds of food, followed by purging the body with laxatives, diuretics, and enemas.

Treatment is a three-stage process:

1. Restoration of normal nutrition. This frequently involves the use of nasogastric tubes or hyperalimentation.
2. Psychotherapy. This involves whole family in a process of psychotherapy, behavior modification, and group therapy.
3. Teaching proper nutritional concepts to the anorectic and her family and helping them clear up misconceptions about nutrition.

REVIEW QUESTIONS

TRUE (A) OR FALSE (B)

Questions 1–25

1. Energy in nutrition is measured by the kilocalorie (kcal).
2. If a person consumed 2,300 kcal/day and expended 3,000 kcal/day, he would have a positive energy balance and could gain weight.
3. The total expenditure of energy involves maintaining the BMR, physical activity, and specific dynamic action.
4. If two people each weigh 180 lb but Mr. A is 6 ft tall and Mr. B is 5 ft 8 in. tall, Mr. A would have a higher BMR.
5. After age 20 a person's BMR is stable and does not change.
6. If a person had a temperature of 102.6°F, his or her BMR will increase by about 10%.
7. The energy required to maintain the BMR in sedentary or moderately active people is very low (10–15%).
8. Ideal body weight figures are not scientifically based but rather are weights that will result in maximum longevity.
9. The so-called ideal weight tables assume that a weight that is ideal at age 25 should be maintained throughout life.
10. Ideally, a person's body weight should consist of as little fat as possible.

11. The body weight of a man is composed of 30% fat; therefore, he is obese.
12. One advantage of determining obesity by body composition (what percentage of the body weight is composed of fat) is that it allows one to distinguish overweight from overfat.
13. When using ideal weight tables, a person is classified as obese if his or her weight is 10% above ideal weight.
14. The factors that can lead to obesity are placed into two categories—metabolic and internal.
15. Children who inherit genes from obese parents are doomed to become obese despite their environment.
16. Three periods when the potential for fat cells to increase in number (hyperplasia) are the last 3 months of fetal development, the first 3 years of life, and adolescence.
17. Hunger is a physiological response to the body's need for food, and appetite is a learned psychological response to food.
18. The majority of obese cases are the result of malfunction of the physiological factors.
19. Most cases of obesity result from insensitivity to internal cues and susceptibility to external cues.
20. A decrease in people's physical activity has been accompanied by better control of the appetite mechanism.
21. The three recommended and proven methods for treatment of obesity are a diet that restricts or includes only a few foods, promises a slow, steady weight loss, and stresses the ease of losing weight.
22. If one needs 2,800 kcal to maintain ideal weight and reduces consumption to 1,800 kcal/day, one will be able to lose 4 lb/week.
23. Anorexia nervosa is a self-starvation disease that is typically found in well educated, middle- to upper-class girls.
24. Two complications of anorexia nervosa are bulimia (eating large quantities of food) and bulimarexia (purging by vomiting or taking laxatives or enemas).
25. The treatment of anorexia nervosa involves restoration of normal nutrition, psychotherapy, and teaching proper nutritional concepts to the anorectic and her family.

MULTIPLE CHOICE

Questions 26–33

26. Which of the following is (are) correct?
    1. The kilocalorie is the amount of energy required to raise the temperature of 1 kg of water 1°C.

2. The calorie is the amount of energy required to raise the temperature of 1 g of water 1°C.
3. The kilocalorie is the correct unit of energy measurement in nutrition.
4. The calorie is the energy measurement used by chemists and physicists.
   A. 1, 2, 3   B. 1, 3   C. 2, 4   D. 4
   E. all of these

27. If a person had an energy intake of 2,900 kcal/day and an energy expenditure of 2,400 kcal/day, the person would _____ per week.
   A. lose 1 lb
   B. gain 2 lb
   C. be in energy balance and gain no weight
   D. gain 1 lb
   E. none of these

28. Which of the following increase the BMR?
   1. increased surface area
   2. increasing age after 30
   3. pregnancy and lactation
   4. fasting
   A. 1, 2, 3   B. 1, 3   C. 2, 4   D. 4
   E. all of these

29. The energy expenditure of the body involves three components: _____ .
   1. appetite
   2. BMR
   3. physical activity
   4. specific dynamic action
   A. 1, 2, 3   B. 1, 3   C. 2, 3, 4   D. 4
   E. all of these

30. An estimate of the total energy requirements for a person who weighs 80 kg and is +30% for energy level and +10% for specific dynamic action is _____ kcal.
   A. 1,920
   B. 2,496
   C. 2,746
   D. 2,857

31. Ideal or desirable weight tables are
   1. very scientifically based
   2. based on a body weight of less than 1% fat
   3. based on the average weight of people in that age and height category
   4. weights for a particular height that result in the longest longevity
   A. 1, 2, 3   B. 1, 3   C. 2, 4   D. 4
   E. all of these

32. The percentage of body weight from fat that indicates obesity for men is _____ and for women is _____ .
   A. 15–20
   B. 25–15
   C. 10–30
   D. 25–30

33. The incidence and causes of obesity are:
   1. 25–30% in adults (obese or overweight).
   2. metabolic factors (genetic, physiological, and hormonal).
   3. regulatory (psychological, social, cultural, and lack of exercise).
   4. more common among women than among men.
   A. 1, 2, 3   B. 2, 4   C. 1, 3   D. 4
   E. all of these

MATCHING

Questions 34–38

___ 34. juvenile-onset obesity
___ 35. adult-onset obesity
___ 36. appetite
___ 37. hunger
___ 38. hypothalamus

A. physiological response to body's need for food
B. region of the brain that interprets hunger and satiety signals
C. learned psychological response to food
D. obesity beginning during any of three critical periods
E. results from hypertrophy of fat cells only

DISCUSSION QUESTIONS

1. Discuss why the term *ideal weight* is a misnomer and what it actually measures.
2. Discuss the four metabolic or internal causes of obesity.
3. Describe the three recommended treatments of obesity.
4. Define underweight. Describe anorexia nervosa, bulimia, and bulimarexia.

REFERENCES

1. C.J.W. Suitor and M.F. Crowley. *Nutrition: Principles and Application in Health Promotion*, 2nd ed. Philadelphia: J.B. Lippincott Co., 1984, pp. 79–81.
2. E.M. Hamilton and E.N. Whitney. *Nutrition: Concepts and Controversies*, 2nd ed. St. Paul, Minn.: West Publishing Co., 1982.
3. E.N. Whitney and C.B. Cataldo. *Understanding Normal and Clinical Nutrition*. St. Paul, Minn.: West Publishing Co., 1983.

4. *Texas Dietetic Association Diet Manual*, 3rd ed., Austin, TX, 1981, p. E-2.

5. F.J. Stare and M. McWilliams. *Living Nutrition*, 4th ed. New York: John Wiley & Sons, 1984, p. 152.

6. "Determining body frame size." *Nutrition and the M.D.*, 9,7, (1983).

7. E.R. Williams and M.A. Caliendo. *Nutrition: Principles, Issues, and Applications*. New York: McGraw-Hill Book Co., 1984.

8. T.B. Van Itallie. "Obesity: Adverse effects on health and longevity." *American Journal of Clinical Nutrition 32*, 2723 (1979).

9. J.H. Hines, "Infant feeding practices and obesity." *Journal of the American Dietetic Association 75*, 122–125 (1979).

10. L.B. Salans. "Natural history of obesity." In *Obesity in America*, G.A. Bray, ed. Public Health Service, National Institutes of Health, Washington, D.C., November 1979, pp. 69–94.

11. J. Hirsch and B. Batchelor. "Adipose tissue cellularity in human obesity." *Clinics of Endocrinology and Metabolism 5*, 299–311 (1976).

12. T.J. Coates and E.C. Thoresen. "Treating obesity in children and adolescents: A review." *American Journal of Public Health 68*, 143–151 (1979).

13. M. Lebow. "Can lighter become thinner?" *Addictive Behaviors 2*, 87 (1977).

14. M. Simonson. "Weight clinic at Johns Hopkins." *The Washington Post*, March 1, 1977, p. A-10.

15. F.I. Ketch and W.D. McArdle. *Nutrition Weight Control and Exercise*. Boston: Houghton Miffin, 1977.

16. R.G. Marks. "Anorexia and bulimia: Eating habits that can kill." *RN*, 47(1), 44–47 (1984).

11 NUTRITION DURING PREGNANCY AND LACTATION

OBJECTIVES

Upon completion of this chapter, you should be able to:

1. Give the RDA values for the following during pregnancy and lactation: energy (kilocalories) protein, iron and folacin, calcium, and phosphorus, plus vitamin D and other minerals.

2. State the function or importance of the above nutrients and energy in pregnancy and lactation.

3. Describe the symptoms of the fetal alcohol syndrome (FAS) and the typical woman who is most likely to have a FAS child.

4. Describe the causes, symptoms, and dietary treatment for nausea and vomiting and pregnancy-induced hypertension.

5. Describe why adolescent or teenage pregnancies are considered high-risk pregnancies.

6. Discuss the major complications of inadequate weight gain by teenagers during pregnancy.

INTRODUCTION

Miscarriage (spontaneous abortion) Interrupted pregnancy before the seventh month.

Premature (preterm) baby Birth of a baby prior to the 38th week of pregnancy.

Low birth weight (LBW) baby A baby that weighs less than 5.5 lb (2500 g.)

Stillborn infant A baby dead at birth.

Pregnancy-induced hypertension (PIH) Formerly called *toxemia of pregnancy* and characterized by proteinuria, hypertension, and edema.

Fetal alcohol syndrome (FAS) Characterized by growth retardation, physical deformities, behavioral defects, and mental retardation in a baby born to an alcoholic mother.

There is no period of a woman's life when nutrition is more important than during pregnancy. The fetus is totally dependent upon the nutritional status of the mother for its development. In addition to the development of the fetus, an optimum diet is important for the mother. Pregnancy brings about many physiological and psychological changes in the mother's body. An inadequate diet during pregnancy may not allow the mother's body to adapt to these changes, which could result in the following problems:

Miscarriage (spontaneous abortion). Interrupted pregnancy before the seventh month.

Premature (preterm) baby. Birth of a baby before the 38th week of pregnancy.

Low birth weight (LBW) baby. A baby that weighs less than 5.5 lb (2,500g).

Stillborn infant. A baby dead at birth.

Pregnancy-induced hypertension. Formerly called *toxemia of pregnancy* and characterized by proteinuria, hypertension, and edema.

Fetal alcohol syndrome (FAS). Characterized by growth retardation, physical deformities, behavioral defects, and mental retardation in a baby born to an alcoholic mother.

Nutrition is important not only during but also before pregnancy. If a woman has been well nourished from childhood through adolescence, she will need to make few changes in her diet during pregnancy, as discussed below.

NUTRITIONAL REQUIREMENTS DURING PREGNANCY AND LACTATION

Lactation Production of milk by the mammary glands.

The nutrient needs of a mother during pregnancy and **lactation** are higher for many nutrients than those of the nonpregnant woman. Table 11-1 presents the Recommended Dietary Allowances (RDAs) for pregnancy and lactation and compares them with those of nonpregnancy.

ENERGY (Kilocalories)

Requirements during Pregnancy

The energy needs of the mother during pregnancy are increased by about 300 kcal/day. Actually, this increase is not really required during the

TABLE 11-1 RECOMMENDED DIETARY ALLOWANCES FOR PREGNANCY, LACTATION, AND NONPREGNANCY

Nutrient	Nonpregnant Adult (23–50 Yr)	Nonpregnant Adolescent (15–18 Yr)	Pregnancy	Lactation
Calories	2,000	2,100	+ 300.0	+ 500.0
Protein (g)	44.0	46.0	+ 30.0	+ 20.0
Vitamin A (μg RE)[a]	800.0	800.0	+ 200.0	+ 400.0
Vitamin D (μg)	5.0	10.0	+ 5.0	+ 5.0
Vitamin E (mg αTE)[b]	8.0	8.0	+ 2.0	+ 3.0
Vitamin C (mg)	6.0	60.0	+ 20.0	+ 40.0
Thiamine (mg)	1.0	1.1	+ 0.4	+ 0.5
Riboflavin (mg)	1.2	1.3	+ 0.3	+ 0.5
Niacin (mg NE)[c]	13.0	14.0	+ 2.0	+ 5.0
Vitamin B_6 (mg)	2.0	2.0	+ 0.6	+ 0.5
Folacin (μg)	400.0	400.0	+ 400.0	+ 100.0
Vitamin B_{12} (μg)	3.0	3.0	+ 1.0	+ 1.0
Calcium (mg)	800.0	1,200.0	+ 400.0	+ 400.0
Phosphorus (mg)	800.0	1,200.0	+ 400.0	+ 400.0
Magnesium (mg)	300.0	300.0	+ 150.0	+ 150.0
Iron (mg)	18.0	18.0	+30–60.0	+30–60.0
Zinc (mg)	15.0	15.0	+ 5.0	+ 10.0
Iodine (μg)	150.0	150.0	+ 25.0	+ 50.0

[a]RE = μg retinol equivalents
[b]TE = mg alpha tocopherol equivalents
[c]NE = mg niacin equivalents
Source: Recommended Dietary Allowances, 9th rev. ed., National Academy of Sciences, Washington, D.C., 1980.

first 2 months of pregnancy.[1] During the first 2 months, the fetal and maternal changes are not as dramatic as they are from the third month through the rest of the pregnancy. The extra 300 kcal are important for the growth of the mother's uterus and **mammary glands,** and increasing blood volume. During the last **trimester,** the extra kilocalories are necessary for the growth of the placenta and fetus.

Mammary glands Specialized glands in the breasts that secrete milk during pregnancy.

Trimester A period of 3 months.

Many authorities recommend that the mother gain between 22–27 lb during pregnancy for the development of a healthy baby. More important than total weight gain is the pattern of gain. An ideal pattern of weight gain is as follows:

• First trimester—2- to 4-lb gain

• Second and third trimesters—$\frac{3}{4}$ to 1-lb gain per week[2]

A weight gain of over 1 lb/week is a clue that the woman is getting more kilocalories than she needs for healthy development of the baby. If this excess weight gain continues, the woman could have a postpregnancy overweight problem.

Requirement during Lactation

Notice that in Table 11-1 the recommended amount of energy for a woman who is lactating is +500 kcal/day compared to +300 kcal/day for pregnancy. The metabolic needs of a mother are actually higher during lactation than during pregnancy, hence the need for the recommended higher level of kilocalories.

The mother's breasts produce about 850 ml (3¾ cups) of milk per day for her nursing infant. The +500 kcal/day is actually not enough to produce the milk; approximately 750 kcal are required. The extra 250 kcal come from the body metabolizing fat that was stored during pregnancy. This stored fat will be used up in about 3 months; therefore, women who breast-feed may need to increase their kilocalorie intake at this point.[3]

PROTEIN

Requirement during Pregnancy

The protein requirement during pregnancy increases by 30 g/day. The increased protein is required for the increased blood volume, enlarged uterus and breasts, and, most importantly, for the synthesis of new tissues in the developing fetus.

Requirement during Lactation

During lactation the protein requirement is +20 g higher than the RDA for a nonlactating woman. The extra protein is important as a normal constituent in milk. Human milk has an average protein content of 1.2 g/dl.

The protein requirement is less for lactation than for pregnancy because fetal and maternal tissue growth is completed with the birth of the child.

IRON AND FOLACIN

Requirement during Pregnancy

Pregnancy results in an increased synthesis of red blood cells (RBCs) (erythropoiesis) in the mother; the fetus produces its own. These changes require increased amounts of iron, with some estimates being as high as 1,000 mg per pregnancy. Many women are iron deficient when they become pregnant. In addition, the average woman absorbs only about 1–2 mg iron per day from her diet, while needing about 3 mg. In order to compensate for the deficiency and the increased needs during pregnancy, the RDA is 30–60 mg of supplemental iron. As indicated, the iron should be in the form of supplementation, since nutritional experts do not feel that diet alone can supply this high level of iron.

Pregnancy requires more folacin than nonpregnancy primarily for increased RBC synthesis. The RDA for folacin during pregnancy is 800 μg, double the 400 μg recommended in nonpregnancy. As with iron, this recommended increase should come from supplements. The reason is that folacin is found primarily in liver, leafy green vegetables, and legumes, which usually cannot be consumed in large enough quantities to supply this high level of folacin.

Folacin and iron are the two nutrients most likely to be lacking during pregnancy. Some studies have shown that folacin-deficient mothers give birth to four times as many LBW infants as mothers with normal amounts of folacin.[4] In addition, studies of women who had moderate to severe iron deficiency during pregnancy had more LBW babies, stillborn babies, and babies who died soon after birth.[5]

Requirement during Lactation

Iron supplementation of 30–60 mg is recommended during lactation, primarily for replacement of iron stores lost during pregnancy. Notice that in Table 11-1 the RDA for folacin during lactation is only $+100\ \mu$g compared to $+400\ \mu$g for pregnancy. After birth, erythropoiesis, and therefore the need for folacin, decreases. The increased folacin during lactation is needed primarily to compensate for the amount secreted in breast milk.

CALCIUM, PHOSPHORUS, AND VITAMIN D

Requirement during Pregnancy

Calcium, phosphorus, and vitamin D are needed in increased amounts for bone formation in the fetus. Since calcium and phosphorus are deposited together in bones, the RDA of $+400$ mg/day is the same for both of them. Likewise, an increase in vitamin D of $+5\ \mu$g is recommended, since it is important for absorption and deposition of calcium and phosphorus.

These nutrients are important not only for the development of the fetal skeleton but also to prevent demineralization of the mother's bones. If the woman's diet is calcium deficient, calcium will be removed from her bones and used by the fetus.

Requirement during Lactation

Notice that in Table 11-1 the requirements for calcium, phosphorus, and Vitamin D during lactation are the same as those during pregnancy. The increased amounts after birth are needed to replace these nutrients that are secreted in breast milk. If the replacement is not accomplished during lactation, demineralization of the mother's skeleton will occur.

OTHER VITAMINS AND MINERALS

Requirement during Pregnancy

Vitamins B_6 and B_{12} are needed in increased amounts. Vitamin B_6 is important for increased protein synthesis in the fetus and mother. Vitamin B_{12} is important for increased RBC production and for the development and maintenance of the nervous system in the fetus and mother.

Increased amounts of vitamin C are important for absorption of iron and for the development of connective tissues and the walls of blood vessels in the fetus and mother. Niacin, thiamin, and riboflavin are required in increased amounts to help provide the increased kilocalories.

Vitamin A is needed in increased amounts for cell development and bone formation in the fetus. Vitamin E is important to help preserve tissue integrity and prevent the breakdown of RBCs.

Zinc in increased amounts is important, since it functions in many important enzyme reactions. The +20 mg of zinc is a higher amount than actually needed during pregnancy, but one must take into account the fact that it is poorly absorbed. Zinc deficiencies in experimental animal studies have resulted in increased fetal malformations.[6]

Iodine is needed in increased amounts of +25 μg for the production of extra thyroxine, which is important for the increased metabolic rate of the mother.

Requirement during Lactation

The RDA of vitamin B_6, like that of folacin, is lower during lactation than during pregnancy. Vitamins A, E, and C, thiamin, riboflavin, niacin, zinc, and iodide are all required in larger amounts during lactation than during pregnancy. The primary reason is their inclusion in breast milk. In addition, the increases in thiamin, riboflavin, and niacin are important for the increased energy needs during lactation.

PROPER DIET FOR PREGNANCY AND LACTATION

The RDAs for most of the previously discussed nutrients can be achieved by following a variation of the basic Four-Food Group Plan, as shown in Table 11-2. Important points about each group are discussed below.

Milk and milk products. Four servings of nonfat or skim milk, as opposed to whole milk, are recommended. They supply calcium and vitamin D.

Protein foods. Two 2-oz servings of animal protein are recommended, as is one serving of plant protein. For example, one cup of legumes supplies more vitamin B_6, folacin, iron, magnesium, and zinc than 2 oz of animal protein.

Fruits and vegetables. One serving of vitamin C–rich fruits and vegetables (e.g., broccoli, cauliflower, tomatoes); one serving of dark green vegetables, which supplies vitamin A and folacin; and one serving of other fruits and vegetables are recommended. Dark yellow fruits and vegetables are excellent sources of vitamin A.

Breads and cereals. Four servings of whole grain breads and cereals are recommended over white or enriched white, since they supply more zinc, magnesium, vitamin B_6, and folacin.

Other foods. Servings of the above foods will supply the RDAs for the essential nutrients but not enough kilocalories. To obtain enough kil-

TABLE 11-2 DAILY FOOD GUIDE FOR PREGNANCY AND LACTATION

Food Group	Number of Servings		
	Nonpregnant Woman	Pregnant Woman	Lactating Woman
Meat and meat substitutes	2	3	3
Milk and milk products	2	4	5
Fruits and vegetables			
Vitamin C and vegetables	1	1	1
Dark green vegetables	1	1	1
Other fruits and vegetables	1	1	1
Grains (breads and cereals)	4	4	4
Other foods	Foods from other groups can be added when above foods have been included. Foods from other groups help achieve the recommended daily kilocalorie level and add variety to meals.		

Source: R.B. Alfin-Slater, L. Aftergood, and J. Ashley, *Nutrition and Motherhood*, Van Nuys, Calif.: PM, Inc., © 1982, pp. 17–20.

ocalories, a person could consume more food from the above groups. In addition, fats, sugars, sweets, and desserts can be consumed.[7]

Most authorities do not feel that a pregnant woman can obtain enough folacin ($+800$ μg/day) and iron ($+30$–60 mg/day) from the diet alone; therefore, supplements are usually recommended. It should be stressed to the patient that iron supplements and pregnancy may cause constipation, which can be reduced by increasing the amount of fiber in the diet. If necessary, a stool softener or bulk-forming laxative may have to be used to alleviate the problem.

ALCOHOL USE DURING PREGNANCY

Much research has been done concerning the effects of alcohol on the development of the fetus during pregnancy. These studies indicate that chronic excess alcohol consumption during pregnancy can result in the fetal alcohol syndrome (FAS). A child diagnosed as having FAS exhibits many abnormalities, such as mental retardation, poor coordination, hyperactivity, facial abnormalities, and abnormal bone formation. FAS children typically are born to women who have had a history of alcoholism for about 7 years.

Much controversy exists about how much alcohol, if any, is safe for a pregnant woman to consume. No absolutely safe level has yet been established. However, consumption of alcohol by pregnant women is common. One study showed that 82% of 587 women consumed alcoholic beverages at least once during pregnancy. More than 10% had consumed 3 oz or more on a single occasion.[8]

Many nutritionists believe that since no absolutely safe level of alcohol consumption has been established, a pregnant woman should avoid alcohol totally during pregnancy.

PROBLEMS AND COMPLICATIONS OF PREGNANCY

NAUSEA AND VOMITING
(Morning Sickness)

Morning sickness Nausea and vomiting experienced by pregnant women.

Nausea and vomiting is often called **morning sickness;** however, it can occur at any time. It is almost unavoidable, since it results from hormonal increases that occur early in the first trimester. Unlike most nausea, relief from morning sickness is achieved by keeping a small amount of food in the stomach. One suggestion is that the meals be small and low in fat content. In addition, eating a few soda crackers or melba toast 15–30 minutes before getting out of bed and confining liquids to between-meal periods help to relieve morning sickness.

PREGNANCY-INDUCED HYPERTENSION (PIH)

Proteinuria The loss of protein in the urine.

PIH is characterized by hypertension, **proteinuria** (loss of protein in urine), edema, and, in severe cases, convulsions or coma. The traditional term for this condition, *toxemia of pregnancy*, is being phased out, since there are no toxins in the blood. There are two stages of PIH:

Preeclampsia Sudden high blood pressure or an increase of 20–30 mmHg in systolic pressure and 10–15 mmHg in diastolic pressure.

Eclampsia High blood pressure accompanied by convulsions and coma.

Preeclampsia. characterized by proteinuria in excess of 5 g in 24 hours and sudden edema in many parts of the body. It usually occurs during the last 20 weeks of pregnancy.

Eclampsia. symptoms of preeclampsia, but also accompanied by convulsions and possibly coma.[9]

Preeclampsia often occurs in women who have diabetes or hypertension. In addition, it is often seen in pregnant teenage girls and women from lower socioeconomic groups. The cause of preeclampsia is unknown, but possible nutritional reasons are low calcium intake, high sodium intake, decreased protein and kilocalorie intake, and general malnutrition.

Preeclampsia problems result from vasoconstriction of arteries, which reduces blood flow through the placenta to the fetus. Decreased blood flow can hinder proper growth and development of the fetus, with an increased risk of premature and stillborn births. This condition can generally be prevented by following an optimum diet for pregnancy.

Dietary treatment for preeclampsia in the acute phase involves parenteral solutions or intravenous infusion of nutrients (see Chapter 17 for details of parenteral nutrition). Women not in an acute phase have been found to benefit from a well-balanced diet somewhat high in protein (75–80 compared to 74 g), plus a high intake of calcium.[10]

TEENAGE PREGNANCY

Teenage pregnancy is considered a high-risk pregnancy. These girls are often characterized by their poor nutritional state when they become pregnant. They may be addicted to drugs, their bodies are still in a state of development, and they have financial and emotional problems that inhibit an optimal nutritional state.

It is ironic that these problems characterize pregnant teenagers, since their nutritional needs are greater than those of adult women, as shown in Table 11-1. Pregnant teenagers frequently do not gain the appropriate amount of weight for pregnancy due to societal pressure to be slim. A major complication of their inadequate weight gain is preeclampsia and LBW infants. In addition to the fact that these problems are higher in pregnant teenagers than older women, these girls have higher rates of premature births and of children born with birth defects and infections after birth.[11]

Pregnant teenagers need intensive and repeated counseling in terms of an optimal diet for the development of their own bodies and, just as importantly, for the proper growth and development of their babies. Vitamin and mineral supplements are especially important for this age group. However, many adolescents do not want to take pills. Therefore, it is essential that they understand that some nutrients cannot be obtained in adequate amounts except in the form of supplements.

OUTLINE

INTRODUCTION

The fetus is totally dependent upon the mother for nutrition during pregnancy.

Inadequate diet can result in the following problems:

- Miscarriage: interrupted pregnancy before the seventh month.
- Premature (preterm) baby: birth of baby before the 38th week of pregnancy.
- Low birth weight (LBW) baby: a baby that weighs less than 5.5 lb (2,500 g) at birth.
- Stillborn infant: a baby dead at birth.
- Pregnancy-induced hypertension (PIH): formerly called *toxemia of pregnancy* and characterized by hypertension, proteinuria, and edema.
- Fetal alcohol syndrome (FAS): characterized by growth retardation, physical deformities, behavioral defects, and mental retardation in a baby born to an alcoholic mother.

NUTRITIONAL REQUIREMENTS DURING PREGNANCY AND LACTATION

Energy (Kilocalories)
Requirement during Pregnancy
A level of +300 kcal/day is recommended above the RDA for the age group; kilocalories are important during the second trimester for growth of the mother's uterus, mammary glands, and increasing blood volume; they are important during third trimester for growth of the placenta and fetus.

The recommended weight gain is 22–27 lb. The pattern of weight gain is as follows:

First trimester: 2–4 lb

Second and third trimesters: ¾- to 1-lb gain per week

Requirement during Lactation
A level of +500 kcal is required for production of milk. Milk synthesis actually requires 750 kcal to produce 850 ml milk per day; the extra 250 kcal come from the body metabolizing fat stored during pregnancy.

Protein
Requirement during Pregnancy
A level of +30 g/day is required. It is important for the mother's increased blood volume, enlarged uterus and breasts, and synthesis of new tissues in the developing fetus.

Requirement during Lactation
A level of +20 g higher than the RDA/day is required. It is important as a constituent in breast milk.

Iron and Folacin
Requirement during Pregnancy
A level of +30 to +60 mg of supplemental iron per day is required. It is important for increased synthesis of RBCs (erythropoiesis) in the mother and fetus.

A level of +800 μg of supplemental folacin per day is required. It is important for erythropoiesis.

These two nutrients are most likely to be lacking during pregnancy. Folacin deficiency may cause mothers to give rise to LBW infants. Moderate to severe iron deficiency during pregnancy may give rise to greater numbers of LBW babies, stillborn babies, and babies who died soon after birth.

Requirement during Lactation
Iron: +30 to +60 mg over the RDA is important for replacement of iron stores lost during pregnancy.

Folacin: +100 μg over the RDA is important for replacement of maternal folacin that is secreted in breast milk.

Calcium, Phosphorus, and Vitamin D
Requirement during Pregnancy
Calcium and phosphorus: +400 mg/day is required. It is important for development of the fetal skeleton.

Vitamin D: +5 μg/day is required. It is important for absorption and deposition of calcium and phosphorus in the bones of the fetus.

Requirement during Lactation
Requirements for all three are the same as for pregnancy. They are important for replacement of the amounts that are secreted in breast milk.

Other Vitamins and Minerals
Requirement during Pregnancy

Vitamin B_6: increased amounts over the RDA are important for increased protein synthesis.

Vitamin B_{12}: this is important for increased RBC synthesis and for development and maintenance of the nervous system in the fetus and mother.

Vitamin C: increased amounts are important for the development of connective tissues and the walls of blood vessels in the fetus and mother.

Niacin, thiamin, and riboflavin: increased amounts are important to help provide increased kilocalories.

Vitamin A: increased amounts are important for cell development and bone formation in the fetus.

Vitamin E: increased amounts help to preserve tissue integrity and prevent breakdown of RBCs.

Zinc: increased amounts are important for many enzyme reactions.

Iodine: it is important for increased synthesis of thyroxine and metabolism.

Requirement during Lactation

Vitamin B$_6$: the RDA is lower during lactation than pregnancy.

Vitamins A, E, and C, thiamin, riboflavin, niacin, zinc, and iodide are all required in larger amounts during lactation than during pregnancy for inclusion in breast milk.

PROPER DIET FOR PREGNANCY AND LACTATION

Table 11-2 presents the number of food servings for the basic Four Food Groups.

- Milk and milk products: three servings of nonfat or skim milk as opposed to whole milk are recommended.
- Protein foods: two servings should be animal protein and one serving should be plant protein.
- Fruits and vegetables: one serving of vitamin C–rich fruits and vegetables (broccoli, cauliflower, and tomatoes), one serving of dark green vegetables, and one serving of other fruits and vegetables are recommended.
- Breads and cereals: four servings of whole-grain breads and cereals are recommended over white or enriched white, since they supply more zinc, magnesium, vitamin B$_6$, and folacin.
- Other foods: servings of other foods supply the necessary kilocalories that the above foods do not provide.

Alcohol Use during Pregnancy

Chronic alcohol consumption can result in fetal alcohol syndrome (FAS); abnormalities of FAS are mental retardation, poor coordination, hyperactivity, facial abnormalities, and abnormal bone formation.

How much alcohol consumption is safe during pregnancy is very controversial. Some professionals recommend no consumption of alcohol at all.

PROBLEMS AND COMPLICATIONS OF PREGNANCY

Nausea and Vomiting (Morning Sickness)

Suggestions that can help alleviate this problem are frequent small meals, eating a few soda crackers or melba toast before getting out of bed, and confining liquids to between-meal periods.

Pregnancy-Induced Hypertension (PIH)

It was formerly called *toxemia of pregnancy*. There are two stages:

- Preeclampsia: sudden high blood pressure, proteinuria in excess of 5 g in 24 hours, and sudden edema in many parts of the body.
- Eclampsia: includes the symptoms of preeclampsia but is also accompanied by convulsions and possibly coma.

Preeclampsia often occurs in women who have diabetes or hypertension, teenage mothers, and women from lower socioeconomic groups.

Problems result from vasoconstriction of arteries, which reduces blood flow through the placenta to the fetus. It can hinder proper growth and development of the fetus, with increased risk of premature and stillborn births.

Dietary treatment in the acute phase involves parenteral or intravenous solutions. Women not in the acute phase have been found to benefit from a well-balanced diet somewhat higher in protein (75–80 g) plus a high intake of calcium.

Teenage Pregnancy

This is considered a high-risk pregnancy. These girls are in a poor nutritional state. They may be addicted to drugs, and their bodies are still in a state of development. Financial plus emotional problems inhibit an optimal nutritional state.

The nutritional needs of teenage mothers are higher than those of older pregnant women. They frequently do not gain an appropriate amount of weight due to pressures to be slim. The major complications of inadequate weight gain in pregnant teenagers are preeclampsia, LBW infants, and higher rates of children born with birth defects, premature births, and infections after birth.

REVIEW QUESTIONS

TRUE (A) OR FALSE (B)

Questions 1–16

1. An ideal pattern of weight gain for a pregnant woman is to gain most of her weight during the first trimester, when the fetus is growing rapidly.
2. A weight gain of over 1 lb/week indicates that a woman is consuming more kilocalories than needed for healthy development of the baby.
3. The recommended kilocalorie intake during

lactation is higher than during pregnancy, since the mother's metabolism is higher in order to produce milk.

4. The RDA for energy (+500 kcal) during lactation is more than adequate for the production of 850 ml of breast milk per day.

5. The purpose of the +30 g of protein per day in the daily diet of a pregnant woman is for the synthesis of new tissues in the fetus.

6. Nutritionists do not feel that a pregnant woman should take iron pills if she consumes a large amount of iron-rich foods.

7. An increased intake of folacin is recommended during pregnancy due to its importance for increased RBC synthesis by the mother and fetus.

8. Increased intake of folacin during lactation is recommended primarily to compensate for the amount the mother secretes in breast milk.

9. Calcium, phosphorus, and vitamin D in increased quantities during pregnancy and lactation help to prevent demineralization of the mother's skeleton.

10. A pregnant teenager who is a vegetarian and does not believe in taking any vitamin tablets should be able to achieve an adequate diet.

11. A proper diet for pregnancy should contain both animal and plant proteins to provide folacin, iron, magnesium, and zinc.

12. In a diet for pregnancy, more servings of milk and milk products are recommended than in a diet for nonpregnant women.

13. FAS children are frequently born to women who consume as little as two drinks daily during pregnancy.

14. Nausea and vomiting (morning sickness) is unavoidable, since it results from hormonal increases in the first trimester of pregnancy.

15. PIH is always a result of excessive sodium and low protein intake.

16. Teenage pregnancies are of low risk, since the mother's body is strong and able to withstand the stress of pregnancy.

MULTIPLE CHOICE

Questions 17–25

17. The recommended increase of +300 kcal/day for a pregnant woman is important for:

1. growth of the uterus
2. growth of the fetus
3. growth of the placenta
4. increasing the strength of the mother's abdominal muscles

A. 1, 2, 3   B. 1, 3   C. 2, 4   D. 4
E. all of these

18. Since the pattern of weight gain is more important than the total amount gained, at the end of the first trimester (3 months) a pregnant woman should have gained _____ .
A. ¾ to 1 lb/week, therefore 12 lb
B. one-third of 22–27 lb, or 7–9 lb
C. 2–4 lb
D. as little as possible

19. The recommended protein increase in a pregnant woman's diet is _____ , which can be partially achieved by _____ _____ servings of protein foods.
A. +20 g—two
B. +50 mg—three
C. +400 μg—four
D. +30 g—three

20. Iron and folacin should be increased in the diet of a breast-feeding mother for the purpose of _____ and are best supplied by _____ .
A. replacing the amounts lost during pregnancy and secreted in breast milk—taking iron and folacin supplements
B. increasing RBC synthesis in the mother and fetus—consuming foods that are rich in iron and folacin
C. increasing the blood volume in the mother—eating liver and leafy green vegetables
D. none of these

21. A proper diet for a pregnant woman is _____ _____
A. milk—four servings
   protein foods—three servings
   fruits and vegetables—three servings
   breads and cereals—four servings
   other foods—enough servings to achieve kilocalorie requirements
B. milk—two servings
   protein foods—two servings
   fruits and vegetables—four servings
   breads and cereals—four servings
   other foods—should not consume foods other than those above

22. FAS children exhibit abnormalities such as _____ .
A. mental retardation
B. hyperactivity
C. facial abnormalities
D. all of these

23. The preeclampsia stage of PIH is characterized by:

1. convulsions
2. proteinuria
3. coma
4. sudden high blood pressure

A. 1, 2, 3   B. 1, 3   C. 2, 4   D. 4
E. all of these

275

24. Dietary treatment for preeclampsia involves
_____ .
   - A. parenteral solutions and a balanced diet high in carbohydrate and fats
   - B. parenteral solutions and a balanced diet high in protein and calcium
   - C. a low-carbohydrate, high-liquid, high-vitamin diet
   - D. none of these

25. Teenage pregnant girls are characterized by:
   1. having nutritional needs greater than those of an adult woman
   2. frequently not gaining an appropriate amount of weight
   3. frequently being in a poor nutritional state at the time they become pregnant
   4. often requiring counseling in regard to an optimal diet for pregnancy
   - A. 1, 2, 3   B. 1, 3   C. 2, 4   D. 4
   - E. all of these

DISCUSSION QUESTIONS

1. Give the RDA values during pregnancy and lactation and the function or importance of energy, protein, iron, and folacin.
2. Give the proper amounts of servings from the Four Food Groups for pregnancy and lactation.
3. Describe the causes, symptoms, and dietary treatment of PIH.
4. Discuss the major complications that may occur if pregnant teenagers fail to gain an adequate amount of weight.

REFERENCES

1. R.M. Pitkin. "Assessment of nutritional status of mother, fetus, and newborn." *American Journal of Clinical Nutrition, 34* (supplement), 658 (1981).
2. R.M. Pitkin. "What's new in maternal nutrition." *Nutrition News, 42,* 5 (1979).
3. W.L. Scheider. *Nutrition: Basic Concepts and Applications.* New York: McGraw-Hill Book Co., 1983, p. 313.
4. "Influences of folic acid on infant birthweight and growth." *Nutrition and the M.D., 3* (6), 1 (1977).
5. E.R. Williams and M.A. Caliendo. *Nutrition: Principles, Issues, and Applications.* New York: McGraw-Hill Book Co., 1984, p. 403.
6. H.A. Kaminetzky and H. Baker. "Micronutrients in pregnancy." *Clinical Obstetrics and Gynecology, 20,* 363 (1977).
7. R.B. Alfin-Slater, L. Aftergood, and J. Ashley. *Nutrition and Motherhood.* Van Nuys, Calif.: PM, Inc., 1982, p. 17.
8. "Alcohol and pregnancy." *Nutrition and the M.D., 10* (8), 3 (1984).
9. "Hypertension in pregnancy." *American Journal of Nursing, 82* (5), 791 (1982).
10. B.G. Morrissey. *Therapeutic Nutrition.* Philadelphia: J.B. Lippincott Co., 1984, p. 405.
11. J.T. Snook. *Nutrition: A Guide to Decision Making.* Englewood Cliffs, N.J.: Prentice-Hall, Inc., 1984, p. 353.

12 NUTRITION DURING INFANCY, CHILDHOOD, AND ADOLESCENCE

OBJECTIVES

Upon completion of this chapter, you should be able to:

1. Discuss the advantages of breast feeding compared to bottle feeding.

2. Describe changes in cow's milk to resemble breast milk more closely.

3. Give two reasons for adding solid foods to a baby's diet and a possible schedule for introduction of solid foods.

4. Discuss food allergies, colic, PKU, and diarrhea in terms of the possible causes and dietary treatment of each.

5. Describe the changes and dietary needs of toddlers, preschoolers, and school-age children.

6. Discuss how kilocalories, protein, and minerals are important in the diet of adolescents.

7. Describe the relationship of acne and diet in adolescents.

8. Discuss obesity, anorexia nervosa, and dental caries in terms of possible causes and dietary treatment in adolescents.

NUTRITION DURING INFANCY

Infancy The period from time of birth through the first year.

Infancy is the period from the time of birth through the first year. An infant grows at a fantastic rate, with the weight usually doubling at 6 months of age and being triple the birth weight by 1 year. In other words a child who weighed 7 lb at birth should weigh 14 lb at 6 months and 21 lb by 1 year. Nutrition is essential for an infant to grow at these rates.

FIRST FOODS FOR THE INFANT

Whether a woman breast-feeds or bottle-feeds the infant, the initial source of nutrients is milk. Many authorities recommend breast feeding as the best means of feeding the infant. Breast milk contains most of the important nutrients in appropriate amounts to support the growth and development of the infant (see Fig. 12-1). Proteins and carbohydrates in breast milk are in a form that allows easier digestion and absorption. Cholesterol is higher in breast milk than cow's milk, which is important for the production of nerve tissue and bile. Vitamin C is higher in breast milk than cow's milk. However, vitamin D is usually less than the Recommended Dietary Allowance (RDA) in breast milk. This deficiency can usually be overcome by exposing the infant to sunlight for short periods of time. However, if the infant is rarely exposed to sunlight because of climate or clothing, a vitamin D deficiency is possible. Vitamin B_{12} can be deficient in breast milk, especially if the mother is a true vegetarian or vegan and is not supplementing her diet.

Calcium and phosphorus are present in breast milk in the more desirable calcium:phosphorus ratio of 2:1 compared to 1:1 to 1:1.5 in many formulas. This ratio is beneficial to the infant's bone and teeth growth, normal cellular functions, and enzymatic reactions.

Besides vitamin D, four other nutrients that are lower in breast milk compared to cow's milk are sodium, potassium, chloride, and iron. Sodium, potassium, and chloride are approximately three times lower in breast milk compared to cow's milk. The advantage is that there is less stress on the infant's kidneys in regulating their level. The lower level of iron in breast milk may seem to be a detriment; however, approximately 49% of this iron is absorbed compared to about 10% of the iron in cow's milk.

One of the most important advantages of breast feeding is the immunologic effects it offers. Breast milk contains antibodies that protect the infant against many infections that invade through the gastrointestinal tract. In addition to having fewer infections, breast-fed infants have fewer allergic reactions even if there is a family history of such disorders.[1]

Some studies indicate that breast feeding prevents infantile obesity. One reason is that a breast-fed baby feeds only when he or she is hungry,

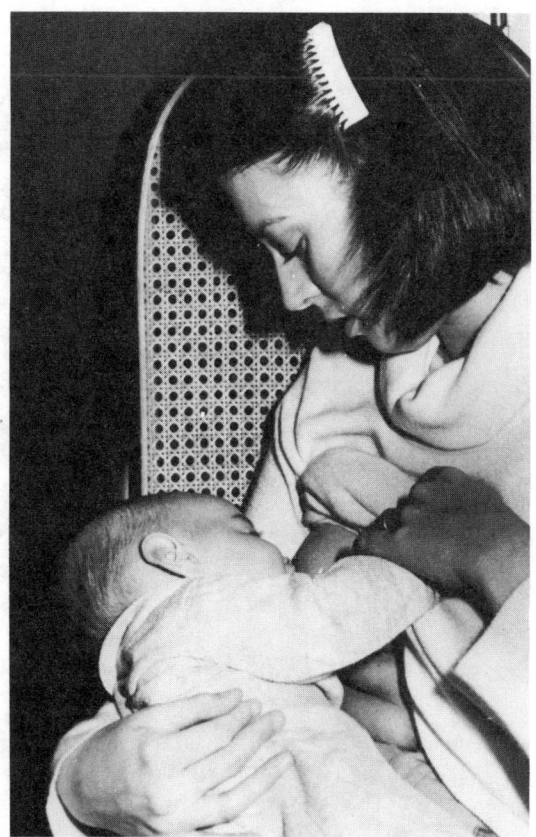

FIGURE 12-1   Breast feeding. (From McFarlane, J.M., Whitson, B.J., and Hartley, L.M. *Contemporary Pediatric Nursing: A Conceptual Approach.* New York: John Wiley & Sons, Inc., © 1980. Reprinted with permission.)

whereas parents often require a bottle-fed baby to consume all of the bottle even though the infant may be already full.

One nonnutritional benefit of breast feeding is the promotion of **bonding** between the mother and child. This psychological value is beneficial to both the mother and the child. However, parents who elect to bottle-feed their infant can also achieve this bonding by holding, kissing, touching, and talking to the infant (see Fig. 12-2).

Breast feeding offers the following advantages to the mother:

Uterine contraction. The enlarged uterus will undergo **involution** more rapidly because breast feeding stimulates the release of **oxytocin,** which promotes uterine contraction.

Weight loss. The loss of weight gained during pregnancy is increased

Bonding   The formation of an emotional link between the mother and the infant.

Involution   The contraction of the enlarged uterus after birth.

Oxytocin   A pituitary hormone that stimulates uterine contractions.

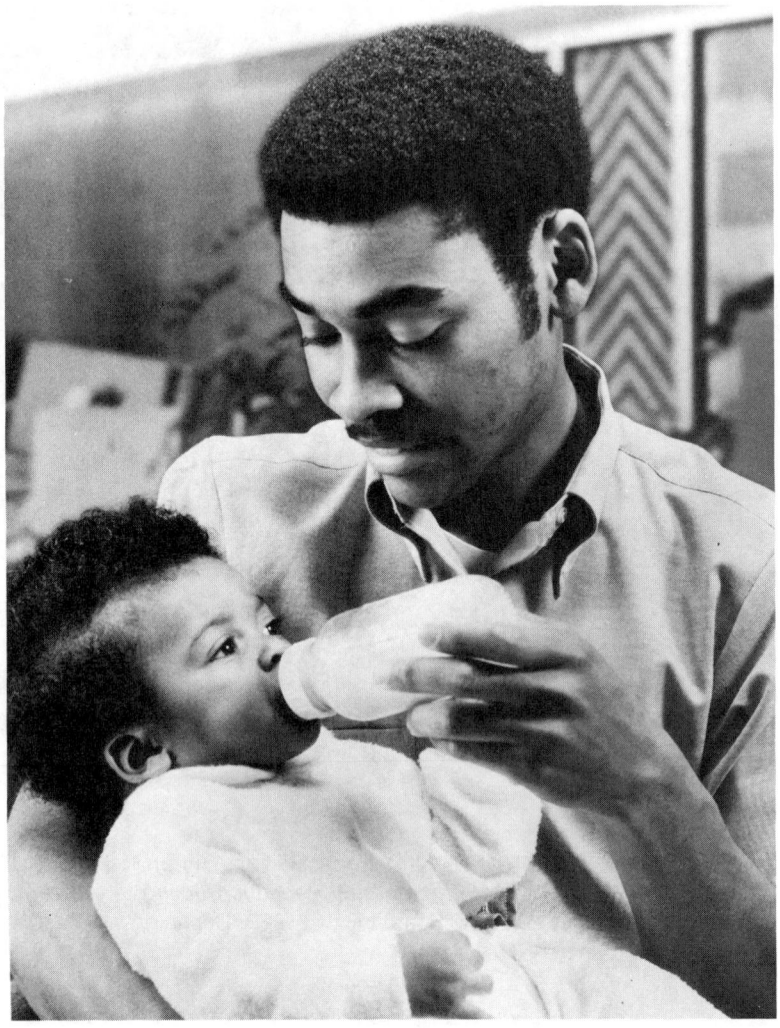

FIGURE 12-2 Bottle feeding. (Courtesy of Gerber Foods.)

by breast feeding, assuming the mother does not consume too many kilocalories, since her metabolic needs are high.

Lower cost. Breast feeding is more economical than buying commercial formulas, despite the fact that the mother must consume more food for milk production.

While breast feeding has many advantages for both the mother and the child, there are some conditions in which it is not advisable. If the mother has a poor nutritional status, her ability to form milk with the proper level of nutrients is hindered.

DDT (dichloro diphenyl trichloroethane) An insecticide that is toxic to insects and humans. It has been found in human breast milk.

Polychlorinated biphenyls (PCBs) Chemicals used in the manufacture of plastics. They are not biodegradable and have been found in breast milk.

Psychotherapeutics Drugs used in the treatment of manic-depressive illness.

If a mother is exposed to large amounts of environmental chemicals such as **DDT** and **polychlorinated biphenyls (PCBs),** she should consider bottle feeding. The reason is that these chemicals have been found in breast milk. In addition, if a lactating woman is on a crash diet, increased fat metabolism and possibly increased release of PCBs from fat tissues will occur.

Women who drink alcohol or consume large amounts of caffeine, nicotine, and **psychotherapeutic** drugs (e.g., lithium) should be aware that these substances will be transmitted in breast milk.

If a mother is overanxious, has no desire, or cannot conveniently breast feed because she is employed outside the home, she may transmit feelings of hostility and anxiety, rather than love, to the infant.

As discussed above, there are certain conditions in which formula feeding is better than breast feeding. Each formula contains cow's milk that has been modified to closely resemble breast milk. For example, proteins have been altered so that they can be more easily digested. In addition, saturated butterfat is replaced by unsaturated vegetable oil. All brands are fortified with vitamins and are available with or without iron fortification.

Some infants are sensitive to protein in formulas; therefore, milk substitute formulas such as soybean preparations are available.

Skim milk should not be used in infant feeding, since it lacks the essential fatty acid linoleic acid and kilocalories.

INTRODUCTION OF SOLID FOODS (Beikost)

Adding solid foods to a baby's diet should be based on two considerations:

• Supplying increasing amounts of nutrients that milk alone cannot supply.
• Supplying the foods in a form the baby is physically able to handle.

Some parents want to introduce solid foods when an infant is only 1 month old. This early introduction of solid food presents several problems. One problem is that babies do not develop voluntary swallowing movements until they are about 3–4 months old. Also, with early introduction of solid foods, salivary amylase for digestion of starches is not present until the second or third month, and the ability of the kidneys to handle an increased level of wastes is not developed until the end of the second month.

Most physicians recommend that solid foods not be introduced until the infant is 4–6 months of age. The Nutrition Committee of the American Academy of Pediatrics recommends that solid foods not be introduced before 3 months of age.[2] One possible schedule for introduction of solid foods is as follows:

Month	Food
4	Cereal
5–6	Strained vegetables
6–7	Strained fruits
6–8	Finger foods (crackers, bananas, etc.)
7–8	Strained meat
10	Strained or mashed egg yolk
10	Bite-sized cooked foods

Cereals are usually introduced first because of their ease of digestion. They are an excellent source of B vitamins and iron (see Fig. 12-3). Rice cereal is a good first choice, since it usually does not cause food allergies. Vegetables are frequently introduced before fruits because they are harder to "learn" to like than the sweeter fruits. When fruits are introduced first, mothers often complain that the baby will not eat vegetables. The reason is that all babies like the sweet taste of fruits and frequently do not care for the taste of vegetables when they are introduced second.

Egg whites are generally not recommended until after 1 year of age.

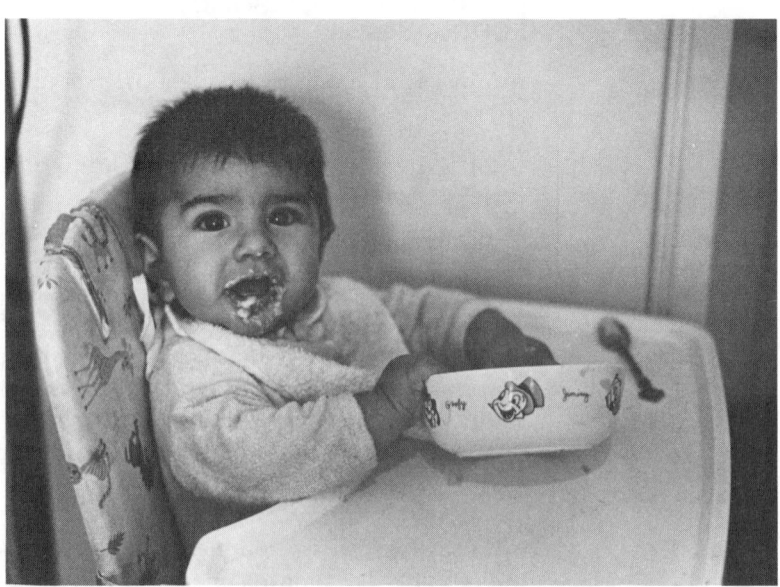

FIGURE 12-3 Cereal is an excellent source of the B vitamins and iron for an infant. (Courtesy of Barbara Rios.)

The reason is that infants are frequently allergic to egg whites but not to egg yolks.

While some parents want to introduce solid foods too early, others delay introduction past the age of 6 months. This situation is more common with breast-fed than bottle-fed children. There are two problems with this delay. First, breast milk is low in iron, especially in comparison to what the infant needs by 6 months of age. Second, breast milk may not contain enough protein for the needs of the infant after 6 months.

INFANT PROBLEMS RELATED TO NUTRITION

Food Allergy

An infant who is allergic to a food develops antibodies to that food. The antibodies are formed by the body to attack and destroy the food, which is the equivalent of an antigen.

Unfortunately, this antigen–antibody response causes serious symptoms in the infant, including **hives** (itching and burning swelling of the skin), **eczema** (redness and small blisters on the skin), **bronchitis, asthma,** coughing, sneezing, diarrhea, and **colic.** It is common for allergic symptoms to appear during the early months of life.

Some of the more common nutrients that infants are allergic to are cow's milk protein, egg protein, wheat protein, and compounds in orange juice. Treatment of allergies involves identification and elimination of the suspected food from the infant's diet. Infants from families with a history of allergies should be breast-fed for the first 4–6 months. Infants who are allergic to cow's milk can be given a milk-free formula such as a soybean formula. Sometimes children outgrow allergies; therefore, the offending food, especially cow's milk, should be reintroduced at a later time.

Colic

Colic, usually seen in infants less than 3 months old, is characterized by profuse crying after eating. Most often the cause is overfeeding with formula. Bacteria often ferment the excess milk, resulting in gas buildup. Dietary adaptations include diluting formula with water, avoiding the use of complex carbohydrates, burping the infant frequently, and experimenting with the temperature of the formula, since an infant sometimes tolerates a cold formula better than a warm one.

Phenylketonuria

Phenylketonuria (PKU) is called a **congenital metabolic disorder** or **inborn error of metabolism.** This means that the infant is born with the

Hives Itching and burning swellings of the skin.

Eczema Redness and small blisters on the skin.

Bronchitis Inflammation of the bronchi, the passageways to the lungs (see Chapter 22).

Asthma A respiratory condition, characterized by recurrent attacks of wheezing, that may be due to bronchitis.

Colic A spasm in an organ accompanied by pain.

Phenylketonuria (PKU) A disorder in an infant caused by the absence of the enzyme phenylalanine hydroxylase, which oxidizes phenylalanine to tyrosine.

Congenital metabolic disorder An inherited metabolic disorder that a child is born with, such as phenylketonuria (PKU).

Inborn error of metabolism The same as a congenital metabolic disorder.

Phenylalanine hydroxylase An enzyme that synthesizes tyrosine from phenylalanine.

Tyrosine A nonessential amino acid.

Phenylalanine An essential amino acid.

problem, which consists of a lack of the enzyme **phenylalanine hydroxylase.** This enzyme functions in the synthesis of the amino acid **tyrosine** from **phenylalanine.** The resulting excess buildup of phenylalanine can result in hyperactivity, irritability, and ultimately mental retardation if left untreated.

The dietary treatment for PKU is a low-phenylalanine diet. Since phenylalanine is an essential amino acid important for tissue synthesis, it cannot be totally eliminated. However, foods rich in phenylalanine such as milk can be reduced in the infant's diet. A milk substitute formula that is 95% free of phenylalanine (Lofenalac) is used in the treatment of PKU. Small amounts of milk are mixed with the formula to provide the needed amount of phenylalanine.

The introduction of solid foods to the diet is done according to phenylalanine exchange food lists. The foods, such as cereals, vegetables, and fruits, provide small amounts of phenylalanine. Meat, fish, poultry, and dairy products are high in phenylalanine and have to be restricted.[3]

Diarrhea

One of the most common causes of diarrhea is overfeeding. Inflammation of the intestinal wall accompanies diarrhea, along with temporary loss of the enzyme lactase, which digests lactose in milk. Because of the loss of lactase, consumption of milk when an infant has diarrhea will only worsen the problem. Dietary treatment of diarrhea in an infant consists of replacement of lost fluids and electrolytes (sodium, chloride, potassium), using a solution such as Pedialyte or Lytren. As the diarrhea subsides, the enzyme lactase reappears, and progression to a dilute formula and finally to a full formula should follow.

Diarrhea can result from many problems, such as allergies and intestinal infections in infants. They should never be taken lightly, since the infant can become dehydrated and even die. If an infant's diarrhea does not improve in approximately 24 hours, a physician should be consulted.

NUTRITION DURING CHILDHOOD

Childhood is the stage of the life cycle that extends from infancy to adolescence and can be subdivided into the toddler, preschool, and school-age periods.

TODDLERS

Toddlers Children from 1 to 3 years of age.

The growth rate of **toddlers** slows down, causing their appetite and consumption of food to decrease. Parents should be aware that these changes are normal and should not be overly concerned that the toddler does not seem to be eating enough.

Although the toddler is not growing as rapidly as during infancy, important muscle changes are occurring. The muscles of the back, buttocks, and thighs are enlarging and strengthening as the toddler begins to stand erect and walk. Much body fat is lost as the muscles increase in size and the bones become harder. The body shape changes from a rather chubby to a more lean appearance.

Muscle control continues to develop, especially fine motor movements. Handling of eating utensils increases, as well as a desire to become independent. As a result, toddlers want to feed themselves but may not be able to do so successfully. The desire for independence is often exhibited by avoiding nutritious foods (e.g., vegetables) and preferring nonnutritious foods such as sweets.

Toddlers tend to imitate adult behavior. Therefore, if parents observe good food habits, they are likely to integrate them into their own behavior.

Diet

The Four-Food Group plan is the basis of dietary planning for toddlers, with a recommended pattern being the following:

Food Group	Number of servings	Portion Size
Milk	3	Cup
Meat and meat substitutes	2	1–2 oz
Fruits/vegetables	4	$\frac{1}{2}$ cup for vegetables $\frac{1}{2}$ cup for fruits
Bread/cereal	4	$\frac{1}{2}$ to 1 slice of bread $\frac{1}{2}$ cup of ready-to-eat cereal $\frac{1}{4}$ to $\frac{1}{2}$ cup of spaghetti and macaroni
Fat	3	Pats of soft margarine
Nutrient-dense snacks		As desired for necessary kilocalories

Milk anemia Anemia that results from feeding older infants only milk that is low in iron.

Milk consumption of more than three cups by toddlers can result in **milk anemia,** since this consumption excludes other foods that are higher in iron. Whole milk rather than skim milk should be consumed until the child is 2 years old, since it contains linoleic acid (essential fatty acid).

Consumption of meat or meat substitutes is important for this group, since their muscles are actively developing. However, if the toddler does not like meat, two glasses of milk and one serving of meat or a substitute will provide an adequate amount of protein.

As with adults, the fruit and vegetable servings should include one serving of a vitamin C–rich fruit or vegetable such as tomato. In addition, one serving of a leafy green or yellow vegetable should be consumed. Toddlers often like raw vegetables served as finger foods.

Iron is frequently low in the diet of toddlers; therefore, it is important that the child be offered iron-enriched cereals. Infant cereals are also a good source of iron. In selecting cereals, parents should consider the amount of sugar and fiber in addition to the amount of iron.

In addition to servings of the above foods, a toddler should get servings of margarine for vitamin A and fats for vitamin E. Since toddlers' stomachs are small, they will not be able to eat all these foods in three meals a day. Instead, they will want to eat food between meals. Parents should recognize that this is a normal pattern. Between-meal snacks can provide essential nutrients that are not necessarily rich in concentrated sweets. Some examples are as follows:

Fruits: apples and oranges cut into small wedges

Vegetables: raw carrots, cucumbers, and celery

Bread: unsalted whole grain crackers

Cheese: small pieces of natural cheese

Peanut butter: spread on small pieces of bread

Sweets: oatmeal, bran, and raisin cookies

It is important for parents to remember that because the toddler's growth rate is slowing down, his or her appetite will be decreased. In addition, the desire to become more independent will cause the toddler to be erratic in his eating habits. If parents are too rigid with the child, it could result in serious appetite problems and nonacceptance of foods.

PRESCHOOLERS

Preschoolers Children from 3 to 6 years of age.

Preschoolers have the same dietary requirement as toddlers. Their growth continues to be slow, and they have little appetite. Permanent food habits are developing during this period; therefore, parents should strive to set a good example by eating the appropriate foods. A preschooler's eating habits are often influenced by those of nursery or preschool peers (see Fig. 12-4).

SCHOOL-AGE CHILDREN

School-age children Children from 6 to 12 years of age.

School-age children tend to grow at a slow, steady rate. A child's body type should be established by now. Some children are athletic and burn up many kilocalories, whereas others are more sedentary.

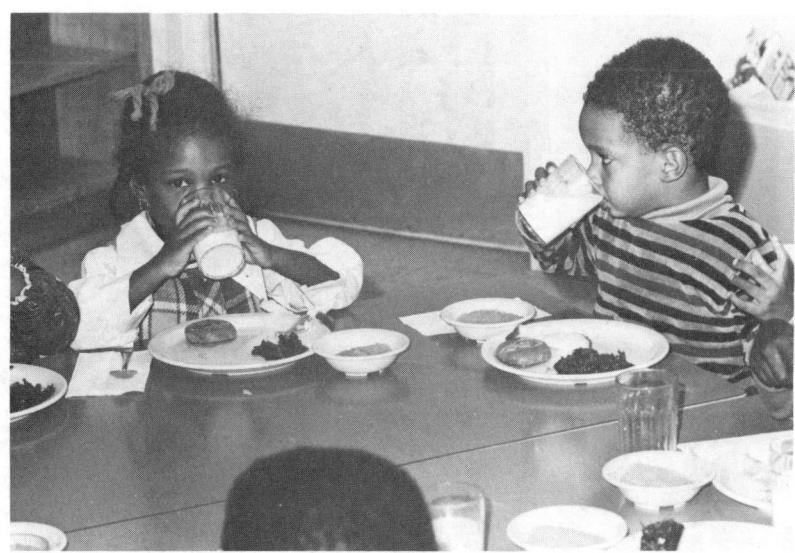

FIGURE 12-4 Preschoolers' eating habits are influenced by their nursery or pre-school peers. (U.S. Department of Agriculture photo.)

Dietary habits are formed by this stage. Snacking is common now, especially after school; therefore, it is important for nutrient-dense snacks to be provided. Breakfast is a very important meal for this age group, since it provides the energy and nutrients for the learning activities that occur before lunch. Since the snacking opportunities for a hungry child before lunch are nonexistent, breakfast should be adequate to last until lunch. Good dietary habits are very beneficial to the child, since parental supervision at lunch is impossible. School lunch programs offer children a nourishing meal and encourage them to consume foods that they might not normally be offered (see Fig. 12-5).

The diet for this group, in terms of the number of servings and portion sizes, is essentially the same as for the preschool child, with modifications based on the child's appetite. Protein intake continues to be important for muscle development. Vitamin A and C deficiencies are common in this group; therefore, emphasis on vegetables and fruits to supply these nutrients or a multivitamin supplement is important.

NUTRITION DURING ADOLESCENCE

DIET FOR ADOLESCENCE

Adolescence The period of life from 12 to about 20 years of age.

Adolescence is the period that bridges childhood and adulthood. It extends from the onset of puberty to the achievement of adult size, or the years from 12 to about 20.

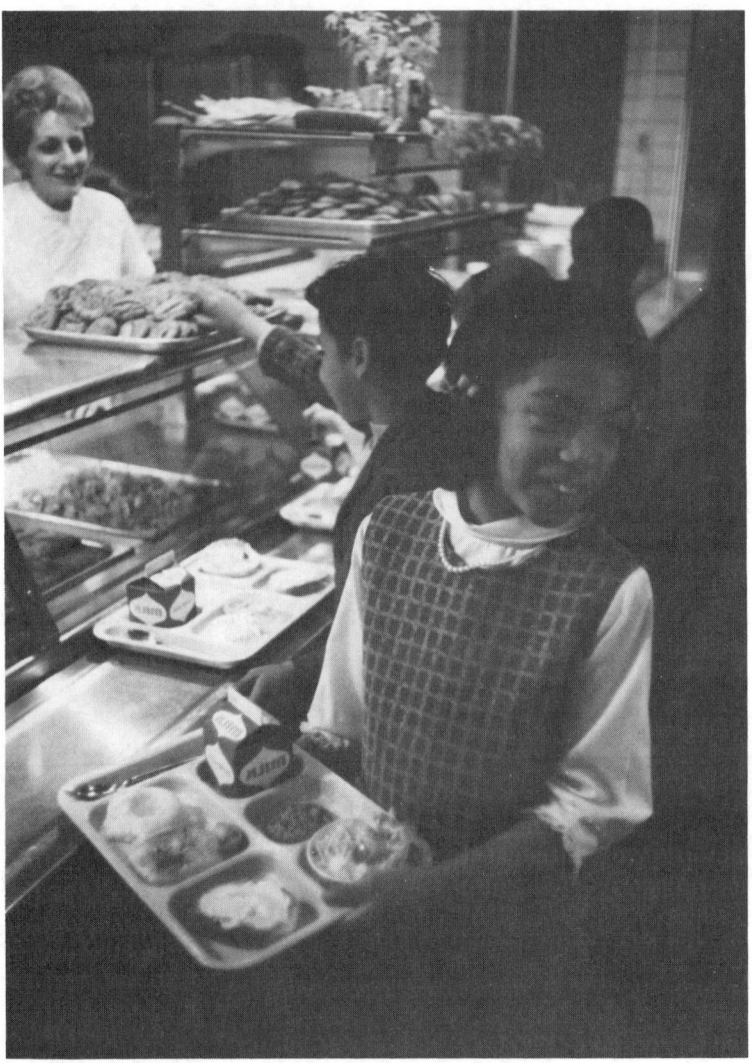

FIGURE 12-5 School lunch programs offer the school-age child a nourishing meal. (Courtesy of the National Dairy Council.)

The rate of growth during adolescence is greater than that of any other period of life except infancy. It is common for boys to grow 4 in. in a year and gain 20 lb. Girls may increase over 3 in. in height and gain somewhat less weight. The growth spurt is accompanied by increased appetite and nutrient needs.

Kilocalories. The RDA for energy of boys during adolescence is, on average, 2,700–2,900 kcal. For girls the average is 2,100–2,200 kcal.

These are average figures and may be considerably higher for some adolescents.

Testosterone The male sex hormone secreted by the testes. It stimulates the development of male secondary sex characteristics.

Estrogen The female sex hormone secreted by the ovaries. It stimulates the development of the female secondary sex characteristics.

Pelvic girdle A ring of bones in the pelvic region composed of two hip bones joined to the sacrum.

Protein. An increase in protein during this period is important in boys for increased muscle mass. During puberty, increased levels of the hormone **testosterone** result in the extensive use of protein for the synthesis of lean muscle tissue and long bone growth. In girls the increased protein, under the influence of the hormone **estrogen,** is used in the synthesis of increased fat tissues in the abdominal area, breasts, and hips. In addition, protein is important in the widening of the **pelvic girdle.** Before the start of puberty, protein is important in girls for long bone growth; this is when most of their increase in height occurs.

Minerals. The RDA for calcium and phosphorus during adolescence is 50% higher than it is during childhood for the increase in bone growth. Teenage girls who diet often eliminate milk and therefore are calcium deficient. Iron requirements are high for both boys and girls. High levels of iron are needed for menstruating girls to replace what they lose in menstrual fluid. In boys, the extra iron is important for expanded blood supply and increased muscle mass.

The Four-Food Group plan is the basis of dietary planning for adolescents. The only modification in the number of servings compared to that of adults is an increase in milk from two to four servings. This increase is essential if adolescents are to achieve the high level of calcium they need. Surveys have found that as many as 50% of adolescent girls are deficient in calcium.[4] Other surveys have found that as many as 80% of girls are deficient in iron.[5]

Sebaceous glands Glands in the skin that secrete the oily substance sebum.

Sebum An oily secretion of the sebaceous glands. It lubricates and waterproofs the skin and hairs.

Blackheads A plug of sebum within a hair follicle.

Pimples Small, elevated areas of pus containing lesions of the skin. They are often called blackheads.

Acne is a problem that affects about 80% of adolescents. The reason it is so prevalent is not related to diet but rather to an increased level of sex hormones that begins at puberty. The **sebaceous glands** are stimulated to secrete more **sebum** by the high level of these hormones. Pores are often blocked by dirt, which causes the sebum to accumulate and form **blackheads** and **pimples.** Bacterial infection of the glands sometimes follows. Diet has no effect on causing or improving acne, despite the myth that foods such as chocolate, fried foods, milk, and sweets cause this condition. While adolescents may wish to restrict their intake of these foods, it should be emphasized that this practice will not necessarily prevent acne.

CHILDHOOD AND ADOLESCENT PROBLEMS RELATED TO NUTRITION

OBESITY

A common nutritional problem in adolescence is obesity, which affects about 15%.[5] Generally, the cause of the problem is lack of exercise rather than excess consumption of kilocalories.

It is very important that adolescents try to lose excess weight before the end of adolescence, since those who do not tend to be obese throughout adult life. Dietary management consists of decreasing the consumption of kilocalories while consuming adequate amount of the essential nutrients. This can generally be accomplished by decreasing the number of snacks, desserts, and second portions. Equally important is encouraging the adolescent to become more physically active.

ANOREXIA NERVOSA AND BULIMIA

The opposite of obesity is anorexia nervosa and bulimia, which are states of self-induced starvation and overeating followed by vomiting, respectively. These disorders are seen in about 1% of adolescent girls and are described in detail in Chapter 10.

DENTAL CARIES

Dental caries is a very common condition in all age groups after infancy. Adolescents have a high level of caries as a result of consuming of sticky, sugar-rich foods. Their problem is often complicated by orthodontic braces, which trap sticky food and makes brushing more difficult. Since most adolescents are conscious about their personal appearance, counseling them about eating good snacks to avoid dental caries and complications with orthodontic appliances can be beneficial.

NUTRITION DURING INFANCY

First Foods for the Infant
Milk is the initial source of nutrients for the infant, whether breast-fed or bottle-fed.

Advantages of breast feeding for the infant
- Nutrient content: breast milk contains high amounts of most nutrients, except vitamin D, sodium, chloride, potassium, and iron; vitamin B_{12} can be deficient, especially if the mother is a strict vegetarian or vegan.

  Calcium and phosphorus are present in the more desirable calcium-to-phosphorus ratio of 2:1 compared to 1:1 to 1:1.5 in formula milk.

  Proteins and carbohydrates are in a form in which they are more readily absorbable.

  Sodium, potassium, and chloride are present in smaller quantities in breast milk, causing less stress to the kidneys; iron is present in smaller quantities in breast milk, but 49% is absorbed compared to about 10% of the iron in cow's milk.
- Immunologic protection: breast milk contributes antibodies that protect the infant against many bacterial infections; breast-fed infants have fewer allergic reactions.
- Possible prevention of infantile obesity: breast-fed infants feed only when hungry, whereas bottle-fed infants may overfeed due to parental pressure to finish the bottle even though the infant is full.
- Bonding between mother and child: breast feeding benefits both mother and child, but bonding can also be achieved if the parents bottle-feed an infant.

Advantages of Breast Feeding for the Mother
- Uterine contraction: the uterus contracts more rapidly due to greater secretion of oxytocin.
- Weight loss: weight loss increases after pregnancy due to the mother's increased metabolic needs.
- Cost: breast feeding is more economical than buying a formula.

Conditions in Which Breast Feeding is not Advisable
- The mother has been exposed to large amounts of DDT and PCB, which will be transmitted to the infant in breast milk.
- Consumption of too much alcohol, nicotine, caffeine or the use of psychoactive drugs (e.g., lithium); these will be transmitted to the infant in breast milk.
- An overanxious mother, or one who does not want to or cannot conveniently breast-feed because she is employed outside the home.

Bottle or Formula Feeding
Milk is modified to resemble breast milk closely; proteins are altered to a form in which they can be more easily digested; saturated butterfat is replaced by unsaturated vegetable oil; all brands are fortified with vitamins and are available with or without iron fortification.

Skim milk should not be used in infant feeding, since it lacks linoleic acid (essential fatty acid) and adequate kcal.

Introduction of Solid Foods (Beikost)
This should be based on two considerations:

- Supplying increasing amounts of nutrients that milk alone cannot supply
- Supplying the foods in a form the baby is physically able to handle

Problems with introducing solid foods are as follows:

- The infant cannot swallow them, since voluntary swallowing is not developed until 3 to 4 months of age.
- Salivary amylase for the digestion of starches is not present until 2 or 3 months of age.
- The ability of the kidneys to handle the increased levels of wastes is not developed until the end of the second month.

A schedule for introduction of solid foods is presented.

Cereals are usually introduced first, because of ease of digestion; they are an excellent source of iron and B vitamins.

Vegetables are introduced before fruits, since they are more difficult to like than the sweeter fruits.

Egg whites should not be introduced until the infant is 1 year of age, since infants frequently develop allergies to protein in egg whites before this age.

Infant Problems Related to Nutrition
Food Allergy
Food allergy is the formation of antibodies to certain foods.

Common symptoms include hives, eczema, bronchitis, asthma, coughing, sneezing, diarrhea, and colic.

Common foods and nutrients that cause allergies are cow's milk protein, egg protein, wheat protein, and compounds in orange juice.

Colic

Colic is usually seen in infants less than 3 months old. It is characterized by profuse crying after eating.

Causes: most often from overfeeding, but it can occur secondary to allergies.

Dietary adaptations: diluting the formula with more water, avoiding the feeding of complex carbohydrates, burping the infant frequently, and possibly using a cold formula.

Phenylketonuria (PKU)

PKU is a congenital metabolic disorder that results from lack of the enzyme phenylalanine hydroxylase. It causes buildup of phenylalanine, which can result in hyperactivity, irritability, and ultimately mental retardation.

Dietary treatment consists of a low-phenylalanine diet. Lofenalac is a formula that is 95% phenylalanine free. Phenylalanine is an essential amino acid; therefore, milk is mixed with the formula to supply the needed amount.

Introduction of solid foods is done according to phenylalanine exchange lists. Cereals, vegetables, and fruits are low in phenylalanine; meat, fish, poultry, and dairy products are high in it.

Diarrhea

A common cause of diarrhea is overfeeding; inflammation of the intestinal wall results in temporary loss of lactase. If milk is consumed, the condition is worsened.

Dietary treatment consists of replacement of lost fluids and electrolytes. Pedialyte or Lytren are two solutions that accomplish this. There should be a progression to dilute formula and finally to full formula.

NUTRITION DURING CHILDHOOD

Toddlers

Children 1–3 years of age have a slower rate of growth than infants, with decreased appetite and consumption of food.

Important muscle changes are occurring. Muscles of the back, buttocks, and thighs are enlarging and strengthening. Much body fat is lost, and the body shape changes from a rather chubby to a more lean appearance.

Toddlers attempt to feed themselves, often unsuccessfully. They exhibit a desire for independence by often not wanting to eat nutritious foods.

Diet

Based on the Four-Food Group plan as given in the chapter.

The toddler should not consume more than three cups of milk, since milk anemia may result. Whole milk should be consumed until 2 years of age in order to obtain its linoleic acid.

Iron is the nutrient that is frequently low in the diet; therefore, it is important to offer the child iron-enriched cereals. One should also consider the amount of sugar and fiber when selecting a cereal.

The child will probably need to eat between-meal snacks, since he or she usually cannot eat all the necessary food at three meals. Examples of nutrient-dense sweets are presented in the chapter.

Preschoolers

Preschoolers, 3 to 6 years of age, have the same dietary requirement as toddlers. Permanent food habits are developing during this time; therefore, parents should set a positive example.

School-Age Children

School-age children, 6 to 12 years old, grow at a slow and steady rate. Dietary habits are formed at this time, and snacking is common.

Breakfast is very important, since the child needs energy to perform well in school before lunch, especially since snacks will be unavailable.

Protein continues to be important for muscle development. Vitamin A and C deficiencies are common; therefore, it is important to emphasize vegetables and fruits or a multivitamin supplement.

NUTRITION DURING ADOLESCENCE

Diet for Adolescence

Adolescence bridges childhood and usually extends from the years 12 to 20. The rate of growth is greater than at any other period of life except infancy. It is common for boys to grow 4 in. in a year and gain 20 lb; girls may increase over 3 in. in height and gain somewhat less weight.

- Kilocalories: the RDA for energy of boys is, on average, 2,700–2,900 kcal; girls have an RDA average of 2,100–2,200 kcal.
- Protein: increased protein in boys is important for the development of muscle mass and long bone growth under the control of testosterone.

  In menstruating girls, increased protein is important in the synthesis of increased fat tissues in the abdominal area, breasts, and hips, and widening of pelvic girdle; before menstruation or puberty, protein is important in girls for long bone growth and when most of their growth in height occurs.
- Minerals: the RDA for calcium and phosphorus during adolescence is 50% higher than it is during childhood for the increase in bone growth; teenage girls are often calcium deficient.

  Iron requirements are high for boys for muscle development; for girls, high iron content is important to replace what they lose during menstruation.

Acne is a problem that affects about 80% of adolescents. The cause is not related to diet but rather to the increased level of sex hormones and sebum production. The diet will not help or worsen the condition.

Childhood and Adolescent Problems Related to Nutrition
Obesity
Found in about 15% of adolescents. It generally results from lack of exercise rather than excess consumption of kilocalories. Dietary treatment of reducing the consumption of kilocalories but not essential nutrients is important. It can generally be accomplished by reducing snacking, second portions, and desserts, and increasing one's physical activity.

Anorexia Nervosa and Bulimia
The opposite of obesity, these problems consist of self-induced starvation and overeating followed by vomiting, and are described in Chapter 10.

Dental Caries
Common in all age groups after infancy. This problem is complicated in adolescents by the presence of orthodontic appliances.

REVIEW QUESTIONS

TRUE (A) OR FALSE (B)

Questions 1–20

1. Not only is breast milk the best source of nutrients for an infant, but the proteins and carbohydrates are in a form that is more easily absorbable.
2. An important advantage of breast milk is the immunologic feature of increased resistance to infections and fewer allergies.
3. A mother who breast-feeds does not have to worry about the infant's diet being deficient in any nutrients.
4. Formulas contain cow's milk that has been modified to make it more absorbable.
5. A mother who bottle-feeds her infant should consider using skim milk rather than whole milk in order to reduce the amount of cholesterol and saturated fat in the infant's diet.
6. A major consideration regarding when to introduce solid foods into the diet of an infant is age, and at 2 months is a good time.
7. Since breast milk is such a good food for infants, a mother should breast-feed the infant until at least the age of 1 year.
8. When introducing solid foods into the infant's diet, one should introduce vegetables before fruits, since vegetables are harder to like.
9. Although whole eggs are an excellent source of nutrients, only the yolk should be introduced before the infant is 1 year old due to a possible allergic reaction to egg white.
10. Allergic reactions in infants usually do not occur until after 1 year of age, and the symptoms are minor ones such as diarrhea and bronchitis.
11. Dietary treatment of PKU consists of complete elimination of the offending amino acid phenylalanine.
12. Dietary treatment for diarrhea consists of feeding milk to the infant in order to replace the lost nutrients as quickly as possible.
13. The growth rate and therefore the appetite of toddlers is greater than during infancy.
14. Milk consumption by toddlers should not exceed about three cups, since excess amounts may lead to milk anemia.
15. Enriched cereals are an excellent source of iron for toddlers.
16. In order to have toddlers develop good eating

habits, parents should prevent them from consuming between-meal snacks.

17. Often a preschooler's rate of growth is slow, and there is little appetite.
18. Increased protein intake is important for adolescent boys due to a great amount of fat deposition.
19. Increased protein intake is important for adolescent girls for protein synthesis in the abdomen and hip regions.
20. There is no relationship between acne and diet in adolescents; rather, acne is a result of increased levels of sex hormones and sebum production.

MULTIPLE CHOICE

Questions 21–25

21. Potential advantages of breast feeding compared to bottle feeding an infant is (are):
    1. immunologic
    2. lower level of cholesterol
    3. possible prevention of infantile obesity
    4. greater amount of iron intake
       A. 1, 2, 3   B. 1, 3   C. 2, 4   D. 4
       E. all of these
22. Adding solid foods to a baby's diet should be based on which of the following considerations?
    A. helping the infant sleep through the night
    B. supplying the foods in a form the baby is physically able to handle
    C. supplying increasing amounts of nutrients that milk alone cannot supply
    D. A, B
    E. B, C
23. Which of the following infant problems and dietary adaptations are correct?
    A. PKU—shift from whole milk to skim milk
    B. colic—substitution of soybean formula for the one causing the problem
    C. diarrhea—increase the feeding of whole milk to get more fat into the gastrointestinal tract
    D. all of these
    E. none of these
24. Which of the following correctly describe the diet during childhood?
    1. toddlers—emphasis on protein for muscle changes but not high levels of kilocalories, since the appetite is decreased
    2. preschoolers—much higher intake of proteins and kilocalories than toddlers due to rapid growth

3. school-age children—dietary habits formed at this time, and breakfast is very important for good performance in classes before lunch
   A. 1, 2, 3   B. 1, 3   C. 2, 3   D. 3
   E. all of these
25. Nutrient needs and their importance during adolescence are:
    1. kilocalories:—boys average 1,700–1,900 kcal; girls average 1,200–1,500 kcal
    2. protein—increased amount is important in girls for the synthesis of fat tissues in the breasts, abdomen, and hips.
    3. minerals—same amounts of calcium and phosphorus are needed as in adults for bone growth
    4. increased iron intake—important in girls to replace the amounts lost during menstruation
       A. 1, 2, 3   B. 1, 3   C. 2, 4   D. 4
       E. all of these

DISCUSSION QUESTIONS

1. Describe four nutrient advantages of breast feeding. Describe three other advantages of breast feeding.
2. Discuss PKU and diarrhea in terms of the causes and dietary treatment of each.
3. Discuss how kilocalories, protein, and minerals are important in the diet of adolescents.
4. Describe the relationship between acne and diet in adolescents.

REFERENCES

1. U.M. Saarinen, A. Backman, M. Kajosarri, and M.A. Siimes. "Prolonged breastfeeding as prophylaxis for atopic disease. *The Lancet* 2 (8135), 163 (1979).
2. *Pediatric Nutrition Handbook*. Evanston, Ill.: Committee on Nutrition, American Academy of Pediatrics. 1979.
3. B.G. Morrissey. *Therapeutic Nutrition*. Philadelphia: J.B. Lippincott Co., 1984, p. 485.
4. D. Marino and J. King. "Nutritional concerns during adolescence." *Pediatric Clinics of North America*, 27 (1), 125 (1980).
5. P.A. Kreutler. *Nutrition in Perspective*. Englewood Cliffs, N.J.: Prentice-Hall, Inc., 1980, p. 547.

13 NUTRITION AND THE ELDERLY

OBJECTIVES

Upon completion of this chapter, you should be able to:

1. Define the term *elderly* and describe their proportion in relation to the rest of the population.

2. Discuss the nutrient needs of the elderly.

3. Discuss why many authorities recommend increased calcium intake for the elderly.

4. Describe the importance of high-fiber diets for the elderly.

5. Discuss protein-calorie malnutrition, delayed wound healing, and undernutrition problems in the elderly.

6. Describe dietary planning for the elderly.

7. Differentiate between nutrition programs for the elderly.

INTRODUCTION

Elderly People who are 65 years of age or older.

The **elderly** are a rapidly increasing age group in the United States as well as worldwide. The proportion of elderly persons in the United States increased from 4% in 1900 to almost 12% in 1980. Many researchers predict that by the year 2025 the number of elderly persons will double to 51 million. These percentages indicate that the elderly are a small percentage of the population; the following figures indicate that they use a considerably higher percentage of the health services provided in the United States. The elderly account for:

29% of the country's health care costs

34% of all days in short-stay hospitals

87% of the occupants in nursing homes

25% of the prescription drugs used

15% of all visits to doctor's offices[1]

There are various reasons why the elderly use a much higher percentage of the health care services compared to their proportion of the population. One reason may be nutrition. Surveys show that the elderly frequently have poorer diets than younger people. Their diets tend to be high in carbohydrates and lacking in fruits, vegetables, milk and dairy products, and meats.[2] High-carbohydrate foods such as bread, crackers, doughnuts, breakfast cereals, sweet rolls, and cookies are consumed in large amounts because they are inexpensive, require little preparation, keep without refrigeration, and are easy to chew.

It is important for health care professionals to understand nutritional needs and deficiencies of the elderly, especially since their number and their use of health care facilities are increasing.

NUTRIENT NEEDS OF THE ELDERLY

Little scientific evidence exists on the nutritional needs of the elderly. Table 13-1 shows that their nutrient needs are included in the 51+ age group. In recent years, studies have been conducted to determine if the nutritional needs of the 65+ age group are different from those of the 51+ age group. One study was conducted by Dr. James S. Goodwin at the University of New Mexico's Department of Medicine and was supported by the National Institute of Aging. The results of the study were not published at the time of this writing. Another study was conducted

TABLE 13-1 RECOMMENDED DAILY DIETARY ALLOWANCES FOR ADULTS

Nutrient	Unit	Allowance, Men			Allowance, Women		
		Age 19–22	23–50	51+	Age 19–22	23–50	51+
Food energy		2,900	2,700	2,400[e]	2,100	2,000	1,800[f]
Protein	g	56	56	56	44	44	44
Fat-soluble vitamins							
Vitamin A	μg RE[a]	1,000	1,000	1,000	800	800	800
Vitamin E	mg α TE[b]	10	10	10	8	8	8
Vitamin D	μg[c]	7.5	5	5	7.5	5	5
Water-soluble vitamins							
Ascorbic acid	mg	60	60	60	60	60	60
Folacin		400	400	400	400	400	400
Niacin	mg equi NE[d]	19	18	16	14	13	13
Riboflavin	mg	1.7	1.6	1.4	1.3	1.2	1.2
Thiamin	mg	1.5	1.4	1.2	1.1	1.0	1.0
Vitamin B_6	mg	2.0	2.0	2.0	2.0	2.0	2.0
Vitamin B_{12}	μg	3.0	3.0	3.0	3.0	3.0	3.0
Minerals							
Calcium	mg	800	800	800	800	800	800
Phosphorus	mg	800	800	800	800	800	800
Iodine	μg	150	150	150	150	150	150
Iron	mg	10	10	10	18	18	10
Magnesium	mg	350	350	350	300	300	300
Zinc	mg	15	15	15	15	15	15

Source: Recommended Dietary Allowances, 9th rev. ed.). Washington, D.C.: National Academy of Sciences, 1980.

[a]Retinol equivalents; 1 retinol equivalent = 1 μg retinol or 6 μg β-carotene.*
[b]α-tocopherol equivalents; 1 mg d-α-tocopherol = 1 TE.**
[c]As cholecalciferol; 10 μg cholecalciferol = 400 IU vitamin D.
[d]1 NE (niacin equivalent) is equal to 1 μg of niacin or 60 μg of dietary tryptophan.
[e]2,050 for men 76+ years of age.
[f]1600 for women 76+ years of age.
 * = Beta carotene.
** = Alpha-tocopherol.

at Tufts University in Boston by the U.S. Department of Agriculture's Human Nutrition Research Center on Aging, with the final results also not published at the time of this writing.

KILOCALORIE NEEDS

The 1980 RDA values given in Table 13-1 show that men and women in the 51+ age group need a 11 and 10% decrease in kilocalories, respectively. This reduction is recommended because of a reduction in the basic metabolic rate (BMR) and the activity level. The reduction in BMR is primarily due to a decrease in muscle and organ tissues. Due to aging, an increased proportion of the body weight is adipose tissue and a decreased proportion is muscle and organ tissues. Elderly people tend to reduce their physical activity. This reduction, combined with the decreased BMR, indicates that their kilocalorie intake should be reduced.

Despite the RDA indicating lower kilocalorie needs for the elderly, many do not reduce their kilocalorie intake. This is evidenced by the fact that the Ten State Nutrition Survey (TSNS) found that 50% of the women and 18% of the men over age 60 were obese.[3] Because obesity is related to many disorders (diabetes and atherosclerosis), it is important for the elderly to watch their kilocalorie intake.

PROTEIN

Table 13-1 shows that the RDA for protein for the elderly is the same as that of their younger counterparts: 56 g for men and 44 g for women, or 0.8 g per kilogram of ideal body weight. However, several studies show that the elderly need a higher protein intake than that indicated by the RDA. The National Academy of Science/National Research Council suggests a minimum intake of 12% of total energy as protein for the elderly.

Some authorities do not agree that the elderly need more protein daily, since they have reduced lean body mass and body protein synthesis. However, the elderly frequently have chronic illnesses that require medications. To counteract these illnesses and the effects of medications, they frequently require increased protein intake. Various surveys, such as the TSNS and the Health and Nutrition Examination Survey (HANES), found that most elderly persons consume protein at or above the RDA level. However, due to economic factors, the protein often is not from high-quality sources such as meat and fish. It should be emphasized to the elderly that dry milk included in cooking is an inexpensive source of high-quality protein. Eggs are also a good source but, due to their high cholesterol level, are not as good as milk.

CARBOHYDRATES AND FAT

The consumption of carbohydrates by the elderly should be the same as that of younger people in that it should compose about 50% of the total kilocalories consumed. The majority of the carbohydrates should come from complex carbohydrates, as opposed to concentrated sweets, which are the major source for many elderly.

Fat intake for the elderly should be basically the same as that for younger people: 30% of total kilocalories, with emphasis on intake of polyunsaturated fats and decreased consumption of saturated fats.

MINERALS

The RDA for calcium for the elderly is 800 mg/day. However, many authorities recommend that this be increased to up to 1,200 mg/day to decrease the potential development of osteoporosis (see Chapter 8 for details). The increased intake of calcium also helps to offset the decreased absorption of calcium that occurs with age. The incidence of osteoporosis in the elderly has been found to be as high as 30% of women over the age of 55 and of men over the age of 60.[4] Increasing consumption of high-calcium foods such as milk may not always be possible, since many elderly persons have a lactase deficiency. Therefore, calcium supplements may be required to reach these elevated levels.

Recommended intake of iron for the elderly is the same as that for younger people. Iron deficiency anemia in the elderly is often not due to dietary deficiency but rather to chronic blood loss, as from ulcers, and to decreased absorption as a result of reduced hydrochloric acid secretion.

VITAMINS

The elderly tend to have vitamin abuse as well as vitamin deficiencies. Many elderly persons consume a vitamin supplement and are predisposed to the various problems of vitamin toxicity. They should be counseled about the unnecessary expense of consuming vitamin supplements if they eat an adequate diet and the problems with vitamin toxicity (see Chapter 6 for details).

The elderly may be deficient in B complex vitamins due to inadequate consumption of fruits and vegetables. Others are deficient because they overuse laxatives or have impaired secretion of bile. Thiamin and riboflavin are two B complex vitamins found in deficient amounts. The lack of these vitamins, plus folic acid and vitamin B_{12}, have been found to cause mental confusion, memory loss, disorientation, and depression.[5] Surveys show that elderly persons who are institutionalized have a lower intake of vitamins than those who are not institutionalized.

FIBER

There are no RDA values for the amount of fiber in the diet. However, most elderly persons need to increase their fiber intake to help alleviate constipation and possibly to reduce the chance of developing colon cancer. As described in Chapter 3, the average American eats about 10–20 g of fiber per day; this must be increased to 25–50 g/day to be beneficial. The elderly should be encouraged to increase their fiber intake by consuming fruits, bread and cereal, and vegetables.

COMMON NUTRITIONAL PROBLEMS
OF THE ELDERLY

Three common problems seen in hospitalized elderly persons are protein-calorie malnutrition (PCM), delayed wound healing, and undernutrition. The characteristics and reasons for these problems will be discussed next.

PROTEIN-CALORIE MALNUTRITION (PCM)

A large proportion of hospitalized patients are elderly, and many of them have PCM. Generally, PCM results from anorexia as a complication of the disease (chronic heart failure, lung disease, renal failure, and liver disease) that caused the hospitalization.

Symptoms and Assessment

A common symptom of PCM is mental confusion, which often results from a low blood protein level and dehydration. Other symptoms are significant weight loss, glossitis, and edema.

Serum albumin A protein in the blood that is important for the regulation of osmotic pressure.

Assessment of PCM is often based on the above symptoms, as well as a careful diet history, a low **serum albumin** level, anemia, and **lymphocytopenia.**[6]

Lymphocytopenia A low level of lymphocytes that help provide immunity.

Treatment

Intensive nutritional treatment is often required to provide an adequate amount of nutrients to correct PCM. This treatment generally requires tube feeding of formulas that supply about 1.0–1.5 kcal/ml (see Chapter 17 for details of tube feeding). Oral feeding is often inadequate because the patient is generally anorexic.

DECREASED WOUND HEALING

One of the major hazards of PCM is decreased wound healing. PCM plus decreased blood flow to tissues, lowered BMR, and deficiencies of certain vitamins and minerals can decrease the rate of wound healing in the elderly. Decreased blood flow to tissues and a lower BMR are natural changes in the elderly. Deficiencies of vitamin A, vitamin C, and zinc are detrimental to wound healing and are reversible.

Vitamin A is especially important for healing of the gastrointestinal tract, skin, and respiratory tract. Vitamin C is important for the synthesis of collagen, which is important for healing of all wounds. Zinc is important in wound healing and for the synthesis of proteins and immunity.

As with the treatment of PCM, the best way to reverse these vitamin and mineral deficiencies for the elderly is to provide food by tube or intravenous feeding.

UNDERNUTRITION

General undernutrition is a common problem in the elderly. Typically, it results from decreased taste sensitivity, dental changes, changes in the gastrointestinal tract, drug–diet interactions, alcoholism, and economic reasons.

Decreased Taste Sensitivity

Decreased taste sensitivity is common in the elderly. The reason why taste sensitivity decreases is not known. Two theories are that the number of taste buds and their sensitivity are reduced. In addition, certain medications can alter the sense of taste.[7] As a result of these changes, the elderly person's appetite is often reduced to the point where adequate amounts of important nutrients are not consumed.

Counseling about the existence of this problem and about which nutrients need to be increased is important. Vitamin and mineral supplements are recommended for people who have markedly low levels of essential nutrients, especially if a chronic disease could further lower these levels.

Dental Changes

Approximately 50% of Americans have lost most of their teeth by age 65 and 75 percent have lost all of their teeth by age 75.[8] The loss of teeth and dry mouth can result in the elderly, altering their diet to the point where they eat only soft, easy-to-chew foods. A major problem with this diet is decreased intake of protein foods, fruits, and fresh vegetables. Counseling the elderly to acquire properly fitting dentures and using a blender to chop up meats, fruits, and vegetables will help to overcome these problems.

Gastrointestinal Tract Changes

Reductions in the secretion of hydrochloric acid and certain enzymes and decreased absorption are common changes that accompany aging. These problems can result in anemia and in decreased digestion and absorption of nutrients. In addition, decreased peristalsis due to weakening of intestinal muscles results in constipation.

While these problems cannot be reversed, counseling as to which foods are high in iron and fiber can help to alleviate some of them.

Drug–Diet Interactions

The elderly use many prescription and nonprescription drugs that, when combined with marginal diets, frequently result in undernutrition. Drugs can interfere with the digestion, absorption, and use of nutrients in a variety of ways (see Chapter 16 for details). Some of the more common groups of drugs and diet problems that the elderly experience are as follows:

Laxatives and cathartics. The elderly frequently take over-the-counter preparations of laxatives and cathartics for relief of constipation, heart-burn, and indigestion. Long-term use of these drugs can result in deficiencies of electrolytes such as sodium, calcium, and potassium, as well as water.

Aspirin. Aspirin is commonly used for arthritis. Prolonged use can result in gastrointestinal tract bleeding and anemia.

Congestive heart failure
A failure of the heart to pump the blood ade-quately to the tissues. It results in an accumula-tion of blood and fluids in the tissues and there-fore causes congestion (see Chapters 21 and 22).

Cardiovascular drugs. Many elderly persons suffer from **congestive heart failure** and other heart problems. The drugs they take often have side effects of anorexia and electrolyte imbalances.

It is very important that the elderly clearly understand the possible nutritional side effects of certain over-the-counter as well as prescription drugs. Health care professionals should ask which drugs the elderly person is taking and should be alert to their side effects. In addition, the elderly should be counseled about which foods they should consume to offset any possible deficiencies or excesses.

Alcoholism

Alcoholism among the elderly is not uncommon. They are susceptible because they are no longer employed, may not have a hobby or recre-ation, and often are alone a great deal. Alcoholism frequently results in inadequate diets. One nutrient that is especially affected by alcohol is thiamin. Thiamin deficiency is common in alcoholics due to interference with absorption and inadequate intake. Thiamin deficiency can result in mental failure, depression, defective memory, and anorexia.[9] In ad-dition, alcohol can interact with medications for heart, kidney, and high blood pressure diseases to cause serious nutritional side effects.

Diet histories often can be used to identify excessive alcohol intake as the underlying cause of undernutrition in the elderly.

Economic Reasons

Poverty frequently determines the adequacy of a person's diet, and some estimates indicate that 25% of America's elderly have incomes below the poverty line. Many elderly persons attempt to save money by buying less expensive foods that are filling and provide energy. These are high-carbohydrate foods such as breads, pastries, and cereals. More expensive foods such as meats, milk, and fresh produce often are reduced, as are their essential proteins, minerals, and vitamins.

DIETARY PLANNING FOR THE ELDERLY

Dietary planning for the elderly is essentially the same as for younger people. It focuses on the Four-Food Group Plan and exchange lists. The elderly need to have a good understanding of these two food guides.

An essential component of dietary planning for the elderly is information about their living conditions (see Fig. 13-1), including whether

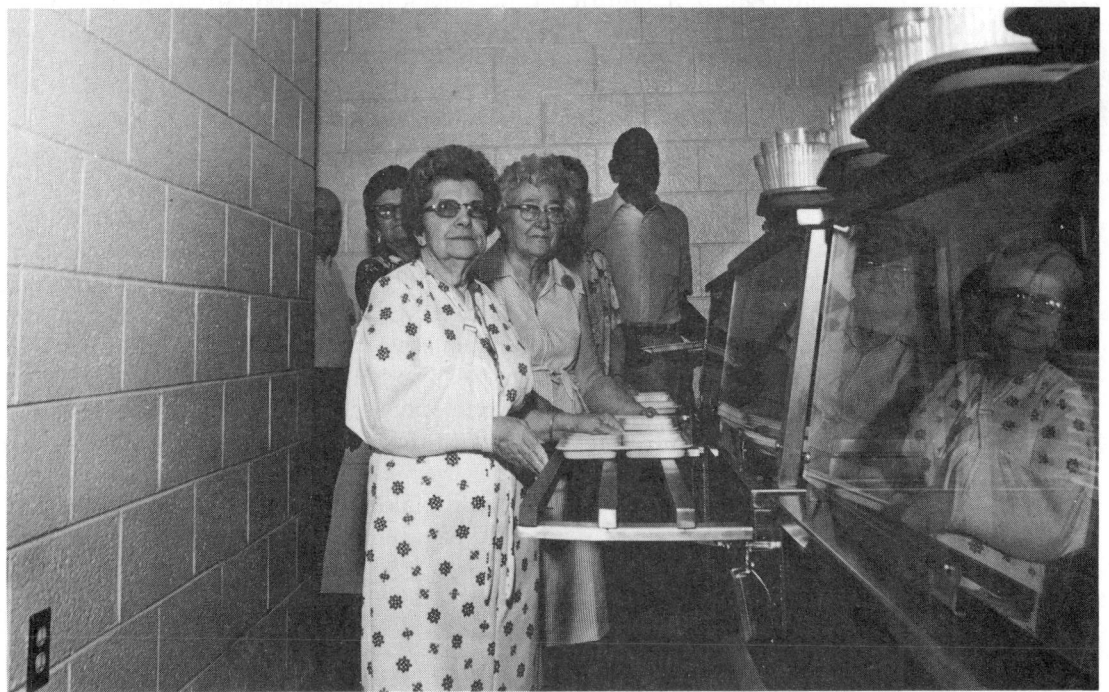

FIGURE 13-1 Elderly persons who live alone are more likely to have an inadequate diet than those who live and eat with others. (Courtesy Coordinating Council for Senior Citizens.)

they live alone, whether they have facilities to store perishable foods, and whether they cook only for themselves or others. Elderly persons who live alone are more likely to have an inadequate diet than those who live and eat with others. Determining the approximate amount of money spent each month on food is important before effective dietary planning can be done.

Once the above information has been obtained, the planning should not impose too many dietary restrictions, cooking restrictions, and changes in shopping habits. Too many restrictions and changes result in less compliance of the elderly with the planning. The more active a role the person has in the dietary planning, the more likely he or she will be to follow the diet plan.

NUTRITION PROGRAMS FOR THE ELDERLY

Several programs have been established to help the elderly alleviate the problems of malnutrition and isolation. It is important for health professionals to be knowledgeable about these programs so that they can refer the elderly if they need aid.

NATIONAL NUTRITION PROGRAM
(Title VII of the Older American Act)

The National Nutrition Program is operated through state agencies on aging or church and school facilities. Its major goals are to provide low-cost, nutritious meals, an opportunity for social interaction, nutritional education, shopping assistance, transportation, and counseling or referral to other social and rehabilitative services.

The meals are served in collective settings to individuals who are 60 years of age or older and to their spouses. They are designed to provide at least one-third of the RDAs for the elderly. The social atmosphere at the sites is almost as valuable as the meals. Elderly persons who associate with others, as opposed to eating alone, tend to be better nourished. The elderly are not required to pay, but they may contribute voluntarily to the meals.

MEALS ON WHEELS

Meals on Wheels is operated on a private, nonprofit, volunteer basis, often through churches. Volunteers usually deliver hot noon meals to homebound elderly, feeble, or handicapped individuals. Frequently, a cold supper is left for those who cannot prepare their own meals.

FOOD STAMP PROGRAM AND
SUPPLEMENTAL SECURITY INCOME

The Food Stamp Program and Supplemental Security Income are not designed specifically for the elderly, but rather for the poor of any age. The food stamp program can be helpful to elderly persons who qualify, enabling them to obtain stamps to buy food which they may not be able to buy otherwise.

Supplemental Security Income helps the very poor by increasing their income to the defined poverty level.

OUTLINE

INTRODUCTION

The proportion of elderly persons is increasing, with predictions that it will double by the year 2025.

The elderly use a much higher percentage of health care facilities than their percentage of the population.

The elderly tend to have poor diets that are high in carbohydrates and low in fruits, vegetables, milk and dairy products.

NUTRIENT NEEDS OF THE ELDERLY

Kilocalorie Needs
Men and women in the 51+ age group should reduce their kilocalorie intake by 11 and 10%, respectively; the reduction is recommended because of the decrease in BMR and activity level.

Protein
The RDA for protein is 0.8 g per kilogram of ideal body weight; some authorities suggest that protein requirements for the elderly be increased above the RDA to a minimum of 12% of the total kilocalorie intake.

Carbohydrates and Fat
The recommended intake of carbohydrates and fat is the same for elderly as younger people: 50% of the total kilocalories from carbohydrates and 30% from fats.

Minerals
The RDA for calcium for the elderly is 800 mg/day. However, since osteoporosis is so prevalent in the elderly (30% of women over age of 55 and of men over age of 60 have it), some authorities recommend a calcium intake of 1,200 mg/day to reduce this risk. The RDA for the other minerals is the same for elderly as for younger people.

Vitamins
The RDA for vitamins for elderly is the same as for younger people.

Some elderly persons exhibit vitamin deficiencies due to inadequate intake of fruits and vegetables. Likewise, some elderly persons exhibit vitamin toxicities due to consumption of excessive amounts of supplements, overuse of laxatives, or impaired secretion of bile.

Thiamin and riboflavin are two common vitamins that the elderly are deficient in. These deficiencies may be the cause of mental confusion, memory loss, disorientation, and depression, which are common in the elderly.

Fiber
No RDA has been established for fiber, but many authorities recommend that the intake be increased to 25–50 g/day, possibly to decrease colon cancer, and constipation. Intake should be encouraged by consuming more fruits, bread and cereal, and vegetables.

COMMON NUTRITIONAL PROBLEMS OF THE ELDERLY

Protein-Calorie Malnutrition (PCM)
Many PCM patients are elderly. PCM generally results from anorexia as a complication of a disease that hospitalized the person.

Symptoms and Assessment
Common symptoms are mental confusion, significant weight loss, glossitis, and edema.

Treatment
Intensive nutritional care often is required, involving tube feeding or parenteral nutrition.

Decreased Wound Healing
Decreased wound healing is caused by PCM, decreased blood flow to tissues, lower BMR, and deficiencies of minerals and vitamins.

It is especially important that deficiencies of vitamins A and C, plus the mineral zinc, be prevented or corrected for effective wound healing.

Undernutrition
Undernutrition generally results from various problems.

Decreased Taste Sensitivity
This problem may result from reduction of taste buds or sensitivity. It reduces appetite to the point where the person consumes inadequate amounts of food.

Dental Changes
A total of 50% of the elderly have lost most of their teeth by age 65 and 75% by age 75. This condition results in change in the diet that cause the person to consume primarily soft, easy-to-chew foods. Dietary changes result in decreased intake of proteins, fruits, and fresh vegetables.

Gastrointestinal Tract Changes
Reduction of hydrochloric acid secretion, enzyme secretion, and decreased peristalsis can result in anemia, constipation, and decreased absorption.

Drug–Diet Interactions
The elderly use many nonprescription and prescription drugs that can interact with nutrients to cause undernutrition. Examples are:

- Laxatives and cathartics: can result in sodium, potassium, and water deficiencies.
- Aspirin: can result in anemia.
- Cardiovascular drugs: can cause anorexia and electrolyte imbalances.

Alcoholism

Alcoholism is fairly common in elderly persons due to no longer working, lack of a hobby or recreation, and often being alone a great deal of the time.

Alcoholism frequently causes thiamin deficiencies, which can result in mental failure, depression, defective memory, and anorexia.

Economic Reasons

Poverty prevents elderly persons from obtaining adequate amounts and types of foods. Some estimates indicate that 25% of America's elderly have incomes below the poverty line.

Diets of poor elderly persons often are high in carbohydrates and low in proteins, vitamins, and minerals.

DIETARY PLANNING FOR THE ELDERLY

Dietary planning for the elderly is essentially same as for younger people in that it is based on the Four-Food Group Plan and exchange lists.

Information about the living conditions of elderly is essential: whether they live alone, have facilities to store perishable foods, and whether they cook only for themselves or for others.

Final dietary plan should not impose too many dietary restrictions, changes in shopping habits, and cooking restrictions. The elderly will not comply with the diet if too many changes and restrictions are imposed.

NUTRITION PROGRAMS FOR THE ELDERLY

National Nutrition Program (Title VII of the Older American Act)

The major goals of this program are to provide low-cost, nutritious meals, an opportunity for social interaction, nutritional education, shopping assistance, transportation, and counseling or referral to other social and rehabilitative services.

Meals on Wheels

Hot noon meals are delivered to elderly persons who are homebound, feeble, or handicapped.

Food Stamp Program and Supplemental Security Income

These programs are designed for the poor of all ages, not just the elderly. They allow qualified people to obtain stamps for food or money in order to increase their income to the defined poverty level.

REVIEW QUESTIONS

TRUE (A) AND FALSE (B)

Questions 1–16

1. The elderly are increasing in numbers as well as using a large percentage of health services.
2. The diet of many elderly persons is high in carbohydrates and lacking in fruits, vegetables, milk and dairy products, and meats.
3. The RDA values for nutrient requirements for the elderly are very different from those of younger people.
4. One bodily change that occurs in the elderly is weight loss, as evidenced by the fact that only a very small percentage of the elderly are overweight.
5. Most nutritional authorities recommend that the elderly decrease their protein consumption to approximately one-half that of the RDA value.
6. Even though elderly persons' bones are not growing, it is recommended that they increase their calcium consumption to reduce the risk of osteoporosis.
7. The elderly almost never exhibit vitamin excesses or vitamin toxicities.
8. Mental confusion, memory loss, disorientation, and depression are common symptoms in the elderly of thiamin and niacin deficiencies.
9. Increasing the fiber intake to 25–50 g/day may help the elderly avoid colon cancer and decrease constipation.
10. PCM in the elderly is almost always a result of cancer.
11. Treatment of PCM in the elderly is primarily by tube feeding, since oral feeding usually is inadequate due to anorexia.
12. Vitamins A and C and zinc are important for wound healing in the elderly.
13. Undernutrition in the elderly often results from natural changes such as decreased taste sensitivity, dental changes, and gastrointestinal tract changes.
14. Alcoholism in the elderly can result in undernutrition, with thiamin deficiency being a common example.
15. The elderly should be placed on very restricted diets to reverse current health problems or prevent problems like colon cancer and constipation.
16. A Meals on Wheels program would be recommended for the elderly to increase their social interaction as well as to provide them with nutritious meals.

MULTIPLE CHOICE

Questions 17–26

17. Which of the following is (are) correct in regard to the elderly?
    1. decreasing in number
    2. many have poor diets
    3. have good diets
    4. use a high percentage of health care services

    A. 1, 2, 3   B. 1, 3   C. 2, 4   D. 4
    E. all of these

18. The nutrient needs of the elderly are _____ .
    1. decreased kilocalories below RDA values
    2. carbohydrates should be 50% of daily kilocalories
    3. increased protein above RDA values
    4. reduction in calcium below RDA values

    A. 1, 2, 3   B. 1, 3   C. 2, 4   D. 4
    E. all of these

19. Increased protein intake in the elderly is important for _____ and _____ .
    A. tissue synthesis—increased peristalsis
    B. counteracting—illness effects of medications
    C. increased—countering mental confusion metabolism
    D. none of these

20. Increased intake of calcium is recommended for the elderly to _____ .
    A. improve the healing of bone fractures
    B. reduce senility
    C. decrease osteoporosis
    D. reduce edema

21. Deficiencies of vitamins _____ and _____ in the elderly can cause mental confusion, memory loss, disorientation, and depression.
    A. A—C
    B. E—K
    C. B_6—D
    D. thiamin—riboflavin

22. Symptoms of PCM in the elderly are
    A. mental confusion
    B. significant weight loss
    C. glossitis
    D. all of these

23. The most effective treatment of PCM in the elderly is _____ .
    A. increased oral consumption of high-protein foods
    B. intensive treatment with tube feedings
    C. increased oral consumption of fats and carbohydrates
    D. none of these

24. Gastrointestinal tract changes that may result in undernutrition are _____ .
    A. decreased mucus secretion
    B. reduced secretion of hydrochloric acid
    C. decreased peristalsis
    D. A, B
    E. B, C

25. The diets of the elderly who have incomes below the poverty line are characterized by _____ .
    A. being high in fruits and vegetables but low in grains and cereals
    B. being low in fats and carbohydrates and high in protein
    C. being high in meats but low in carbohydrates
    D. being high in pastries, breads, and cereals

26. Dietary planning for the elderly involves _____ .
    A. the Four-Food Group Plan, exchange lists, and few restrictions
    B. extensive changes in nutrient intakes, shopping habits, and food preparation
    C. the Geriatic Food Plan, exchanges for the elderly, and dietetic foods
    D. none of these

DISCUSSION QUESTIONS

1. Discuss the nutrient needs of the elderly in terms of kilocalories, protein, carbohydrates, fat, minerals, vitamins, and fiber.
2. Discuss why increased calcium intake is recommended for the elderly.
3. Discuss three groups of drugs commonly taken by the elderly and dietary problems related to their consumption.

REFERENCES

1. C. Lecos. "Diet and the elderly." *FDA Consumer*, September 1984, p. 22.
2. Kohrs M.B. O'Hanlon. "Dietary studies of older Americans." *American Journal of Clinical Nutrition*, 31, 1257 (1978).
3. U.S. Department of Health, Education and Welfare. *Ten State Nutrition Survey, 1968–1970*, Vols. 1–5. DHEW Publication No. (HSM) 72-8130–8133. Washington, D.C., 1974.
4. J. Jowsey. "Prevention and treatment of osteo-

porosis." In M. Winick (ed.), *Nutrition and Aging.* New York: John Wiley & Sons, Inc., 1976.

5. R.B. Weg. *Nutrition and the Later Years.* Los Angeles: University of Southern California Press, 1978.

6. C.O. Mitchell and D.A. Lipschitz. "Detection of protein calorie malnutrition (PCM) in the elderly." *American Journal of Clinical Nutrition, 35,* 398 (1982).

7. "Nutrition for the elderly." *Nutrition in Practice, 2* (5), 10 (February–March 1983).

8. C.S. Kart, E.S. Metress, and J.F. Metress. *Aging and Health: Biologic and Social Perspectives,* Menlo Park, Calif.: Addison-Wesley Publications, 1978.

9. F.L. Iber, J.P. Blass, M. Brin, et al. "Thiamin in the elderly—Relation to alcoholism and to neurological degenerative disease." *American Journal of Clinical Nutrition, 36,* 1067 (1982).

14 NUTRITION AND PHYSICAL FITNESS

OBJECTIVES

Upon completion of this chapter, you should be able to:

1. Discuss what a person needs to do to increase muscle size besides increase the consumption of protein.

2. Give and discuss five disadvantages of a high-protein diet for athletes.

3. Discuss the use of carbohydrates as a muscle fuel.

4. Describe why complex carbohydrates are a better source of muscle fuel than simple sugars.

5. Describe the two phases of glycogen loading and the advantage of this process.

6. Discuss two disadvantages of glycogen loading.

7. Discuss the importance of water to an athlete during competition and why electrolyte replacement beverages are not as beneficial as plain cold water.

8. Discuss the disadvantages of a high-protein, high-fat diet and describe the advantages of an ideal preevent meal.

9. Describe the composition of a weight-gaining diet that will increase the composition of lean tissue.

10. Discuss the procedure an athlete needs to follow in order to determine whether his weight gain is primarily lean or adipose tissue.

INTRODUCTION

Recently, there has been an increased interest in physical fitness. In addition, interest in nutrition has increased as a way for the person to improve physical performance. Unfortunately, much of the nutritional information that professional and recreational or part-time athletes receive is a mixture of tradition, supersition, and fact. The purpose of this chapter is to dispell the myths and to present the correct nutritional information that an athlete needs to know.

IMPORTANCE OF PROTEIN IN MUSCLE DEVELOPMENT AND ATHLETIC PERFORMANCE

One of the oldest myths is that athletes need a diet high in protein. This myth contends that high protein levels are needed to build bigger and stronger muscles and to replace the muscle tissue that is broken down during exercise. While it is true that athletes frequently have larger and stronger muscles than nonathletes, this result is not due strictly to protein. The composition of muscle tissue is 30% protein and 70% water. Therefore, the amount of protein in muscle tissue is less than many people believe. In addition, simply forcing more protein on the muscles without increasing their activity will not increase their size or strength. Muscles increase their uptake of nutrients and therefore their size when they are exercised to a greater extent. In other words, muscle cells will take up the amount of nutrients needed to meet the demands placed on them.

If a teenage athlete wants to increase the size of his muscles, then he needs to exercise them more and consume protein at the rate of about 1.3–1.5 g/day per kilogram of body weight.[1] This level of protein consumption can be achieved without consuming liquid or powdered protein supplements. All that is needed is to increase the consumption of food.

Adult athletes, unless they are subject to repeated trauma (e.g., football players), do not need any more than the protein RDA of 0.8 g per kilogram of body weight. However, some studies have found that the American athlete's diet contains. 1.7–2.4 g per kilogram of body weight or two to three times the protein RDA.[2]

DISADVANTAGES OF A HIGH-PROTEIN DIET

There are definite potential adverse effects that can result from a diet that is higher in protein than the above-mentioned amounts:

Increase in fat tissue. Protein consumption of more than the recommended amounts can result in increased fat tissue. As discussed in Chapter 5, excess protein consumption can result in synthesis of fat tissue.

Dehydration. High protein intake results in increased urea production, thereby increasing urination and water loss.

Increased salt loss. Increased water loss often result in increased loss of sodium, possibly resulting in **hyponatremia**.

Hyponatremia Low blood sodium level.

Decreased consumption of carbohydrates. A high-protein diet reduces consumption of carbohydrates, which are very important energy nutrients for muscles.

Increased risk of atherosclerosis. A high-saturated-fat intake often accompanies a high-protein diet. If this high-saturated-fat intake occurs over a prolonged period, the person has a greater risk of developing atherosclerosis than if he or she is consuming protein at the RDA level.

The myth that a high-protein diet is needed to replace protein that was used for energy during exercise is just that—a myth. Amino acids can feed into the citric acid cycle (see Fig. 5-13) and result in the synthesis of ATP; however, the extent of this reaction is minimal. The major energy sources for muscles are glucose and fat, as described below.

IMPORTANCE OF FAT IN PHYSICAL ACTIVITY

Some myths state that athletes should avoid all fats, fried foods, and oily dressings, since they will increase the adipose fat tissue and interfere with performance. An athlete should consume the recommended amount of fat, which is 30% percent of daily kilocalories. If the caloric intake is not excessive, this level of fat consumption will not lead to increase adipose tissue. Likewise, athletes should not consume extra fat for increased energy needs. While it is true that muscles do burn fats for energy during moderate exercise, the amount normally present in the body and consumed in a preevent meal should be adequate. Like nonathletes if athletes want to lose weight, they need to reduce their consumption of all nutrients, not just fat.

IMPORTANCE OF CARBOHYDRATES IN PHYSICAL ACTIVITY

Carbohydrates are very important to an athlete in two ways—to aid in the synthesis of muscle tissue and to function as a clean-burning fuel in muscles. If athletes wish to increase their lean or muscle tissue, they need to consume enough carbohydrates to spare proteins for this goal. A major problem with the athletic myth that a high-protein, low-carbohydrate diet is best to build lean tissue is that much of the protein will be burned for energy. To spare proteins, an athlete should consume the recommended amount of carbohydrates, 50–55% of the daily kilocalories. In summary, if an athlete wants to increase his or her lean tissue, this is best accomplished by consuming the recommended amounts of nutrients:

- Protein: 0.8 g per kilogram of body weight for adults and 1.3–1.5 g per kilogram of body weight for teenagers
- Fats: 30% of daily kilocalories
- Carbohydrates: 50–55% of daily kilocalories

In addition, the athlete needs to increase his or her kilocalorie intake and the demands on the muscles.

USE OF CARBOHYDRATES AS A MUSCLE FUEL

Carbohydrates are the most efficient muscle fuel. The reason is that the only waste products from the metabolism of carbohydrates are carbon dioxide and water, whereas urea and ketones result from the metabolism of protein and fat, respectively. Excretion of carbon dioxide and water is accomplished with less stress to the organs than excretion of urea and ketones.

Muscles use carbohydrates from blood glucose and glycogen stored in their own cells as well as in the liver. Two-thirds of the body's glycogen is stored in the muscles and one-third in the liver. Glycogen is first broken down to glucose and then metabolized. During moderate activity, the muscles use glucose and fatty acids as fuel, both of which require oxygen. While the fatty acids are not the most efficient fuel, their use spares glycogen for more intensive exercise and, more importantly, ensures that glucose is available for the central nervous system. During intensive exercise, glucose is used only because oxygen cannot be supplied fast enough to use fat as a fuel.[3]

CARBOHYDRATE IN THE DIET

The best source of carbohydrates in the diet to replace glycogen is complex carbohydrates such as starches. Brown rice and pasta are two examples. One might think that simple sugars would be a better source, since all the muscle cells would have to do is to absorb them and synthesize glycogen. However, studies have found that simple sugars are mainly converted to fatty acids and stored as fats rather than as glycogen.[4]

A common myth of athletes is that consumption of "quick-energy foods" (candy, honey, and concentrated sugar drinks) shortly before they compete will give them quick extra energy. Actually, consumption of these foods may hurt their performance. One reason is that concentrated sugars will stimulate an increase in the plasma insulin level, which lowers the level of fatty acids available to muscle cells. (Refer to Chapter 18 for details of the relationship between insulin and fatty acids.) In addition, concentrated sugars increase the osmotic pressure in the intestines, which shifts large amounts of water into them. As a result of this shift, the athlete may experience nausea, stomach cramps, and dehydration during endurance events.

Another myth is that consumption of "electrolyte replacement" beverages will help replace an athlete's fluids and provide extra energy. These commercial beverages often contain glucose, salts, and water, but they have been found to enter the blood more slowly than a dilute glucose solution (2% or less).[5] The dilute solution not only enters the blood more quickly but also does not increase the plasma insulin concentration significantly.

CARBOHYDRATE OR GLYCOGEN LOADING

Carbohydrate loading is a technique used by many athletes to increase the level of muscle glycogen above the normal level. Athletes who participate in endurance events may extend their capacity for prolonged, severe exertion from 30 minutes to 3 hours as a result of glycogen loading. Glycogen loading is usually done in two phases:

Phase 1. This phase is characterized by depletion of glycogen in the muscles. This result is achieved by exercising to exhaustion while at the same time consuming a low-fat, high-protein, low-carbohydrate (50–75 g) diet. The small amount of carbohydrate helps to prevent ketosis. Table 14-1 presents an example of the number of exchanges needed to achieve this diet. This phase should be initiated about a week before an event and continues for approximately 3–4 days. The athlete may experience fatigue, irritability, and nausea.

Phase 2. This phase is characterized by a sharp reduction in activity level while consuming large amounts of carbohydrates (450–500 g). It is important that the carbohydrates be complex, such as

TABLE 14-1 EXCHANGE PATTERN FOR GLYCOGEN LOADING

Exchange Group	Period 1 (g of carbohydrate)	Period 2 (g of carbohydrate)
Milk	1 cup (12)	2 cups (24)
Vegetable	2 exchanges (10)	4 exchanges (20)
Fruit	2 exchanges (20)	20 exchanges (200)
Bread	2 exchanges (30)	14 exchanges (210)
Meat	12 exchanges (0)	6 exchanges (0)
Fat	20 exchanges (0)	6 exchanges (0)
Total carbohydrates	72 g	454 g

breads, pasta, rice, cereals, fruits, and vegetables. Protein and fat consumption remains about the same as in phase 1. Table 14-1 shows an example of an exchange pattern to achieve this diet. The large consumption of carbohydrates replenishes the glycogen supply and increases it to above-normal levels. The athlete needs to reduce his or her training activities in order to conserve glycogen. This phase will last for about 3 days.[6]

Carbohydrate loading can be quite effective for continuous, endurance-oriented activities that last for 1 hour or more, such as running 15–30 miles, riding a bicycle 50–70 miles, or swimming 2–4 miles. A normal mixed diet should be used instead of carbohydrate loading for athletes who compete in golf, tennis, handball, or short runs or swims.

DRAWBACKS OF CARBOHYDRATE LOADING

While carbohydrate loading can be quite effective, it also has some drawbacks. One problem with an increase in glycogen stores is increased retention of water. For every gram of glycogen increase, 2.7 g of water are stored. In addition to gaining weight, the athlete may feel sluggish and muscle stiffness.[1]

A major drawback of carbohydrate loading is the necessity to decrease training intensity for 3 or 4 days before the event. In addition, an athlete will experience a deterioration in performance during phase 1 when the consumption of carbohydrates is lowered and he or she exercises to exhaustion.

To avoid these drawbacks, some experts recommend elimination of phase 1. This practice increases the total level of glycogen but allows the athlete to train more before the event. It is recommended that glycogen loading be practiced no more than three times a year.[6]

FLUID AND ELECTROLYTES IN PHYSICAL ACTIVITY

The most important nutrient for an athlete is water. The belief that drinking water immediately before or during an event may cause cramps is not true. Water functions in the biochemical reactions that supply the muscles with needed energy and transport nutrients to the cells. It also removes waste products from the body.

Athletes frequently do not realize how much water they lose through sweating. A loss of 3% of body weight through sweating can seriously hinder an athlete's performance. A 3% loss in a 150-lb man would amount to 4.5 lb, which is not unusual during a vigorous training session.[1] It is important for the athlete to replace this lost water during the athletic event or training session as opposed to afterward. The replacement ideally consists of frequent intake of small amounts of plain cold water (at refrigerator temperature) (see Fig. 14-1). As mentioned above, electrolyte replacement beverages frequently contain 5% sucrose, which reduces the rate at which water is absorbed. The salts in these beverages also slow absorption and are not as important to the athlete as water. The electrolytes are replaced at the first meal after the activity.

Some experts recommend that athletes force fluids during the increased activity period rather than waiting until they feel thirsty. The

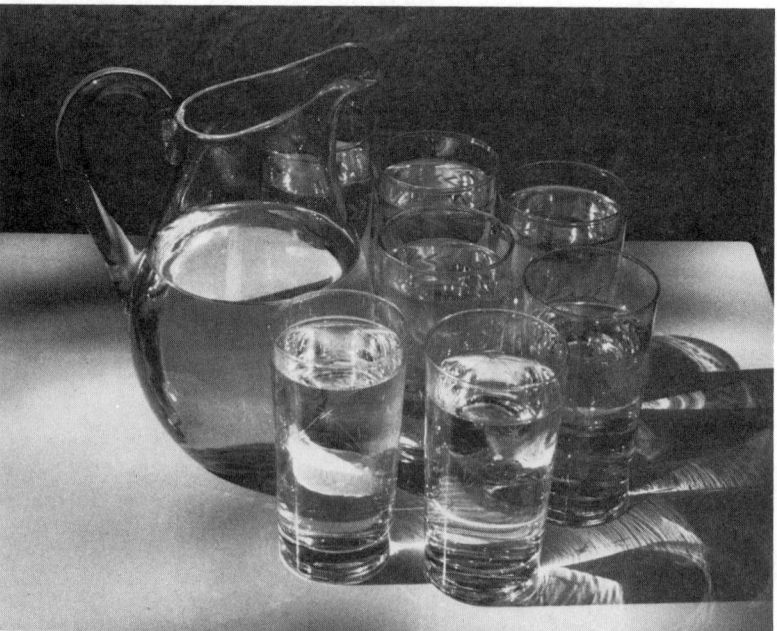

FIGURE 14-1 In order to replace fluid lost during an event, an athlete should drink small amounts of plain cold water.

reason is that the thirst mechanism is blunted compared to the actual fluid needs. The athlete should consume a small amount of cold water approximately every 15 minutes.

PREEVENT MEAL

The meal on the day of the athletic event is important, and much misinformation concerning this meal exists among coaches and athletes. An old myth is that this meal should consist of steak, eggs, and other high-protein, high-fat foods. The theory is that this meal supplies a large amount of protein and energy, giving the athlete a competitive advantage. However, fat delays the emptying of food from the stomach, thereby increasing the chances of nausea and vomiting. Increased protein results in an increased level of urea and strain on the kidneys. Neither condition contributes to the synthesis of glycogen. The only advantage of this meal is a psychological one. Many athletes have been taught that this is a beneficial meal; therefore, it can be psychologically uplifting.

The ideal preevent meal consists of the following:

High-carbohydrate, low-residue foods. Examples are fruit juices, fruit jello salad, sherbert, and sugar cookies. These foods are digested and absorbed quickly, while increasing blood glucose.

Low-fat, low-protein, complex carbohydrates. Examples are chicken, whole wheat bread, beef noodle soup, fruits, and pasta (see Fig. 14-2).

High level of fluids. The athlete should drink water beyond his or her thirst level. This is one of the most important parts of the diet, since hydration of the muscles is very important to a successful performance.

Schedule the meal 3–4 hours in advance of the event. Scheduling the meal this far in advance of the event allows emptying of the stomach, thereby reducing the chances of nausea and vomiting. In addition, if the above foods are consumed, their absorption and transformation into glycogen should be completed by the time of the event.[7]

In addition to the above examples, an alternative is a liquid meal that is high in carbohydrates. It can achieve the above-mentioned goals. One must be certain, however, that the liquid meal is low in osmolality. A high-osmolality fluid tends to pull fluids into the stomach and intestines.

Consumption of concentrated sugars, honey, candy, and soft drinks has been recommended for athletes during the hour preceding endurance exercise. However, these foods do not provide any advantage and

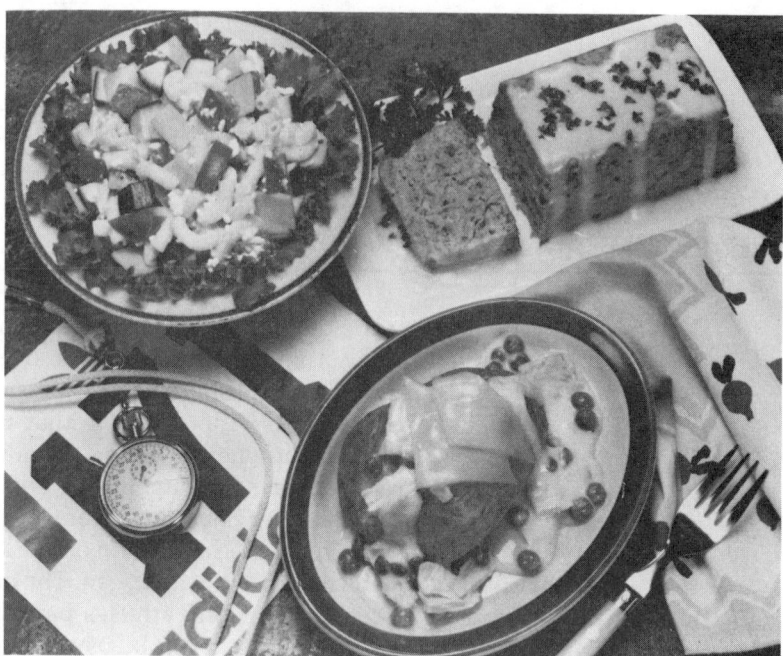

FIGURE 14-2 Preevent meals should consist of foods that contain low fat, low protein, and complex carbohydrates.

can actually hinder performance. Insulin secretion is stimulated by sugar, which lowers blood sugar quickly. In addition, insulin lowers the level of fatty acids in the blood, which results in a lower level of fuel for moderate exercise. Lastly, these foods may result in dehydration, since their high osmolality pulls large amounts of fluids into the intestines.

WEIGHT-GAIN DIET

Athletes who want to gain weight have to be careful that their gain is primarily lean muscle as opposed to fat tissue. As mentioned earlier, a gain in lean muscle tissue can be achieved without a high-protein diet. Instead, the level for teenage athletes should be about 1.3–1.5 g of protein per kilogram of body weight per day. Adults can gain lean muscle tissue by consuming 0.8 g of protein per kilogram of body weight. In addition, the key to increasing lean muscle tissue is for the diet to supply an additional 1,000 kcal/day. This level of kilocalorie increase will result in an increase of approximately 2 lb/week. The distribution of the kilocalories, other than protein, should be like that of a normal diet—30% from fat and 55–60% from carbohydrates.

If the above suggestions are followed but weight training and increased demand are not placed on the muscles, the weight gain will be fat as opposed to lean tissue. Athletes cannot determine whether their weight gain is primarily lean or fat tissue by simply measuring body weight and looking in the mirror. Instead, periodically they need to measure the triceps skinfold thickness with calipers. This measurement involves determining the thickness of the skin at points like the tricep brachii muscles. Since approximately 50% of body fat is stored under the skin, or subcutaneously, this measurement indirectly assesses the amount of body fat. If body fat increases, the athlete can increase the demand on the muscles or decrease the kilocalorie intake.

USE OF ANABOLIC STEROIDS

Anabolic steroids Male hormones that are naturally secreted in large quantities during sexual maturity.

Spermatogenesis The production of sperm cells in the testes.

Testicular degeneration Degeneration of the testes.

Some athletes have used **anabolic steroids** to help them gain lean muscle tissue. The steroids increase muscular development in males; this is the reason why some athletes take steroid supplements. Studies have found that steroids are no more effective than increasing the food intake and exercise level. There are also hazards associated with their use. In older athletes, steroids have been found to interfere with **spermatogenesis** and to cause **testicular degeneration**. In younger athletes, they have been found to cause premature fusion of vertebrae, thereby stunting growth.[8]

WEIGHT-LOSS DIET

Athletes who want to lose weight should not do so by resorting to sauna baths, diuretics, induced vomiting, or starvation diets. These quick-loss techniques can result in dehydration, loss of lean tissue, depletion of glycogen stores, and even abnormal heart rhythms.[9] In addition to these problems, the person may have actually decreased the fat tissues very little.

A sound weight loss diet consists of reducing kilocalorie consumption by 1,000–1,500 kcal/day. If this is done along with increasing the exercise level, the person can lose approximately 2–3 lb/week.

OUTLINE

IMPORTANCE OF PROTEIN IN MUSCLE DEVELOPMENT AND ATHLETIC PERFORMANCE

There is a myth that athletes need a high-protein diet to increase the size and strength of their muscles.

Forcing protein on muscles without increasing the demand on them will not increase lean tissue but rather fat tissue.

Teenage athletes need approximately 1.3–1.5 g protein per kilogram of body weight per day. Adult athletes need the RDA for protein, 0.8 g per kilogram of body weight per day.

Disadvantages of a High-Protein Diet

- Increased fat tissue
- Dehydration
- Increased salt loss
- Decreased consumption of carbohydrates
- Increased risk of atherosclerosis

IMPORTANCE OF FAT IN PHYSICAL ACTIVITY

Athletes should not totally avoid fats, nor should they consume large amounts for energy purposes.

IMPORTANCE OF CARBOHYDRATES IN PHYSICAL ACTIVITIES

Carbohydrates are important in two ways: they aid the synthesis of muscle tissue by sparing proteins and they function as a clean-burning fuel in muscles.

Use of Carbohydrates as a Muscle Fuel

Carbohydrate is the most efficient muscle fuel, since it produces only carbon dioxide and water as end products, whereas proteins produce urea and ketones, respectively.

Muscles burn both glucose and fatty acids during moderate exercise. During intensive exercise only glucose is used, since oxygen cannot be supplied fast enough to use fat as a fuel.

Carbohydrate in the Diet

The best source of carbohydrates in the diet to replace muscle glycogen is complex carbohydrates such as starches; examples are brown rice and pasta.

Simple sugars are not a good source of glycogen, since they are primarily converted to fatty acids and stored as fats.

There is a common myth that quick-energy foods (candy, honey, and concentrated sugar drinks) give the athlete quick extra energy; these foods actually can hurt performance for two reasons:

- Concentrated sugars increase the release of insulin, which lowers the level of fatty acids to muscle cells (a major muscle fuel).
- Concentrated sugars increase osmotic pressure in the intestines, which shifts large amounts of water into them, causing the athlete to experience nausea, stomach cramps, and dehydration.

Another myth is that consumption of electrolyte replacement beverages will help replace an athlete's fluids quickly and give quick energy. Evidence shows that these fluids enter the blood more slowly than water or a dilute (2% or less) glucose solution.

Carbohydrate or Glycogen Loading

This is used by athletes to extend the capacity for prolonged, severe exertion from 30 minutes to 3 hours. It consists of two phases:

Phase 1. Depletion phase, characterized by depletion of glycogen by means of vigorous exercise and low carbohydrate intake. It should be initiated about a week before the event and continued for about 3–4 days.

Phase 2. Characterized by a sharp reduction in activity while consuming large amounts of carbohydrates (450–500 g).

Drawbacks of Carbohydrate Loading

- Increased retention of water: for each 1 g of glycogen synthesized, 2.7 g of water are stored.
- Decreased training intensity: the major drawback is the decreased training 3 to 4 days before the event.

To avoid these drawbacks, some experts recommend eliminating of phase 1 and following only phase 2.

FLUID AND ELECTROLYTES IN PHYSICAL ACTIVITY

The most important nutrient is water, which is important in biochemical reactions that supply muscles with needed energy and transport nutrients to the cells and remove wastes.

Loss of 3% of body weight through sweating can hinder performance. Experts recommend that athletes consume small amounts of plain cold water while exercising. Electrolyte replacement fluids are not recommended, since they slow the absorption of water.

PREEVENT MEAL

There is a myth that an athlete should consume a preevent meal that is high in protein and fat; these foods decrease emptying of the stomach, increase the level of urea and the strain on kidneys, and do not contribute to the synthesis of glycogen. The only advantage is a psychological one.

The ideal preevent meal consists of the following:

- Select high-carbohydrate, low-residue foods
- Low-fat, low-protein, and complex carbohydrates.
- High level of fluids
- Schedule the meal 3–4 hours before the event

If liquid meals are consumed, they should be high in carbohydrates but low in osmolality.

Consumption of concentrated sugars, honey, candy, and soft drinks sometimes is recommended to athletes to obtain more energy for exercising. This can result in loss of water from the muscles, increased secretion of insulin, and therefore hypoglycemia.

WEIGHT-GAIN DIET

Athletes who want to gain weight that will be primarily lean muscle tissue should consume protein at a rate of 1.3–1.5 g per kilogram of body weight (teenage athlete) or 0.8 g per kilogram of body weight (adult athlete).

An increase of 1,000 kcal/day will result in a weight gain of approximately 2 lb/week. The 1,000 extra kcal should be distributed in a ratio of 30% from fat and 55–60% from carbohydrates, plus the amount of protein recommended above.

In addition to the above recommendations, the athlete has to place more demands on the muscles, or the weight gain will be primarily fat.

Use of Anabolic Steroids

Some athletes take steroids to increase the amount and strength of muscle tissue.

Studies have found them to be no more effective than consuming increased amounts of foods and increasing demands on muscles.

Hazards associated with steroid use are decreased spermatogenesis and testicular degeneration in older athletes. In younger athletes they have been found to cause premature fusion of vertebrae, thereby stunting growth.

WEIGHT-LOSS DIET

Athletes should not resort to sauna baths, use of diuretics, induced vomiting, or starvation diets. These techniques can result in dehydration, loss of lean tissue, depletion of glycogen stores, and even abnormal heart rhythms.

REVIEW QUESTIONS

TRUE (A) OR FALSE (B)

Questions 1–14

1. Skeletal muscles are composed primarily of protein; therefore, to increase muscle mass, athletes should consume large amounts of protein.
2. An increase in lean muscle tissue will occur with a high-protein diet and no change in activity level.
3. Possible disadvantages of a high-protein diet to an athlete include an increase in fat tissue, dehydration, increased salt loss, and increased risk of atherosclerosis.
4. Carbohydrates are important to an athlete in two ways; they aid in the synthesis of muscle tissue and they function as clean-burning fuel in muscles.
5. During moderate activity the muscles use glycogen only as a source of fuel, whereas during intensive exericse they use both glucose and fatty acids.
6. Simple sugars are not as good a source of energy for muscles as complex carbohydrates, since simple sugars stimulate secretion of a large amount of insulin, with a resulting decrease in fatty acid levels.
7. Another reason why simple sugars are not a good fuel for athletes, compared to complex carbohydrates, is that they increase the osmotic pressure and draw a large amount of fluid into the intestines.
8. Electrolyte replacement beverages are not as effective in replacing fluids in muscles as water alone.
9. Glycogen loading is a very effective way for all athletes to increase their energy level for any competition.
10. In phase 2 of glycogen loading, the athlete exercises to exhaustion and then consumes a very small amount of carbohydrates.
11. One drawback of glycogen loading is that it results in retention of 2.7 g of water for each 1 g of glycogen synthesized.

12. An athlete should not consume water during an athletic event, since it can result in cramps.
13. The best preevent meal is one that consists of steak, gravy, potatoes, and eggs or high protein and fat.
14. A weight gain of 5 lb in an athlete can be assumed to be all lean muscle tissue, despite the person's activity level.

MULTIPLE CHOICE

Questions 15–22

15. In reference to the importance of protein to muscle development in athletes:
    1. a high-protein diet is absolutely essential for best performance
    2. there are no disadvantages to a high-protein diet for athletes
    3. adult athletes need even higher protein intakes than a teenage athlete
    4. use of protein as an energy source for muscles is minimal
    A. 1, 2, 3
    B. 1, 3 C. 2, 4
    D. 4
    E. all of these
16. The importance of carbohydrates in physical activity is (are):
    A. to aid in the synthesis of muscle tissue
    B. to aid in the breakdown of fats
    C. to increase the amount of body fat
    D. to function as a clean-burning fuel
    E. A, D
17. _____ carbohydrates are the best source of carbohydrate to replace glycogen because _____.
    A. Simple—they can be quickly absorbed and changed to glycogen
    B. Complex—they supply more energy per gram than glucose
    C. Simple—they increase the level of insulin, thereby increasing the level of fatty acids
    D. Complex—they are converted to glycogen more readily than simple carbohydrates
18. The drawbacks of completing phases 1 and 2 carbohydrate loading are _____.
    A. storage of large amount of water, sluggishness, and lost days of training
    B. excess level of energy, dehydration, and weight gain
    C. edema, fatigue, and weight loss
    D. none of these
19. In reference to fluid and electrolytes in physical activity:
    1. drinking water immediately before or during an athletic event can cause cramps

2. water is the most important nutrient to an athlete
3. electrolyte replacement beverages are the best for an athlete to replace water and electrolytes
4. plain cold water is absorbed faster by muscles than are electrolyte beverages
   A. 1, 2, 3 B. 1, 3 C. 2, 4 D. all of these
20. An ideal preevent meal consists of _____ _____.
    1. high-carbohydrate, low-residue foods
    2. low fat, low protein, and complex carbohydrates
    3. high levels of fluids
    4. a meal eaten 3–4 hours before the event
    A. 1, 2, 3   B. 1, 3   C. 2, 4   D. 4
    E. all of these
21. A teenage athlete who wants his or her weight gain to be primarily lean muscle tissue should _____.
    A. consume a diet consisting of 30% protein, 30% fat, and 40% carbohydrate
    B. consume protein at a high level (3.5 g per kilogram of body weight per day), 15% from fat and 70% from carbohydrates
    C. consume protein at a rate of 1.3–1.5 g of protein per kilogram of body weight, 30% from fat, 55–60% from carbohydrates, and increase the demand on the muscles.
    D. exercise to exhaustion and then consume a diet that is high in protein, low in fat, and high in carbohydrates and take protein supplements
22. Anabolic steroids are _____ and their use by athletes _____.
    A. male hormones—have been proven to be very effective in increasing muscle mass with no side effects
    B. stimulants—increases the rate of synthesis of muscle tissue
    C. synthetic proteins—provide more protein for muscle synthesis, but with possible side effects
    D. male hormones—have not been proven more effective than increased food intake and exercise

DISCUSSION QUESTIONS

1. List and discuss five disadvantages of a high-protein diet to athletes.
2. Discuss the differences in the use of carbohydrates and fatty acids as a muscle fuel in moderate compared to intensive exercise.
3. Discuss why complex carbohydrates are a better source of muscle fuel than simple sugars.
4. State the importance of water to an athlete dur-

ing competition and state why electrolyte replacement beverages are not as beneficial as plain cold water.
5. Discuss two possible disadvantages of glycogen loading.
6. Describe the composition of a weight-gain diet that will increase the amount of lean tissue.

REFERENCES

1. G.R. Hagerman. "Nutrition in part-time athletes." *Nutrition and the M.D.*, 7(8), 1–2 (1981).
2. W. McArdle, F. Katch and V. Katch. *Exercise Physiology-Energy, Nutrition, and Human Performance*. Philadelphia: Lea & Febiger, 1981.
3. E.R. Buskirk, L. Hermansen, L. Hultman, et al. "Muscle fuel for competition." *Physician and Sportsmedicine*, 7, 47 (1979).
4. D.L. Costill, W.M. Sherman, W.J. Fink, et al. "The role of dietary carbohydrates in muscle glycogen resynthesis after strenous running." *American Journal of Clinical Nutrition*, 34(9), 1831 (1981).
5. "Nutrition and athletic performance." *Seminars in Nutrition*, 3(6), 12 (June–July 1984).
6. M. Moore. "Carbohydrate loading: Eating through the wall." *Physician and Sportsmedicine*, 9(10), 97 (1981).
7. N.J. Smith. "Nutrition game plans for athletes." *Professional Nutritionist*, 14(4), 1 (1982).
8. N.J. Smith. "Gaining and losing weight in athletics." *Journal of the American Medical Association*, 236, 149–151 (1976).
9. "Nutrition and athletic performance." *Dairy Council Digest*, 46, 2, (1976).

PART III

THERAPEUTIC NUTRITION

15. INTRODUCTION TO DIET THERAPY

16. DRUG–FOOD (NUTRIENT) INTERACTIONS

17. ENTERAL-PARENTERAL NUTRITION

18. DIABETES MELLITUS AND HYPOGLYCEMIA

19. DISEASES OF THE GASTROINTESTINAL TRACT

20. DISEASES OF LIVER, GALLBLADDER, AND PANCREAS

21. DISEASES OF THE CARDIOVASCULAR SYSTEM

22. DISEASES OF THE RESPIRATORY SYSTEM

23. DISEASES OF THE KIDNEYS

24. NUTRITION AND CANCER

25. PRE- AND POSTOPERATIVE NUTRITION

26. NUTRITION AND MENTAL HEALTH

15 INTRODUCTION TO DIET THERAPY

OBJECTIVES

Upon completion of this chapter you should be able to:

1. Give the principle and purposes of diet therapy.

2. Give the four key components of nutritional assessment.

3. State the importance of the anthropometric measurements—triceps skinfold thickness and midarm muscle circumference.

4. State what specific nutrients are measured by serum albumin, creatinine height index, serum transferrin, and hemoglobin-hematocrit laboratory tests.

5. Name the three ways in which a diet history is important to patients.

6. Discuss the advantages and disadvantages of the dietary methods—24-hour recall, usual intake pattern, food frequency record, and food diary.

7. Recognize and list the characteristics, underlying causes, anthropometric and laboratory measurements, and length of time to develop marasmus and kwashiorkor.

8. Give the four components of a problem-oriented medical record.

9. State and describe what the letters of the acronym SOAP stand for in relation to progress notes in a problem-oriented medical record.

10. Describe the four possible modifications of normal diets.

11. Name the four ways in which hospital diet manuals are important.

12. Name the steps involved in the implementation of a nutritional care plan.

13. Describe the components involved in the evaluation of a nutritional care plan.

INTRODUCTION

Diet therapy The use of modified diets to help a person overcome or cope with an illness or inter-related illnesses.

In Part I, we discussed the basic principles of nutrition in relation to the human body. We also examined changes in nutritional needs during the human life span. Part III covers the nutritional needs of people when they are ill.

The chapters discuss the application of basic nutritional principles in clinical care. Readers must comprehend normal nutrition and metabolism before the principles of **diet therapy** will be clear, so they may need to refer back to the chapters on normal nutrition.

It should be emphasized that information in this chapter refers to hospitalized patients; however, these principles also apply to people in nursing homes, private practice, community centers, outpatient clinics, and their own homes.

PRINCIPLE AND PURPOSE OF DIET THERAPY

PRINCIPLE

Therapeutic nutrition Nutritional care that is used to help a person cope with an illness.

Therapeutic nutrition is based on modification of the nutrients in a normal diet to help a patient overcome or cope with a specific illness or interrelated illnesses. It is essential that a student have a good foundation in normal nutrition and metabolism.

PURPOSE

The basic purpose of therapeutic nutrition (diet therapy) is to help restore homeostasis in a patient. Diet therapy is used in three ways to achieve this purpose:

- As a major means of treatment
- To prevent further illness
- In conjunction with other treatments

The care of hospitalized patients takes into account five factors that can affect their nutritional status:

Physiological. Almost any illness affects the physiological functions of the body. A therapeutic diet is designed to help correct physiological malfunctions.

Psychological. Hospitalization itself is a psychological stress that may cause people to become depressed or withdrawn. Children, (particularly very young ones who cannot communicate well), need special help in their psychological adjustment to a therapeutic diet.

Cultural. People's cultural, ethnic, and religious background directly affects their values and attitudes about food as well as their reaction to illness and medical treatment. All of these factors have to be considered if a therapeutic diet is to be successful.

Social. Hospitalization takes people away from their family and friends and the sociability of meals with them. The food pattern and time of meals in the hospital probably differ from what they normally experience. Input and support from family and friends for a therapeutic diet may play a major role in the patient's adjustment.

Economic. Worries about the cost of the hospital bill, lost income from the job, or concern about when the person will be able to go back to work can affect his or her appetite and acceptance of a therapeutic diet.

By recognizing the many factors that affect a hospitalized patient, the health team and patient can work together to plan a therapeutic diet that meets his or her unique needs.

IDENTIFYING AND PROVIDING NUTRITIONAL CARE TO PATIENTS

Two tools are used most frequently in identifying and providing nutritional care to patients: the clinical care process and the problem-oriented medical record (POMR). In addition to these processes, there are many specific tools that can be used, such as food exchange tables, food composition tables, and height–weight charts.

CLINICAL CARE PROCESS

Clinical care process A series of activities (assessment, planning, implementation, and evaluation) used by health professionals to identify and meet patients' needs.

The **clinical care process** is identical to the four steps described in Chapter 1: assessment, planning, implementation, and evaluation. Table 15-1 presents a summary of these four steps.

ASSESSMENT

Assessment, the first step in providing nutritional care, involves a detetermination of the nutritional status of the patient. It includes four key

TABLE 15-1 SUMMARY OF THE FOUR STEPS IN THE CLINICAL CARE PROCESS

Assessment
Identification of the nutritional status of a patient
  Collection of data by historical data, physical examinations, anthropometric measurements, and laboratory tests,
Statement of the problem

Planning
Establishment of goals, objectives, and specific activities for correcting nutritional problems
Nutritional care plan

Implementation
Putting the nutritional care plan into action
Providing an adequate normal or modified diet
Providing nutrition education and counseling

Evaluation
Measurement of the patient's progress
Evaluation of the effectiveness of the nutritional care plan
Modification of the plan based on the evaluation

Source: Adapted from C.J.W. Suitor and M.F. Crowley. *Nutrition: Principles and Application in Health Promotion,* 2nd ed. Philadelphia: J.B. Lippincott, 1984, p. 298

components: historical data, physical examinations, anthropometric measurements, and laboratory tests. The data from each component are difficult to interpret, but when the components are put together, a complete picture of the person's nutritional status emerges. The individual components of nutritional assessment will now be discussed in detail.

Historical Data

The first component of nutritional assessment involves collecting subjective historical data. The person's medical, diet, and drug history, when combined with the other three components, helps to complete the picture of his or her nutritional status.

In this chapter, the only historical data that will be discussed in detail is diet. Drug history and interactions with nutrients will be discussed in Chapter 16.

Medical history. The person's medical history (for example, any recent major illness or surgery) basically consists of the medical record or chart. When an examiner reviews this history, he or she is looking for important risk factors that can have either long- or short-term effects on the patient's nutritional status. Risk factors can affect nutrition by interfering with ingestion, digestion, absorption, metabolism, or excretion of nutrients.[1]

Antibiotics Chemical substances produced by bacteria, yeasts, and molds that are damaging to other cells such as disease-producing bacteria.

Anticonvulsants Agents that suppress convulsions; the drug Dilantin is an example of an anticonvulsant.

Antihypertensive agents Agents that reduce high blood pressure.

Antineoplastic agents Cancer-fighting drugs.

Catabolic steroids Steroid hormones that promote catabolism.

Subjective Conditions or changes perceived by the patient rather than by a health examiner.

24-hour recall A recounting of the kinds and amounts of food consumed during the 24 hours preceding the interview.

Drug history. In the last few years, the importance of drugs and their interactions with foods have been recognized. Details of drugs and their interactions are discussed in Chapter 16. Some general classifications of drugs that may influence the nutritional status of a patient are **antibiotics, anticonvulsants, antihypertensive agents, antineoplastic agents** (cancer-fighting drugs), **catabolic steroids,** and oral contraceptives.

A professional performing an assessment should inquire whether the patient is or has been taking any of these types of drugs. The amount and length of time should be noted on the drug history portion of the patient's medical record.

Diet history. The patient's history is important for three reasons. First, it identifies the patient who is at high risk of having or developing a nutritional problem. Second, it reveals which foods are acceptable to the patient in order to plan a therapeutic diet he or she will follow. Third, it serves as a check on the findings of the clinical examination and laboratory tests.

Assessing the patient's diet history involves gathering **subjective** data on the quality and quantity of the diet, indicating history inadequacies or excesses. The interviewing skill of the history taker and the cooperation and memory of the patient are critical to the accuracy of the data gathered.

Several methods are used to determine food intake:

24-hour recall. This is the most commonly used method and involves the person, or parent of a child, remembering the kinds and amounts of food consumed during the 24 hours preceding the interview. Table 15-2 is an example of a 24-hour recall form that can be filled out by a patient or by an interviewer for an illiterate person.[2]

Advantages

- It can be done quickly
- It is less frustrating to the patient to recall the diet for only 24 hours as opposed to a longer period of time

Disadvantages

- It relies on the patient's memory; therefore, accuracy varies
- The previous day's intake may not be usual
- It does not provide a good estimate of the quantity of food eaten, since it is difficult for many people to estimate quantities

TABLE 15-2 A 24-HOUR RECALL FORM

24-Hour Recall

Name:
Date and time of interview:
Length of interview:
Date of recall:
Day of the week of recall:
  1-M 2-T 3-W 4-Th 5-F 6-Sat 7-Sun

I would like you to tell me everything you (your child) ate and drank from the time you (he) got up in the morning until you (he) went to bed at night and what you (he) ate during the night. Be sure to mention everything you (he) ate or drank at home, at work (school), and away from home. Include snacks and drinks of all kinds and everything else you (he) put in your (his) mouth and swallowed. I also need to know where you (he) ate the food. Now let us begin.

What time did you (he) get up yesterday?

Was it the usual time?

When was the first time you (he) ate or had anything to drink yesterday morning? (List on the form that follows.)

Where did you (he) eat? (List on form that follows.)

Now tell me what you (he) had to eat and how much?

(Occasionally the interviewer will need to ask):
When did you (he) eat again? or, Is there anything else?
Did you (he) have anything to eat or drink during the night?

Was intake unusual in any way?   Yes   No
(If answer is yes)   Why?
                        In what way?

What time did you (he) go to bed last night?

Do(es) you (he) take vitamin or mineral supplements?
        Yes   No
(If answer is yes)   How many per day?
                        Per week?

What kind? (Insert brand name if known.)
Multivitamins
Ascorbic acid
Vitamins A and D
Iron
Other

TABLE 15-2 *(Continued)*
Suggested Form for Recording Food Intake

Time	Where eaten	Food	Type and/or preparation	Amount	Food code*	Amount code*

Code
  H = Home
  R = Restaurant, drug store, or lunch counter
  CL = Carried lunch from home
  CC = Child-care center
  OH = Other home (friend, relative, baby-sitter, etc.)
  S = School, office, plant, or work
  FD = Food dispenser
  SS = Social center, eligible senior citizen, etc.
*Do not write in these spaces.

Source: Barbara Luke, *Principles of Nutrition and Diet Therapy,* pp. 369–370. Copyright © 1984 by Barbara Luke. Reprinted by permission of Little, Brown and Company.

Usual intake pattern A recounting of the foods that a person first eats or drinks during the day.

Usual intake pattern. This method is similar to the 24-hour recall in that a person is asked to recall the first thing he or she usually eats or drinks during the day. Similar questions are asked until a typical pattern is established.

Advantages

• It gives a more long-term picture of food intake
• It is useful in verifying food intake when the past 24-hours have been atypical

Disadvantages

• *The same as for 24-hour recall.*

Food frequency record. This method is used to determine how many times per day, week, month, or year a person consumes specific foods from the basic four food groups (Table 15-3).[1] The data are analyzed by a computer and translated into an average daily nutritional intake. The data can then be analyzed to determine whether the person is consuming the proper amounts of food from the four food groups or whether the diet is inadequate.

Advantages

• It helps pinpoint nutrients that are excessive or deficient in the diet

Disadvantages

• It is very time-consuming
• It requires a trained interviewer
• It requires a computer or hand-calculated analysis

Food diary. This method involves the person's keeping a written record of the food consumed for a specified period of time and the factors associated with intake (time of day, place eaten, mood, etc.) (Figure 10-9). A 3-day diary is usually appropriate for people whose intake does not vary significantly from day to day (infants, school-aged children, and most adults). A 7-day or longer diary may be needed for people whose intake is more variable (obese people and adolescents).

Advantages

• The diary keeper plays an active role and may begin to see and understand his or her own food habits
• Professionals get a good idea of the patient's lifestyle and factors that influence his or her diet
• It helps determine the foods to which the person has allergies

Disadvantages

• There is poor compliance with recording of information
• It yields qualitative rather than quantitative data
• The patient can unconsciously change his or her eating habits during the time the diary is kept.

TABLE 15-3 A FOOD FREQUENCY RECORD

Date: _____

Name: _____
Age: _____ Sex: _____

Below is a list of foods. It is called a "food frequency" record because you are asked how *often* you eat these foods.

Directions:
- Write how often you eat each food (or group of foods). Each food may be eaten by itself or as a main ingredient in a mixed dish (e.g., beans in navy bean soup, or beef in beef stew).
- Complete each square with a numerical response.
- If you do not know the answer, or if it does not apply to you, leave it blank.
- Make a check if the food is a favorite food.
- There will probably be foods you eat regularly that are not on the list. If so, write them in the blank spaces at the end, and answer as before.

Example:

1. If you drink 2 cups of low-fat milk per day, your response is:

Daily	Weekly	Monthly	Favorite
2			

Milk: _____

2. If you have 2 eggs during the week for breakfast, and an omelette (with 2 eggs) on the weekend two times per month, your response is:

Daily	Weekly	Monthly	Favorite
	3		

Eggs: _____

Foods	Daily	Weekly	Monthly	Favorite
Chicken, turkey				
Beef, hamburger				
Pork, lamb				
Venison, rabbit, quail, other game				
Liver				
Cold cuts, sausage, bacon				
Heart, kidney, tongue, tripe				
Eggs				
Peanut butter				
Fish, tuna, seafood				
Shellfish				
Sardines, salmon (with bones), oysters				
Nuts and seeds (e.g., almonds, pecans, Walnuts, peanuts, sunflower or Pumpkin seeds)				
Legumes (e.g., kidney beans, lima beans, Black-eyed peas, soybeans)				
Soy milk				
Tofu				
Milk (name type)				
Cottage cheese				
Cheese (all types except cottage and cream Cheese)				
Yogurt, keifer				
Custard, pudding				
Ice cream, ice milk				

TABLE 15-3 *(Continued)*

Foods	Daily	Weekly	Monthly	Favorite
Beet, mustard, or turnip greens, collards, Kale, spinach				
Carrots				
Sweet potatoes, yams				
Pumpkin				
Corn, peas, green beans, eggplant, zucchini				
Apricot, plums				
Peaches				
Cantaloupe, watermelon				
Papaya, mango				
Broccoli				
Bean or alfalfa sprouts, parsley				
Tomatoes, tomato juice				
Oranges, orange juice				
Tangerines				
Grapefruit, grapefruit juice				
Vitamin C-fortified juice				
Strawberries				
Other berries				
Asparagus, okra, artichoke, Brussel sprouts				
Cabbage, sweet green pepper				
Cauliflower				
Turnip, rutabaga, radish				
Lettuce, celery, cucumber				
Prunes, dates, raisins				
Bananas				
Apples, pineapples, grapes				
Whole-grain bread, rolls, bagels, cereal, Noodles				
Bulger, bran, wheat germ				
Popcorn, corn tortillas				
Brown rice				
Enriched bread, rolls, bagels, cereal, Noodles, crackers, rice, tortillas, grits, Pancakes, waffles				
Sorgum, blackstrap molasses				
Cake, doughnuts, sweet rolls, cookies, pie, Pastries				
Potato chips, fried potatoes, other chips, Pretzels				
Avocado, olives				
Butter, cream cheese, sour cream, heavy cream, gravy, cream sauce				
Margarine, vegetable oil, salad dressing Mayonnaise				

TABLE 15-3 *(Continued)*

Foods	Daily	Weekly	Monthly	Favorite
Soy sauce, meat sauce, catsup, barbeque Sauce				
Sugar, honey, jam, jelly, syrup				
Candy, jello____ Chocolate____				
Soda pop (regular, not diet)____ Fruit drink, Kool-Aid, Hi-C, lemonade				
Diet soda pop____ Coffee, tea____ Wine, beer____ Liquor: scotch, bourbon, gin, rum, vodka				
Other foods not listed that you eat Regularly____ Vitamin or mineral supplement name:____ Other supplements (e.g., protein powders, Brewer's yeast) name:____				

Source: Adapted from Wisconsin State Department of Health, 1979.

Analysis of Dietary Data. Once dietary information has been gathered, it has to be compared to standards such as laboratory and anthropometric data. The standards in this case are the recommended nutrient intakes, which in the United States are the recommended dietary allowance (RDA) and the Four-Food Group Plan (see Chapter 2 for details on these standards).

The easiest assessment is to compare the patient's food intake with the Four-Food Group Plan. It is more difficult to compare the person's intake with the RDA values, since this comparison frequently involves converting household portion sizes to a weighed amount. Failure of a person's diet to meet RDA standards does not necessarily mean that malnutrition exists. The reason, as discussed in Chapter 2, is that RDAs are calculated to be above-average physiological requirements for each nutrient except kilocalories. Remember, also, that nutritional standards were developed for healthy people and nutrient needs are sometimes different for people who are ill.

Should Each Patient Be Assessed? Should each patient be assessed? The answer is, not necessarily. After reviewing the medical, diet, and drug histories of a patient, the professional should determine if any factors exist that will place the patient at high risk for nutrient deficiencies.

If it is determined that a patient should be assessed and if the measurements described earlier were done on every patient, the process would be very expensive, time-consuming, and impractical. In order to reduce these disadvantages, the American Public Health Association published guidelines for minimal, midlevel, and in-depth nutritional assessment of various age groups. Table 15-4 presents information on the level of nutritional assessment for an adult.[2] This same type of information is available for infants and children, adolescents, and the elderly.

See the following discussion concerning the correct assessment of nutritional status in relation to cost-effectiveness measures.

Physical Examinations

A physical examination involves observing and examining a patient. The observations are carried out in an orderly manner, focusing on one area of the body at a time. The purpose is to detect **overt** nutritional deficiencies or potential difficulties with ingestion, absorption, digestion, or excretion.

Overt Open and observable.

An examiner looks for physical signs and symptoms associated with malnutrition. Examination of the skin, hair, mouth, and eyes is particularly important. The reason is that physical signs of malnutrition appear most rapidly in body structures with a rapid turnover of cells. Table 15-5 lists areas of the body, their normal appearance, and signs associated with malnutrition.[5]

If suggestive physical findings and historical data are recorded, they should be pursued further by laboratory tests, anthropometric measurements, and dietary assessments.

Anthropometric Measurements

Anthropometric measurements, the third component of nutritional assessment, involves measurements of **body size** (height, weight) and **body composition** (fat, muscle, water). These measurements are relatively **objective** and are simple and inexpensive methods of assessing, in particular, the patient's protein and calorie reserves. In order to determine whether or not anthropometric measurements for an individual are normal, they must be compared with standards specific for sex and age. Some of these standards are presented in this text.

Body size Height and weight.

Body composition The percentage of total body weight that is composed of fat, muscle, and water.

Objective Observable or measurable phenomena.

Anthropometric measurements can be used in two ways:

- They can be used to compare an individual's nutritional status with that of the population as a whole.

- Repeated measurements over a period of time can provide record of changes in the individual's nutritional status.[6]

TABLE 15-4 LEVELS OF NUTRITIONAL ASSESSMENT FOR ADULTS

Level of Approach	History — Dietary	History — Medical and Socioeconomic	Clinical Evaluation	Laboratory Evaluation
Minimal	Present food habits Meal patterns "Empty calories" Dietary supplements	Name, age, sex Address Socioeconomic level Number in family Brief medical history (including family)	Height, weight Blood pressure	Hemoglobin A simplified Dipstix evaluation, which would identify presence of protein and glucose in blood, urinary pH
Midlevel	Semiquantitative determination of food intake	Sequential history: present health, history, review of history, review of systems, family history, social history (e.g., Cornell Medical Index), smoking history	Anthropometric measurements (skinfold thickness, etc.), brief examination by physician or physician's assistant, chest x-ray as indicated	Evaluations for serum cholesterol, vitamin A, vitamin C, and folic acid; urine excretion of thiamin
In-depth	Household survey data Quantitative 24-hour recall Dietary history Diet patterns as they might influence lipogenic characterics	All of the above Personal interview by physician Family history of cardiovascular disease	Comprehensive health status evaluation by an appropriate health team, by or under supervision of a physician	Serum triglyceride level, plus nutrients in midlevel Urine or serum evaluation of pyridoxine status (vitamin B_6 nutriture) Evaluation of protein nutriture by height, weight, and chronologic age indices Serum essential and nonessential amino acid ratios Evaluation of vitamin B_{12} nutriture by serum analysis Serum iron and serum iron-binding capacity Adipose tissue aspiration and fatty acid analysis by gas-liquid chromatography

Source: G. Christakis, *Nutritional Assessment in Health Programs,* Washington: American Public Health Association, 1973.

DIAGNOSIS-RELATED GROUPS (DRGs) AND NUTRITIONAL CARE

During the 1970s, Yale University developed a system of disease classification based on Diagnosis-Related Groups (DRGs) for the Department of Health Education and Welfare. This system, called the Medicare Prospective Payment System (PPS), categorizes all possible disease diagnoses. It became effective on April 20, 1983, when President Ronald Reagan signed Public Law 98-21 as a component of the Social Security Amendments of 1983.

Within the Prospective Payment System, there are 467 DRGs. Each patient whose hospital expenses are being paid through Medicare (a form of health care insurance provided by the U.S. government to the elderly, disabled, and people enrolled in the end-stage renal disease program) is classified by DRG based on the primary diagnosis. The hospital is then reimbursed by the government, not according to the patient's length of stay, but at a flat rate. The reimbursement rate is determined by the DRG classification. If the hospital can provide the same services at a lower cost and the patient can be discharged within a shorter time, the hospital will have a profit left after receiving its reimbursement. Likewise, if the hospital costs exceed the DRG reimbursement, it loses money.[3]

Effects of DRGs on Nutritional Care

Malnutrition is classified as a comorbidity or complicating condition (CC) under DRGs. When a patient is initially assessed, if malnutrition is diagnosed, this condition can result in increased DRG payments. It is believed that malnutrition is currently underdiagnosed. As a result, these patients stay in the hospital longer and cost the hospital more. If malnutrition is correctly diagnosed when a patient is assessed and if complications associated with malnutrition can be avoided, the hospital will make money.[4]

In summary, the effects of DRGs on nutritional care will be more emphasis on health professionals to diagnose malnutrition initially and then to try to reduce related complications. The end result will be cost effective health programs and assurance that the quality of health care is not compromised.

TABLE 15-5 PHYSICAL SIGNS INDICATIVE OR SUGGESTIVE OF MALNUTRITION

Body Area	Normal Appearance	Signs Associated with Malnutrition
Hair	Shiny; firm; not easily plucked	Lack of natural shine; hair dull and dry; thin and sparse; fine, silky, and straight; color changes; can be easily plucked
Face	Skin color uniform; smooth, pink, healthy appearance; not swollen	Skin color loss; skin dark over cheeks and under eyes; lumpiness or flakiness of skin of nose and mouth; swollen face; enlarged parotid glands; scaling of skin around nostrils
Eyes	Bright, clear, shiny; no sores at corners of eyelids; membranes a healthy pink and moist; no prominent blood vessels or mounds of tissue or sclera	Eye membranes are pale or red; redness and fissuring of eyelid corners; dryness of eye membranes; dull appearance of cornea; softness of cornea; scar on cornea; ring of fine blood vessels around cornea
Lips	Smooth; not chapped or swollen	Redness and swelling of mouth or lips, especially at corners of mouth
Tongue	Deep red; not swollen or smooth	Swelling; scarlet and raw tongue; purplish color of tongue; smooth tongue; swollen sores; hyperemic and hypertrophic papillae; atrophic papillae
Teeth	No cavities; no pain; bright	May be missing or erupting abnormally; gray or black spots; cavities
Gums	Healthy; red; do not bleed; not swollen	"Spongy" and bleed easily; recede
Glands	Face not swollen	Thyroid enlargement (front of neck); parotid enlargement (cheeks become swollen)
Skin	No signs of rashes, swellings, dark or light spots	Dryness of skin; sandpaper feel of skin; flakiness of skin; skin swollen and dark; red swollen pigmentation of exposed areas; excessive lightness or darkness of skin; black and blue marks due to skin bleeding; lack of fat under skin
Nails	Firm; pink	Nails are spoon-shaped; brittle, ridged nails
Muscular and skeletal systems	Good muscle tone; some fat under skin; can walk or run without pain	Muscles have "wasted" appearance; baby's skull bones are thin and soft; round swelling of front and side of head; swelling of ends of bones; small bumps on both side of chest wall (on ribs)—beading of ribs; baby's soft spot on head does not harden at proper time; knock knees or bow legs; bleeding into muscle; person cannot get up or walk properly
Internal Systems Cardiovascular	Normal heart rate and rhythm; no murmurs or abnormal rhythms; normal blood pressure for age	Rapid heart rate; enlarged heart; abnormal rhythm; elevated blood pressure

TABLE 15-5 (Continued)

Body Area	Normal Appearance	Signs Associated with Malnutrition
Gastrointestinal	No palpable organs or masses (in children, however, liver edge may be palpable)	Liver enlargement; enlargement of spleen (usually indicates other associated diseases)
Nervous	Psychological stability; normal reflexes	Mental irritability and confusion; burning and tingling of hands and feet; loss of position and vibratory sense; weakness and tenderness of muscles (may result in inability to walk); decrease and loss of ankle and knee reflexes

Source: Reprinted with permission from Eschleman, M.M. *Introductory Nutrition and Diet Therapy.* Philadelphia: Lippincott/Harper & Row, 1984.

Some of the more common measurements and what they measure are as follows:

Height and weight. These two measurements are the most useful indicators of nutritional status, especially underweight, overweight, and obesity (see Chapter 10 for standards).

Recent weight loss exceeding 10% of the usual weight indicates a need for extensive nutritional assessment and possibly aggressive measures of nutritional support.[7] In order to determine this 10% weight loss, a valuable measurement is the **percent usual body weight (% UBW):**

Usual body weight (UBW) The normal or usual weight of a person.

$$\% \text{ UBW} = \frac{\text{actual weight}}{\text{usual weight}} \times 100$$

which determines what is normal for each individual. This is an especially important measurement for obese people, since malnutrition may be overlooked if weight measurements are based on ideal body weight only.

In addition to measuring height and weight in children, head and chest circumference measurements are important in determining growth.

Triceps skinfold thickness Measurement of skin thickness over the triceps brachii muscle, a good indicator of overall fatness.

Triceps skinfold thickness. This is an indirect measurement of body fat or calorie reserves. It is considered to be a good indicator of overall fatness, since about 50% of body fat is located subcutaneously. The technique involves the use of calipers and is illustrated in Figure 10-3. The measurements can be compared with standards to determine if a person is normal, overweight, or obese.

One important difference between the skinfold measurement and body weight is that it measures actual gain or loss of body fat. A change in body weight frequently is the result of water loss or retention, and not necessarily a change in the amount of body fat.

Midarm muscle circumference (MAMC) A measurement of the circumference of the arm. Usually done approximately midway between the shoulder and elbow. Using the formula, it is a good indicator of lean body or muscle mass.

Midarm Muscle Circumference (MAMC). This measurement is an indirect indicator of lean body or muscle mass. The contribution of the underlying fat tissue is then determined by using the following formula:

$$\text{MAMC} = \text{arm circumference (cm)} - (3.14 \times \text{skinfold}) \text{ (cm)}$$

Again, these measurements should be compared to standard values or plotted on reference graphs.

Anthropometry in Children. Anthropometric measurements are especially useful in children to detect abnormal growth patterns. The rate of change in body stature or structure occurs more rapidly and makes detection of the problem easier.

In severely malnourished children, a radiographic examination of the hand and wrist aids in determining the biologic age of the child, since malnutrition can severely retard the biologic age.

Laboratory Assessment

Laboratory tests, the last component of assessment, provide current information about the nutritional status inside the body, whereas anthropometric measurements concern changes that have already occurred. Laboratory tests measure the level of nutritional, excretory, and **intrinsic** substances in blood and urine.

Intrinsic Functional substances in blood or urine.

The main purpose of laboratory assessment is to detect marginal nutritional deficiencies before the onset of overt clinical signs. Laboratory tests today are very important in detecting protein-calorie malnutrition (PCM). Interpretation of test results must be done very carefully and can be used with more confidence when supportive information such as diet history, clinical symptoms, and anthropometric measurements are available.

Some of the more common laboratory measurements and comments about them are listed below.

Nutrient Measured	Test	Comments
Protein visceral	Serum albumin	Useful indicator of prolonged protein depletion
		Can decrease significantly in 10 days or less in patients in catabolic stress who are receiving only 5% dextrose
		Decreases in albumin levels can also occur in liver disease, renal disease, and congestive heart failure

Nutrient Measured	Test	Comments
Skeletal muscle mass	**Creatinine height index**	Reflects amount of skeletal muscle mass
		Reliable test assumes normal renal function, since renal disease lowers amount of creatinine excreted in urine
		Not a very practical test for nutritional screening, since a 24-hour urine collection is needed
		Decrease in creatinine with loss of lean body mass accompanies PCM
Protein that transports iron	**Serum transferrin**	Main function of this protein is transport of iron
		Considered to be a more sensitive indicator of PCM than the serum albumin test
		Elevated values occur in iron deficiency, pregnancy, **hypoxia**, and chronic blood loss
		Decreased values occur in pernicious anemia, chronic infection, liver disease, protein malnutrition, and iron overload[6,8]
Iron	Hemoglobin and hematocrit	Both measure the level of iron, with hemoglobin being a more direct measurement of iron deficiency than hematocrit
		Decreased values occur in **hemorrhage**, anemia, and PCM
		Elevated values occur in dehydration and **polycythemia**

Creatinine height index
A laboratory test that measures the amount of creatinine excreted in the urine. Creatinine results from muscle metabolism; therefore, it is indicative of the skeletal muscle mass.

Serum transferrin test
A test that measures the amount of globulin protein that transports iron; a sensitive indicator of PCM.

Hypoxia A decreased amount of oxygen available to the tissues.

Other laboratory tests that can be used to assess nutritional status are as follows:

Minerals: iron, calcium, and iodine

Blood lipids: cholesterol, triglycerides

Enzymes implicated in heart disease and liver disease

Blood-forming nutrients: folic acid, vitamins B_6, and B_{12}

Water-soluble vitamins: thiamin, riboflavin, niacin, and ascorbic acid

Fat-soluble vitamins: A, D, E, and K

Stool tests for occult blood and fat

Tests for immunologic function[2]

Laboratory assessment definitely has advantages in determining the nutritional status of a patient, but there are some disadvantages as well. One disadvantage is the high cost of laboratory tests. These expenses need to be considered in the context of maintaining a reduced cost of health care for the general population. Another disadvantage is the danger of a negative reaction by the patient to having blood drawn and possible infection.

Nutritional Status of Hospitalized Patients and Iatrogenic Malnutrition

Iatrogenic malnutrition Physician-induced malnutrition.

Practitioners over the years have not done a detailed assessment of their patients' nutritional status, nor have they considered the effect of nutrition in increasing recovery time. Therefore, many hospitalized patients have experienced **iatrogenic malnutrition**. This term should not be interpreted as malicious intent or as a disregard for the patient's welfare. It generally results from a reduced emphasis on principles of nutrition, with an accompanying overemphasis on medical technology or pharmacologic treatment.

Malnutrition may occur in hospitalized patients in as little as 2 weeks, as evidenced by a 20 to 79% decrease in vitamins A and C, serum albumin level, hemoglobin, hematocrit, weight loss, and midarm muscle circumference. Often patients have been found to have a decreased nutritional status at the time of hospital discharge.

Protein-Calorie Malnutrition (PCM). Studies of hospitalized patients performed during the last 10 years have revealed the presence of PCM in one-fourth to one-half of the medical-surgical populations. The major complications produced by PCM include slow wound healing and increased chances of infection. If a high priority is placed on identification, treatment, and prevention of PCM, it is possible to prevent a long, unnecessary hospital stay. The characteristics of patients who are at a high risk of developing PCM are listed in Table 15-6.[9]

Some factors contributing to PCM include the following:

- Surviving long trauma that contributes to exhausted nutritional reserves

- Failure to assess the patient's ability to heal and resist complications

- Premature dependence on antibiotics, discounting the body's ability to resist infections

There are three main types of PCM (see Chapter 5 for details on the symptoms of these conditions):

TABLE 15-6 CHARACTERISTICS OF PATIENTS AT RISK OF DEVELOPING PCM

1. Below 80% or above 120% of standard body weight
2. Rapid weight loss of 10% or more
3. Long periods on simple intravenous solutions without oral nutrient intake
4. Alcoholism
5. Conditions contributing to nutrient loss, such as:
   Malabsorption syndromes
   Short-gut syndromes and fistulas
   Renal dialysis
   Draining abcesses
6. Hypermetabolic conditions such as:
   Burns
   Infection
   Trauma
   Prolonged fever
7. Drug/nutrient interactions, particularly with:
   Steroids
   Antitumor agents
   Immunosuppressants
8. Clear liquid diet for more than 5 days
9. Recent surgery/impending surgery
10. Obesity
11. Illness of 3 weeks' duration or more
12. Patient N.P.O. (nothing by mouth) restricted for diagnostic tests

Marasmus. This type generally takes months or even years to develop, since it involves both fat and muscle wasting. A long-term kilocalorie deficit is the underlying cause. This deficit initially results in depletion of the body's fat stores, followed by depletion of protein in order to supply enough kilocalories.

Laboratory findings are not altered significantly, and assessment is based primarily on decreases in anthropometric measurements such as triceps skinfold thickness (less than 3 mm) and MAMC (less than 15 cm).

Since this problem is more chronic than acute, the treatment needs to be started slowly in order to allow readaptation of the intestinal and metabolic functions. Mortality is low.

Kwashiorkor. This type of PCM is different from marasmus in that the primary underlying cause is a very low intake of protein but not necessarily a low intake of kilocalories. It frequently occurs in hospitalized patients with poor protein intake (such as those on intravenous, clear-liquid or full-liquid diets for a long period) in the presence of stress such as illness or surgery. This protein deficiency condition

TABLE 15-7 COMPARISON OF MARASMUS AND KWASHIORKOR

	Marasmus	Kwashiorkor
Underlying cause	Long-term kilocalorie deficits	Low protein intake
Time course of development	Months to years	Weeks
Anthropometric measurements	Triceps skinfold thickness <3 mm MAMC <15 cm	Not important, since person generally looks fairly normal
Laboratory measurements	Not important, since generally not changed from normal	Decreased serum albumin level, <2.8 g/dl Decreased lymphocyte count, <1,200 cells/mm^3
Physical signs	Starved appearance	Edema Easily pluckable hair
Mortality	Low	High

is an acute problem and can develop in 2 weeks, as opposed to a chronic problem like marasmus (see Table 15-7 for a comparison of the characteristics of marasmus and kwashiorkor).

Unlike marasmus, with kwashiorkor laboratory tests are the primary component of assessment. Sharp declines in serum albumin levels (less than 2.8 g/dl) and lymphocyte count (less than 1,200 cells/mm^3) are two examples. The major reason why anthropometric measurements are not significant in assessing this condition is due to edema, which results from lowered serum albumin levels. Edema causes the person to have a fairly well-nourished appearance. Other signs indicating kwashiorkor include delayed wound healing and scalp hair that is easily pluckable.

Marasmic kwashiorkor. The combined state of marasmic kwashiorkor may occur when a malnourished patient is threatened by the stress of illness or surgery. This condition is life-threatening. The patient usually has a body weight that is less than 60% of the standard, edema, and a severely depleted weight-for-height standard. The patient runs a high risk of infection and other serious complications.[9]

PLANNING

As mentioned in Table 15-1, once assessment is completed, planning involves the establishment of goals, objectives, and specific activities for correcting nutritional problems. The end result of planning is a nutritional care plan.

Goal A statement of the desired outcome in a patient.

Objective A statement of a short-term specific step to be used to help achieve a goal.

Normal A diet that consists of any and all foods and provides the RDAs and adequacy by means of the Four Food Group Plan.

Modified (therapeutic) A normal diet that has modifications of nutritional components.

High-fiber diet A diet that contains large amounts of fiber, (greater than 40 g) such as fresh fruits, vegetables, and bran cereals.

Clear liquid diet A diet limited to liquids such as broths, Jello, and strained fruit juices.

Low-residue diet A diet low in residue and fiber; it is also called a *low-fiber diet.*

Soft diet A diet modified in consistency that includes high-protein liquid foods and solid foods low in fiber.

High-potassium diet A diet that contains foods that are rich in potassium such as bacon, bran, instant coffee, and oatmeal.

Low-sodium diet A diet that allows no salt in cooking or at the table; all cured and canned meats are also eliminated.

Hiatal hernia A condition in which the stomach protrudes through an opening in the diaphragm through which the esophagus passes.

A **goal** is a statement of the desired outcome in a patient and is written in general terms. An **objective** is a statement of a specific short-term step to be taken to help achieve the goal. Examples of each are as follows:

Goal: gradual weight gain until desirable body weight is achieved

Objective: weight gain of 1 lb/week by increasing the patient's daily diet by 500 kcal/day.

The purpose of a goal is to provide a general direction to the health care team for correction of the patient's problems. Objectives, however, help the team to decide what specific steps need to be taken in order to accomplish the goal.

After the goal and objectives have been determined, the specific diet for meeting the patient's needs is written in the medical record.[10]

Types of Diets

A physician will write a specific diet order based on assessment data. The diet will be one of two types:

Normal (regular, house, standard): This is the most frequently used diet. The only modification is a frequent reduction in kilocalories due to the patient's inactivity.

Modified (therapeutic). There are four possible modifications to normal diets:

Texture. Consistency and fiber content are altered. **High-fiber, clear liquid, low-residue,** and **soft diets** are examples. The main purpose is to provide ease of chewing, swallowing, or digestion in order to rest affected organs. Gastrointestinal, postsurgery, and cardiovascular patients are examples of patients who commonly receive this diet.

Nutrient level. Reduced or high-kilocalorie, low-fat, **high-potassium, low-sodium,** and high-protein diets are examples. Patients who commonly are prescribed this type of diet are those with elevated serum lipid levels and kidney diseases.

Frequency of meals. Three meals a day may be replaced by six small meals to reduce stress to the organ systems. Patients with ulcers and **hiatal hernia** receive this type of diet.

Exclusion of certain foods. Foods containing lactose, wheat, and purines are examples. People who have lactose intolerance, **gluten-induced enteropathy,** and gout often receive this type of diet.[5]

Initiation and Nomenclature of Diets

A physician orders a specific diet based on the assessment of the patient. The name of the diet should correspond to the name given in the hospital's diet manual. The diet order should describe exactly the nutrient modifications as opposed to being written in general terms. As an example, instead of a diet order reading "low sodium, high protein, and high kilocalories," it is much better if it read "500 mg sodium, 120 g protein, and 3,000 kcal."

The actual formulation of the diet is done according to information in the hospital's diet manual. The manual generally describes which foods are allowed and not allowed together with the rationale for and adecequacy of the diet. A sample menu is often included as well. In some hospitals the manual is compiled by the dietitians, physicians, and nurses and approved by the administrators. Other hospitals may adopt a manual from an association such as a state dietetic association. Hospital diet manuals are important in four ways:

- As a guide for the physician in prescribing a diet
- As a reference for the nurses
- As a procedural tool for the dietitian
- As a teaching tool for new health team members[11]

Common therapeutic diets appear in Chapters 18 through 25.

IMPLEMENTATION

The next step in the clinical care process after planning is implementation. As Table 15-1 indicates, implementation involves putting the nutritional care plan into action, providing an adequate normal or modified diet, and providing nutritional education and counseling.

Providing an Adequate Normal or Modified Diet

Providing an adequate normal or modified diet is dependent upon the interaction of the patient, nurses, and dietary department of the hospital or health care facility. The success of any diet depends upon how well a patient accepts and eats it. In order to enhance success, it is very important that the nurses and dietitians determine what foods are acceptable to the patient within the guidelines of the prescribed diet. In large hospitals, this is frequently done by giving menus that allow patients to select food from three or more food items within the categories of appetizer, entree, vegetable, salad, bread, dessert, and beverage. Sometimes a diet may have to be individualized for a patient due to his or her social, cultural, religious, or ethnic background.

Providing Nutritional Education and Counseling

Education of a patient is an essential part of implementing the new diet. A dietitian is the most qualified person to provide nutritional education;

however, the nurse has more contact with the patient and therefore plays a major role in education. There are many times when patient teaching can take place: at the bedside, during a treatment, or even in the community. Some important suggestions for educating a patient are as follows:

Treat the patient as an individual. Each person has different eating habits, knowledge about nutrition, and the ability to learn. The teacher must be a good listener and assess these points.

Help the patient see how the information is relevant to his or her goals. Most people will not learn nutrition information unless it is relevant to their daily or long-term goals. As an example, a boy who is active in sports may learn and accept his diet better if he understands it may improve his athletic performance.

Emphasize the patient's good food habits. Positive reinforcement of good eating behavior is more likely to be repeated than emphasis on bad eating habits.

Choose the right time to teach the patient. Patients cannot concentrate on teaching if they are under stress or upset. If possible, let patients decide when the teaching sessions will occur or tell them the schedule in advance so that they will be prepared.

Try to involve the patient actively. Nutritional information is retained better if a patient is actively involved in the learning as opposed to just listening to a lecture. As an example, a diabetic may learn more from being involved in the planning of an exchange diet as opposed to listening to a lecture.

Teach small amounts of material at a time. Most people can learn material better if only one or two points are covered in 15- to 30-minute sessions as opposed to several points in an hour-long session.

Teaching Aids and Materials

A patient generally will learn more if the teaching is enhanced with nutrition education materials or teaching aids. Many health agencies have printed and audiovisual materials that present nutritional information at different age and education levels.

The printed material often includes meal plans, exchange lists, diet teaching sheets, and schedules that are valuable to patients not only in the hospital but especially when they go home. It is particularly important for a patient who is recieving a therapeutic diet to be able to take home a written diet plan prepared by a health agency or the hospital.[10]

EVALUATION

Evaluation is the last of the four steps in the clinical care process. As mentioned in Table 15-6, this step involves measurement of a patient's progress, evaluation of the effectiveness of the nutritional care plan, and modification of the plan based on the evaluation.

Measurement of a Patient's Progress

Measurement of a patient's progress involves essentially many of the same anthropometric, laboratory, and physical measurements that are performed during assessment. An evaluation of how much a patient has learned about his or her diet and condition can also be made. Some examples are as follows: Has the patient lost the amount of weight that was prescribed? Is a diabetic's blood sugar under control, and does this person have a general understanding of the prescribed exchange diet and injection of insulin? Has a sodium-restricted diet lowered blood pressure, and does the patient show a knowledge of foods that are low in sodium?[5]

PROBLEM-ORIENTED MEDICAL RECORD (POMR)

Problem-oriented medical record (POMR) A communication tool that focuses on a patient's health problems and the structuring of a cooperative health care plans to cope with the identified problems.

The **POMR** is the second general tool used by many hospitals and professionals in identifying nutritional problems and providing nutritional care to patients. This type of medical record provides a logically organized method for recognizing a patient's problems. It provides a patient-centered problem-solving approach to care, one that all health disciplines contributing to the care of the patient can use together.

There are four basic components of a POMR:

Defined data base. This includes the nursing history, assessment, physician's history, and physical examination.

Problem list. This list consists of problems that demand attention of a diagnostic, therapeutic, or educational nature. The problems can be socioeconomic, **demographic**, psychologic, and physiologic in nature.

Demographic The study of human populations in terms of size, growth, density, and other vital statistics.

Plans. A care plan is established for each problem and should include further data that need to be collected, therapeutic measures to be implemented, and education of the patient and his or her family.

SOAP Subjective, objective, assessment, and planning. This is a format in which progress notes are written.

Progress notes. These are narrative notes made by all members of the health team that describe the patient's progress in dealing with his or her problems. The format for writing progress notes is known as **SOAP**, which stands for Subjective, Objective, Assessment, and Planning.

- Subjective data: record of how the patient feels, his or her concerns and his symptoms.
- Objective data: facts such as physical findings, laboratory data, and the patient's response to treatments and education.
- Assessment: professional interpretation of the subjective and objective data.
- Plans: revision of the initial plans or initiation of new ones based on subjective, data, objective data, and assessment.[12]

EXAMPLE OF A NUTRITIONAL ASSESSMENT WRITTEN FROM HOSPITAL ADMITTING NOTES

The material on pp. 353–354 are hospital admitting notes and an example of a nutritional assessment. As you read and study this material, pay close attention to the following:

- Separation of the data into objective and subjective categories
- The analysis of the patient's daily diet
- How the plans are related to the subjective, objective, and assessment information

The following questions and comments are based on the information presented on pages 353 and 354. What subjective data indicated to the professional that this patient needed a more thorough nutritional assessment? If you look back at previous information in the chapter, you will see that the data are a loss of 22 lb (10 kg) in the last 2 months, diarrhea, and poorly fitting dentures.

What objective data indicated the need for a more thorough assessment? Again, a review of the previous information shows that the patient's current weight is 16% below his usual body weight and that he has poorly fitting dentures.

What specific anthropometric measurements would be important to verify the assessment of possible PCM? Since the patient's height and weight have already been measured, triceps skinfold thickness and MAMC are important to help assess this problem. If these measurements are well below normal, which laboratory measurements do you think should be ordered in order to reinforce the anthropometric measurements? Serum albumin level, transferrin, hematocrit, and hemoglobin are all good indicators of PCM.

Under plans of the SOAP chart, the suggestion of a high-calorie, high-protein diet is not nearly specific enough (as discussed in the chapter). If the anthropometric and laboratory measurements did verify the assessment of PCM, the attending physician would write specific orders about the diet and treatment.

For further practice and review of assessment and SOAP charts, please consult the review questions at the end of this chapter.

Name: Mr. XY   Age: 69 years   Sex: Male

1. Height: 5′ 11″ (177 cm)

2. Present weight: 132 lb (60 kg)
   Normal weight: 154 lb (70 kg), patient statement.

3. Lost 22 lb (10 kg) in the past 2 months, patient statement.

4. Upper and lower dentures fit loosely as a result of weight loss.

5. Likes all foods. "It's been hard to eat with my dentures slipping. I must eat softer foods now with my dentures, and I have diarrhea." Allergic to nuts, shellfish, coconut, chocolate.

6. Breakfast—0600   1 cup oatmeal with 1 tsp sugar, $\frac{1}{4}$ cup whole milk
                     2 slices white toast with 1 tsp margarine on each
                     2 cups black coffee

   Lunch—1200 $\frac{1}{2}$ cup cottage cheese
                     2 canned peach halves
                     1 glass water

   Dinner—1700   1 cup macaroni and cheese (frozen, heated up)
                     $\frac{1}{2}$ cup applesauce
                     2 cups tea with 1 tsp sugar in each
                     "I know I should be eating better, but I don't have much energy to fix much food. Nothing tastes very good right now when I know I'll be losing it in a few hours."

7. Does not use alcohol or tobacco.

8. Problems with chewing and keeping dentures in place.

Decubiti Bed sores or skin ulcers that result from interference with blood circulation to the skin.

9. Thin; bones are prominent, with some **decubiti** forming on the pressure points; pale; **lethargic**; dry skin and hair; numerous bruises.

10. No history of therapeutic diet.

Lethargic Sluggishness, slowness, and sleepiness that often result from drugs.

11. Stools—four to five per day for the past 2 months, very loose, black, foul odor; no pain on elimination.

12. Inactive, stays in room; very weak; afraid to go beyond living quarters with diarrhea.

13. Lives in an efficiency retirement apartment partially federally funded; a widower, no children; stove/oven, sink with running water, refrigerator; the building provides a housekeeper to come in once a week to clean; receiving pension and social security.

14. No previous operations or hospitalization.

15. No medications, vitamins, antacids, aspirin.

From the above patient information, the professional prepares the following SOAP chart for the POMR.

SOAP Chart

S: Subjective
Patient states he has lost 10 kg in the past 2 months because of severe diarrhea and no appetite. "Nothing tastes very good right now when I know I'll be losing it in a few hours." He states that the stools are loose, black, and have a foul odor. "It's been hard to eat with my dentures slipping. I know I should be eating better, but I don't have much energy to fix much food."

O: Objective
Very thin—5' 11", 132 lb, therefore 26 lb (16%) below usual body weight.

$$\%UBW = \frac{\text{actual weight (132)}}{\text{usual weight (158)}} \times 100$$
$$= 84\% \text{ or } 16\% \text{ below UBW}$$

Decubiti forming on pressure points, numerous bruises.
Poorly fitting dentures.
Stool specimen is dark, tarry.

A: Assessment
1. Cachetic (general ill health and malnutrition), possible PCM.

2. From stated dietary recall, the patient's diet is deficient in all the Basic Four Food Groups except the bread and cereal group.

P: Plans
1. Order a dietary consultation (an interview of the patient by a dietitian) to do a more thorough nutritional assessment, including anthropometric measurements.

Mechanical soft diet
Same as a soft diet.

2. Suggest a high-calorie, high-protein, **mechanical soft diet** with six to seven small feedings a day after diarrhea is under control. Until the diarrhea stops, suggest seven cans of a commercial milk-based nutritional supplement diet (Ensure, Sustacal, Isocal, etc.) every 24 hours, alternating flavors to meet patient's likes.

3. Multivitamin supplement.

4. Ascorbic acid.

Etiology Cause.

5. Hold iron medication until the **etiology** of the dark, tarry stools has been determined.[13]

PRINCIPLES AND PURPOSES OF DIET THERAPY

Principle
Therapeutic nutrition is based on modifications of the nutrients in a normal diet to help a patient overcome a specific illness or interrelated illnesses.

Purpose
The purpose is to help restore homeostasis in a patient; five factors that affect the nutritional status of a patient are physiological, psychological, cultural, social, and economic.

IDENTIFYING AND PROVIDING NUTRITIONAL CARE TO PATIENTS

CLINICAL CARE PROCESS

Assessment
This includes four key components: physical examinations, anthropometric measurements, laboratory tests, and historical data.

Historical Data
- Medical history: important for revealing risk factors that can have either long- or short-term effects on nutritional status; risk factors can affect nutrition.
- Drug history: antibiotics, anticonvulsants, antihypertensive agents, antineoplastic agents, catabolic steroids, and oral contraceptives can influence the nutritional status of a patient.
- Diet history: important in three ways: to identify patients who are at high risk of having or developing a nutritional problem, to find out which foods are acceptable to a patient, and serve as a check on the findings of the clinical examination and lab tests.

Examples of dietary methods used to determine food intake:

- 24-hour recall
- Usual intake pattern
- Food frequency record
- Food diary

Physical Examinations
The purpose is to detect overt nutritional deficiencies or potential difficulties with ingestion, absorption, digestion, or excretion. Table 15-5 lists physical signs associated with malnutrition and the nutrient deficiencies.

Anthropometric Measurements
These are measurements of body size and composition.

- Height and weight: most useful indicators of nutritional status; head and chest circumference measurements in addition to height and weight are important in children.
- Triceps skinfold thickness: indirect measurement of body fat or calorie reserves.
- Midarm muscle circumference (MAMC): indirect indicator of lean body or muscle mass.

Laboratory Assessment
The main purpose is to detect marginal nutritional deficiencies before the onset of overt clinical signs.

- Protein
  Visceral: serum albumin level, a useful indicator of prolonged protein depletion.
  Muscle mass: creatinine height index; reflects skeletal muscle mass; a decrease in creatinine level accompanies PCM.
  Iron transport: serum transferrin, a more sensitive indicator of PCM than albumin level.
- Iron
  Hemoglobin and hematocrit; decreased values occur in PCM.

Nutritional Status of Hospitalized Patients and Iatrogenic Malnutrition
Protein-Calorie Malnutrition (PCM)
  PCM may be present in one-fourth to one-half of medical-surgical populations; major complications are slow wound healing and increased chances of infection. Table 15-6 presents characteristics of patients that are at high risk of developing PCM.
Types of PCM
  Marasmus: characterized by fat and muscle wasting; major indicators are declining skinfold thickness and MAMC and decreased serum albumin level. Table 15-9 compares and contrasts the characteristics of marasmus and kwashiorkor.

  Kwashiorkor: acute exhaustion of the protein mass of the internal organs; frequently occurs in patients who are on intravenous therapy for long periods; major indicators are a sharp decline in serum albumin level and a decreased lymphocyte count; major signs are edema, delayed wound healing, and easily pluckable hair.

  Marasmic kwashiorkor: may occur when a malnourished patient is threatened by stress of illness or surgery; signs are a body weight that is less than 60% of standard, edema, and a severely reduced weight-for-height standard.

Planning
Planning involves the establishment of goals, objectives, and specific activities for correcting nu-

tritional problems; the end result is a nutritional care plan.

Types of Diets
Normal (regular, house, standard)
   Most frequently used diet; consists of any and all foods and provides RDAs of foods from the Four Food Groups.
Modified (Therapeutic)
   Normal diet with modifications of nutritional components. Four possible modifications to normal diets:

- Texture: consistency and fiber content are altered.
- Nutrient level: reduced or increased kilocalories, low-fat, high-potassium, and low-sodium diets are examples.
- Frequency of meals: three meals may be replaced by several small meals to reduce stress to the organ systems.
- Exclusion of certain foods: foods containing lactose, wheat, and purines are examples.

Initiation and Nomenclature of Diets
The name of a diet should correspond to the name given in the hospital's diet manual; hospital diet manuals are important:

- As a guide for the physician in preparing a diet
- As a reference for the nurses
- As a procedural tool for the dietitian
- As a teaching tool for new health team members

Implementation
This step involves putting the nutritional care plan into action, providing an adequate normal or modified diet, and providing nutritional education and counseling.

Providing an Adequate Normal or Modified Diet
This involves interaction of the patient, nurses, and dietary department; sometimes the diet may have to be individualized due to a patient's social, cultural, religious, or ethnic background.

Providing Nutritional Education and Counseling
Education of a patient is an essential part of implementing the new diet.
   Important suggestions for educating a patient are these: treat the patient as an individual; help the patient see how the information is relevant to his or her goals; emphasize the patient's good food habits; choose the right time to teach the patient; try to involve the patient actively, teach small amounts of material at a time.

Teaching Aids and Materials
Patients generally learn more if the teaching is enhanced with teaching aids—meal plans, exchange lists, diet teaching sheets, and schedules; these aids are important not only while patients are in the hospital but especially important when they go home.

Evaluation
This is the last of the four steps involved in the clinical care process and includes measurement of a patient's progress, evaluation of the effectiveness of the nutritional care plan, and modification of the plan based on evaluation.

Measurement of a Patient's Progress
Involves essentially many of the same anthropometric, laboratory, and physical measurements that are performed during assessment.

Planning

PROBLEM-ORIENTED MEDICAL RECORD (POMR)

This tool is used in identifying and providing nutritional care to patients. It is composed of four components—a defined data base, problem list, plans, and progress notes. The SOAP format is used in writing progress notes.

REVIEW QUESTIONS

TRUE (A) OR FALSE (B)

Questions 1–18

1. The clinical care process, used in identifying and providing nutritional care to patients, consists of four steps—assessment, planning, implementation, and evaluation.
2. In assessing the nutritional status of a patient, all that is required is to determine his or her dietary background.
3. When doing a physical examination to detect nutritional deficiencies, an examiner is most interested in examining regions of the body where the turnover of cells is very slow.
4. Anthropometric measurements are important for determining body size and composition.
5. Triceps skinfold thickness is an anthropometric measurement of body fat or calorie reserves.
6. Midarm muscle circumference (MAMC) is an indirect measurement of stored body fat.
7. Laboratory tests measure changes that have

already occurred, whereas anthropometric measurements measure the current nutritional status of the body.

8. Serum albumin level and creatinine height index are both laboratory indicators of the quantity of iron in the blood.

9. The serum transferrin laboratory test is a more sensitive indicator of PCM than the serum albumin level.

10. Hemoglobin and hematocrit laboratory values tend to be decreased in PCM.

11. The fourth and final component of nutritional assessment is historical data, which involves medical, diet, and drug histories.

12. A 24-hour recall form, in determining the diet history of a patient, has the disadvantages of taking a long time to fill out and estimates the quantity of food eaten as opposed to the quality.

13. A food frequency record in the diet history of a patient has the advantages of giving a picture of a person's lifestyle and food habits to a professional as well as determining to which foods a person has allergies.

14. Iatrogenic malnutrition means physician-induced malnutrition and generally results from overemphasis on medical technology or pharmacologic treatment.

15. The primary underlying cause of marasmus is long-term kilocalorie deficits, and assessment is based primarily on skinfold thickness and MAMC.

16. Kwashiorkor is a malnutrition problem seldom seen in hospitalized patients, since they have an abundance of protein available.

17. There are four basic components of a problem-oriented medical record (POMR)—a defined data base, a problem list, plans, and progress notes.

18. Progress notes in a POMR are written in whatever format the professional chooses.

MULTIPLE CHOICE

Questions 19–27

19. The components of a nutritional assessment include:
   1. physical examination
   2. anthropometric measurements
   3. dietary planning
   4. laboratory tests
   A. 1, 2, 3   B. 1, 3   C. 2, 4   D. 4
   E. all of these

20. Which of the following anthropometric measurements and comments is (are) correct:
   1. triceps skinfold thickness: a good indicator of body fat or calorie reserves.

2. height and weight: recent weight loss exceeding 10% of the usual weight is indicative of a need for nutritional assessment.
3. midarm muscle circumference: indirect indicator of lean body or muscle mass.
4. anthropometry in children: not important, since they grow so rapidly.
   A. 1, 2, 3   B. 1, 3   C. 2, 4   D. 4
   E. all of these

21. Which of the following laboratory tests and comments is (are) correct:
   1. serum albumin: indicator of prolonged protein depletion
   2. creatinine height index: indicates the status of visceral protein in the body
   3. serum transferrin: protein that transports iron and is a sensitive indicator of PCM
   4. stools: examined for the presence of water and fat-soluble vitamins
   A. 1, 2, 3   B. 1, 3   C. 2, 4   D. 4
   E. all of these

22. Which of the following are ways in which a dietary history is important for a hospitalized person?
   1. identifies the patient who is at high risk of having or developing a nutritional problem.
   2. finds out which foods are acceptable to the patient.
   3. serves as a check on the findings of the clinical examination.
   4. indicates the patient's current dietary deficiencies.
   A. 1, 2, 3   B. 1, 3   C. 2, 4   D. 4
   E. all of these

23. Which of the following is (are) correct concerning methods used to determine food intake?
   1. 24-hour recall: good estimate of the quantity of food eaten
   2. usual intake pattern gives a good picture of short-term food intake
   3. food frequency record: very easy to do and less frustrating for the patient than 24-hour recall
   4. food diary: the person may begin to see and understand his own food habits
   A. 1, 2, 3   B. 1, 3   C. 2, 4   D. 4
   E. all of these

24. PCM can result from _____?
   A. protein deficits
   B. kilocalorie deficits
   C. surviving a long trauma that exhausts the person's nutritional reserves
   D. A, B
   E. A, B, C

25. Which of the following types of PCM and accompanying comments is (are) correct?

357

1. marasmus: can develop within 2 weeks, and the underlying cause is very low protein intake
2. kwashiorkor: can take months or years to develop, and the underlying cause is kilocalorie deficits
3. marasmic kwashiorkor: characteristic of people who are obese but suddenly are not consuming adequate amounts of protein
   A. 1, 2, 3   B. 1, 3   C. 2, 3   D. 3
   E. None of these

26. The components of a problem-oriented medical record (POMR) are:
    1. progress notes   3. plans
    2. defined data base   4. problem list
       A. 1, 2, 3   B. 1, 3   C. 2, 4   D. 4
       E. all of these

27. The format for writing progress notes includes:
    1. subjective data   3. assessment
    2. objective data   4. plans
       A. 1, 2, 3   B. 1, 3   C. 2, 4   D. 4
       E. all of these

MATCHING

Questions 28–31

___ 28. subjective data   A. iron deficiency anemia

___ 29. objective data   B. decrease daily milk intake and increase intake of iron-containing foods

___ 30. assessment   C. 17-month-old girl appears pale to mother recently

___ 31. plans   D. hemoglobin value low for 17-month-old girl; height and weight for age are only 75% of normal

DISCUSSION QUESTIONS

1. Name and briefly describe the four key components of nutritional assessment.
2. Discuss what triceps skinfold thickness and midarm muscle circumference measurements measure.
3. Compare the advantages and disadvantages of a 24-hour recall with those of a food diary.
4. Name and briefly describe the four possible modifications of normal diets.
5. Compare marasmus with kwashiorkor in terms of underlying causes and laboratory measurements.

REFERENCES

1. E.N. Whitney and C.B. Cataldo. *Understanding Normal and Clinical Nutrition.* St. Paul, Minn.: West Publishing Co., 1983, pp. 700–726.
2. B. Luke. *Principles of Nutrition and Diet Therapy.* Boston: Little, Brown, 1984, pp. 354–361.
3. American Medical Association. *Diagnosis-Related Groups and the Prospective Payment System: A Guide for Physicians.* Chicago: American Medical Association, 1984.
4. S. Hull. "Nutrition support is profitable and cost effective in the DRG era." Columbus, Ohio: Ross Laboratories, 1984.
5. M.M. Eschleman. *Introductory Nutrition and Diet Therapy.* Philadelphia: J.B. Lippincott, 1984.
6. A. Grant. *Nutritional Assessment Guidelines,* 2nd ed. Seattle: A. Grant, 1979, pp. 5–42.
7. R.A. Hooley. "Clinical nutritional assessment: A perspective." *Journal of the American Dietetic Association,* 77, 682 (1980).
8. S.M. Tilkian and M.H. Conover. *Clinical Implications of Laboratory Tests.* St. Louis: C.V. Mosby Co., 1975, pp. 1–3.
9. R.L. Weinsier and C.E. Butterworth. *Handbook of Clinical Nutrition.* St. Louis: C.V. Mosby Co., 1981, pp. 7–10.
10. C.J.W. Suitor and M.F. Crowley. *Nutrition: Principles and Application in Health Promotion,* 2nd ed. Philadelphia: J.B. Lippincott, 1984, pp. 340–354.
11. M. Green and J. Harry. *Nutrition in Contemporary Nursing Practice.* New York: John Wiley & Sons, 1981, pp. 560–561.
12. B.Kozier and G.L. Erb. *Fundamentals of Nursing: Concepts and Procedures.* Menlo Park, Calif.: Addison-Wesley Publishing Co., 1979, pp. 309–311.
13. F.L. Bower. *Nutrition in Nursing.* New York: John Wiley & Sons, Inc., 1979, pp. 68–71.

16 DRUG–FOOD (NUTRIENT) INTERACTIONS

OBJECTIVES

Upon completion of this chapter, you should be able to:

1. Give the two general mechanisms by which drugs and foods (nutrients) interact.

2. Give the names of specific nutrients that interact and inhibit the absorption of specific drugs.

3. Describe the ways in which foods increase the absorption of drugs

4. Discuss the effects of foods (nutrients) on the metabolism of drugs.

5. Give examples of the effects of food (nutrients) on the excretion of drugs.

6. Discuss ways in which specific drugs decrease the ingestion of food.

7. Describe ways in which specific drugs decrease the absorption of nutrients.

8. Give examples of ways in which specific drugs alter the metabolism of nutrients.

9. Discuss how specific drugs increase the excretion of nutrients.

10. Describe some of the drug–nutrient interactions that elderly persons have with cardiovascular, pulmonary, gastrointestinal, rheumatoid, and diabetes diseases, plus depression.

INTRODUCTION

Drugs Chemical sub-
stances that are intended
to have a therapeutic ef-
fect on a patient.

The therapeutic use of **drugs** to maintain or restore health has increased
tremendously during the past 20 years.[1] Since foods and nutrients interact with drugs and their use is increasing, it is important that health
professionals anticipate and correct nutritional imbalances caused by
their use.

Not all people are affected equally by the drug–food (nutrient) interactions we will discuss. People who must take drugs over a long period
of time are more susceptible to problems. Elderly patients are the largest
group of drug users; therefore, due to changed dietary habits and physiologic changes, the elderly are very likely to develop adverse drug–food
(nutrient) interactions.

WAYS IN WHICH DRUGS AND FOODS
(NUTRIENTS) INTERACT

There are two general mechanisms by which drugs and foods (nutrients)
interact:

• Drugs plus foods (nutrients) = altered drug effects
• Drugs plus foods (nutrients) = altered nutritional balance

In other words, drugs can interact with a diet to affect the nutritional
status of a person. Likewise, a person's diet can interact with drugs to
affect their therapeutic functions. In each case there are specific methods
and mechanisms involved in the interactions, which will be discussed
below. When specific drugs are discussed, both their **generic** and trade
names (given in parentheses) will be given. If a drug is usually known
by only one name, such as digitalis or phenobarbital, only that name
will be used.

Generic Chemical name
of a drug.

DRUGS + FOODS (NUTRIENTS) = ALTERED
DRUG EFFECTS

In order for drugs to act, they must be present in appropriate amounts
at sites where drug–cell interaction takes place. There are a number of
factors that affect the action of a drug and, therefore, its effect on the

body. Four of these factors are absorption of the drug, movement of the drug through the blood, metabolism or biotransformation of the drug, and excretion. Absorption, metabolism, and excretion will be discussed in terms of how foods and nutrients interact with these factors.

EFFECTS OF FOODS (NUTRIENTS) ON ABSORPTION OF DRUGS

Motility Spontaneous movement. The contractions of the gastrointestinal tract are an example.

Absorption of drugs after oral administration is regulated by a variety of factors in the gastrointestinal tract: pH, **motility**, and secretions. In general, foods and beverages other than water delay drug absorption.

Ways in Which Foods (Nutrients) Decrease Absorption of Drugs

Tetracycline An antibiotic that is effective against microorganisms such as gram-positive and gram-negative bacteria.

Food causes increased secretion of hydrochloric acid in the stomach, which can result in destruction of certain oral penicillin antibiotics, such as penicillin G potassium (G-Recillin, Pentids, Pfizerpen).[2] It is advised that penicillin be taken 1 hour before or 3 hours after meals.

Calcium in milk and dairy products tends to bind with **tetracycline** antibiotics such as tetracycline hydrochloride (Sumycin) to form nonabsorbable compounds, thereby causing a loss of the drug in stools.[3] Iron salts such as ferrous sulfate can also bind with and result in loss of tetracycline antibiotics. Therefore, at least 2 hours should pass between iron salt ingestion and tetracycline administration.

Phenothiazine tranquilizers A group of major tranquilizers used in the treatment of severe mental illnesses.

Since food delays gastric emptying and decreases gastric motility, **phenothiazine tranquilizers** such as promazine hydrochloride (Sparine) are more subject to degradation by gastric enzymes. Table 16-1 summarizes the effects of nutrients that interfere with drug absorption.

TABLE 16-1 NUTRIENTS THAT INTERFERE WITH DRUG ABSORPTION

Nutrient	Drug	Effects
All nutrients	Pencillin G potassium (G-Recillin)	All nutrients increase the amount of HCl in the stomach, which can destroy pencillin
Calcium	Tetracycline antibiotics (Sumycin)	Calcium binds to the drug and decreases absorption
Iron salts	Tetracycline antibiotics (Sumycin)	Iron binds to the drug and decreases absorption
All nutrients	Phenothiazine tranquilizers such as promazine hydrochloride (Sparine)	Food delays gastric emptying, thereby allowing degradation by gastric enzymes

Ways in Which Foods Increase Absorption of Drugs

Acid-resistant Something that is resistant to acid but susceptible to bases. An example is the enteric coating on some drugs.

Enteric Pertains to the small intestine. An enteric coat prevents the release and absorption of the drug until it reaches the small intestine.

Antifungal An agent that destroys or checks the growth of fungi.

Time-release drugs contain an **acid-resistant** (base-susceptible) **enteric** coating that enables them to pass through the acid stomach into the alkaline small intestine before being absorbed. Administration of these drugs with food, which increases gastric acidity, may result in loss of the protective coat and thereby in rapid release and absorption of the drug. Aspirin and erythromycin (E-mycin) are two drugs commonly administered in an enteric-coated form that may be administered mistakenly with meals.[4] Aspirin without an enteric coat should be taken with meals or fluids to reduce gastric irritation.

Griseofulvin (Fulvicin) is an antibiotic and **antifungal** drug whose absorption is increased when taken with foods that are high in fat.

Iron supplements such as ferrous sulfate (Entron, Feosol) are absorbed better when taken with ascorbic acid or foods rich in vitamin C such as fruit juices. It was stated in Chapter 9 that ascorbic acid aids in the conversion of ferric iron (Fe^{3+}) to ferrous (Fe^{2+}), which is the more absorbable form. Table 16-2 summarizes the effects of nutrients on increasing the absorption of drugs.

EFFECTS OF FOODS (NUTRIENTS) ON METABOLISM OF DRUGS

Pharmacologic doses Doses of a nutrient that exceed the normal requirements to the point where drug-like effects are observed.

Pharmacologic effect A drug-like effect.

The metabolism of drugs usually refers to inactivation or detoxification by enzyme systems in the liver and other organs. Some nutrients can interfere with these enzyme systems, which decreases inactivation of certain drugs.

One example of nutrients interfering with metabolism of drugs is administration of vitamins in **pharmacologic doses**. When any nutrients (vitamin B_6 and folacin are two examples) are given in doses that exceed normal requirements, they might produce a **pharmacologic effect**. Pharmacologic doses of folacin can cause a lowering of the levels of diphen-

TABLE 16-2 NUTRIENTS THAT INCREASE ABSORPTION OF DRUGS

Nutrient	Drug	Effects
All nutrients	Enteric-coated drugs such as aspirin, erythromycin (E-mycin)	Consumption of food increases gastric acidity, which destroys the enteric coat and results in rapid absorption of the drug
Fats	Griseofulvin (Fulvicin)	Fat increases absorption
Vitamin C (ascorbic)	Ferrous sulfate (Entron, Feosol)	Vitamin C transforms the ferric to the more absorbable ferrous form

TABLE 16-3 NUTRIENTS THAT DECREASE METABOLISM OF DRUGS

Nutrient	Drug	Effects
Vitamin B_6 Folacin	Diphenylhydantoin (Dilantin)	Vitamins interfere with enzymes that metabolize the drug
Vitamin K	Dicumarol	Vitamin K interferes with chemical reactions of dicumarol in preventing blood clotting

ylhydantoin (Dilantin) and phenobarbital, which are used in treating epilepsy and emotional stress.

Pharmacologic doses of vitamin K can interfere with the chemical reactions of dicumarol (anticoagulant) in such a way as to hinder its effectiveness in preventing blood clotting. Table 16-3 summarizes how nutrients decrease the metabolism of drugs.

EFFECTS OF FOODS (NUTRIENTS) ON EXCRETION OF DRUGS

Acidic An acid-forming substance. Some foods cause an acidic pH in the urine (see Chapter 23).

Basic A base-forming substance. Some foods cause a basic pH in the urine (see Chapter 23).

Some foods, when metabolized, can render the pH of the urine more **acidic** or **basic**, thereby affecting the excretion of drugs. When the excretion of a drug is changed, so is the duration of its effects. As an example, if the excretion of a drug is decreased, more of it will be reabsorbed into the blood and its effects will be prolonged. The pH of the urine and the acid-base character of a drug determine how much will be excreted, as summarized below:

Drug Character	Urine pH Change	Change in Drug Excretion
Acidic	More basic	Increased elimination
Acidic	More acidic	Decreased elimination
Basic	More basic	Decreased elimination
Basic	More acidic	Increased elimination

The information above shows that whatever the pH of a drug, an identical urine pH change results in decreased elimination. As an example, if a drug has an acidic character and the urine becomes more acidic due to the diet, less excretion or more retention of the drug will occur. Likewise, if the urine becomes more basic, more excretion of the acidic drug will occur.

Ascorbic acid (vitamin C) acidifies urine, thereby reducing elimination of acidic drugs like phenobarbital and aspirin. If an antibiotic is given for a urinary tract infection, decreasing elimination by acidifying the urine may be the best approach. Likewise, a case in which a change in

TABLE 16-4 NUTRIENTS THAT AFFECT EXCRETION OF DRUGS

Nutrient	Drug	Effects
All nutrients	Drugs with acid or basic character	Foods with same pH as a drug decrease excretion; foods with opposite pH of a drug increase excretion
Vitamin C	Phenobarbital, aspirin	Acidifies urine and reduces excretion of acidic drugs like phenobarbital and aspirin

Ventricular arrhythmias Abnormal rhythms in the contractions of the ventricles in the heart.

Atrial arrhythmias Abnormal rhythms in the contractions of the atria in the heart.

urine pH can result in decreased elimination and possible toxicity is quinidine sulfate (Cin-Quin), a cardiac drug used to treat **ventricular** and **atrial arrhythmias**. Quinidine has a basic pH, and if the urine becomes more basic, decreased elimination can lead to quinidine intoxication. An alkaline pH can result from a vegetarian diet and a high intake of antacids. Table 16-4 summarizes how nutrients influence the excretion of drugs.

DRUGS + FOODS (NUTRIENTS) = ALTERED NUTRITIONAL BALANCE

The interaction of drugs on nutrients to the point of causing an altered nutritional balance is more subtle and long-term in development than the effects of food on drugs. In addition, nutritional deficiencies are unlikely to develop unless a patient's nutritional status is initially borderline.

DECREASED INGESTION OF FOOD DUE TO DRUGS

Taste and appetite are frequently decreased by drugs, thereby reducing the amount of food a person consumes. Drugs whose side effects include nausea and vomiting cause a decrease in appetite. Cancer chemotherapeutic agents, antineoplastic agents such as methotrexate (Amethopterin), and anticonvulsants such as phenytoin sodium (Dilantin) are examples of drugs that decrease appetite.

Antihistamines Drugs that counteract inflammation or allergies.

Antihistamines such as diphenhydramine hydrochloride (Benadryl) can decrease saliva production.

Some oral contraceptives such as medroxyprogesterone acetate (Provera) have been found to increase appetite. Table 16-5 summarizes the effects of drugs on ingestion of food.

TABLE 16-5 DRUGS THAT DECREASE INGESTION OF FOOD

Drug	Nutrient	Effects
Cancer chemotherapeutic agents such as methotrexate (Amethopterin)	All	Decrease appetite
Antihistamines such as diphenhydramine hydrochloride (Benadryl)	All	Decrease secretion of saliva
Oral contraceptives such as medroxyprogesterone acetate (Provera)	All	Increase appetite

DECREASED ABSORPTION OF NUTRIENTS DUE TO DRUGS

Luminal effects Changes that occur in the lumen of the small intestine.

Mucosal effects Changes that occur in the mucosal lining of the gastrointestinal tract or inactivation of enzyme systems.

Lumen The inside of a tube.

Drugs have two basic effects on nutrient absorption—**luminal** and **mucosal**. Luminal effects are changes that occur in the **lumen** of the small intestine such as changing motility, altering pH, or binding with nutrients. Mucosal effects are changes in the mucosal lining of the gastrointestinal tract or in the inactivation of enzyme systems.[5]

Examples of Drugs That Have Luminal Effects

Laxative-cathartic drugs are taken to increase defecation by increasing the motility of the gastrointestinal tract. However, they cause the nutrients to be moved through the intestines so rapidly that some cannot be absorbed. Phenolphthalein and bisacodyl (Dulcolax) are two laxatives especially prone to cause decreased absorption of water, potassium, and sodium. Repeated use of these drugs can result in hypokalemia, **hyponatremia**, and dehydration.

Hyponatremia Deficiency of sodium in the blood.

Some drugs that bind with nutrients and reduce their absorption can have both beneficial and harmful effects. Cholestyramine (Questran) is a drug that is administered to people with **hyperlipidemia**. Its beneficial effect is to lower cholesterol levels indirectly by binding with bile salts and decreasing their absorption. The liver cells remove cholesterol from the blood and convert it to bile. The end result is that the blood cholesterol level is lowered. However, the harmful effect of cholestyramine is the decreased absorption of fat-soluble vitamins, folacin, calcium, iron, and vitamin B_{12}.

Hyperlipidemia High levels of blood cholesterol.

Aluminum hydroxide (Kolantyl) is a drug that benefits the body by decreasing the absorption of phosphorus. Renal failure frequently results in **hyperphosphatemia**, and aluminum hydroxide helps to lower it.

Hyperphosphatemia An excess of phosphate in the blood.

Antacids such as aluminum hydroxide, magnesium hydroxide, and calcium carbonate have a very basic pH and, when taken for an upset stomach, decrease the acidity of the stomach. When the gastric pH becomes less acidic, iron absorption is decreased. An acidic gastric pH is required to change ferric iron $(3+)$ to the more absorbable ferrous $(2+)$ form.

Examples of Drugs That Have Mucosal Effects

A drug that affects the mucosal lining of the intestine is colchicine (Colsalide), an **anti-inflammatory agent** used in the treatment of gout and arthritis. The intestinal irritation produced by colchicine can result in reduced absorption of vitamin B_{12}, fat, lactose, and carotene. To reduce the irritation, colchicine should be administered immediately before or after meals.

A drug that inactivates cell enzyme systems is phenoformin, a **hypoglycemic agent**. It interferes with enzymes that catalyze the interaction of vitamin B_{12} with the intrinsic factor. Since the intrinsic factor is required for absorption, phenoformin can result in malabsorption of vitamin B_{12} problems such as **megaloblastic anemia**. Table 16-6 summarizes the effects of drugs on the absorption of nutrients.

Anti-inflammatory agent An agent that counteracts inflammation.

Hypoglycemic agent A drug that decreases blood glucose levels.

Megaloblastic anemia Anemia characterized by large, immature, nucleated red blood cells called *megaloblasts*.

ALTERED METABOLISM OF NUTRIENTS DUE TO DRUGS

Most of the problems with drugs interfering with nutrients occurs during absorption: however, some drugs interfere with nutrient metabolism.

TABLE 16-6 DRUGS THAT DECREASE ABSORPTION OF NUTRIENTS

Drug	Nutrient	Effects
Laxative-cathartic drugs such as phenolphthalein and bisacodyl (Dulcolax)	Water, sodium, potassium	Increase motility of gastrointestinal tract so that nutrients cannot be absorbed effectively
Cholestyramine (Questran)	Cholesterol, fat-soluble vitamins, folacin, calcium, iron, and vitamin B_{12}	Cholesterol level is intentionally reduced by binding with bile acids; the harmful effects are the decreased absorption of the other listed nutrients
Aluminum hydroxide (Kolantyl)	Phosphorus, iron	Phosphorus absorption is decreased intentionally; reduced iron absorption is a side effect and results from gastric pH becoming too basic
Colchicine (Colsalide)	Vitamin B_{12}, fat, lactose, and carotene	Irritation of the intestinal mucosa reduces absorption of indicated nutrients
Phenoformin	Glucose, vitamin B_{12}	Glucose is intentionally reduced; vitamin B_{12} reduction results from interference of drug with intrinsic factor

TABLE 16-7 DRUGS THAT AFFECT METABOLISM OF NUTRIENTS

Drug	Nutrient	Effect
Anticancer drugs such as methotrexate (Amethopterin)	Folacin	Drug displaces folacin in the metabolic pathway; kills cancer cells but is detrimental to healthy cells
Anticonvulsants such as phenytoin sodium (Dilantin)	Vitamin D	Drug interferes with enzymatic conversion of inactive form of vitamin D to active form

This interference can occur when a drug that is similar in structure to a vitamin displaces a vitamin in a metabolic pathway. One example is methotrexate (Amethopterin) and the vitamin folacin. Methotrexate is an antineoplastic drug that kills cancer cells by displacing folacin. However, the healthy cells also are prevented from metabolizing folacin, with the end result being macrocytic anemia.

The anticonvulsant phenytoin sodium (Dilantin) interferes with the enzymes in the kidney that convert the inactive form of vitamin D, calcidiol, to the active form, calcitriol. People undergoing long-term treatment with Dilantin may experience bone changes such as osteomalacia. Table 16-7 summarizes the effects of drugs on metabolism of nutrients.

INCREASED EXCRETION OF NUTRIENTS AS A RESULT OF DRUGS

Hepatic cirrhosis The degeneration of liver cells with the formation of fibrous scar tissue.

Diuretics frequently are taken to correct edema resulting from congestive heart failure, **hepatic cirrhosis**, and renal disorders. While they are successful in reducing the excess water level in the body, they also result in the excretion of large amounts of potassium and magnesium. Patients chronically treated with thiazide diuretics such as hydrochlorothiazide (HydroDIURIL) are often encouraged to increase their intake of foods high in potassium such as bananas and orange juice. Table 16-8 summarizes the effects of drugs on excretion of nutrients.

TABLE 16-8 DRUGS THAT INCREASE EXCRETION OF NUTRIENTS

Drug	Nutrient	Effect
Thiazide diuretics such as hydrochlorothiazide (HydroDIURIL)	Potassium, magnesium, water	Decrease absorption of indicated nutrients

FOOD (NUTRIENTS)–DRUG INTERACTION IN THE ELDERLY

Elderly people are the largest group of drug users. They purchase two and a half to three times as many drugs as the nonelderly population because chronic disease is present in about 70% of the elderly. Elderly people are very susceptible to drug–nutrient interactions. Their susceptibility results from the high amounts of drugs they consume and to the decreased activity of their organ systems, especially the liver and kidneys.[6]

Some of the more common diseases or disorders suffered by the elderly, drugs prescribed, and drug–nutrient interactions will be discussed next.

CARDIOVASCULAR DISEASE

Congestive heart failure is often treated with the diuretic digoxin (Lanoxin), which renders elderly persons very vulnerable to potassium and magnesium imbalances. To counter these imbalances, they should be encouraged to eat more potassium- and magnesium-rich foods. However, elderly persons who are taking spironolactone (Aldactone) or triamterene (Dyrenium) should not be encouraged to increase their consumption of potassium and magnesium, since these are potassium-sparing diuretics.

PULMONARY DISEASE

Chronic obstructive pulmonary disease (COPD) A chronic, persistent obstruction of the air flow into the bronchi of the lungs. Asthma, bronchitis, and emphysema are the main causes of this condition (see Chapter 22).

Elderly patients who have **chronic obstructuve pulmonary disease** and are being treated with theophylline (Slo-Phyllin) should be advised to eat normal amounts of protein and carbohydrates. High protein intake will delay the action of theophylline, whereas high carbohydrate intake will speed it up. Stimulant beverages such as those containing caffeine (coffee, tea, and cola) should be avoided while taking theophylline since they will enhance the effects of the drug.

GASTROINTESTINAL DISEASE

Common gastrointestinal symptoms experienced by the elderly include constipation, heartburn, and indigestion. As a result of these symptoms, they frequently consume excessive amounts of laxatives, cathartics, and antacids.

Elderly persons should be advised that habitual use of laxative-cathartic preparations can result in decreased absorption of potassium, sodium, and water. Low levels of these nutrients can result in hypokalemia, hyponatremia, and dehydration.

Many elderly persons take over-the-counter antacids that are high in either aluminum or magnesium hydroxide. Aluminum hydroxide antacids, such as Amphojel or Nutrajel, if taken in large doses continuously, can result in constipation. Likewise, magnesium hydroxide antacids, such as Mag-Ox or Oxabid, can result in diarrhea. To avoid these problems, many preparations combine magnesium and aluminum hydroxides, with Kolantyl and Maalox being two examples. Some of these preparations are high in sodium, which can be a problem for elderly persons who are on a low-sodium diet. Magaldrate Riopan is an example of an antacid that is low in sodium.

RHEUMATOID DISEASE

Rheumatoid Disease A disease the results in inflammation and degeneration of the connective tissues around joints.

Aspirin is used widely by elderly persons for the treatment of **rheumatoid disease.** Chronic use of aspirin can cause gastric irritation followed by gastric bleeding and can result in iron deficiency anemia and increased urinary losses of vitamin C and potassium. The elderly should be advised that gastric distress can be reduced if aspirin is taken with food, milk, crackers, or a full glass of water. Also, it should be emphasized that consumption of alcohol along with aspirin will increase gastric irritation.

Severe gastrointestinal distress can occur in elderly rheumatoid patients who are treated with anti-inflammatory drugs such as phenylbutazone (Butazolidin) and indomethacin (Indocin). These drugs are not normally used for relief of minor pain, but only when the patient does not respond to less toxic agents. Phenylbutazone can cause sodium retention; therefore, if edema occurs, a low-sodium diet may need to be prescribed.

DEPRESSION

Tricyclic antidepressants A group of drugs used in the treatment of depression. The drugs are thought to work by increasing the amount of norepineprhine and serotonin.

Epigastric distress Pain and discomfort in the epigastrium region, which is the upper central region of the abdomen.

Esophageal reflux Backward and upward flow of food through the esophagus (see Chapter 19).

Prolonged depression in the elderly is often treated with **tricyclic antidepressants** such as amitriptyline (Elavil) and imipramine (Tofranil). The levels of these drugs in the blood of the elderly tend to increase more than they do in the young due to decreased detoxification by the liver. Side effects that can result from the increased levels of these drugs are dry mouth, sour or metallic taste, **epigastric distress,** and constipation. Other side effects of these antidepressants are nausea, vomiting, anorexia, and **esophageal reflux..**

DIABETES

Some non-insulin-dependent diabetics treated with oral hypoglycemic agents such as tolbutamide (Orinase) or chlorpropamide (Diabinese) have reported episodes of nausea. A major concern with the use of oral hypoglycemic agents is hypoglycemic episodes. These episodes may be caused by inadequate or irregular food intake; warning signs include excited, nervous behavior, rapid, shallow breathing, and hunger. Diabetics need to be counseled on the importance of adequate and regular food intake. In addition, it should be strongly emphasized to patients who take oral hypoglycemic agents that consumption of alcohol can result in side effects such as facial flushing, nausea and vomiting, rapid heart beat, and headache.[7]

OUTLINE

INTRODUCTION

A drug (medication) is a chemical substance intended to have a therapeutic effect on a person.

WAYS IN WHICH DRUGS AND FOODS (NUTRIENTS) INTERACT

- Drugs + foods (nutrients) = altered drug effects
- Drugs + foods (nutrients) = altered nutritional balance

DRUGS + FOODS (NUTRIENTS) = ALTERED DRUG EFFECTS

Four factors that affect the action of a drug: absorption of a drug, movement of a drug through the blood, metabolism or biotransformation of a drug, and excretion; absorption, metabolism, and excretion will be discussed.

Effects of Foods (Nutrients) on Absorption of Drugs

Factors in the gastrointestinal tract that affect absorption of drugs are pH, motility, and secretions.

Ways in Which Foods (Nutrients) Decrease Absorption of Drugs

- Increased secretion of HCl in the stomach, which can cause destruction of certain penicillin antibiotics
  Examples: penicillin G potassium (G-Recillin, Pentids). Best for penicillin to be taken 1 hour before or 3 hours after meals.
- Calcium and iron salts bind with tetracycline antibiotics to decrease absorption
  At least 2 hours should pass between consumption of milk and iron salts before tetracycline administration.
- Food in the stomach increases the degradation of phenothiazine tranquilizers
  Example: promazine hydrochloride (Sparine)

Ways in Which Foods Increase Absorption of Drugs

- Increased acidity of the stomach increases absorption of enteric coated drugs
  Examples: aspirin and erythromycin (E-mycin) are often administered in enteric form.
- High fat level increases absorption of griseofulvin (Fulvicin), an antibiotic and antifungal drug.
- Acidity increases absorption of iron supplements

Examples: ascorbic acid or foods rich in vitamin C increase absorption of ferrous sulfate (Entron, Feosol).

EFFECTS OF FOOD (NUTRIENTS) ON METABOLISM OF DRUGS

Some nutrients interfere with deactivation or metabolism of drugs in the liver.

Example: pharmacologic doses of folacin can cause lowering of the level of diphenylhydantoin (Dilantin) and phenobarbital, which are used in treating epilepsy and emotional stress.

Pharmacologic doses of vitamin K can interfere with chemical reactions of dicumarol (anticoagulant) to prevent blood clotting.

Effects of Food (Nutrients) on Excretion of Drugs

Foods can change the pH of urine, thereby affecting the excretion of drugs; affecting the excretion of a drug also affects the duration of its effects (for example, decreasing the excretion of a drug increases its effects).

Whatever the pH character of a drug, an identical change in urine pH results in decreased elimination. For example, if a drug has an acidic character and the urine becomes more acidic, less excretion or more retention of the drug will occur. Likewise, if the urine becomes more basic, more excretion of the acidic drug will occur.

Example: ascorbic acid (vitamin C) acidifies urine, thereby reducing the elimination of acidic drugs like phenobarbital and aspirin.

DRUGS + FOODS (NUTRIENTS) = ALTERED NUTRITIONAL BALANCE

Decreased Ingestion of Food Due to Drugs

- Drugs that decrease taste and appetite
  Examples: cancer chemotherapeutic agents or antineoplastic agents; methotrexate (Amethopterin) and anticonvulsants such as phenytoin sodium (Dilantin).
- Drugs that decrease saliva production
  Example: antihistamines such as diphenhydramine hydrochloride (Benadryl).

Decreased Absorption of Nutrients Due to Drugs

Drugs affect nutrient absorption in two ways: Luminal: changes that occur in the lumen of the small intestine (changing motility, altering pH, or binding with nutrients).

Examples of Drugs That Have Luminal Effects

Phenolphthalein and bisacodyl (Dulcolax) are two laxatives that can increase motility, thereby decreasing absorption of water, potassium, and sodium.

Cholestyramine (Questran) binds with bile acids, preventing its absorption, thereby reducing the level of cholesterol, since it is a component of bile acids. This reaction is detrimental to the body because it decreases absorption of fat-soluble vitamins, folacin, calcium, iron, and vitamin B_{12}.

Aluminum hydroxide (Kolantyl) decreases absorption of phosphorus, which can be beneficial in hyperphosphatemic conditions, which are often caused by renal failure.

Mucosal: changes in the mucosal lining of the gastrointestinal tract or inactivation of enzyme systems.

Examples of Drugs That Have Mucosal Effects

Cochicine (Colsalide), an anti-inflammatory agent, reduces absorption of vitamin B_{12}, fat, lactose, and carotene by irritating the mucosal lining of the gastrointestinal tract; to reduce irritation, colchicine should be administered immediately before or after meals.

Phenoformin (a hypoglycemic agent) interferes with enzymes that catalyze the absorption of vitamin B_{12}, thereby possibly resulting in megaloblastic anemia.

Altered Metabolism of Nutrients Due to Drugs

Some drugs interfere with nutrients by displacing the nutrient in a metabolic pathway.

Examples: methotrexate (Amethopterin), an anticancer or antineoplastic drug, displaces folacin, thereby possibly resulting in megaloblastic anemia.

Phenytoin sodium (Dilantin) prevents the activation of the inactive form of vitamin D, calcidiol, to the active form, calcitriol; long-term treatment with Dilantin may result in osteomalacia.

Increased Excretion of Nutrients as a Result of Drugs

Diuretics frequently are taken to reduce edema, but they also result in the excretion of large amounts of potassium and magnesium.

Examples: thiazide diuretics, hydrochlorothiazide (HydroDIURIL).

FOOD (NUTRIENTS)–DRUG INTERACTION IN THE ELDERLY

The elderly (people 65 years of age or older) are the largest group who purchase and use drugs in the United States. Some of the more common diseases or disorders suffered by the elderly, drugs prescribed, and drug–nutrient interactions are as follows:

Cardiovascular Disease

- Digoxin (Lanoxin): diuretic, can cause potassium and magnesium imbalances.
- Spironolactone (Aldactone) or triamterene (Dyrenium): potassium- and magnesium-sparing diuretics.

Pulmonary Disease

Theophylline (Slo-Phyllin), taken for chronic obstructive pulmonary disease, is hindered by a high protein intake, whereas a high carbohydrate intake will increase speed of the drug.

Gastrointestinal Disease

The elderly frequently experience constipation, heartburn, and indigestion and frequently consume laxatives, cathartics, and antacids, to achieve relief.

Example: laxative-cathartic preparations can result in decreased absorption of potassium, sodium, and water.

Antacids that are high in aluminum or magnesium hydroxide, such as Amphojel or Nutrajel, can result in constipation; Mag-Ox or Oxabid can result in diarrhea.

Some laxative-cathartic compounds are high in sodium.

Rheumatoid Disease

Aspirin: is used widely for rheumatoid disease and can cause gastric irritation, bleeding, iron deficiency anemia, and urinary losses of vitamin C.

Phenylbutazone (Butazolidin) and indomethacin (Indocin): drugs used when arthritis is severe and does not respond to aspirin; can cause sodium retention.

Depression

Antidepressant drugs such as amitriptyline (Elavil) and imipramine (Tofranil) can result in dry mouth, sour or metallic taste, epigastric distress, constipation, nausea, vomiting, anorexia, and esophageal reflux.

Diabetes

Non-insulin-dependent diabetics who take oral hypoglycemic agents such as tolbutamide (Orinase) or chlorpropamide (Diabinese) can experience nausea and hypoglycemic episodes; those who take it with alcohol can experience facial flushing, nausea, rapid heartbeat, and headache.

TRUE (A) OR FALSE (B)

Questions 1–14

1. All people are equally affected by drug–food (nutrient) interactions.
2. Four important factors that affect the action of a drug and its effects on the body are type of food eaten, amount of food eaten, number of meals consumed, and number of kilocalories in the meals.
3. Food causes decreased secretion of hydrochloric acid in the stomach, which can result in destruction of some oral penicillin antibiotics such as penicillin G potassium (G-Recillin).
4. Enteric-coated drugs like aspirin should not be administered with food, since increased acidity will break down the coat, resulting in rapid release and absorption.
5. Foods rich in vitamin C (ascorbic acid) increase absorption of iron by changing it from the ferric to the ferrous form.
6. Metabolism of drugs refers to their effects on the tissues.
7. Vitamin K can interfere with the chemical reactions of dicumarol and thereby hinder it from preventing blood clotting.
8. If a drug has an acidic character and the urine becomes more acidic, more excretion and less retention of the drug will occur.
9. Cancer chemotherapeutic agents such as methotrexate (Amethopterin) have been found to increase the appetite.
10. Drugs have two basic effects on nutrient absorption: decomposition of food and increased mucus secretion, so that absorption is decreased.
11. Some drugs that reduce absorption of nutrients can be beneficial, such as cholestyramine, which lowers blood cholesterol levels.
12. Phenoformin, a hypoglycemic agent, can reduce the absorption of vitamin B_{12} by interfering with enzymes that catalyze the interaction of intrinsic factor with the vitamin.
13. The anticonvulsant phenytoin sodium (Dilantin) affects enzymes in the kidneys so that more vitamin D is activated.
14. Elderly persons are more susceptible than younger persons to drug–nutrient interactions because of the amount of drugs taken and the decreased activity of their organ systems.

MULTIPLE CHOICE

Questions 15–25

15. Absorption of drugs after oral administration is governed by the following factors in the gastrointestinal tract:

    1. pH   3. secretions
    2. motility   4. length of the tract
       A. 1, 2, 3   B. 1, 3   C. 2, 4   D. 4
       E. all of these

16. In general, foods and beverages other than water delay drug absorption. Which of the following drugs and inhibition mechanisms is (are) correctly paired:
    A. penicillin G potassium (G-Recillin)—calcium binds with and decreases absorption of penicillin
    B. tetracycline hydrochloride (Sumycin)—increased HCl in stomach destroys and decreases absorption of tetracycline drugs
    C. promazine hydrochloride (Sparine) tranquilizers—increase motility of the gastrointestinal tract and decrease absorption of promazine tranquilizers
    D. all of these
    E. none of these

17. Enteric-coated drugs such as _____, when administered with foods, result in _____.
    A. griseofulvin (Fulvicin) and ferrous sulfate (Entron)—increased alkalinity and decreased absorption
    B. aspirin and erythromycin—increased alkalinity and increased absorption
    C. griseofulvin (Fulvicin) and ferrous sulfate (Entron)—increased acidity and increased absorption
    D. aspirin and erythromycin—increased acidity and increased absorption

18. Iron supplements such as ferrous sulfate (Entron, Feosol) are absorbed better when taken with _____ due to _____.
    A. base-forming foods—increased basicity changing ferric iron to the more absorbable ferrous form
    B. acid-forming foods—increased acidity changing iron from the ferrous to the more absorbable ferric form
    C. base-forming foods—increased basicity changing iron from the ferrous to the more absorbable ferric form
    D. acid-forming foods—increased acidity changing iron from the ferric to the more absorbable ferrous form

19. The excretion of an acidic drug like phenobarbital is _____ by the urine pH becoming more _____.

A. decreased—acidic
B. increased—basic
C. decreased—basic
D. A, C
E. A, B

20. Laxative-cathartic drugs such as phenolphthalein and bisacodyl (Dulcolax) can cause decreased absorption of
A. water
B. potassium
C. sodium
D. A, B, C
E. A, C

21. Cholestyramine (Questran) binds with nutrients and benefits the body by decreasing absorption of _____ but hurts the body by preventing absorption of _____.
A. bile—fat
B. cholesterol—fat-soluble vitamins, folacin, calcium, iron, and vitamin B_{12}
C. carbohydrate—water-soluble vitamins, vitamin B_6, and cholesterol
D. protein—fats and carbohydrate

22. The anticancer drug methotrexate (Amethopterin) displaces _____ from its metabolic pathway with the end result being _____.
A. vitamin B_{12}—microcytic anemia
B. vitamin D—osteomalacia
C. folacin—macrocytic anemia
D. vitamin C—scurvy

23. Many elderly persons take antacids containing aluminum and magnesium hydroxide. Large doses of aluminum hydroxide can result in _____ and magnesium hydroxide can result in _____.
A. constipation—diarrhea
B. dehydration—gastric ulcers
C. decreased iron absorption—macrocytic anemia
D. none of these

24. Elderly persons frequently take aspirin for rheumatoid arthritis and, when taken chronically without meals, it can result in _____.
A. gastric irritation
B. gastric bleeding

C. iron deficiency anemia
D. none of these
E. all of these

25. Noninsulin diabetics who take oral hypoglycemic agents such as tolbutamide (Orinase) need to be counseled to _____.
A. consume a low-carboyhydrate diet.
B. consume an adequate and regular diet.
C. be aware that consumption of alcohol can result in facial flushing, nausea, and vomiting.
D. A, C
E. B, C

DISCUSSION QUESTIONS

1. Name three ways in which food can decrease the absorption of drugs and give an example of a drug in each category.
2. Discuss the luminal and mucosal effects of drugs, with an example of each, on decreased absorption of nutrients.
3. Discuss some of the food–drug interaction problems that the elderly have with digoxin, Amphojel, aspirin, and tolbutamide medications.

REFERENCES

1. B. Luke. *Principles of Nutrition and Diet Therapy.* Boston: Little, Brown and Co., 1984, p. 619.
2. R.R. Levine. *Pharmacology: Drug Actions and Reactions,* 3rd ed. Boston: Little, Brown and Co., 1983, pp. 299–301.
3. D.A. Roe. *Handbook: Interactions of Selected Drugs with Nutrients in Patients.* Chicago: American Dietetic Association, 1982.
4. L.H. Bodinski. *The Nurse's Guide to Diet Therapy.* New York: John Wiley and Sons, 1982, p. 339.
5. J.C. Scherer. *Introductory Clinical Pharmacology,* 2nd ed. Philadelphia: J.B. Lippincott Co., 1982, p. 91–96.
6. K.A. Conrad and R. Bressler. *Drug Therapy for the Elderly.* St. Louis: C.V. Mosby Co., 1982.
7. "Nutrition and the elderly: Food and drug interactions." *Nutrition and the M.D.,* 8(11), 1–2 (1982).

17 ENTERAL-PARENTERAL NUTRITION

OBJECTIVES

Upon completion of this chapter, you should be able to:

1. Distinguish between enteral and parenteral nutrition.

2. Give four advantages of enteral nutrition.

3. Describe three common types of liquefied formulas used in tube feedings.

4. Discuss three complications associated with tube feeding.

5. Describe the benefits of parenteral nutrition.

6. Describe the kilocalories, grams of nutrients, and importance of D_5W, crystalline amino acid (3.5%), and 10% fat emulsion solutions.

7. Define total parenteral nutrition (TPN).

8. Distinguish between peripheral TPN and central vein TPN in terms of who can benefit from each and the basic differences in the solutions infused by each method.

9. Describe catheter and metabolic complications of central vein TPN.

INTRODUCTION

Enteral Nutrition The movement of nutrients through the intestine into the blood.

The majority of hospital patients receive oral diets. In some cases, they may have to receive nutrients through a tube. In either case, they are receiving **enteral nutrition.** Some patients cannot receive nutrients except directly into their veins; these patients are receiving **parenteral nutrition.**

Parenteral Nutrition The movement of nutrients that bypass the intestine and are infused directly into the veins.

ENTERAL NUTRITION

Enteral feeding has the following advantages:

Intraluminal effect. The presence and absorption of nutrients help to prevent **atrophy** of the intestinal mucosa.

Atrophy A decrease in the size of a normally developed organ.

Safety. There is less chance of infection and fluid-electrolyte imbalance if the gastrointestinal tract is used as opposed to direct infusion of the nutrients into the veins.

Normal insulin-glucagon ratio. Absorption of carbohydrates through the intestines helps to keep the blood levels of glucagon and insulin normal.

Reduced cost. Feeding by the enteral route requires less staff and equipment than parenteral nutrition.[1]

Oral feeding is always the first choice in terms of enteral nutrition if the person is able to take food orally. If the person is not able to consume food orally but the gastrointestinal tract is functional, the next choice of enteral nutrition is tube feeding.

TUBE FEEDING

Nasogastric Referring to a tube of soft rubber or plastic that is inserted through a nostril into the stomach. It is used to instill liquid foods or withdraw gastric contents.

People who have extreme anorexia, lesions of the mouth, inability to swallow, severe burns, or cancer of the gastrointestinal tract require feeding through a tube. The tube is inserted into the stomach or small intestine through various routes. The most common route is **nasogastric** (see Fig. 17-1), since no incision is required. Over a long period of time, this route can lead to irritation of the mucous membranes of the nose and throat. Therefore, for long-term tube feeding, an **esophagotomy,** a gastrostomy, or jejunostomy is preferred.

Esophagotomy Introduction of a tube through the skin into the esophagus.

The food administered is liquefied so that it can be easily digested and absorbed. Most hospitals use commercially prepared formulas that are composed of purified or synthetically made nutrients and are called

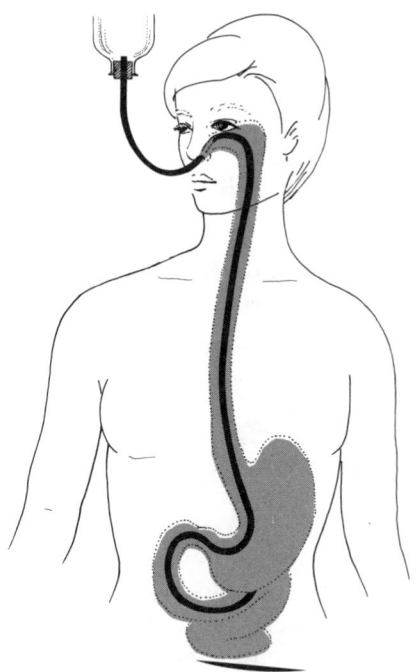

FIGURE 17-1   A nasogastric tube for enteral feeding.

Chemically Defined (Elemental) Diets Formulas that are composed of purified or synthetic nutrients.

Viscosity The tendency for a fluid to resist flowing.

chemically defined or elemental diets. There are three basic types of tube feedings; they differ in osmolality, digestibility, kilocalories, lactose content, **viscosity**, and fat content.

Isotonic formula. This formula contains proteins, fats, and carbohydrates. It has a high molecular weight and an osmolality equal to that of the body (300 mOsm). Normal digestion is required for protein and fat. Isocal and Osmolite are two examples. They supply 1 kcal/ml. These two formulas are lactose free and are therefore appropriate for lactose-intolerant patients.

Elemental formula. This formula contains monosaccharides and amino acids but is almost totally deficient in triglycerides. It requires minimal gastrointestinal function and causes minimal pancreatic stimulation. Vivonex and Vivonex HN are two examples. They supply 1 kcal/ml. Due to the hypertonic concentration, elemental formula should be started at half strength or less and gradually increased to full strength.

Fluid restriction formula. This is a highly concentrated source of kilocalories and is beneficial for patients who have fluid restrictions. Magnacal is an example; it supplies about 2 kcal/ml. Due to the hypertonicity of the formula, it should be started at half strength and gradually increased to full strength.[2]

Bolus Feeding Intermittent feeding of a formula as meals.

Gravity-Drip method A method by which liquid formulas flow slowly by gravity through a nasogastric tube.

These formulas may be fed as a **bolus feeding** or continuously by the **gravity-drip method.** The latter method has been found to be better tolerated, with fewer complaints of abdominal discomfort. Generally, about 1,000–1,500 ml (1,000–1,500 kcal) is given daily to maintain nutritional balance. Additional water is needed by most patients in addition to that in the formula.

COMPLICATIONS ASSOCIATED WITH TUBE FEEDING

Patients sometimes experience complications due to tube feeding. Some of the more common complications and the reasons for them are as follows:

Diarrhea. This is the most common complication associated with tube feeding and is generally due to the formula being hypertonic or being administered too rapidly. Hypertonic formulas tend to pull large amounts of water into the intestines (remember that water moves from low-osmotic to high-osmotic fluids). Diarrhea can be reduced by initial dilution of hypertonic formulas followed by a gradual increase in the concentration as the small intestine adapts to the formula. Continuous feeding by the gravity-drip method also allows the intestine to adapt to the formula.

Lactose intolerance is a condition in which the body does not digest and absorb lactose, resulting in a hypertonic condition in the intestines. Lactose intolerance is common in adults and in certain postsurgical patients. In some populations, such as blacks, Indians, Mexican-Americans, Jews, and Orientals, the incidence may be as high as 95%.[3] Some drugs can cause diarrhea. Therefore, drugs that do not cause diarrhea can be considered, or antidiarrheal drugs such as kaloin and pectin (Donnagel) can be administered.

Dehydration. Diarrhea can result in dehydration as well as hyperglycemia. Formulas that are high in carbohydrates can cause hyperglycemia, resulting in "spillage" of sugar into urine and large losses of water. The loss of water is due to the great hypertonicity of the urine as a result of the high sugar content. Diabetics are very susceptible to this problem. Administration of insulin and feeding by the gravity-drip method introduce carbohydrates slowly and lower blood glucose levels, thereby reducing dehydration.

Aspiration Pneumonia Regurgitation of the stomach contents and inhalation into the lungs.

Regurgitation Backup of stomach contents through the esophagus.

Aspiration pneumonia. This problem results from **regurgitation** (backup) of the stomach contents and inhalation into the lungs. Unconscious, comatose, or severely debilitated patients are most likely to experience this problem. Reduction of aspiration is accomplished by elevating the head of the bed by 30 degrees during feeding. Gravity-drip feeding and introduction of the tube by gastrostomy or jejunostomy reduce the chance of developing aspiration pneumonia.

PARENTERAL NUTRITION

As defined previously, parenteral nutrition involves nutrients bypassing the small intestine and entering the blood directly. Parenteral nutrition is used in the following situations:

Unwillingness of the patient to eat. Anorexia nervosa patients frequently have to be fed by parenteral nutrition.

Inability to eat. Patients who are in shock or postoperative generally have to be fed parenterally.

Inadequate oral intake or absorption. Some conditions prevent patients from consuming enough food orally or absorbing the nutrients. Cancer patients undergoing treatment that interferes with gastrointestinal tract functions, people who have been severely burned, and patients who will not receive food for 7–10 days after treatment are examples of people who need parenteral nutrition.[4]

If possible, physicians like to use enteral and parenteral feedings simultaneously in order to prevent atrophy of the intestinal mucosa.

Parenteral nutrition is accomplished by use of a **peripheral** or **central vein.**

PERPHERAL VEIN

The radial, basilic, and cephalic veins are the peripheral veins most commonly used. The veins on the **dorsum** of the hand and the **dorsal plexus** of the foot are also used if they are large enough (see Fig. 17-2).

Advantages and Disadvantages

The primary advantage of using peripheral veins is one of safety. It is safer to infuse nutrients into peripheral veins than into a central vein like the superior vena cava or subclavian. The size of the **catheter** inserted into a central vein and entrance into the **thoracic cavity** increases the chances of infection compared to peripheral vein infusion. A disadvantage of using peripheral veins is that hypertonic solutions cannot be infused without causing complications like **phlebitis, thrombosis,** and **sclerosis.** Therefore, peripheral solutions can help most patients meet

Peripheral Vein A vein near the skin surface in the arm and forearm.

Central Vein A vein located in the center or midline of the body; an example is the superior vena cava.

Dorsum The back or posterior surface of a body or part.

Dorsal Plexus A network of veins located near the dorsal surface of the foot.

Catheter A slender, flexible tube of rubber or plastic that is inserted into a channel such as a vein.

Thoracic Cavity Chest cavity.

Phlebitis Inflammation of a vein.

Thrombosis Blood clot formation.

Sclerosis Hardening of a vein.

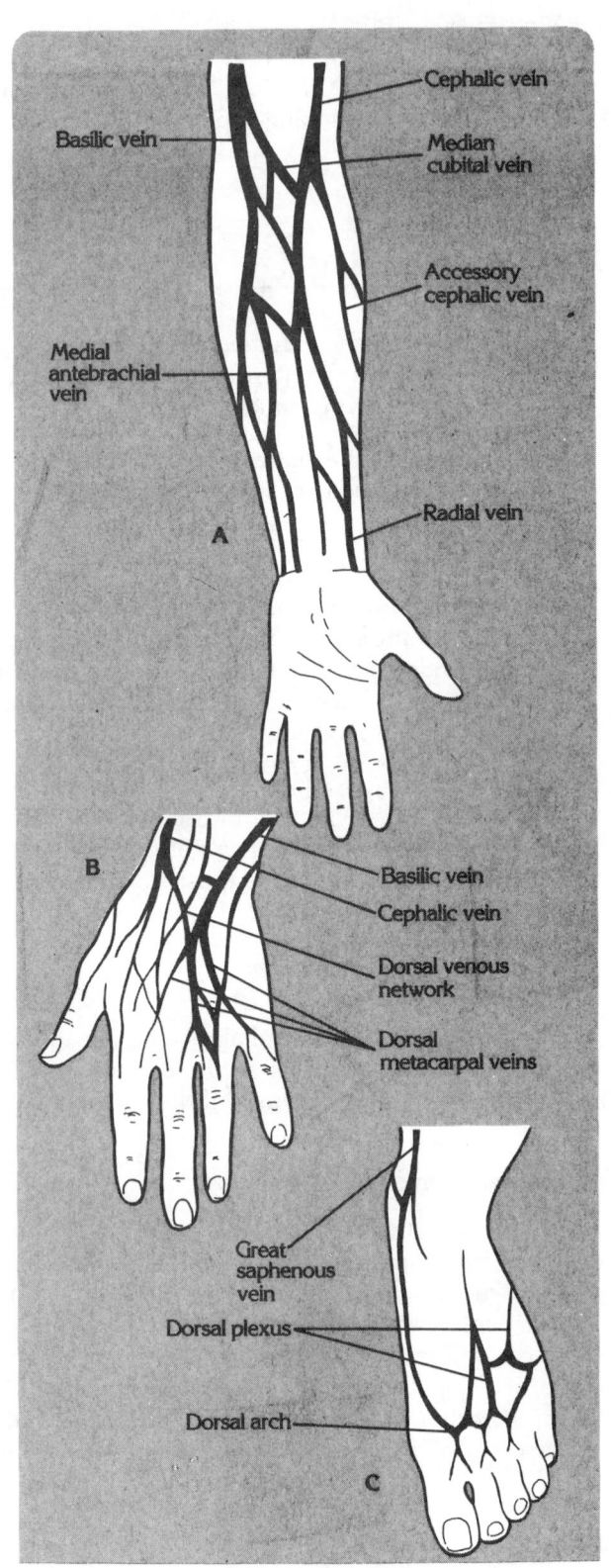

Cephalic vein

Basilic vein

Median cubital vein

Accessory cephalic vein

Medial antebrachial vein

Radial vein

A

B

Basilic vein

Cephalic vein

Dorsal venous network

Dorsal metacarpal veins

Great saphenous vein

Dorsal plexus

Dorsal arch

C

only their maintenance energy needs, not their repletion needs. Central vein infusion is indicated for patients who need more than 2,500 kcal for tissue repletion, such as those with major burns, trauma, and infection.

PERIPHERAL VEIN SOLUTIONS

Two common types of solutions infused into peripheral veins are **protein-sparing** and **total parenteral nutrition (TPN)**.

Protein-Sparing Solution

A protein-sparing solution is beneficial for patients who have minimal or no protein deficits and are not **hypermetabolic**. Obese people have their protein stores protected but do not receive excess kilocalories. Specific examples of protein-sparing solutions are as follows:

D₅W. This solution contains 5% dextrose (glucose) in water or 50 g dextrose per liter (1,000 ml) water. The dextrose (glucose) used in parenteral solutions is **monohydrous** rather than the **anhydrous** form that is typically found in foods.

Monohydrous dextrose supplies 3.4 kcal/g rather than the usual 4.0 kcal/g. Therefore,

$$\frac{50 \text{ g dextrose}}{\text{liter}} \times \frac{3.4 \text{ kcal}}{\text{g}} = 170 \text{ kcal/liter}$$

As the calculation shows, for every liter of solution infused, a person receives only 170 kcal. Since 3 liters is the maximum amount of fluid that can be infused safely in a 24-hour period, a person would be getting only $3 \times 170 = 510$ kcal. However, 1,600 kcal/day is the basic requirement for an adult on bed rest. This figure is increased by fever and hypermetabolism.[5] This deficit of approximately 1,100 kcal can result in the oxidation of tissue proteins for energy and a negative nitrogen balance. In other words, a kwashiorkor-type malnutrition may result from prolonged use of this type of solution.

The 10 and 20% dextrose solutions, which are hypertonic, are frequently infused along with an **intralipid** solution (see intralipid solutions below) to increase the kilocalorie intake and reduce the osmolality of the dextrose solution. Dextrose solutions with concentrations higher than 20% should not be infused through a peripheral vein.

Protein-Sparing Solution A solution that supplies the needed kilocalories so that proteins can be spared as a source of kilocalories.

Total Parenteral Nutrition (TPN) Infusion of solutions composed of dextrose for energy, amino acids for tissue synthesis, fats for energy, and essential fatty acids plus vitamins and minerals.

Hypermetabolic A high metabolic rate following problems like major trauma or burns.

Monohydrous Containing one water molecule; an example is monohydrous dextrose, which contains one water molecule connected to a dextrose molecule.

Anhydrous Lacking water molecules; an example is anhydrous dextrose, which is found in food.

Intralipid A fat emulsion solution that is administered intravenously to supply essential fatty acids and kilocalories.

FIGURE 17-2 Peripheral veins used in parenteral nutrition. *(a)* Arm and forearm; *(b)* dorsum of the hand; *(c)* dorsal plexus of the foot. (Reprinted with permission from B. Kozier, and G.L. Erb. *Fundamentals of Nursing: Concepts and Procedures.* Menlo Park, Calif: Addison-Wesley Publishing Company, Inc., 1979.)

Crystalline amino acid solution (3.5%). This solution supplies a nitrogen source to help achieve a nitrogen balance. Achieving a nitrogen balance is very important in patients stressed by severe trauma, burns, and **sepsis** (pathogenic bacteria in the blood), since more than 75 g of tissue protein and 12 g of nitrogen (6.25 g protein = 1 g nitrogen) are broken down per day for energy.

The recommended intake of amino acids for adults varies from 0.8 g/kg/day for nondepleted postoperative patients to 2.0 g/kg/day for hypermetabolic patients (with severe trauma or burns).[6] A 70-kg man would need 56–140 g amino acids, depending upon his condition. *Crystalline amino acid solutions yield 1 g of nitrogen for every 5.9 g of amino acids rather than 1 g of nitrogen for every 6.25 g of protein.*

A 3.5% solution of amino acids supplies the following:

$$\frac{35 \text{ g amino acids}}{\text{liter}} \times \frac{4 \text{ kcal}}{\text{g}} = 140 \text{ kcal/liter}$$

$$\frac{35 \text{ g amino acids}}{\text{liter}} \times \frac{1 \text{ g nitrogen}}{5.9 \text{ g amino acids}} = 5.9 \text{ g nitrogen per liter}$$

Amino acid solutions are also supplied in 5.5% (220 kcal/liter), 8.5% (340 kcal/liter), and 10% (400 kcal/liter).

Enough amino acids should be given to help achieve a positive nitrogen balance but not so much that **azotemia** (excess nitrogen in blood) occurs.

10% fat emulsion. Fat in parenteral solutions is a mixture of soybean oil (Intralipid) or safflower oil (Liposyn), egg yolk, phospholipid, and glycerol. *A fat emulsion looks like milk and supplies 11 kcal/g, whereas in food 1 g of fat supplies 9 kcal/g.*

A 10% fat emulsion supplies the following:

$$\frac{100 \text{ g fat}}{\text{liter}} \times \frac{11 \text{ kcal}}{\text{g fat}} = 1,100 \text{ kcal/liter}$$

Three reasons for including fat emulsions in parenteral solutions are that they supply concentrated kilocalories in an isotonic solution; supply linoleic acid and prevent essential fatty acid deficiency; and they enable fat-soluble vitamins to be absorbed.

Fat emulsions can be infused with dextrose and amino acid solutions simultaneously. However, fat emulsions cannot be mixed with dextrose and amino acid solutions in the same container.* Remember, fats are insoluble in water; therefore, they would break down and

---

*In 1985 the Food and Drug Administration (FDA) approved mixing intralipid or fat emulsions with dextrose and amino acid solutions. However, many hospitals still do not mix them. (*Mixed-up About Mixing I.V.S.*, Nursing 85, 15, Sep. 1985. p. 12.)

clog up the tube. To avoid this problem, fat emulsions are infused from separate containers through separate tubing. The tubing from the fat emulsion is connected to the amino acid and dextrose solution by a Y connector just before it enters a vein (see Fig. 17-3).

Some patients have adverse reactions to intravenous fat solutions such as chills, fever, backache, chest pain, vomiting, headache, and blurred vision. In anticipation and elimination of these problems, a patient's liver functions, blood count, and plasma lipid levels are evaluated before infusion. Once infusion begins, electrolyte, **blood urea nitrogen (BUN),** serum triglyceride, and cholesterol levels should be measured regularly.[7]

Blood Urea Nitrogen (BUN) Nitrogenous waste product formed in the liver when amino acids are deaminized (see Chapters 20 and 23).

Peripheral Total Parenteral Nutrition (TPN)

As mentioned above, intralipid and dextrose solutions can be infused simultaneously. In addition, electrolytes and vitamins can be mixed with dextrose and amino acid solutions. These mixtures meet all the body's needs or supply total parenteral nutrition, rather than just supplying kilocalories and sparing proteins.

TPN via a peripheral vein is suitable for patients who require nutritional maintenance for about 7–10 days. An example of a TPN solution

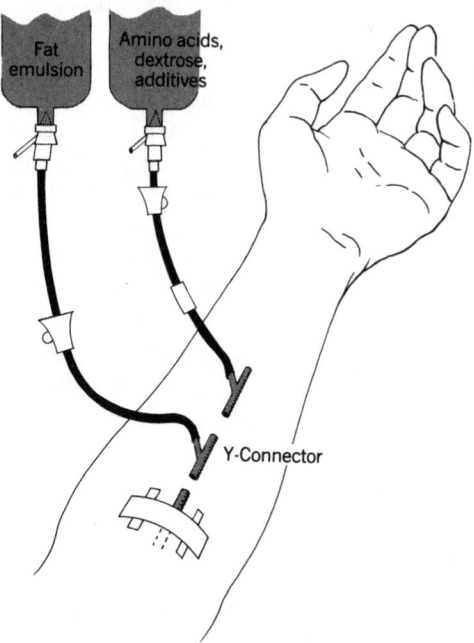

FIGURE 17-3 Tubing from a fat emulsion connected to amino acids, dextrose, and additives solution by a Y connector.

infused through peripheral veins for a stable, nonhypermetabolic adult weighing 70 kg is as follows:

Solution	Nutrients	Kilocalories
1 liter crystalline amino acid solution (7%)	70 g amino acids, (11.8 g nitrogen)	280
1 liter dextrose solution (20%)	200 g carbohydrates	680
1 liter fat emulsion (10%)	100 g fats	1,100
Electrolytes and minerals in appropriate amounts[4]		2,060

An analysis of this TPN diet shows that 2,060 kcal is adequate to maintain a nonhypermetabolic 70 kg person. The 70 g of protein is higher than the minimum of 56 g (70 g × 0.8/kg/day). The fat emulsion supplies essential fatty acids. Appropriate amounts of electrolytes and minerals are also provided.

In essence, the diet should allow for maintenance of the person's tissues. However, if the person were hypermetabolic and needed **repletion**, as a burn patient would, the diet would need to be increased in kilocalories and amino acids.

Electrolytes and Vitamins. The major electrolytes (sodium, potassium, calcium, magnesium, chloride, and phosphate) must always be a part of any complete parenteral nutritional support solution, regardless of the duration of therapy. Ideally, they should be added and decreased according to the individual's needs. Additionally, all the essential vitamins, minerals, and trace elements should be added to the solution just before infusion. In severe stress, the requirements for vitamins and minerals may be three times the recommended daily allowances (RDAs). Vitamins and minerals not added to the solution just before infusion are vitamin K, folic acid, vitamin B_{12}, and iron. They are not added because they interact with other vitamins or minerals, causing nutrient imbalances, or they precipitate with other vitamins and minerals and impair availability. They should be administered **intramuscularly**.

CENTRAL VEIN TOTAL PARENTERAL NUTRITION (TPN)

Central vein TPN refers to infusion of nutrients through a catheter into the **subclavian vein** and guided into the **superior vena cava** (see Fig. 17-4). In this chapter, the term *total parenteral nutrition* refers to any intravenous solution that contains dextrose, amino acids, and fats, plus

Repletion Restoration of body composition.

Intramuscularly Within a muscle.

Central Vein Total Parenteral Nutrition Infusion of nutrients through a catheter into the subclavian vein and their guidance into the superior vena cava.

Subclavian Vein A vein in the shoulder region that is often used for insertion of a TPN catheter.

Superior Vena Cava A vein that carries blood from the upper part of the body into the heart. A TPN catheter is guided into this vein from the subclavian vein.

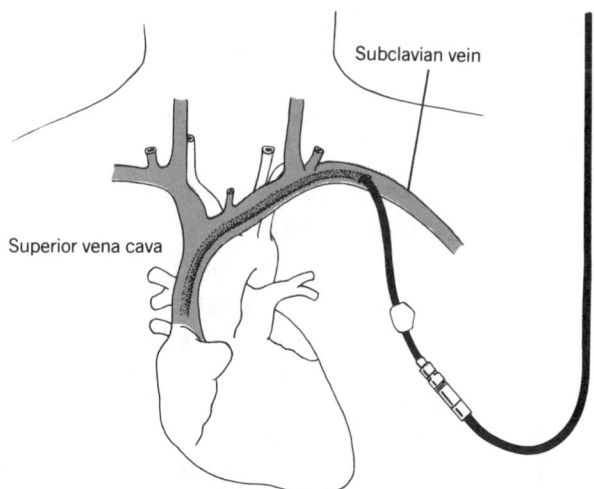

Subclavian vein

Superior vena cava

FIGURE 17-4 A central vein TPN catheter inserted into the subclavian vein and guided into the superior vena cava.

Hyperalimentation Feeding by hypertonic solutions (frequently 2,000 mOsm) that are infused through the central vein.

vitamins and minerals, and can be infused into peripheral or central veins. Traditionally, when this term is used alone, it usually refers to central vein TPN. The term **hyperalimentation** is frequently used interchangeably with TPN.

Hypertonic solutions are infused so that a large number of kilocalories in a small volume of fluid can be introduced. A central vein is used for infusion, since it is large in diameter and the large volume of blood flowing through it quickly dilutes hypertonic solutions. Dilution of the solutions is important to reduce the chance of developing phlebitis, thrombosis, and other venous complications.

Who Should Receive Central Vein TPN?

Infusion of hypertonic fluids is important to achieve a positive nitrogen balance. In other words, these high-kilocalorie fluids permit both maintenance of tissues and repletion. Examples of patients who can benefit from central vein TPN are the following:

• Patients with severe burns

• Patients who require long-term parenteral nutrition

• Patients with protein-kilocalorie malnutrition

• Postoperative patients who cannot receive oral intake for several days

• Patients who have prolonged vomiting

• Patients who have prolonged diarrhea

Anabolism A metabolic process whereby large molecules are synthesized from small ones.

The main advantage of central vein TPN, compared to peripheral TPN, is that it can be continued over a longer period of time. It is not usually initiated for periods of less than 2 weeks. In addition, it enables a person to achieve **anabolism** or repletion.

Central Vein TPN Solution and Administration

An example of a solution that may be infused through a central vein is 500 ml D_5W plus 500 ml of amino acid solution (8.5%). The kilocalorie content is 850 plus 170, respectively, for a total of 1,020 kcal. The reason for using 500 ml of dextrose and amino acids, as opposed to 1 liter of each, is to dilute the solution. During the first 24 hours, the dilute solution is infused, allowing the person to adapt to the high glucose concentration and osmolality. After the first 24 hours, the kilocalorie intake is increased by 1,000 until, by the third day, the person is getting fat emulsion and full-strength dextrose solutions for a total of approximately 3,000 kcal per 24 hours. The final solution also includes vitamins and minerals, and possibly insulin if hyperglycemia occurs.

Catheter and Metabolic Complications of Central Vein TPN

Aseptic Free from infection or infectious material.

Hemothorax Presence of blood in the chest.

Superior Vena Cava Thrombosis A blood clot in the superior vena cava.

Air Embolism Air bubbles in the blood as a result of air leaks through a catheter.

Hydrothorax Fluid in the chest.

Pneumothorax Air or gas in the chest.

Hyperammonemia High blood ammonia levels.

The potential for complications with central vein TPN is very great. One major reason is that the catheter must be surgically inserted through the skin into the subclavian vein and then left in place for an extended period of time. A second reason is that the hypertonic, high-kilocalorie, high-fat solutions can cause metabolic imbalances. Sepsis is potentially one of the most serious complications. Septic complications are inversely proportional to careful monitoring and attention to **aseptic** catheter insertion, catheter dressing changes, and changes of IV tubing. Some complications related to catheter insertion and care are **hemothorax**, **superior vena cave thrombosis**, **air embolism**, **hydrothorax**, and **pneumothorax**.

Metabolic complications are also very possible. Examples are as follows:

Hyperglycemia. A temporarily elevated blood glucose level is common the first few days but then clears as the efficiency of glucose removal increases. Persistence of hyperglycemia suggests the possibility of diabetes, sepsis, and stress.

Hypoglycemia. A low blood glucose level usually results from interruption of TPN infusion.

Hyperammonemia. A high blood ammonia level results from impairment of liver functions.

Hypophosphatemia Low blood phosphorus levels.

Hypophosphatemia. A low blood phosphorus level usually results from inadequate inorganic phosphate in TPN solutions.

Azotemia. Excess nitrogen in the blood may follow amino acid infusion that is excessive in terms of anabolic needs.

These complications are controlled when central vein TPN is closely monitored by a nutritional support service or team.[2]

TRANSITIONAL FEEDINGS

The interval when a patient changes from one form of feeding to another is termed the *transitional feeding* period. During this period, a patient's nutritional status can usually be maintained by overlapping the two feeding methods. As an example, if a patient has been receiving tube feeding, it should be gradually decreased as the oral intake of food increases.

Patients who have received central vein TPN for an extended period of time may have to proceed first to tube feeding and then to oral feedings. They are gradually weaned from one type of feeding to the other as their tolerance for each increases.[7]

OUTLINE

INTRODUCTION

Enteral nutrition is the movement of nutrients through intestine into blood. Parenteral nutrition is the bypassing of the intestine by nutrients and their infusion directly into the blood.

ENTERAL NUTRITION

Advantages

- Intraluminal effect
- Safety
- Maintenance of normal insulin-glucagon ratio cost reduced

Tube Feeding

People who cannot ingest food through their intestine can benefit from tube feeding. A tube is inserted into the stomach through the nasogastric route, through the skin into the stomach (gastrostomy), or through the skin into the esophagus (esophagotomy).

Three common types of liquified formulas are administered:

- Isotonic: contains proteins, fats, and carbohydrates; supplies 1 kcal/ml; Isocal and Ensure are examples.
- Elemental: contains amino acids and monosaccharides; supplies 1 kcal/ml; Vivonex and Sustacal are examples.
- Fluid restriction: highly concentrated kilocalories with a minimum of water needed; supplies 2 kcal/ml; Magnacal is an example; important for patients who have fluid restrictions.

Formulas may be fed by bolus (intermittent meals) or by the continuous gravity-drip method.

Complications Associated with Tube Feeding

- Diarrhea: can be caused by too rapid administration of the formula, lactose intolerance, and some drugs.
- Dehydration: diarrhea and hyperglycemia can both result in dehydration; diabetics are especially susceptible.
- Aspiration pneumonia: regurgitation (backup) of stomach contents and inhalation into lungs. Unconscious, comatose, and severely debilitated patients are most likely to suffer this problem. Elevating the head of the bed by 30 degrees, gravity-drip feeding, and introduction of tubes directly into the stomach or jejunum help decrease the chances of developing this problem.

PARENTERAL NUTRITION

People who benefit from parenteral nutrition are those who cannot absorb nutrients through the intestine, cannot ingest food orally, or need more kilocalories for repletion of tissues than they can get from tube feeding. Some examples of patients who can benefit from parenteral nutrition are those with:

- Anorexia nervosa
- Shock
- Postoperative status
- Cancer
- Severe burns

Peripheral Vein

Nutrients are introduced through peripheral veins (radial, basilic, and cephalic).

Advantages and Disadvantages

Advantages: safer in that there is less chance of infection compared to central vein TPN.
Disadvantages: complications from hypertonic solutions such as phlebitis, thrombosis, and sclerosis.

Peripheral Vein Solutions

There are two common types:

Protein-Sparing Solution

This is beneficial for patients who have minimal or no protein deficits and are not hypermetabolic. Examples:

- D_5W: contains 50 g dextrose per liter; supplies 170 kcal/liter; 10 and 20% dextrose solutions are also infused, along with intralipid solutions.
- Crystalline amino acid (3.5%): supplies a source of nitrogen, which is important for severe trauma, burns, and sepsis; supplies 140 kcal/liter and 5.9 g nitrogen per liter.
- 10% fat emulsion: supplies concentrated kilocalories in an isotonic solution; important for supplying kilocalories, supplying essential fatty acids, and enabling absorption of fat-soluble vitamins; cannot be mixed with dextrose and amino acid solutions before infusion; supplies 1,100 kcal/ml.

Peripheral Total Parenteral Nutrition (TPN)

A TPN solution is one that contains dextrose, amino acids, fats, vitamins, and minerals. TPN can be infused through peripheral or central veins. It is suitable for patients who require nutritional maintenance for about 7–10 days.

Central Vein Total Parenteral Nutrition (TPN)

A TPN solution is infused into a central vein (subclavian into the superior vena cava).

The solutions are very hypertonic and are quickly diluted by the large volume of blood flowing through the superior vena cava.

Who Should Receive Central Vein TPN?
Examples of patients who can benefit are those with:

- Severe burns
- Long term parenteral-nutritional care
- Protein-kilocalorie malnutrition
- Prolonged vomiting
- Prolonged diarrhea

Central Vein TPN Solution and Administration
Hypertonic solutions are administered half strength for 24 hours and then approximately 1,000 kcal are added every 24 hours until 3,000 kcal/day are infused.

Catheter and Metabolic Complications of Central Vein TPN
Complications related to catheter care and insertion are:

- Hemothorax
- Superior vena cava thrombosis
- Air embolism
- Hyrothorax
- Pneumothorax

Metabolic complications are:

- Hyperglycemia
- Hypoglycemia
- Hyperammonemia
- Hypophosphatemia
- Azotemia

TRANSITIONAL FEEDINGS
The interval during which a patient changes from one form of feeding to another is termed *transitional feeding*. The nutritional status of the patient is maintained by overlapping two feeding methods until the person's tolerance to the new method is established.

REVIEW QUESTIONS

TRUE (A) OR FALSE (B)

Questions 1–15

1. Enteral nutrition involves the movement of nutrients through the intestine into the blood.
2. Two advantages of enteral nutrition are increased insulin secretion and decreased thickness of the intestinal mucosa.
3. An isotonic tube feeding includes proteins and fat, which require normal digestion, whereas an elemental formula contains monosaccharides and amino acids, which require minimal digestion.
4. The advantages of the fluid restriction formula Magnacal are that it is an isotonic formula and supplies 1 kcal/liter.
5. Constipation is a common complication of tube feeding due to hypotonic formulas pulling water out of the intestines.
6. Tube feedings high in carbohydrates can result in hyperglycemia and dehydration.
7. Hyperglycemia and dehydration can be reduced by bolus feeding and decreased administration of insulin.
8. Parenteral nutrition is tube feeding introduced directly into the stomach or jejunum.
9. The primary advantage of using peripheral veins for parenteral nutrition is that they are more accessible and hypertonic fluids can be easily infused.
10. A D_5W solution is a protein-sparing solution that contains 50 g dextrose and supplies 170 kcal/liter.
11. A 3.5% amino acid solution supplies 35 g amino acids and 5.9 g nitrogen per liter, which is important for severe trauma, burns, and sepsis patients.
12. A 10% fat emulsion provides 100 g fat per liter and 900 kcal.
13. A 10% fat emulsion cannot be infused simultaneously with dextrose and amino acid solutions because it makes the solution hypertonic and increases the kilocalorie level excessively.
14. A total parenteral nutrition (TPN) solution is always infused through a central vein.
15. The main advantage of central vein TPN over peripheral TPN is that it can be continued over a longer period of time and can help achieve repletion of tissues.

MULTIPLE CHOICE

Questions 16–25

16. The advantages of enteral nutrition are
    1. the intracellular effect
    2. a normal insulin-glucagon ratio
    3. infusion of hypertonic solutions
    4. safety
    A. 1, 2, 3   B. 1, 3   C. 2, 4   D. 4
    E. all of these
17. Which of the following is (are) not correctly paired for tube feedings?

A. elemental formula—contains proteins, fats, and carbohydrates; isotonic and supplies 1 kcal/ml.
   B. isotonic formula—contains monosaccharides and amino acids that require digestion; hypertonic.
   C. fluid restriction formula—highly concentrated source of kilocalories; hypertonic and supplies 2 kcal/ml.
   D. A, B, C
   E. A, B

18. Conditions that can benefit from parenteral nutrition are
   1. anorexia nervosa
   2. shock
   3. cancer of the gastrointestinal tract
   4. malabsorption
      A. 1, 2, 3   B. 1, 3   C. 2, 4   D. 4
      E. all of these

19. A D$_5$W solution is characterized by:
   1. 50 g dextrose per liter
   2. protein-sparing solution
   3. 170 kcal/liter
   4. 200 kcal/liter
      A. 1, 2, 3   B. 1, 3   C. 2, 4   D. 4
      E. all of these

20. Three important reasons for including fat emulsions in parenteral solutions are:
   A. they provide concentrated kilocalories in a hypertonic solution; they provide essential amino acids; they enable fat-soluble vitamins to be absorbed.
   B. concentrated kilocalories in an isotonic solution; they provide essential fatty acids; they enable absorption of fat-soluble vitamins.
   C. they provide nitrogen for tissue repletion; they provide linoleic acid; they enable absorption of water-soluble vitamins.
   D. none of these

21. A TPN solution is composed of the following nutrients:
   A. dextrose, cholesterol, proteins, vitamins, and minerals.
   B. starch, fatty acids, proteins, minerals, and water
   C. sucrose, linoleic acid, proteins, minerals, and vitamins
   D. dextrose, fatty acids, amino acids, vitamins, and minerals

22. A TPN solution composed of amino acids (5.5%; 55 g/liter), 10% fat emulsion (100 g/liter), and dextrose (20%; 200 g/liter) contains a total of _____ kcal.
   A. 1,920
   B. 2,305

C. 2,200
   D. 2,000

23. TPN solutions infused into peripheral veins differ from those infused into central veins by _____.
   A. containing amino acids, dextrose, fatty acids, vitamins, and minerals.
   B. containing fewer kilocalories and having a lower osmolality.
   C. containing more kilocalories and having a higher osmolality.
   D. containing dextrose only.

24. Two advantages of central vein TPN compared to peripheral TPN are _____ and _____.
   A. continued over a longer period of time—achieve repletion of tissues
   B. use of a less concentrated solution—less chance of hyperglycemia
   C. less chance of infection—easier access to veins
   D. none of these

25. Metabolic complications from the use of central vein TPN are:
   1. hypoglycemia
   2. hyperammonemia
   3. azotemia
   4. hyperglycemia
      A. 1, 2, 3   B. 1, 3   C. 2, 4   D. 4.
      E. all of these

DISCUSSION QUESTIONS

1. Discuss four advantages of enteral nutrition.
2. Discuss three complications associated with tube feeding.
3. Describe the kilocalories, grams of nutrients, and importance of the D$_5$W, crystalline amino acid (7.0%), and 10% fat emulsion solutions.
4. Distinguish between peripheral TPN and central vein TPN in terms of who can benefit from each and the basic differences between solutions infused by each method.
5. Give four possible catheter complications and four possible metabolic complications of central vein TPN.

REFERENCES

1. C.J.W. Suitor and M.F. Crowley. *Nutrition: Principles and Application in Health Promotion*, 2nd ed. Philadelphia: J.B. Lippincott Co., 1984, p. 390.
2. U. Cllbon and C.P. Page. *Adult Nutrition Assessment and Support, An Information Manual*.

Galveston: The University of Texas Medical Branch, 1982.

3. J.D. Welsh. "Diet therapy in adult lactose malabsorption: Present practices." *American Journal of Clinical Nutrition*, 31, 592–596 (1978).

4. B.G. Morrissey. *Therapeutic Nutrition*. Philadelphia: J.B. Lippincott Co., 1984, p. 55.

5. L.H. Bodinski. *The Nurse's Guide to Diet Therapy*. New York: John Wiley and Sons, 1982, p. 309.

6. B. Luke. *Principles of Nutrition and Diet Therapy*. Boston: Little, Brown and Co., 1984, p. 600.

7. M. Ament. "Home total parenteral nutrition." *Nutrition and the M.D.*, 9(6), 2–3 (1983).

18

DIABETES MELLITUS AND HYPOGLYCEMIA

OBJECTIVES

Upon completion of this chapter, you should be able to:

1. Define diabetes mellitus and describe its prevalence.

2. Describe the genesis or cause of insulin-dependent diabetes mellitus (IDDM).

3. Discuss the functions of insulin when there is a normal or increased amount and what happens when there is a deficiency of insulin.

4. Name and give the reasons for the symptoms associated with IDDM.

5. Describe the blood tests and values that are used to diagnose diabetes.

6. Give two advantages of the glycolysated hemoglobin (HbA_{1c}) test for checking diabetes control.

7. Name and give the peak period of activity for the three different types of insulin.

8. Define hypoglycemia, give four causes and five symptoms, and discuss how to correct it.

9. Describe the sequence of steps in diabetic ketoacidosis (DKA) that can ultimately result in death.

10. State what percent of the daily kilocalories should come from carbohydrate, pro-

tein, and fat in a diet for a person with IDDM.

11. Discuss the importance of distributing kilocalories and carbohydrate grams throughout the day according to the type of insulin used.

12. Describe the importance of a high-fiber diet to a diabetic.

13. Describe the general characteristics of non-insulin-dependent diabetes mellitus (NIDDM).

14. Discuss the genesis or cause of NIDDM.

15. Describe the sequence of steps that result in hyperglycemic hyperosmolar non-ketotic coma (HHNK) and state how it differs from diabetic ketoacidosis.

16. Describe the dietary treatment of IDDM.

17. Discuss diet and insulin modifications for a pregnant diabetic.

18. Define fasting and functional hypoglycemia and compare the causes, symptoms, and treatment of each.

19. Name five drugs that cause an increase and five drugs that cause a decrease in blood glucose level.

INTRODUCTION

Two common metabolic disorders involving altered blood glucose level are diabetes mellitus and hypoglycemia. Diabetes mellitus is the more common disorder; hypoglycemia can occur as a complication. However, hypoglycemia can occur in nondiabetics and will be discussed at the end of the chapter.

DIABETES MELLITUS

DEFINITION AND PREVALENCE

Diabetes mellitus is defined as a group of disorders that have a variety of genetic causes but that have in common hyperglycemia. It is a complex disease involving biochemical and anatomic abnormalities that will be discussed in detail in this chapter.

The term *diabetes* (excessive urine excretion) *mellitus* (honey sweet) literally means excessive excretion of urine with a sweet taste. Another type of diabetes is **diabetes insipidus** (without taste), caused by inadequate secretion of antidiuretic hormone; it is discussed in Chapter 23. The shortened term *diabetes* will be used in this chapter and text to refer to diabetes mellitus only.

It is estimated that 10 million Americans, or 5% of the population, may have diabetes. Studies also estimate an approximate 6% growth yearly due to the increased longevity of the population. Due to its complications (heart disease, **stroke**, and kidney failure), diabetes is the third leading cause of death after cardiovascular diseases and cancer. The potential for diabetics to develop severe problems, compared to nondiabetics, is tremendous. Examples show that diabetics have a rate of blindness 25 times higher, kidney disease 17 times higher, gangrene 5 times higher, and heart disease 2 times higher than nondiabetics.[1]

TYPE I: INSULIN-DEPENDENT DIABETES MELLITUS (IDDM)

General Characteristics

Approximately 15% or less of diabetics have **insulin-dependent diabetes mellitus (IDDM)** or require injections of insulin to help control their diabetes. Some of the former terms for IDDM are *juvenile diabetes, juvenile-onset diabetes,* and *ketosis-prone diabetes.* The term *juvenile-onset diabetes* was used because it typically has an onset before the age of 20, with the

---

Diabetes insipidus A type of diabetes that is caused by inadequate secretion of the antidiuretic hormone (ADH).

Stroke A rupture or blockage of a blood vessel in the brain, resulting in loss of consciousness, paralysis, or other symptoms; it is also called a *cerebrovascular accident.*

Insulin-dependent diabetes mellitus (IDDM) A type of diabetes in which the person does not secrete enough insulin to control the blood glucose level.

average age being 12. (*See Case Study: Insulin-Dependent Diabetes at end of chapter, for reinforcement of information on insulin-dependent diabetes.*)

The onset of IDDM is sudden and occurs more often in children who have recently had a viral infection such as the mumps or flu. Apparently, the virus results in the destruction of **beta cells** in the pancreas, which secrete insulin. Hyperglycemia is a constant problem and can be controlled only by injection of an **exogenous** source of insulin.

A complication of hyperglycemia is **ketoacidosis**, which can result in a person going into a coma and even dying if the condition is not corrected.

Beta cells Cells in the pancreas that secrete insulin. These cells are often damaged in IDDM, causing an insulin deficiency.

Exogenous Outside of the body.

Ketoacidosis High blood level of ketones (acids).

Genesis or Cause

Much research shows that IDDM results from genetic factors (as mentioned in the definition of diabetes). The genetic factors indicate that some individulas have **genes** on chromosome 6 (a total of 46 **chromosomes** are present in each human cell) that produce certain types of **human lymphocyte antigens (HLA)**.

The function of HLAs is, first, to recognize foreign material (e.g., bacteria and protein) and, second, to initiate the formation of antibodies, which attach to and neutralize the bacteria, thereby preventing infection. In other words, the HLAs help to provide immunity.

Certain HLAs specifically HLA-B8 and HLA-B15, have been found in higher quantities in IDDM patients than in the general population. In addition, high levels of **islet cell antibodies** have been found, which attack the beta cells of the **islets of langerhans** in the pancreas (see Fig. 18-1). Beta cells secrete insulin; therefore, their destruction and the ensuing insulin reduction result in hyperglycemia and the symptoms of IDDM (discussed below).

There is much controversy as to what influences the development of islet cell antibodies. Some researchers believe that it may be due to viruses such as coxsackie B-4 (which causes upper respiratory tract infections) and mumps viruses. One possible sequence of events that may ultimately result in IDDM is the following (see Fig. 18-2):

Genes The portion of DNA molecules that contains information necessary to synthesize an enzyme.

Chromosomes Rod-like structures that appear in the nucleus of the cell during mitosis. The chromosomes contain genes.

Human lymphocyte antigens (HLA) A lymphocyte (a type of white blood cell) that has an antigen attached to its surface.

Islet cell antibodies Antibodies formed in response to islet of Langerhan cell fragments.

Islets of Langerhans Irregular microscopic structures scattered throughout the pancreas. They are composed of alpha cells that secrete glucagon and beta cells that secrete insulin.

1. Coxsackie B-4 or mumps virus invades the beta cells of the islets of Langerhans.

2. Slightly degraded tissue from the beta cells is released into the blood.

3. HLAs recognize the degraded tissue as foreign and initiate the formation of islet cell antibodies.

4. Islet cell antibodies attack and destroy the beta cells.

5. Destruction of the beta cells results in decreased secretion of insulin followed by IDDM.

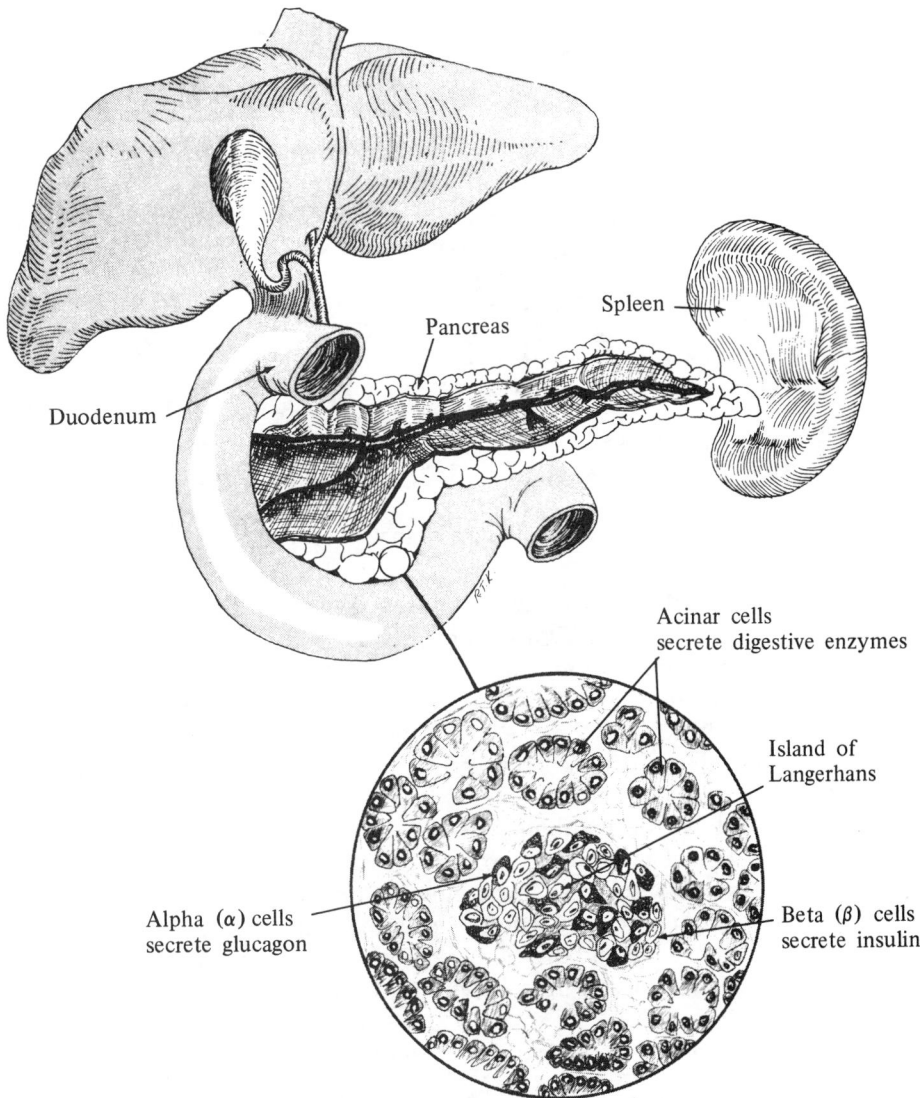

FIGURE 18-1 Pancreas with alpha and beta cells. (From T. Randall Lankford, *Integrated Science for Health Students,* 3rd ed. 1984. Reprinted by permission of Reston Publishing Company, a Prentice-Hall Company, 11480 Sunset Hills Road, Reston, VA 22090.)

It should be emphasized that this is just one possible sequence of events. Some investigators have different theories as to how the HLAs and islet cell antibodies result in decreased insulin secretion.

Autoimmunity A condition in which the body forms antibodies against its own tissues.

Most researchers state that IDDM is a result of **autoimmunity**. IDDM persons form islet cell antibodies against their own beta cells, hence the reason for calling it an example of autoimmunity.[2]

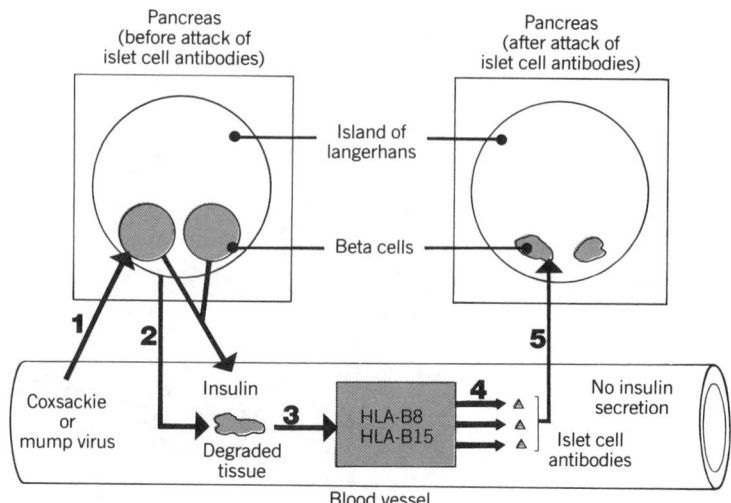

FIGURE 18-2   Five events, in sequence, that may result in IDDM.

Functions of Insulin and Results of Deficiencies. The hyperglycemic problem of IDDM patients is due to inadequate secretion of insulin. To understand the symptoms of IDDM, one needs to know the metabolic functions of insulin and the metabolic changes that result from an insulin deficiency.

The main function of insulin is to promote the transfer of glucose across certain cell membranes so that it can be oxidized for energy. However, insulin is also secreted to facilitiate the uptake, use, and storage of fat and amino acids. The action of insulin takes place in three principal tissues: liver, muscle, and fat. These tissues are also the sites of much activity when there is an insulin deficiency. The effects of insulin in normal and deficient amounts on the levels of glucose, fat, and amino acids in liver, muscle, and fat tissues are summarized below.

Normal or increased amounts of insulin:

↓ blood glucose *results from* ↑ uptake of glucose and ↑ synthesis of glycogen in liver and skeletal muscles

↓ blood fatty acids *result from* ↑ uptake of fatty acids and synthesis of fats by fat cells.

↓ blood amino acids *result from* ↑ uptake of amino acids and synthesis of proteins by muscle cells.

Deficient amounts of insulin:

↑ blood glucose *results from* ↑ breakdown of glycogen and release of glucose by liver; ↓ uptake of glucose and conversion to glycogen by skeletal muscles; ↓ uptake of glucose and conversion to fat in fat cells.

↑ blood fatty acids and ketones *result from* ↑ breakdown of stored fats and release of fatty acids; the liver has ↑ metabolism of fatty acids with ↑ ketones as a by-product. The increased ketones are the reason for the ketacidosis condition that IDDM individuals are prone to develop.

The increased release of fats is partially the reason why IDDM individuals have an increased risk of atherosclerosis.

↑ amino acids *result from* ↑ degradation of proteins in muscles and release of amino acids. This metabolic change is partially the reason why IDDM individuals frequently are underweight when initially diagnosed.[3]

When there is a deficiency of insulin, proteins and fats are degraded to supply energy for the cells. Normally, glucose is used as the energy source, but with an insulin deficiency, not enough glucose can be moved into the cells.

Clinical Symptoms and Complications

The clinical symptoms of IDDM progress from simple complaints at the beginning to potentially very serious complications if the condition is untreated and uncontrolled. The progression through the following symptoms can be very rapid. In fact, the symptoms frequently develop secondary to a viral infection or severe emotional stress; therefore, the parents of an IDDM child may associate the symptoms directly with the infection or stress. It is not uncommon for the initial diagnosis of IDDM to occur when a child is brought to the hospital in a coma due to ke-toacidosis.

The symptoms and the underlying cause for each are as follows:

Initial complaints

Polyuria Increased uri-nation.

Polyuria. When the level of glucose in the blood increases above about 170 mg/dl, it begins to spill into the urine. The osmotic pressure of the urine increases due to the high level of glucose, which pulls a great deal of water into the urine and increases urination.

Polydipsia Increased thirst.

Polydipsia. Increased urination results in dehydration of the tissues.

Polyphagia Increased hunger.

Polyphagia. Glucose is not being properly metabolized; therefore, the cells start metabolizing fat and protein for energy. The result is an increased need for food.

Weight loss. This condition results from the fact that the body does not use glucose properly for energy, but instead starts breaking down fat and protein tissues.

Later complaints

Blurred vision. One of the complications of IDDM is damage to blood vessels in the retina of the eye.

Pruritis vulvae Itching of the external genitalia of the female.

Skin itching or infection. Skin itching in women is particularly noticeable around the external genitalia (**pruritus vulvae**). This condition results from the excessive excretion of urine that is high in glucose.

Loss of strength (weakness)

Life-threatening symptom

Diabetic ketoacidosis (DKA) A buildup of ketones in the blood that results from uncontrolled IDDM.

Diabetic ketoacidosis (DKA). If IDDM is not properly controlled with insulin and diet, a buildup of ketones in the blood results from the oxidation of fats as the primary source of energy. Ketones are acids, and their increase, combined with hyperglycemia, sets into motion a series of changes shown in Figure 18-3. This sequence of changes can ultimately result in coma and death. Some of the symptoms of ketoacidosis are discussed later in relation to insulin deficiency problems.

Gangrene Death of body tissue due to a loss of the vascular supply, followed by bacterial invasion and putrefaction.

Large-vessel disease The development of atherosclerosis in various arteries.

Small-vessel disease (microangiopathies) A thickening of small vessels such as arterioles, venules, and capillaries.

Chronic Complications

Previously, it was mentioned that diabetics often suffer from complications such as blindness, **gangrene**, and cardiovascular disorders. It is because of these complications that diabetes is the third leading cause of death.

The complications can be divided into **large-vessel disease, small-vessel disease,** and susceptibility to infection.

Large-Vessel Disease. Large-vessel disease is essentially the development of atherosclerosis in various arteries. Diabetics are more prone to

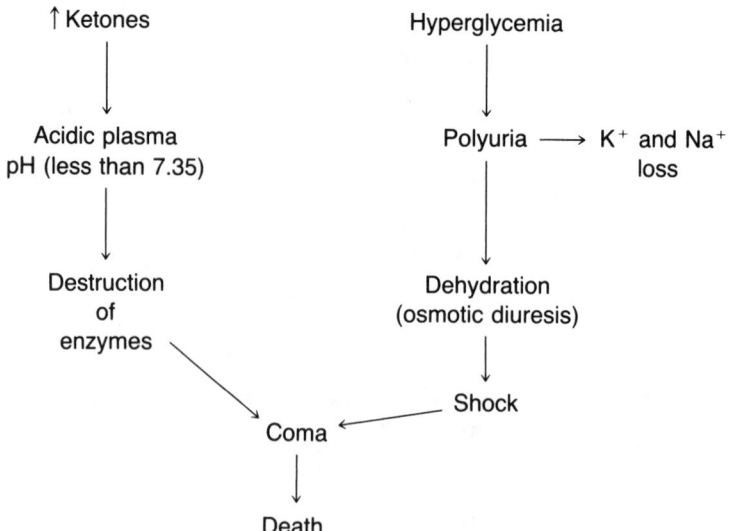

FIGURE 18-3 Sequence of changes that result in diabetic ketoacidosis (DKA).

this problem than nondiabetics, since they often have a large amount of fat circulating in the blood. Large vessels supplying blood to the brain, kidneys, heart, and lower extremities are places where atherosclcerotic plaques frequently develop.

Atherosclerosis reduces the supply of blood to the above-mentioned organs and regions of the body, leading to the problems of stroke in the brain, kidney failure, heart attack, and gangrene in the lower extremities.

Small-Vessel Disease. Small vessels consist of the microscopic arterioles, venules, and capillaries, and therefore, are the source of the term *microangiopathies*. Apparently, the increased glucose and fat circulating through these vessels causes a thickening of the capillary basement membrane.

Diabetic retinopathy Damage to the retinal blood capillaries as a result of diabetes.

Diabetic nephropathy Kidney disease caused by damage to blood vessels that results from diabetes.

The capillaries most commonly affected are those supplying the retina of the eye and the kidney, with **diabetic retinopathy** and **diabetic nephropathy**, respectively, being examples of the resultant diseases. As indicated earlier, diabetics have a rate of blindness 25 times higher, kidney disease 17 times higher, gangrene 5 times higher, and heart disease 2 times higher than those of nondiabetics. These statistics show that these diabetic complications are very prevalent; therefore, one of the goals of diabetic therapy (discussed later) is to prevent or delay the onset or progression of the associated complications.

Susceptibility to Infection. Diabetics are more susceptible to infections than nondiabetics, since the bacteria multiply and grow in the high-glucose environment.[4] Therefore, all injuries, cuts, and blisters, especially on the lower extremities, should be treated meticulously.

Diagnosis and Monitoring of Diabetes

Two common methods of diagnosing and monitoring diabetes are tests of urine and blood samples.

Reagent A substance that is used to produce a chemical reaction.

Urine Testing. Urine is commonly tested for sugar and ketones during a routine physical examination. At home, diabetics monitor their diabetes by checking it sometimes as often as four times daily, before meals and at bedtime. The second-voided specimen is the one that is always tested. The glucose and ketones in urine can be measured by dipping indicator paper strip or **reagent** strips into urine. A color change results that can be compared to a color chart to determine the concentration of glucose in percentages, with 0–0.25% indicating adequate diabetic control. Glucose present in greater quantities in the urine of a person receiving a physical examination suggests the need for blood tests to check for diabetes more thoroughly. Ketones are checked in the same manner.

Blood Testing. If urine tests indicate a high level of glucose, two types of blood tests can be performed to give a definite diagnosis of diabetes.

Fasting blood glucose /Sugar (FBG/FBS). This test is performed on a persons blood after an overnight fast. If the test results show a glucose concentration higher than 140 mg/dl on two separate occasions, the test is positive.

Fasting blood glucose/ sugar (FBG or FBS) A blood glucose test performed on a person's blood after an overnight fast.

Oral glucose tolerance test (OGTT). This test is performed on a person's blood after an overnight fast and then the person is given a measured amount of glucose in an oral glucose drink. The amount of glucose for children is calculated as 1.75 g per kilogram of ideal body weight up to a maximum of 75 g, which is the common amount for adults. The person continues to fast and blood samples are taken and analyzed at $\frac{1}{2}$, 1 hour, and 2 hours. If two of the samples show a blood glucose level equal to or greater than 200 mg/dl (see Fig. 18-4), this finding is diagnostic of diabetes. Some physicians may run a second OGTT, since stress, drugs, and inactivity may affect the results. Home monitoring of the blood glucose level by a diabetic is performed by pricking a fingertip, using reagent strips and color changes to determine the amount of glucose present. The tests typically are performed before and 1 hour after meals and at bedtime or when symptoms of hyperglycemia or hypoglycemia occur. Some diabetics may measure their blood glucose level by using a **reflectance photometer** (Glucometer, Glucochex).[5]

Oral glucose tolerance test (OGTT) A blood glucose test in which a person fasts overnight and is then given a measured amount of glucose in an oral glucose drink.

Reflectance photometer A special device that measures the intensity of light reflected through urine and thereby the amount of glucose that is present.

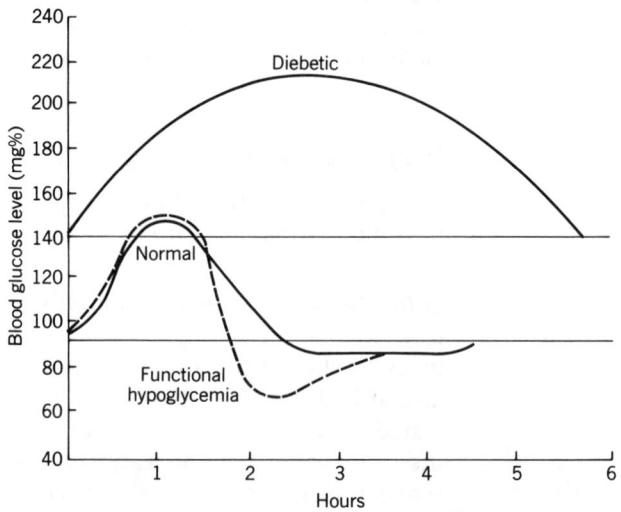

FIGURE 18-4 Glucose curve showing the amount of blood glucose in a diabetic, normal, and functional hypoglycemic person after consumption of a glucose drink. (From S.M. Hunt, J.L. Groff, and J.M. Holbrook, *Nutrition: Principles and Clinical Practice.* New York: John Wiley & Sons, Inc., © 1980. Reprinted by permission.)

Glycolysated hemoglobin (HbA₁c) A test that measures the amount of hemoglobin to which glucose is attached.

Glycolysated Hemoglobin (HbA$_{1c}$). The amount of glycolysated hemoglobin in nondiabetics is about 4–8% of the total hemoglobin. In diabetics, glycolysated hemoglobin may compose 10–28% of the total hemoglobin. Since the amount of HbA$_{1c}$ varies with the blood glucose level, this test can measure blood glucose control.

One advantage of performing this test is that it can be done in a nonfasting state. Also, since the life of glycolysated hemoglobin is about 120 days, a physician can determine how successful diabetes control has been over the past 2–4 months. This factor is important, since some diabetics may have had poor control for a lengthy period but can have a normal urine and blood test by starving or increasing their insulin intake the day before being tested. In addition, the test results are not affected by the time of day, stress, exercise, or food intake.[6]

Treatment of Insulin-Dependent Diabetics

Successful treatment of insulin-dependent diabetics involves coordination of the diet to provide adequate kilocalories for growth and weight gain and to help avoid hypoglycemic or hyperglycemia attacks. The diet must also provide kilocalories for the high activity level of the young diabetic. A key component of successful treatment is injection of the appropriate amounts of exogenous insulin.

Recombinant DNA DNA in bacteria that has genes spliced into the normal molecule. Frequently, human genes that produce insulin are spliced, thereby forming recombinant DNA insulin; it is also called *artificial human insulin.*

Insulin. The primary sources of exogenous insulin are the pancreas of cattle and pigs, commonly called *beef insulin* and *pork insulin,* respectively. New insulins have been recently marketed that are purer than older ones. Even **recombinant DNA** human insulin is now available under the name Humulin.

There are three types of insulin: rapid acting (e.g., regular), intermediate acting (for example, NPH, Lente), and prolonged acting (for example, PZI). Table 18-1 presents information on the three types.

The exact type, amount injected, and time of injection are determined by a physician. These determinations are based on the stage of growth, activity patterns, eating habits, and individual responses of the diabetic. Hyperglycemia and hypoglycemia (the warning signs of each are presented in Table 18-2) are two complications that result if the diabetic gets too little or too much insulin, respectively.

U100 insulin 100 units per milliter of insulin.

Two basic criteria determine the amount of insulin a diabetic needs: the stage of growth and the activity level. Since these criteria are always changing, so will the amount of insulin a diabetic needs. Basically, a diabetic needs 0.5–1.0 unit of insulin per kilogram of body weight. Insulin is available in the **U100**, strength. Interestingly, increased activity increases the glucose needs of the body but decreases the amount of insulin actually required by the diabetic. This relationship results from

TABLE 18-1 TYPES OF INSULIN AND THEIR ACTIVITY

Kind of Insulin	Preparation	Onset of Action (hr)	Maximal Action (hr)	Total Duration of Action (hr)
Short-acting	Regular[a]	0.5–1	2–4[b]	4–6
	Semilente	1–2	3–6	8–12
Intermediate-acting	NPH[c]	3–4	10–16	20–24
	Lente	3–4	10–16	20–24
Long-acting	PZI[d]	6–8	14–20	>32
	Ultralente	6–8	14–20	>32

[a]Also called *crystalline zinc insulin (CZI)*.
[b]In some patients, the action of regular insulin may peak later than indicated here (between 4 and 8 hours) and last considerably longer. Therefore, addition of regular insulin to intermediate-acting insulin may cause afternoon hypoglycemia in these patients.
[c]Neutral protamine Hagedorn.
[d]Protamine zinc insulin.

Source: M.B. Davidson, *Diabetes Mellitus: Diagnosis and Treatment.* New York: John Wiley & Sons, Inc., © 1981. Reprinted by permission.

the fact that exercise increases the number of insulin receptors on muscles, thereby increasing the efficiency of insulin. Exercise tends to lower the blood glucose level; therefore, if the amount of insulin is not lowered during increased exercise, a diabetic will become hypoglycemic.

Injection sites for insulin are surfaces of the arms, thighs, abdomen, and buttocks. Areas that are about to be exercised should be avoided, since the insulin will be absorbed at a faster rate, resulting in hypoglycemia. As an example, a jogger probably would not want to inject himself in the thighs just before jogging. The injection site can also influence when the peak activity of an insulin is achieved. Regular, short-acting insulin peaks fastest when injected into the **deltoid muscle**. Injections into the anterior thigh and the buttocks yield the slowest and lowest peaks, respectively.

Deltoid muscle Triangular-shaped muscle at the cap of the shoulder. It is frequently used as a site of injections.

A diabetic may have side effects from the use of some types of insulin. Some of the side effects are as follows:

• Allergy: appears as a hive-like rash at the injection site.

Lipoatrophy Loss of fat at the injection site, resulting in indentation.

• **Lipoatrophy**: loss of fat at the injection site, resulting in indentation.

• **Hypertrophy**: buildup of a mound of fat tissue at the injection site.

Hypertrophy A buildup of a mound of fat tissue at the injection site.

• **Insulin resistance**: deactivation of much of the insulin by the body causing the person to take 200 units or more per day.

Insulin resistance The deactivation of insulin.

Most of these problems are eliminated by a taking the purified forms of insulin. To avoid lipoatrophy and hypertrophy, a diabetic should be encouraged to rotate injection sites.

Timing of insulin injections needs to be coordinated with meals so that insulin is available when glucose is absorbed into the blood. Some diabetics absorb insulin over a 24-hour period and need only one injec-

TABLE 18-2 WARNING SIGNS OF HYPOGLYCEMIC AND HYPERGLYCEMIC REACTIONS

Hypoglycemic Reaction (Insulin Reaction)	Warning Signs	Hyperglycemic Reaction (Diabetic Coma)
Sudden	Onset	Gradual
Pale, moist, perspiring	Skin	Flushed, hot, dry
Excited, nervous, trembling, weak, irritable, confused faint, blurred vision	Behavior	Drowsy, weak
Normal	Breath	Fruity odor (acetone)
Normal to rapid shallow	Breathing	Deep, labored
Absent	Vomiting	Present with nausea
Moist, numb, tingling	Tongue	Dry
Present	Hunger	Absent
Absent	Thirst	Present (dehydration)
Headache	Pain	Abdominal
Normal, slight sugar	Urine	Frequent with large amounts of sugar; ketones present
Unconsciousness	Consciousness	Unconsciousness leading to coma
Too much insulin Undereating Vomiting or diarrhea Delayed meal Excessive exercise	Cause	Not enough insulin Overeating Infection Illness Surgery Stress Nausea or vomiting
Orange juice (100 ml) Coke Hard candy (Lifesavers, 4–5) Glucagon if unconscious	Treatment	Check urine Go to bed Keep warm Force fluids Take usual or increased dose of insulin Call doctor

Source: M.L. Green and J. Harry, Nutrition in Contemporary Nursing Practice. New York: John Wiley & Sons, Inc., © 1981. Reprinted by permission.

tion (usually 1 hour before breakfast) of intermediate-acting insulin (NPH or Lente) per day. A few diabetics absorb insulin in less than 24 hours and need two injections of intermediate-acting insulin per day (usually one before breakfast and one 12 hours later). Some diabetics need a mixture of rapidly absorbed insulin (Regular or Semilente) and intermediate-acting insulin before breakfast.

Some diabetics wear an insulin pump. The pump is a small, light-weight machine (about the size of a beeper) that is worn externally. Insulin is contained in a syringe or reservoir in the pump and is delivered into the body through tubing. The tubing is attached to a needle that is inserted under the skin, usually in the abdominal area. Insulin is delivered to the diabetic on a continuous basis, and the amount can be altered in relation to the meals and the blood glucose level of the individual. The main advantage of the pump is elimination of the jolt to the body caused by daily injections of insulin. It may also decrease the damage to the eyes and kidneys that result from daily injections of insulin.

Insulin shock (insulin reaction) A condition caused by a blood glucose level below 50 mg/dl.

Insulin Shock or Hypoglycemia. **Insulin shock** or insulin reaction should be considered synonymous with hypoglycemia (a blood glucose level below 50 mg/dl), since a low blood glucose level precipitates it.

Four basic situations that may cause hypoglycemia are an overdose of insulin, excessive exercise, undereating or skipping meals, and vomiting or diarrhea. The daily activities of a young diabetic may inadvertently increase to the point where he or she forgets to eat. In a nondiabetic, these changes probably would not cause a problem, but a diabetic may start to develop symptoms of an insulin reaction. Diabetics should learn to recognize the symptoms of hypoglycemia, which are summarized in Table 18-2. The onset of the symptoms is sudden, and the diabetic should immediately eat some form of readily absorbed glucose (dextrose). Approximately 10 g of glucose is needed to reverse the symptoms; examples of foods that supply this amount are 4 oz fruit juice, ½ cup of a regular (not sugar-free) soft drink, four to five Life Savers, and two large sugar cubes. After the diabetic has responded to the quick-acting glucose, foods containing either a disaccharide or starch should be eaten. These carbohydrates will be digested and absorbed more slowly, which helps to maintain the blood glucose level, restores liver glycogen, and prevents secondary hypoglycemia.

In severe cases, a diabetic may be so agitated that he spits out food given to him and spills juice. Trying to give food orally in this situation is not advisable. Instead, glucagon should be given subcutaneously, intramuscularly, or intravenously. Glucagon is a hormone whose action is opposite to that of insulin. It stimulates the liver to break down glycogen and release glucose into the blood. The body always releases glucagon from the alpha cells of the pancreas whenever a hypoglycemic condition occurs. Therefore, injection of glucagon enhances the normal response of the body to hypoglycemia. The blood glucose level should rise enough in 5–20 minutes so that food can be given orally until the diabetic is seen by a physician. A diabetic should be encouraged to have glucagon available in the home, and the family should know how to inject it.

Another alternative in emergencies is to use a commercial glucose product (Instant Glucose, Glutol, Glutose) that is glue-like in consistency. This material can be squeezed into the mouth and will be quickly absorbed through the oral tissues into the blood. If neither glucagon nor the commercial products are available, honey placed on the tongue in amounts up to 2 tsp can be used.

Hyperglycemic Reaction. A second potential problem with insulin treatment is hyperglycemia. This problem can result from insufficient injection of insulin or from conditions that require more insulin. Whenever a person is in a stressed state (infection, illness, surgery, injury), the body secretes the stress hormones **cortisone** and epinephrine. These hormones help the body overcome the stress condition by stimulating the liver to break down glycogen and release glucose, thereby, providing more energy to combat stress. If a stress condition occurs in a diabetic, the person must inject more insulin to counter the increased blood glucose level. Table 18-2 compares the symptoms of hyperglycemia and hypoglycemia.

Cortisone A hormone secreted from the cortex region of the adrenal glands. It increases the blood glucose level.

Dietary Treatment of IDDM

The goal of treatment of children with diabetes is to provide a diet that permits normal growth and activity and that controls the disease. The following variables must be considered when planning a diet for these individuals: timing of meals, diet composition, energy content, and level of physical activity.

Timing of Meals. An insulin-dependent diabetic needs to eat regular meals that are evenly spaced. Timing of meals should be planned so that they are 5 hours apart. If a diabetic starts skipping or delaying meals, hypoglycemia or an insulin reaction may result. Tight control of a diabetic's blood glucose level depends on regular eating.

Typically, six meals a day are advised—breakfast, a mid-morning snack, a noon meal, a mid-afternoon snack, an evening meal, and a bedtime snack.

Diet Composition. Carbohydrates should account for 50–60% of the total daily kilocalories. Concentrated sweets or simple carbohydrates should be kept to a minimum. Instead, diabetics should consume complex carbohydrates such as rice, corn, bread, and potatoes, which take longer to metabolize and absorb. This diet will help to supply the blood with glucose in a slow, steady manner. However, recent research has found that some of the traditionally recommended complex carbohydrates, such as bread and potatoes, cause a greater rise in blood glucose level than foods containing simple carbohydrates, such as ice cream.[7] These same studies have found that, in general, carbohydrates from legumes (e.g., beans, peas) and carbohydrates that have been minimally processed (e.g., whole rice as opposed to ground rice) cause a smaller rise in glucose levels when eaten than other carbohydrate sources.

Protein requirements for a diabetic should meet the Recommended Dietary Allowance (RDA) values for the IDDM person's body size and age. The protein allowance should be about 20% of the total kilocalorie intake for young growing diabetics. As IDDM persons complete their growth, their protein requirements decrease, and so should the total percentage of their daily kilocalories from protein. As with a nondiabetic, the protein should be of high quality in order to provide enough essential amino acids.

Fats should compose about 30% of the total kilocalories, with approximately one-third coming from saturated fat and two-thirds from polyunsaturated fats such as soft margarine, corn oil, and safflower oil. Foods high in cholesterol such as eggs, shellfish, and liver should be consumed in small amounts. No more than 300 mg of cholesterol per day should be consumed because of the increased susceptibility of diabetics to cardiovascular disease. See Table 18-3 for an example of a calorie-controlled diet.

Energy Content. The number of kilocalories for young diabetics need to be adequate for their growth and physical activity. The most accurate way to determine this kilocalorie value is to refer to the RDA table for energy intake (Table 10-1) for the child's weight, height, and age. One method for calculating the kilocalorie value is to allow 1,000 kcal for 1 year of age and add 100 kcal for every additional year. According to this method, a 5-year-old child needs 1,600 kcal, whereas a 12-year-old requires 2,200.

TABLE 18-3 CALORIE-CONTROLLED DIETS

Purpose:	Achieve and maintain desirable body weight and near-normal blood glucose levels, and reduce hyperglycemia, glycosuria, and other complications of diabetes mellitus.
Use:	Used for people with either insulin-dependent diabetes mellitus, non-insulin-dependent diabetes mellitus, or for weight reduction and maintenance.
Examples of foods:	Basically a general diet with calculated amounts of carbohydrates, proteins, and fats and the reduction of concentrated sweets.
Adequacy:	Diet is adequate; however, diets with less than 1200 kcal may be inadequate in some nutrients and therefore a multi-vitamin supplement is recommended.

Source: Chicago Dietetic Association, *Manual of Clinical Dietetics*, 2nd ed. Philadelphia, W.B. Saunders Company, 1981. Reprinted by permission.

The actual kilocalorie requirement will vary from child to child, since their growth rates and physical activity are different. When children know that their activity level will be higher than normal, they need to increase their carbohydrate and kilocalorie consumption. A rule of thumb in this respect is to consume an extra 10–15 g (approximately one fruit or bread exchange) of carbohydrate per hour of moderate exercise. For each hour of strenuous activity (running or playing basketball), a person needs an extra 20–30 g of carbohydrate per hour.

Distribution of Kilocalories and Carbohydrates. It is very important that a diabetic's diet be planned so that there is a distribution of carbohydrate and kilocalories to coincide with the type of insulin being used. As an example, if a diabetic injects a mixture of NPH insulin (peak activity of 8–14 hours) and rapid-acting insulin (peak activity of 2–4 hours) at 6:30 A.M., he or she will need to consume more carbohydrate and kilocalories at the noon meal than at the 10 A.M. snack in order to avoid a hypoglycemic reaction. A common distribution of kilocalories and carbohydrate for NPH and rapid-acting insulin is as follows:

Breakfast	4/18 (22%)
Morning snack	2/18 (11%)
Lunch	4/18 (22%)
Afternoon snack	1/18 (5.5%)
Dinner	5/18 (27.5%)
Bedtime snack	2/18 (11%)

Other popular distribution options are in tenths, 2/10ths to 4/10ths of total kilocalories and carbohydrates at each main meal and 1/10th for each snack, 2/7ths for each of the three main meals and 1/7th for a bedtime snack, and 2/5ths for breakfast and evening plus 1/5th for the lunch meal. See the following material on how to calculate a diabetic diet and distribute the kilocalories and carbohydrates using the exchange system.

A young diabetic and his or her parents should be taught how to use the exchange lists. Copies of exchange lists for meal planning and exchange lists for fast foods are available from the American Diabetes Association (see the reference at the end of the chapter for the address). These lists make it possible for diabetics to enjoy eating with their friends and still adhere to their diet. It should be emphasized that diabetics can eat normal foods and do not have to consume expensive dietetic foods for diabetics.[8]

Dietary Fiber and Diabetes. Research shows that increasing the amount of fiber in the diet of some diabetics can help keep blood glucose levels

How to Calculate A Diabetic Diet Using Exchange Lists

The following steps can be used to plan a diabetic diet for both IDDM and NIDDM diabetics.

As an example, let's take a 12-year-old boy who is 59 in. tall and weighs 90 lb.

Step 1. Determine desirable body weight in pounds

A. Adults
Consult a desirable body weight chart (Table 10-3) for the desirable weight based on height, frame, and sex.

B. Children
Consult a growth pattern on a graph. These growth patterns are readily available at health facilities and in Appendix J. The child's growth pattern should be charted every 3–6 months.

Our 12-year-old boy is on about the 50th percentile for his height and weight; therefore, his height and weight are normal for his age.

Step 2. Determine the total kilocalorie needs

A. Adults

1. Kilocalories for basal metabolism:
   desirable body weight (lb) $\times$ 10 = _____ kcal

2. Kilocalories for activity level:
   - Sedentary:
     desirable body weight (lb) $\times$ 3 = +_____ kcal
   - Moderate:
     desirable body weight (lb) $\times$ 5 = +_____ kcal
   - Strenuous:
     desirable body weight (lb) $\times$ 10 = +_____ kcal

3. Pregnancy:
   Add 300 kcal/day to gain
   23 lb in 9 months   = +_____ kcal

4. Lactation:
   Add 500 kcal/day   = +_____ kcal

5. Weight loss:
   Subtract 500 kcal/day to
   lost 1 lb/week   = −_____ kcal
   Total kcal needed   = _____ kcal

B. Children

The above steps will not work for estimating total kcal needs for children. Their needs are calculated from Mean Heights and Weights and Recommended Energy Intakes (Table 10-1). When we look up the kcal needs for our 12-year-old, we find he needs 2700 kcal. Total kcal needed = 2700 kcal.

Step 3. Divide the kilocalories into grams of protein, carbohydrate, and fat

For this example, we will use 20% of total kilocalories from protein, 50% from carbohydrate, and 30% from fat.

Protein:

$$2{,}700 \text{ kcal} \times 20\% = 540 \text{ kcal} \times \frac{g}{4 \text{ kcal}} = 135 \text{ g}$$

Carbohydrate:

$$2{,}700 \text{ kcal} \times 50\% = 1{,}350 \text{ kcal} \times \frac{g}{4 \text{ kcal}} = 338 \text{ g}$$

Fat:

$$2{,}700 \text{ kcal} \times 30\% = 810 \text{ kcal} \times \frac{g}{9 \text{ kcal}} = 90 \text{ g}$$

Step 4. Calculate the meal plan in exchanges

Dietary manuals in health facilities have examples of exchange patterns based on the total number of kilocalories and grams of protein, carbohydrate, and fat. An example of our 2,700-kilocalorie meal plan is as follows:

Exchange group	Number of Exchanges	Carbohydrate (g)	Protein (g)	Fat (g)
1. Milk, nonfat	4	48	32	0
2. Vegetables	4	20	8	0
3. Fruit	6	60	0	0
4. Bread	14	210	28	0
5. Meat, low fat	10	0	70	30
6. Fat	12	0	0	60
		Total 338	138	90

The actual meal plan for the 12-year-old will depend on his likes and dislikes of certain foods. It is important to stress that the number of kilocalories and grams of protein, carbohydrate, and fat are probably adequate now for this 12-year-old; however, when he becomes a teenager, these values may need to be changed, since this is a period of rapid growth.

Step 5. Determine how many kilocalories and carbohydrate grams will be consumed at each meal

Let us assume that our 12-year-old needs six meals a day, with 4/18ths to 5/18ths of the kilocalories and carbohydrate grams for each major meal and 1/18th to 2/18ths for the three snacks. The distribution might look like this:

$$2700 \text{ kcal} \times 1/18 \text{ } (5.5\%) = 149 \text{ kcal}$$
$$338 \text{ g carbohydrate} \times 1/18 \text{ } (5.5\%) = 19 \text{ g carbohydrate}$$

	Breakfast (4/18)	Mid-morning snack (2/18)	Lunch (4/18)	Mid-afternoon snack (1/18)	Dinner (5/18)	Bedtime snack (2/18)
Energy (kcal)	596	298	596	149	745	298
Carbohydrate (g)	76	38	76	19	95	38

from rising sharply after a meal. Fiber can also reduce the amount of insulin needed by some diabetics who are taking oral drugs or receiving less than 30 units. Insulin-dependent diabetics taking high doses of insulin receive the least benefit from the increased fiber in the diet.[9] How an increase in fiber can reduce the amount of insulin a diabetic needs and lower the blood glucose level is not clear. Some theorize that the increased rate at which food moves through the gastrointestinal tract decreases the amount of glucose absorbed.

A high-fiber diet is one in which the dietary fiber content exceeds 40 g/day. Diabetics should be advised to increase their fiber intake gradually until they are consuming about 45 g/day. Chapter 5 presents the food groups and specific foods that contain approximately 2 g of fiber per serving. Also, Appendix B lists common foods and their fiber content per serving.

Before a diabetic begins to increase the amount of fiber in the diet, he or she should be cautioned about some of the adverse effects—abdominal fullness, flatulence, and diarrhea. Most of these symptoms, except flatulence, subside with time if the amount of fiber is increased gradually.

TYPE II: NON-INSULIN-DEPENDENT DIABETES MELLITUS (NIDDM)

General Characteristics

Non-insulin-dependent diabetes mellitus (NIDDM) A type of diabetes mellitus that is not caused by an insulin deficiency but rather by the ineffectiveness of insulin in moving glucose into the cells.

Maturity-onset diabetes of youth (MODY) NIDDM that occurs in people under 40.

Non-insulin-dependent diabetes mellitus (NIDDM) was previously called *adult* or *maturity-onset diabetes*. In a few cases, it occurs in younger people and is called **maturity-onset diabetes of youth (MODY)**. This type is much more prevalent, with about 90% of all diabetics being NIDDM. It is usually milder and progresses more slowly than IDDM. NIDDM typically develops later in life, usually after age 40; about 80% of those affected are over age 50.

As the name implies, these diabetics generally do not have an insulin deficiency. Rather, they have a normal amount or even, in some cases, an insulin surplus. However, their insulin is ineffective in moving glucose into cells. From 60 to 90% of NIDDM people are obese, which may be part of the reason why their insulin is ineffective, as described below. Most NIDDM patients can be controlled by a weight loss diet, increased exercise, and decreased stress.

Hyperosmolar hyperglycemic nonketotic coma (HHNK) A complication of type II or non-insulin-dependent diabetes mellitus. Hyperglycemia causes a loss of fluids and electrolytes that can result in coma and death.

NIDDM patients are not ketoacidosis prone, but they are prone to **hyperosmolar hyperglycemic nonketotic coma (HHNK)**. They usually have less vascular damage to small vessels but more atherosclerosis, possibly due to age. (*See Case Study: Non-Insulin-Dependent Diabetes at end of the chapter, for application, and reinforcement of information on non-insulin-dependent diabetes mellitus.*)

Genesis or Cause

There are two basic theories concerning the cause of NIDDM. One theory is that the number of insulin receptors is decreased in obese people (see Fig. 18-5). When they lose weight, the number of insulin receptors returns to normal. Insulin must combine with a receptor before its functions can begin. As a result of the decreased number of receptors, the cells are less responsive to insulin and hence less capable of using glucose.

A second theory is that the problem is within the target cells after insulin binds to the receptors. The biochemical changes within the cell, normally initiated by attachment of insulin to receptors, do not occur. The consequence is less use of glucose.[1]

No relation to the HLA antigens exists in NIDDM people, and they rarely show an elevated level of islet cell antibodies.

Symptoms and Complications

The symptoms of NIDDM are the same as those of IDDM: polyuria, polydipsia, and hyperglycemia. Diagnosis is based on glucose tolerance test results.

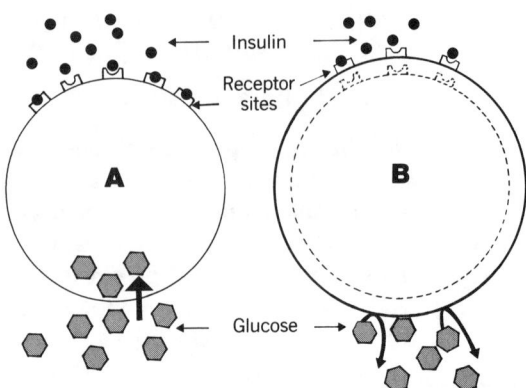

FIGURE 18-5 Cause of NIDDM. (*a*) The number of insulin receptors and the permeability of the cell to glucose are shown in the nonobese condition. (*b*) A reduced number of insulin receptors and a decreased permeability to glucose are shown in the obese condition.

As described earlier, NIDDM people do not have as many of the chronic cardiovascular complications as IDDM people, except for atherosclerosis. One very serious complication of NIDDM is HHNK. This problem is very similar to diabetic ketoacidosis (DKA) in that it is initiated by a hyperglycemic condition and the sequence of changes shown in Figure 18-6 occur. If you compare this sequence of changes with that of DKA, you will see that there is no increase in ketones; therefore, the

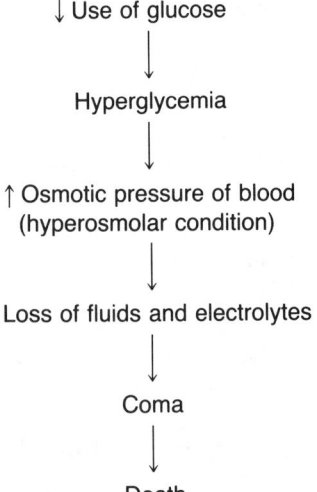

FIGURE 18-6 Sequence of changes that result in hyperosmolar hyperglycemic nonketotic coma (HHNK).

blood does not become acid. No ketones are formed because the body secretes enough insulin to avoid the breakdown of fats but not enough to prevent hyperglycemia. The coma is the result of both dehydration and hyperosmolarity.

HHNK is diagnosed by a high blood glucose value, a high level of glucose in urine, and the lack of a corresponding increase in ketones (e.g., acetone) in urine. While insulin is the key to treating DKA together with fluid and electrolyte replacement, only the latter is important in treating HHNK. In fact, giving ample amounts of water may be the key to preventing this syndrome. The mortality of HHNK (60–70%) is higher than that of DKA (as low as 0%) because the patients are older and often have serious complications (pneumonia, **pancreatitis**, thrombosis, and **cerebrovascular accidents**).[10]

Pancreatitis Inflammation of the pancreas.

Cerebrovascular accidents Same as stroke.

Treatment

The goal of treatment for NIDDM patients is the same as that of IDDM patients. The main difference between the two is that NIDDM people can usually control their blood glucose level with diet alone, since they have insulin that is circulating but not being used. Since 60–90% of NIDDM diabetics are obese, they need to be on a weight loss diet to achieve and maintain a desirable body weight. This diet requires a reduction of total daily kilocalories to below their normal needs. Some NIDDM diabetics may have to use drugs in addition to diet.

Dietary Treatment. As mentioned above, the diet for most NIDDM diabetics is a low-kilocalorie weight loss diet. At first, their intake per day may be as low as 600 kcal in order to lower their blood glucose to an acceptable level. A weight loss of 5–10 lb should provide considerable improvement in their blood glucose level. The basic reason is that as they lose weight, the number of insulin receptors increases greatly, thereby improving the effectiveness of their insulin. Once their blood glucose level has been lowered, the number of kilocalories they should be consuming daily to lose weight at a rate of 1–2 lb/week needs to be determined. A procedure for doing this is shown in the box titled "How to Calculate a Diabetic Diet Using Exchange Lists." A reduction of 500 kcal/day from the diabetic's normal intake will result in a deficit of 3,500 kcal/week and a loss of 1 lb. Frequently, though, diabetics are placed on a 1,000 to 1,200 kcal/day diet.

NIDDM diabetics need to be taught how to use the exchange lists. Usually, only three meals a day are recommended. The timing and distribution of the kilocalories are not critical.

Exercise. Exercise is one of the most important aspects of treatment for NIDDM diabetics. Increasing exercise lowers the blood glucose and fatty acid levels. Exercise has also been found to raise the levels of high density lipoproteins (HDL), which benefit the diabetic by lowering cholesterol and triglyceride levels.

Exercise can be risky for some diabetics who have cardiac disease or other diabetic complications. Diabetics whose blood glucose level is uncontrolled (over 300 mg/dl) or who have ketones in their urine should not begin to exercise until control has been established.

A diabetic should exercise when the blood sugar level is at its peak (after a meal) rather than when the insulin or oral hypoglycemic dose is having its peak effect.

Oral Hypoglycemic Drugs. Some NIDDM diabetics cannot control their blood glucose level by diet and exercise alone. These people may be required to take oral hypoglycemic drugs or insulin. The effects of insulin were discussed earlier in the chapter.

Oral hypoglycemics are not a form of oral insulin. Insulin is a protein that, if taken orally, would be digested or broken down into individual amino acids by the stomach. Oral hypoglycemics stimulate the beta cells of the pancreas to secrete more insulin and to increase the affinity of insulin receptors in peripheral tissues.[2]

The oral hypoglycemics currently approved by the Food and Drug Administration are known as *sulfonylurea drugs.* Common examples are tolazamide (Tolinase), tolbutamide (Orinase), and chlorpropamide (Diabinese). The possible side effects of these drugs are as follows:

Hypoglycemia. Reduction of the blood glucose level is what these drugs are designed to accomplish. However, a combination of these drugs and certain conditions (reduction in kidney or liver functions, infection, surgery, or other stress conditions) can cause the blood glucose level to drop into the hypoglycemic range (below 50 mg/dl).

Gastrointestinal irritation. The symptoms are usually mild and may involve only nausea and occasional vomiting or diarrhea.

Allergic skin reactions

Alcohol sensitivity. Some diabetics who consume alcohol and oral drugs may have a reaction that makes them appear drunk—stumbling and slurring of words. They may also experience facial flushing and a pounding headache.[4]

The most likely candidates for oral therapy are diabetics who are ketoacidosis resistant or who have NIDDM, cannot control their blood glucose level by diet and exercise alone, and generally need fewer than 40 units of insulin per day. The biggest advantages of oral therapy are ease of administration and acceptance. Use of oral drugs, as opposed to insulin, has allowed some diabetics to keep jobs whose working hours are highly irregular (construction workers, railroad workers, etc.).

DIABETES AND PREGNANCY

The goals of care for a pregnant diabetic are two:

- To prevent diabetes from adversely affecting the pregnancy
- To prevent pregnancy from adversely affecting the diabetes

To accomplish these two goals, there must generally be some modifications in the diabetic's diet and insulin therapy.

Diet Modifications

There is an increased need for glucose and kilocalories during pregnancy to meet the needs of the developing fetus and the diabetic mother. The RDA during pregnancy is +300 kcal and +30 g of protein. The fetus requires about 50 g of glucose per day; to meet this requirement and help supply the increased kilocalories, the American Diabetes Association recommends no less than 200 g of carbohydrate per day. It is important that the carbohydrate be evenly distributed throughout the day. Weight gain of the diabetic during pregnancy is not as rigidly controlled.

Insulin Therapy

Insulin requirements during pregnancy probably will fluctuate. During the first trimester, insulin requirements frequently decrease. This decrease results from the movement of glucose from the mother to the fetus, thereby lowering her blood glucose level.

During the second and third trimesters, the mother's insulin requirements generally increase. This increase results from hormones secreted by the placenta (estrogen, **progesterone**, and **placental lactogen**) functioning as antagonists to insulin. The possibility of developing ketoacidosis is greater during the second and third trimesters. This condition is not only potentially harmful to the mother but, more importantly, may cause brain damage to the fetus.[11]

Most authorities do not recommend the use of oral hypoglycemic drugs during pregnancy. These compounds do not control hyperglycemia as well as insulin. Also, they pass through the placenta into the fetus, in whom they can cause prolonged hypoglycemia and possibly death.

Progesterone A female hormone that is important in the menstrual cycle and in pregnancy.

Placental lactogen A hormone secreted by the placenta that enhances lactation and inhibits insulin activity in the mother.

DRUGS THAT CAN INTERFERE WITH DIABETES CONTROL

Many drugs that a diabetic may take can affect diabetes control by either raising or lowering the blood glucose level. Tables 18-4 and 18-5 list the major drugs known to affect diabetes control. However, these drugs do

SWEETENERS FOR DIABETIC DIETS

Diabetics have to be careful in choosing sweeteners to consume and to avoid. In general, they need to be encouraged to substitute low-calorie sweeteners for natural ones in order to enhance palatibility of foods while reducing kilocalorie intake. The advantages and disadvantages of various types of sweeteners are discussed below.

Sweeteners can be divided into two varieties: nutritive and nonnutritive.

Nutritive

Nutritive sweeteners contain 4 kcal/g as does sucrose. Fructose, sorbitol, and xylitol are examples.

Fructose. One advantage of using fructose is that it does not require insulin for absorption and metabolism. In addition, fructose is 15–80% sweeter than sucrose; therefore, it can provide the same degree of sweetness with fewer kilocalories.

The main disadvantage of fructose is that it is not lower in kilocalories than sucrose and therefore is not an aid for type II diabetics who need to lose weight.

Sorbitol. This nutritive sweetener is only half as sweet as sucrose. It is commonly found in sugar-free gums and candies. Like fructose, it does not require insulin to be absorbed.

Due to its reduced sweetness and same kilocalorie level as sucrose, this sweetener is not of much aid in weight loss. Another disadvantage is that consumption of 30–50 g/day can result in osmotic diarrhea.

Xylitol. The advantages of xylitol are the same as those of sorbitol. However, several animal species have developed tumors as a result of xylitol consumption. Therefore, food manufacturers have voluntarily curtailed the use of xylitol until further research on this relationship can be determined.[12]

Nonnutritive

Nonnutritive sweeteners are often known as artificial and low-calorie sweeteners, since they contain very few kilocalories. The term *nonnutritive* also stems from the fact that they contribute almost no energy.

Aspartame (Nutra Sweet). One teaspoon equals one-tenth of 1 kcal; in comparison, 1 tsp of sucrose contains approximately 20 kcal.

Nutra Sweet is used extensively in soft drinks, presweetened cold cereals, instant puddings, gelatins, dessert toppings, and chewing gum. In addition, Nutra Sweet is present in Equal, a low kilocalorie tabletop sweetener.

This product is not recommended for people with phenylketonuria and may be toxic to those with liver disease.

Saccharin. Saccharin is 300–500 times sweeter than sucrose and contains no kilocalories. It is controversial in that it has been determined to cause cancer in laboratory rats. This relationship in humans has not been definitely established; however, saccharin is banned in Canada.

Saccharin is added to baked goods and is sold as a tabletop sweetener.

Sweet 'n Low. This sweetener is a blend of lactose, saccharin, and cream of tartar. One package has the sweetening power of 2 tsp of sugar. While it is low in kilocalories, the lactose can be metabolized to glucose, thereby raising the blood glucose level of a diabetic.[13]

not cause control problems for all diabetics. Also, even if a drug does affect a diabetic's blood glucose level, the physician can probably help the patient integrate it into the diabetes management plan.

In Tables 18-4 and 18-5 the generic or chemical name of the drug is given first, followed in parentheses by its brand or trade name.

TABLE 18-4 DRUGS THAT INCREASE BLOOD GLUCOSE LEVEL[13]

Drug	Normal Functions
Corticosteroid[a] (Prednisone, Decadron, Kenalog, Cortisone)	Relieve inflammation, redness, irritation, and swelling associated with asthma, arthritis, and multiple sclerosis
Diazoxide[a] (Hyperstat, Proglycem)	Hyperstat treats high blood pressure; Hyperstat and Proglycem are the same drug.
	Proglycem treats low blood glucose levels caused by insulin-producing pancreatic tumors
Diuretics[a] (Diuril, HydroDIURIL, Esidrix)	Treat high blood pressure and congestive heart failure.
Phenytoin[a] (Dilantin)	Treat epilepsy

[a]These drugs are especially prone to interact with oral hypoglycemics.

TABLE 18-5 DRUGS THAT DECREASE BLOOD GLUCOSE LEVEL[13]

Drug	Normal Functions
Chloramphenicol[a] (Chloromycetin)	Antibiotic used in treating infections; affects only diabetics who use oral hypoglycemics
Phenylbutazone[a] (Butazolidin)	Anti-inflammatory used in treating arthritis; affects only diabetics who use oral hypoglycemics
Propranolol (Inderal)	Treats angina pectoris and unsteady heartbeats; can prevent some hypoglycemic symptoms
Sulfa drugs[a] (Gantrisin, Septra, Bactrim)	Antibiotics that treat infections; affects only diabetics who use oral hypoglycemics
Aspirin[a]	Treats headache or temporary fever; small amounts do not cause a problem, but large

[a]These drugs are especially prone to interact with oral hypoglycemics.

HYPOGLYCEMIA

The discussion that follows refers only to hypoglycemia that occurs in people who do not take insulin injections or oral hypoglycemic drugs. Hypoglycemia is defined as a blood glucose level below 50 mg/dl and is divided into two main types: **fasting** and **functional**.

Fasting hypoglycemia A type of hypoglycemia that occurs either long after a meal, in the middle of the night, or before breakfast.

Functional hypoglycemia A type of hypoglycemia that occurs 3–4 hours after eating or in response to a meal.

Insulinoma A small noncancerous pancreatic tumor that causes secretion of an excessive amount of insulin.

FASTING HYPOGLYCEMIA

Fasting hypoglycemia typically occurs long after a meal (fasting state), usually 8 hours later, in the middle of the night or before breakfast. In other words, this type of hypoglycemia does not occur as a response to a meal. The typical symptoms include mental dullness, fatigue, confusion, amnesia, headache, convulsions, and loss of consciousness. These symptoms result essentially from an insufficient supply of glucose to the brain.

A basic reason for this condition is secretion of too much insulin.

A common cause of excessive insulin secretion is **insulinoma**. Diseases that prevent the liver from working properly (cirrhosis, severe hepatitis, and cancer of the liver) can also cause this problem. Glucose-raising hormones (glucagon and epinephrine) normally stimulate the breakdown of glycogen in the liver in a hypoglycemic condition; therefore, when the liver is not functioning properly, these hormones cannot raise the blood glucose level.

Treatment

The source of the problem must be diagnosed (e.g. pancreatic tumor, malfunction of the liver, etc.) and the disorder must be treated. Dietary treatment is only a secondary consideration.

FUNCTIONAL (REACTIVE) HYPOGLYCEMIA

Functional or reactive hypoglycemia typically occurs 3–4 hours after eating or in response to a meal. The most common symptoms are irritability, sweating, palpitations, shakiness, and anxiety. These symptoms are not caused by a low blood glucose level but rather result from an increase in the level of the glucose-raising hormones, epinephrine and norepinephrine. These hormones not only stimulate the breakdown of glycogen but also increase the activity of various organs and glands, causing the symptoms.

People who have functional hypoglycemia typically release insulin and absorb glucose normally. Therefore, the hypoglycemia may be a side effect of gastrectomy or may result from excessive intake of alcohol, crash dieting, or stress.

A **partial gastrectomy** frequently results in a **dumping syndrome** (Chapter 19), with hypoglycemia being one of the symptoms. Alcohol is a hypoglycemic substance in that it inhibits the liver's output of glucose.

Partial gastrectomy An operation in which a portion of the stomach is removed. The remaining section is joined to the duodenum (see Chapter 19).

Dumping syndrome A number of physical problems (nausea, vomiting, sweating, and palpitations) that develop from a gastrectomy. The problems develop when the stomach contents enter the duodenum too rapidly and large amounts of fluid shift out of the blood into the duodenum (see Chapter 19).

Treatment

Functional hypoglycemia can be treated by diet modifications that cause a slow, gradual release of insulin, thereby decreasing the possibility of a rapid drop in the blood glucose level.

A functional or reactive hypoglycemic should consume high levels of complex carbohydrates (approximately 75–100 g/day) and very small amounts of simple sugars. In addition, they should consume about 70–130 g protein per day. The rest of their daily kilocalories should come from fat. See table 18-6 for a functional hypoglycemia diet.

Complex carbohydrates are broken down and absorbed slowly, causing a gradual secretion of insulin. This amount of carbohydrate is less than the minimum (100–125 g) required to avoid ketosis. However, the body converts enough of the protein to glucose to make up the deficiency. The advantage of obtaining glucose in this manner is that it causes minimal stimulation of insulin secretion. Hypoglycemics should eat five or six small meals per day, which helps to distribute the carbohydrates throughout the day.[1] See the following sample menu for a functional (reactive) hypoglycemia diet.

SAMPLE MENU FOR FUNCTIONAL (REACTIVE) HYPOGLYCEMIA

Exchange		C (g)	F (g)	P (g)
	Breakfast			
2 fat	2 slices bacon	—	10	—
2 medium-fat meat	2 eggs or substitute	—	10	14
½ bread	½ slice toast	7.5	—	2
2 fat	2 tsp margarine	—	10	—
½ milk	½ cup skim milk	6	—	4
	1 cup decaffeinated coffee			
		13.5	30	20
	Mid-Morning Snack	C	F	P
3 high-fat meat	3 slices cheddar cheese	—	24	21
½ bread	3 saltine crackers	7.5	—	1
½ milk	½ cup skim milk	6	—	4
		13.5	24	26
	Lunch	C	F	P
3 lean meat	3 oz broiled chicken	—	9	21
½ bread	¼ hamburger bun	7.5	—	2
½ fruit	1 medium fresh apricot	5	—	—
2 fat	2 tsp margarine	—	10	—
	lettuce salad	—	—	—
2 fat	2 tbsp french dressing	—	10	—
	1 cup decaffeinated coffee	—	—	—
	artificial sweetener	—	—	—
		12.5	29	23
	Mid-Afternoon Snack	C	F	P
2 high-fat meat	2 oz cold sliced beef	—	16	14
½ bread	½ slice bread	6	—	4
½ milk	½ cup skim milk	6	—	4
		12	16	22

	Dinner	C	F	P
3 high-fat meat	3 oz baked country-style ham	—	24	21
½ bread	¼ cup mashed potatoes	7.5	—	1
1 vegetable	½ cup spinach	5	—	2
	lettuce salad	—	—	—
1 fat	2 tsp salad dressing, mayonnaise type	—	5	—
2 fat	2 tsp margarine	—	10	—
	1 cup decaffeinated coffee	—	—	—
	artificial sweetener	—	—	—
		12.5	39	24

	Evening Snack	C	F	P
½ milk	½ cup skim milk	6	—	4
2 lean meat	½ cup cottage cheese	—	6	14
½ bread	1 graham cracker	7.5	—	1
1 fat	1 tsp margarine	—	5	—
		13.5	11	19

Analysis and Comments

- An analysis of the menu shows that it contains 2 milk, 1 vegetable, ½ fruit, 3 bread, 15 meat, and 12 fat exchanges.

- Notice that the 78 g of carbohydrate are distributed quite evenly throughout the six meals. This distribution is important to provide a slow, constant absorption of carbohydrate into the blood, thereby preventing overstimulation of insulin. This low level of carbohydrates is increased by the conversion of the proteins and fats, as described below.

- The 134 g of protein and 149 g of fat do not stimulate secretion of insulin as they are absorbed. After absorption, they are converted to glucose slowly, thereby providing needed kilocalories.

- Notice that there are no simple sugars, as evidenced by the use of artificial sweeteners, no miscellaneous foods high in simple sugars, and only 2 milk exchanges, thereby reducing the disaccharide lactose to a very low level.

Source: Menu adapted from the Chicago Dietetic Association, *Manual of Clinical Dietetics*, 2nd ed. Philadelphia: W.B. Saunders Company, 1981. Reprinted by permission.
Key: Carbohydrate (C), Fat (F), Protein (P)

TABLE 18-6 FUNCTIONAL (REACTIVE) HYPOGLYCEMIA

Purpose:	To correct postprandial (after a meal) reactive hypoglycemia caused by oversecretion of insulin.
Use:	To raise blood glucose level from a low level (below 50 mg/dl) into the normal range of 80–120 mg/dl.
Examples of foods:	High in complex carbohydrate (usually limited to 75–110 g/day), high in protein and fat, with small, frequent feedings.
Adequacy:	Diet is adequate.

Source: Chicago Dietetic Association, *Manual of Clinical Dietetics*, 2nd ed. Philadelphia, W.B. Saunders Company, 1981. Reprinted by permission.

CASE STUDY: INSULIN-DEPENDENT DIABETES

Billy, an 11-year-old boy, has recently been diagnosed as an insulin-dependent diabetic. He is 5 ft 5 in. tall and weighs 78 lb (his ideal weight should be 105–114 lb). His condition was diagnosed after he was brought to the hospital unconscious. The symptoms he exhibited at the time of admission included deep, labored breathing, polyuria, and flushed, hot, dry skin. His laboratory data and medications are as follows:

Laboratory Findings		Normal values
Serum glucose	325 mg/100 ml	70–110 mg/dl
Urine ketones (acetone)	4+	none
Blood pH	7.1	7.35–7.45
Serum sodium	130 mEq/liter	136–145 mEq/liter
Blood urea nitrogen (BUN)	74 mg/dl	10–20 mg/dl

$$\% \text{ ideal body weight (IBW)} = \frac{\text{actual weight (78 lb)}}{\text{ideal weight (105 lb)}} \times 100 = 68\%$$

Medications
Insulin-NPH   32 units/day

1. Billy's symptoms at the time of admission indicated that he was unconscious due to a _____ reaction.
   A. hypoglycemic
   B. hyperglycemic
2. According to Billy's ketone and pH values, his condition could also be described as _____ .

    A. ketoacidosis

    B. HHNK

3. The elevated BUN level and UBW only 68% of normal indicate that glucose is not being properly used for energy; therefore, _____ _____ .

    A. protein digestion and absorption are being decreased.

    B. increased metabolism of tissue proteins and formation of urea.

    C. there is decreased fat digestion and metabolism.

    D. none of these

Billy's diet includes the following number of exchanges:

1. milk (skim)	4
2. vegetable	3
3. fruit	5
4. bread	9
5. meat	8
3 lean	
5 medium	
6. fat	6

Using the information in Table 2-5, calculate the answers to questions 4–8.

4. The number of grams of carbohydrate in the diet is _____ .

    A. 153

    B. 205

    C. 248

    D. 303

5. The number of grams of protein in the diet is _____ .

    A. 112

    B. 92

    C. 83

    D. 164

6. The number of grams of fat in the diet is _____ .

    A. 34

    B. 55

    C. 48

    D. 64

7. The total number of kilocalories in the diet is _____ .

    A. 1,816

    B. 1,978

C. 2,016

D. 2,278

8. The percentages of kilocalories due to carbohydrate (C), protein (P), and fat (F) are _____ .

A. C—40%
   P—30%
   F—30%

B. C—60%
   P—30%
   F—10%

C. C—50%
   P—20%
   F—30%

Billy's diet plan includes between-meal snacks, with 20 g of carbohydrate in the morning and 20 g before bedtime. Which of the following exchanges and foods can he consume and achieve the 20 g of carbohydrate? Use the information in Table 2-5 to answer questions 9–13.

Key: a = food and exchange can be consumed
     b = food and exchange cannot be consumed

9. _____ 1 bread + ½ fruit; example: 2 graham crackers + ½ apple

10. _____ 2 fruits; example: 1 whole banana

11. _____ ½ milk + 1 bread; example: ½ cup milk and ¾ cup unsweetened cereal

12. _____ 1 meat + 1 bread; example: 1 slice cheese + 6 crackers

13. _____ 2 meats: example: 2 boiled eggs

Billy plays soccer and basketball and runs track at his school. Would the snacks given above provide Billy with enough extra carbohydrate for 1 hour of these strenuous activities?

A. Yes, all of them would.

B. No, none of them would, since he would need more than a minimum of 20 g of extra carbohydrate per hour of increased activity.

C. Yes, examples 9, 10, and 11 would, since 20 g of extra carbohydrate should be adequate per hour of increased activity.

D. none of these

CASE STUDY: NON-INSULIN-DEPENDENT DIABETES

Mr. N is a 34-year-old man with NIDDM. he is 6 ft 3 in. tall, with a medium frame, and weighs 245 lb (recommended weight, 167–182 lb). He works in an office and recently began having spells of extreme thirst, headache, dizziness, blurred vision, abdominal pain, labored breathing and rapid pulse. Mr. N. admitted that he had not been following his diet or taking his medications properly, and frequently had been drinking excessive amounts of beer.

His laboratory data and medications are as follows:

Laboratory Findings		Normal Values
Serum glucose	310 mg/dl	70–110 mg/dl
Serum triglycerides	525 mg/dl	10–200 mg/dl
Blood pressure	152/97	90–140/50–90
% ideal body weight (IBW) $= \dfrac{\text{actual weight (245 lb)}}{\text{ideal weight (182 lb)}}$ $= 135\%$ over ideal weight		
Medications		
tolbutamide (Orinase)	500 mg tablets	four times a day

1. Is Mr. N. obese, since 115–120% of IBW is indicative of obesity?
   A. No
   B. Yes

2. How many kilocalories should Mr. N be required to consume in order to allow weight loss but still be adequate?
   A. 2,000 kcal
   B. 1,800 kcal
   C. 900 kcal
   D. 1,500 kcal

3. What other steps besides dietary restriction should be taken to control Mr. N's diabetes?

   1. diet alone should be adequate
   2. he should begin a moderate, regular exercise program
   3. he should reduce or omit alcohol
   4. he should take his oral hypoglycemic medication regularly

   A: 1, 2, 3   B. 1, 3   C. 2, 3, 4   D. 3, 4   E. all of these

Occasionally, when stressful events occur at work, Mr. N. experiences episodes of hypoglycemia. Which of the following would supply approximately 10 g of glucose and therefore be most suitable to correct his hypoglycemia?

Use the following key to answer questions 4-9.

Key: a = suitable
        b = unsuitable

4. _____ 1 cup milk

5. _____ ½ cup pineapple juice

6. _____ ½ cup diet cola

7. _____ 4 or 5 Life Savers

8. _____ go for a brief walk

9. _____ consume small packet of honey

10. How many meals should Mr. N consume per day?

    A. any number would be suitable
    B. three, with a snack when hypoglycemia occurs
    C. six are essential to control his diabetes
    D. only one in order to facilitate weight loss

11. What nutrient distribution is recommended for Mr. N.?

    A. 20% protein, 30% carbohydrate, 50% fat
    B. 10% protein, 50% carbohydrate, 40% fat
    C. 20% protein, 50% carbohydrate, 30% fat
    D. none of these

12. If Mr. N. consumes beer while taking his tolbutamide (Orinase) tablets, which of the following possible side effects might he experience?

    1. stumbling   3. facial flushing
    2. slurring of words   4. pounding headache
        A. 1, 2, 3   B. 1, 3   C. 2, 4   D. 4   E. all of these

OUTLINE

DIABETES MELLITUS

Definition and Prevalence

Diabetes is a group of disorders that have a variety of genetic causes, but that have in common hyperglycemia (a high blood glucose level).

A total of 10 million people, or 5% of the population, are estimated to have diabetes; this number is increasing by 6% per year.

Type I: Insulin-Dependent Diabetes Mellitus (IDDM)

General Characteristics

Approximately 15% or less of diabetics have IDDM. Typically, the onset is before age 20, with a mean age of 12.

The onset is sudden, often in children who have had a recent viral infection with mumps and flu.

Ketoacidosis is a mjaor complication.

Genesis or Cause

Research shows that IDDM individuals have increased levels of human lymphocyte antigens (HLA): HLA-B8 and HLA-B15. HLAs are found only in individuals who have genes that produce them.

Some researchers believe that islet cell antibodies result from viruses that have invaded and altered the beta cells of the pancreas; islet cell antibodies attack and destroy the beta cells, resulting in insulin deficiency; autoimmunity is a condition in which the body forms antibodies against its own tissues.

Functions of Insulin and Results of Deficiencies

Normal or increased amounts of insulin result in increases of the following: uptake of glucose and synthesis of glycogen, uptake of fatty acids and synthesis of fats by fat cells; uptake of amino acids and synthesis of proteins. As a result of these increases, there are decreases in blood glucose, fatty acid, and amino acid levels.

A deficiency of insulin results in increased levels of the following: blood glucose, fatty acids and ketones, and amino acids.

Clinical Symptoms and Complications

The symptoms of IDDM include polyuria, polydipsia, polyphagia, weight loss, obesity, blurred vision, skin itching or infection, loss of strength, and diabetic ketoacidosis (DKA).

Chronic Complications of IDDM

Divided into large-vessel and small-vessel disease and susceptibility to infectious complications.

Large-vessel disease: primarily atherosclerosis in blood vessels supplying the brain, kidneys, heart, and lower extremities.

Small-vessel disease (microangiopathies): increased glucose and fat circulating through the capillaries, arterioles, and venules, causes a thickening of the capillary basement membrane and thereby decreasing the amount of nutrients reaching certain tissues. The capillaries most often affected are those supplying the retina of the eye and the kidney, with retinopathy and nephropathy, respectively, being examples of the problems that arise from damage to these vessels.

Susceptibility to infection: very high in diabetics due to the growth and multiplication of bacteria in the high blood glucose environment.

Diagnosis and Monitoring of Diabetes

Urine Testing. Urine is tested for the presence of glucose and ketones to both diagnose and monitor diabetes. A glucose level greater than 0.25% in the urine is indicative of possible diabetes, and a blood test should be performed for definitive diagnosis. Diabetics can monitor the progress of their diabetes by measuring the glucose level in their urine, with 0–0.25% indicating adequate control.

Blood Testing. Two types of tests are performed to diagnose diabetes:

- Fasting blood glucose/sugar (FBG/FBS). This test is done on blood after an overnight fast, with a value greater than 140 mg/dl on two different occasions being positive for diabetes.
- Oral glucose tolerance test (OGTT). The person consumes a measured amount of glucose after an overnight fast. Blood tests are run at $\frac{1}{2}$, 1, and 2 hours; if two of the samples show a blood glucose level equal to or greater than 200 mg/dl, this result is diagnostic of diabetes.

Glycolysated Hemoglobin (HbA$_{1c}$. This test is not used to diagnose diabetes but rather to check how well it is being controlled. The advantages are that it can measure control over the past 2–4 months, can be performed on a diabetic in a nonfasting state, and is not affected by the time of the day, stress, exercise, and food intake.

Treatment of Insulin-Dependent Diabetics

Insulin. Three basic types of insulin are available for diabetics- rapid, intermediate, and prolonged acting.

The exact type, amount injected, and time of injection are based on the stage of growth, activity patterns, eating habits, and individual responses of the diabetic.

Some side effects of insulin are allergy, lipoatrophy, hypertrophy, and insulin resistance.

Some diabetics absorb insulin over 24 hours and need only one injection per day (usually 1 hour before breakfast). Some need two injections per day (one before breakfast and one 12 hours later). Some need a mixture of rapidly absorbed and intermediate-acting insulin before breakfast.

An insulin pump is worn by some diabetics. It is about the size of a beeper and is usually injected through tubing into the abdomen on a continual basis; the diabetic can control the amount injected and the time of injection.

Insulin shock or hypoglycemia. A blood glucose level below 50 mg/dl that is definition of hypoglycemia. Four causes are overdose of insulin, excessive exercise, undereating or skipping meals, and vomiting or diarrhea. The symptoms of hypoglycemia are summarized in Table 18-2.

With the onset of hypoglycemic symptoms, the diabetic should consume 10 g of readily absorbable glucose; examples are 4 oz fruit juice, one-half cup of a regular soft drink, four to five Life Savers, and two large sugar cubes.

In situations where glucose cannot be consumed orally, glucagon (a glucose-increasing hormone) should be given subcutaneously, intramuscularly, or intravenously. Another alternative is to use a commercial glucose product that is absorbed rapidly through the oral tissues of the mouth.

Hyperglycemic reaction. This results from injection of insufficient insulin situations in which insulin conditions require more insulin, such as infection, illness, surgery, and injury. Symptoms of hyperglycemia are compared with those of hypoglycemia in Table 18-2.

Dietary Treatment of IDDM

Timing of meals is very important; a diabetic should consume food at least every 5 hours in order to avoid a hypoglycemic reaction. Many juvenile diabetics consume six meals a day—breakfast, a mid-morning snack, a noon meal, a mid-afternoon snack, an evening meal, and a bedtime snack.

Carbohydrates should account for 50–60% of the total daily kilocalories. The majority of the carbohydrates should be complex, not simple. Carbohydrates from legumes (beans, peas) and those that have been minimally processed (whole rice as opposed to ground rice) cause less of a rise in blood glucose than other carbohydrate sources.

Protein should compose about 20% of the kilocalorie intake for growing young diabetics; the number of grams of protein should be the RDA for the diabetic's age and sex.

Fats should compose about 30% of the total kilocalories, with the majority being polyunsaturated. No more than 300 mg of cholesterol should be consumed due to the increased susceptibility of diabetics to cardiovascular disease.

The total kilocalorie intake should be adequate for the young diabetics growth and physical activity; this can be determined by referring to the RDA table for energy intake (Table 10-1); it can be estimated by allowing 1,000 kcal for 1 year of age and adding 100 kcal for every additional year of age.

It is important for kilocalories and carbohydrate grams to be distributed througout the day according to the type of insulin being used. A common distribution for diabetics who consume six meals a day is 4/18ths to 5/18ths of kilocalories and carbohydrates at the three main meals and 1/18th to 2/18th for each of the three snacks. Diabetics and their parents should be taught how to use exchange lists for meal planning and eating out.

Increasing the amount of fiber in the diet, along with exercise, has been found to decrease the amount of insulin needed by diabetics. The diabetic should increase the amount of fiber in the diet until he or she is consuming about 45 g/day. Chapter 5 presents the food groups and specific foods that contain approximately 2 g of fiber per serving.

Type II: Non-Insulin-Dependent Diabetes Mellitus (NIDDM)

General Characteristics

This is the more common type, with about 90% of all diabetics being NIDDM. It develops later in life, usually after age 40; about 80% of patients are over age 50. They generally do not have an insulin deficiency, and some even have an insulin surplus.

The NIDDM patient is not ketoacidosis prone but is prone to hyperosmolar hyperglycemic nonketotic coma (HHNK). There is less vascular damage to the small vessels but more atherosclerosis.

Genesis or Cause

One theory is that the number of insulin receptors is decreased in obese people, with the end result being that less glucose is taken up by the cells. The number of insulin receptors returns to normal when the person loses weight.

A second theory is that the target cells in obese people do not bring about the proper biochemical changes in glucose after it is absorbed.

Symptoms and Complications
The symptoms of NIDDM are the same as those of IDDM: polyuria, polydipsia, and hyperglycemia. Diagnosis is based on the same glucose tolerance test results as IDMM.

A life-threatening complication is HHNK. This problem is almost identical to diabetic ketoacidosis (DKA) in the way it is initiated and the sequence of events that occur. A major difference between the two is that there is no increase in ketone levels with HHNK.

Treatment
The goals of treatment are identical to those of IDDM. The main difference between the two is that NIDDM diabetics can usually control their blood glucose level with diet alone; most NIDDM diabetics are obese, and therefore need to be on a weight loss diet.

Initially, the kilocalorie intake on a weight loss diet may be as low as 600 in order to lower the blood glucose to an acceptable level. Once the blood glucose level is lowered, the number of kilocalories needed to lose 1–2 lb/week should be determined; frequently, it may be 1,000–1,200 kcal/day.

Exercise decreases blood glucose and fatty acid levels; it also raises the levels of high-density lipoproteins (HDL), which benefits the diabetic by lowering the cholesterol and triglyceride levels.

Some NIDDM diabetics need to take oral hypoglycemic drugs, in addition to diet and exercise, to lower their blood glucose level. Oral drugs increase the output of insulin from the pancreas and increase the affinity of insulin receptors in peripheral tissues.

Possible side effects of the use of oral drugs are hypoglycemia, gastrointestinal tract irritation, allergic skin reactions, and alcohol sensitivity.

Diabetes and Pregnancy
Diet Modifications
There is an increased need for glucose and kilocalories during pregnancy. The RDA during pregnancy is +300 kcal and +30 g of protein. The American Diabetes Association recommends no less than 200 g of carbohydrate per day.

Insulin Therapy
Insulin requirements generally decrease during the first trimester, since a large amount of glucose shifts into fetus from the mother. Insulin requirements generally increase during the second and third trimesters, since placenta hormones (estrogen, progesterone, and lactogen) act as insulin antagonists.

Most authorities do not recommend the use of oral hypoglycemic drugs during pregnancy, since they are not as effective in controlling glucose levels as insulin; also, they can cause hypoglycemia in a fetus and possibly death.

Drugs That Can Interfere with Diabetes Control
Diabetics need to be aware that some drugs can lower or raise their blood glucose level, therefore affecting their ability to control their condition. Some drugs can also interfere with the action of oral hypoglycemic agents.

Drugs that can increase blood glucose levels are given in Table 18-3, and drugs that decrease blood glucose levels are given in Table 18-4.

HYPOGLYCEMIA

Fasting Hypoglycemia
Hypoglycemia is a blood glucose level below 50 mg/dl. This type occurs long after a meal or when a person is in a fasting state. Symptoms include mental dullness, fatigue, confusion, amnesia, headache, convulsions, and loss of consciousness.

The main reason for this problem is secretion of too much insulin.

Tumors of the pancreas (insulinoma) often result in secretion of too much insulin. Cirrhosis, severe hepatitis, and cancer of the liver can result in hypoglycemia due to a deficiency of glycogen.

Treatment
Treatment involves diagnosis and appropriate medical steps; dietary treatment is only secondary.

Functional (Reactive) Hypoglycemia
This condition typically occurs 3–4 hours after eating or in response to a meal. Common symptoms

are irritability, sweating, palpitations, shakiness, and anxiety.

Typical causes are side effects of surgery on the stomach (gastrectomy), excessive intake of alcohol, crash dieting, and stress.

Treatment

Treatment involves dietary modifications designed to cause a slow, gradual release of insulin. The diet should be high in complex carbohydrates (75–100 g/day), with 70–130 g of protein per day. The rest of the kilocalories should come from fat.

REVIEW QUESTIONS

TRUE (A) OR FALSE (B).

Questions 1–38.

1. Diabetes is not a genetic but rather a biochemical problem.
2. Diabetes, although a serious problem, is not a leading cause of death.
3. Insulin-dependent diabetes mellitus (IDDM) is the most common type of diabetes and is caused by early-onset obesity in children.
4. IDDM people almost always have a higher level of human lymphocyte antigens HLA-B8 and HLA-B15, plus islet cell antibodies.
5. Many researchers believe that IDDM is an example of autoimmunity, since the body forms islet cell antibodies against its own pancreas tissue.
6. Normal or increased amounts of insulin result in increased amounts of blood glucose, blood fatty acids, and blood amino acids.
7. The symptoms of IDDM develop very rapidly, usually secondary to a viral infection or severe emotional stress.
8. The symptoms of IDDM are polyuria, polydipsia, polyphagia, skin itching, and diabetic ketoacidosis (DKA).
9. DKA is characterized by a high plasma pH, hypoglycemia, edema, shock, and coma.
10. Retinopathy and nephropathy result from too much fat damaging the walls of the microscopic vessels supplying the retina and kidney, respectively.
11. A fasting blood glucose (FBG) test result of 120 mg/dl and two oral glucose tolerance test values of 140 mg/dl are indicative of diabetes.
12. The advantages of glycolysated hemoglobin

(HbA$_{1c}$) tests are that it allows a physician to check how successful diabetes control has been over the past 2–4 months and can be performed on a person in a nonfasting state.
13. As the exercise level of a diabetic increases, the need for insulin decreases.
14. Insulin should not be injected into areas of the body that are about to be exercised, since it will be absorbed faster and result in hypoglycemia.
15. Situations that may cause a hypoglycemic or insulin shock reaction are lack of exercise, overeating, and stress.
16. Symptoms of a hypoglycemic reaction are drowsy, weak, deep, labored breathing and vomiting.
17. In a severe insulin shock reaction, glucagon may be given to increase glucose by breaking down glycogen.
18. In a stress condition, the diabetic should increase the amount of insulin injected to counter the increased blood glucose level.
19. An IDDM diet should be low in carbohydrates and high in protein, with a medium amount of fat.
20. The diet mentioned in question 19 is high in protein so that the excess can be converted to carbohydrates without stimulating the release of insulin.
21. Recent research has shown that complex carbohydrates such as bread and potatoes cause a greater rise in blood glucose level than foods containing simple carbohydrates such as ice cream.
22. Carbohydrates from legumes (e.g., beans, peas) and carbohydrates that have been minimally processed cause less of a rise in glucose level than other carbohydrate sources.
23. The kilocalorie level of IDDM diabetics should be low, since these persons are usually obese.
24. It is very important that the distribution of kilocalories and grams of carbohydrates for IDDM diabetics coincide with the type of insulin being used.
25. All diabetics can keep their blood glucose levels from rising sharply by increasing their dietary fiber intake up to 45 g/day.
26. A high-fiber diet supposedly reduces that rapid rise in blood glucose level following a meal because fiber prevents the digestion of carbohydrates to glucose.
27. NIDDM diabetics have hyperglycemia because obesity reduces the number of insulin receptors.
28. One very serious possible complication of

NIDDM diabetes is hyperglycemic hyperosmolar nonketotic coma (HHNK).

29. The major difference between DKA and HHNK is that the latter does not result in an increase in ketone levels.

30. A weight loss diet for an NIDDM diabetic should be low enough in kilocalories that the person loses weight at a rate of 5 lb/week until the recommended weight is achieved.

31. Some NIDDM diabetics must take oral insulin such as tolazamide (Tolinase), tolbutamide (Orinase), and chlorpropamide (Diabinese) to control their blood glucose level.

32. A pregnant diabetic needs an extra 300 g of protein and 30 kcal/day for her increased needs and those of the fetus.

33. During the first trimester of an IDDM pregnancy, the insulin requirements generally decrease, since a large amount of glucose shifts from the mother into the fetus.

34. Oral hypoglycemics generally are not recommended during pregnancy, since they may cause prolonged hypoglycemia and possibly death of the fetus.

35. Fasting hypoglycemia typically occurs 8 hours after a meal and is characterized by irritability, sweating, palpitations, shakiness, and anxiety.

36. The symptoms of functional hypoglycemia result from an increased level of insulin.

37. Functional hypoglycemia can be treated by a diet that includes 75–100 g complex carbohydrates and 70–130 g protein per day.

38. The diet in question 37 is designed to convert some of the protein to glucose with a minimal stimulation of insulin secretion.

MULTIPLE CHOICE

Questions 39–50

39. A possible sequence of events that could lead to the development of IDDM is:
    1. recognition of degraded pancreas tissue by HLA cells
    2. islet cell antibodies attack and destroy beta cells
    3. virus invades and causes the release of degraded pancreas beta cell tissue
    4. decreased secretion of insulin followed by IDDM
    A. 1, 2, 3   B. 3, 2, 1, 4   C. 3, 1, 2, 4
    D. 2, 3, 1, 4

40. Which of the following is (are) correctly paired when a person has an increased secretion of insulin?
    A. decreased blood glucose—increased uptake of glucose and synthesis of glycogen in the liver
    B. increased blood fatty acids—increased breakdown of stored fats
    C. decreased blood amino acids—increased uptake of amino acids and synthesis of proteins by muscle cells
    D. A, C
    E. A, B

41. The following changes can occur when an IDDM diabetics has DKA. Select the one answer that presents the changes in the correct order.
    1. destruction of enzymes
    2. acidic plasma
    3. coma
    4. increase in ketone level
    A. 2, 4, 1, 3   B. 4, 1, 2, 3   C. 4, 2, 1, 3
    D. 2, 1, 4, 3

42. Which of the following tests are indicative of diabetes or inadequate diabetic control?
    1. fasting blood glucose level of 130 mg/dl on two separate occasions
    2. 1% glucose level in urine
    3. oral glucose tolerance test (OGTT) values of 150 mg/dl at 1 hour and 130 mg/dl at 2 hours
    A. 1, 2, 3   B. 2   C. 2, 3   D. 1, 3
    E. 3

43. Two basic criteria determine the amount of insulin an IDDM diabetic needs: _____ and _____.
    A. stage of growth—activity level
    B. age—weight
    C. basal metabolic rate—age
    D. time of meals—total kilocalorie intake

44. Four situations that might cause hypoglycemia or an insulin reaction are:
    1. overdose of insulin
    2. lack of exercise
    3. undereating
    4. edema
    A. 1, 2, 3   B. 1, 3   C. 2, 4   D. 4
    E. all of these

45. Symptoms of hypoglycemia are:
    1. agitation, nervousness, trembling
    2. vomiting
    3. normal to rapid shallow breathing
    4. lack of hunger
    A. 1, 2, 3   B. 1, 3   C. 2, 4   D. 4
    E. all of these

46. A diet composition for an IDDM might be _____ percent of the total daily kilocalories.

A. carbohydrates 50–60; proteins, 20; fats 30
B. carbohydrates, 30–40; proteins, 30; fats 30
C. carbohydrates, 10–15; proteins, 50; fats 40
D. none of these

47. The benefit to a diabetic from a high-fiber diet is to _____ and a high-fiber diet is defined as dietary fiber that exceeds _____ _____ g/day.
   A. help prevent hypoglycemia—20
   B. prevent a rapid rise in—40
      the glucose level after a meal
   C. prevent hyperglycemia—30
   D. prevent colon cancer—50

48. One theory as to why obesity can result in NIDDM is that _____.
   A. fat infiltration into the pancreas destroys beta cells.
   B. fat prevents the liver from synthesizing glycogen.
   C. the number of insulin receptors attached to cells is reduced.
   D. none of these

49. The treatment of NIDDM consists of the following:
   1. low-kilocalorie weight loss diet
   2. increased exercise
   3. oral hypoglycemic drugs for some NIDDM people
   4. eating large amount of dietetic foods
   A. 1, 2, 3   B. 1, 3   C. 2, 4   D. 4
   E. all of these

50. Which of the following correctly compare fasting and functional (reactive) hypoglycemia:
   Fasting Hypoglycemia—Functional Hypoglycemia
   1. does not occur as a response to a meal—occurs as a response to a meal
   2. causes: pancreas tumor, liver disease—side effect of stomach surgery, excessive alcohol intake, crash dieting
   3. treatment: dietary only—treatment: diagnosis and correction of the medical problem; dietary treatment secondary
   A. 1, 2, 3   B. 1, 2   C. 2, 3   D. 3
   E. all of these

MATCHING

Questions 51–54. Match the function in colume B with the drug in column A.

Column A

51. diazoxide (Hyperstat, Proglycem)
52. phenylbutazone (Butazolidin)
53. chloramphenicol (Chloromycetin)
54. diuretics (Diuril, HydroDIURIL)

Column B

a. increase blood glucose level
b. decrease blood glucose level

DISCUSSION QUESTIONS

1. Discuss the effects of a deficient amount of insulin on the levels of blood glucose, blood fatty acids and ketones, and amino acids.
2. Give four symptoms of IDDM and the underlying causes of each.
3. Describe the blood tests and values that are used to diagnose diabetes.
4. Describe the sequence of changes that result in DKA.
5. Discuss the importance of distributing kilocalories and carbohydrate grams throughout the day according to the type of insulin used.
6. Discuss the cause of NIDDM.
7. Describe the sequence of changes that result in HHNK.
8. Compare and contrast fasting hypoglycemia and functional hypoglycemia in terms of the causes, symptoms, and treatment of each.

REFERENCES

1. A.L. Notkins. "The causes of diabetes." *Scientific American*, 241, 62–73. (November 1979).
2. H.L. Little, A. Patz, R.L. Jack, and P.H. Forsham. *Diabetic Retinopathy*. New York: Thieme-Stratten, Inc., 1983, pp. 3–9.
3. C.H. Robinson, and M.R. Lawler. *Normal and Therapeutic Nutrition,* 16th ed. New York: Macmillian Publishing Co., Inc., 1982, p. 603.
4. *Diabetes Mellitus*, 8th ed. Indianapolis: Eli Lilly, 1980.
5. B.G. Morrissey. *Therapeutic Nutrition*. Philadelphia: J.B. Lipincott Co., 1984, pp. 182–183.
6. "Current status of diet therapy in the management of diabetes mellitus." *Nutrition in Practice, 1*(3), 4–20 (1981).

7. P.A. Crapo. The Relationship Between Food and Blood Sugar, *Nutrition and the M.D.*, *10* (7), 1–4 (1984).
8. "Exchange Lists for Meal Planning." New York, American Diabetes Association, Inc., 1976.
9. "Dietary Filler and Diabetes." *Nutrition and the M.D. 10*(10), 3–4 (1984).
10. *Managing Diabetes Properly.* Horsham, Pa: Intermed Communications, 1977, pp. 141–153.
11. L.H. Bodinski. *The Nurse's Guide to Diet Therapy.* New York: John Wiley and Sons, 1982, p. 309.
12. J.M. Olefsky and P. Crapo. "Fructose, xylitol, and sorbitol." *Diabetes Care*, *3*(2), 390–393 (1980).
13. B.G. Morrissey. *Therapeutic Nutrition.* Philadelphia: J.B. Lippincott Co., 1984, pp. 223–224.
14. R.K. Campbell, and P.D. Hansten. "Use with caution!" *Diabetes Forecast*, 1982.

19 DISEASES OF THE GASTROINTESTINAL TRACT

OBJECTIVES

Upon completion of this chapter, you should be able to:

1. Describe the structure and function of the esophagus.

2. Give the cause, symptoms, and diet therapy for hiatal hernia.

3. List four functions of the stomach.

4. Recognize the cause, symptoms, and diet therapy for acute gastritis.

5. Give the cause, symptoms, and diet therapy for a peptic ulcer.

6. Describe the symptoms of and reasons for the dumping syndrome.

7. Give the dietary treatment of dumping syndrome.

8. Describe the long-range nutritional problems after a subtotal gastrectomy.

9. Give three functions of the small intestine.

10. Recognize the cause, symptoms, and diet therapy for nontropical sprue (celiac disease).

11. Describe the cause, symptoms, and diet therapy for lactose intolerance.

12. Give the cause, symptoms, and diet therapy for Crohn's disease.

13. Recognize three functions of the large intestine.

14. Give the cause, symptoms, and diet therapy for diverticulosis and diverticulitis.

15. Give the cause, symptoms, and diet therapy for ulcerative colitis.

INTRODUCTION

Alimentary canal A muscular tube that extends from the mouth to the anus.

The **alimentary canal** is the muscular tube (see Fig. 19-1) into which one ingests food, digests it, and absorbs it and from which feces are excreted. The canal is specialized in certain regions for particular functions. In this chapter, we will study the esophagus, stomach, and small and large intestinal regions in terms of their functions and therapeutic nutrition for disorders of these areas.

ESOPHAGUS

Bolus A round mass of food.

Peristaltic contractions Rhythmic waves of smooth muscle contractions.

The esophagus (Fig. 19-1) begins at the base of the pharynx, extends through the thorax, posterior to the trachea, continues through the diaphragm, and finally joins the stomach. It functions as the passageway for food from the pharynx to the stomach. It moves a **bolus** into the stomach by **peristaltic contractions** of the muscular wall (Fig. 19-2). A sphincter-type valve is present at the entrance of the stomach. It opens to allow food into the stomach and closes to prevent regurgitation.

DISORDERS

Hiatal Hernia

The most common form of a hiatal hernia is one in which the esophagus–stomach junction slides through the diaphragm when the person lies down (see Fig. 19-3).

Cause. Hiatal hernia can result from a congenital weakness of the diaphragm muscle as well as from aging, obesity, pregnancy, and tight-fitting clothes.

Pyrosis Heartburn.

Reflux Regurgitation.

Dysphagia Difficulty in swallowing.

Symptoms. The most common complaint is **pyrosis,** which results from a **reflux** of stomach contents. Other complaints are **dysphagia,** substernal pain, and vomiting.

Diet Therapy. The primary goal of the diet is to prevent reflux. The diet is bland, with small, frequent feedings. Antacids are frequently taken to help neutralize the acidity in the stomach. Foods should not be eaten for 3–4 hours before bedtime. It is important that the patient avoid physical activity that requires stooping forward after eating. The head of the bed should be elevated to avoid reflux.[1] A weight reduction diet

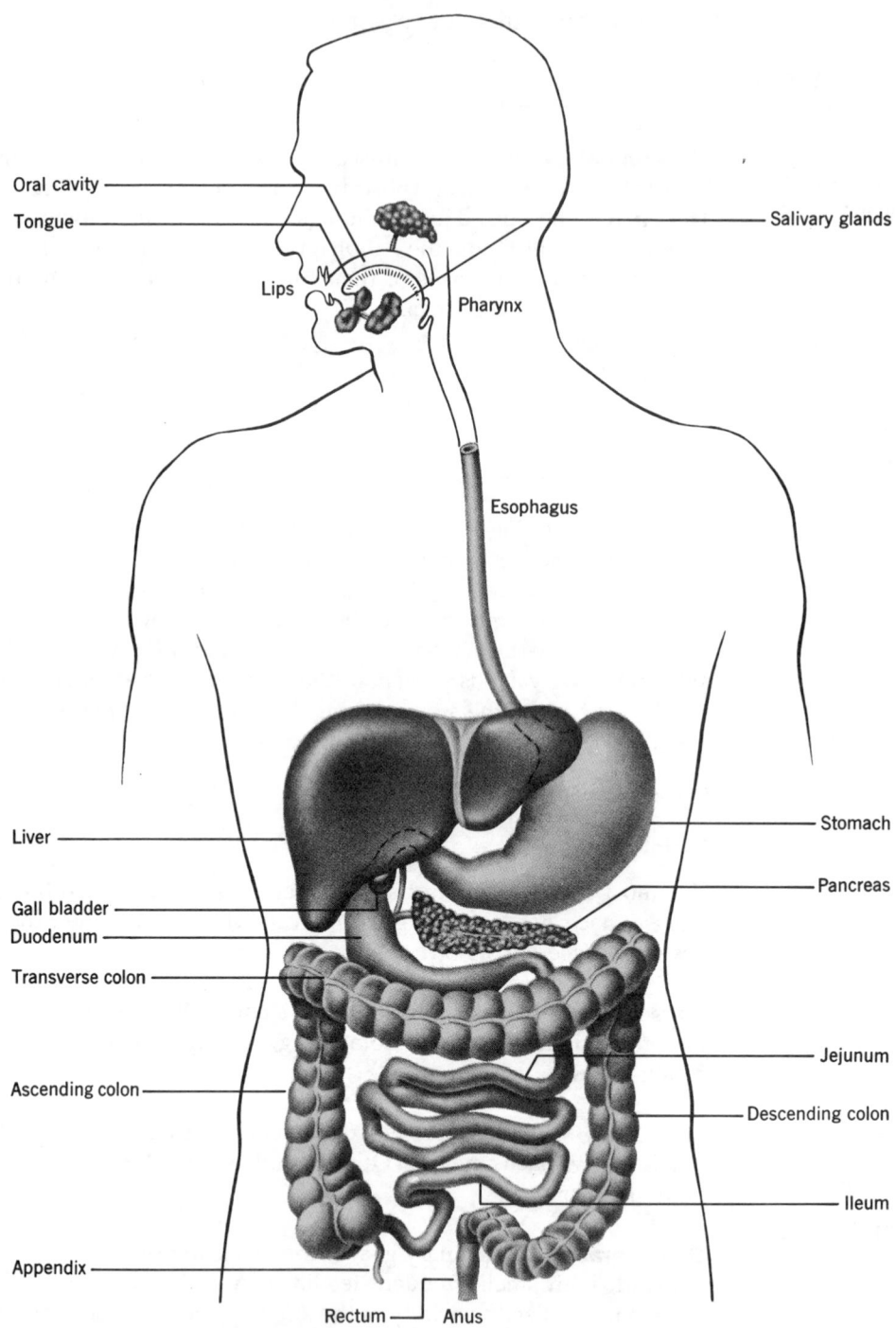

FIGURE 19-1 Alimentary canal and specialized regions. (From S.R. Burke, *Human Anatomy and Physiology for the Health Sciences,* 2nd ed. New York: John Wiley & Sons, Inc., © 1985. Reprinted by permission.)

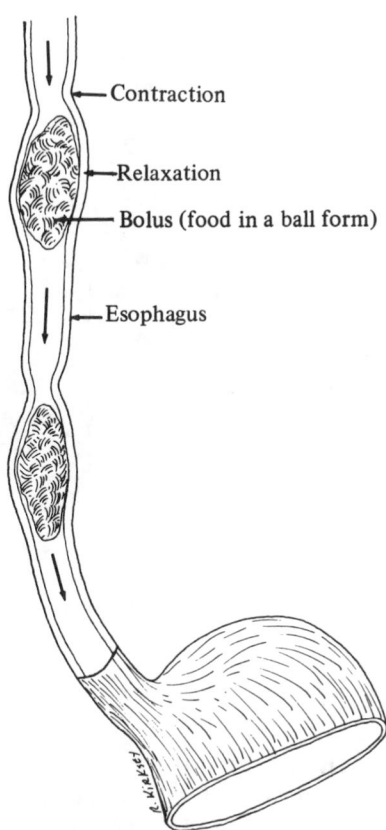

FIGURE 19-2 Peristaltic contractions of the esophagus that move a bolus of food from the pharynx to the stomach. (From T. Randall Lankford, *Integrated Science for Health Students,* 3rd edition, 1984. Reprinted by permission of Reston Publishing Company, a Prentice-Hall Company, 11480 Sunset Hills Road, Reston, VA 22090.

may be appropriate for hiatal hernia, since many people with this condition are obese. The principles of a restricted bland diet are provided in Table 19-1. Table 19-2 gives a summary of the above information.

STOMACH

Chyme Semifluid mass of food that is formed in the stomach and released into the duodenum.

The stomach (see Fig. 19-4) has four basic functions:

Storage. It temporarily stores **chyme,** which is released to the duodenum for further digestion.

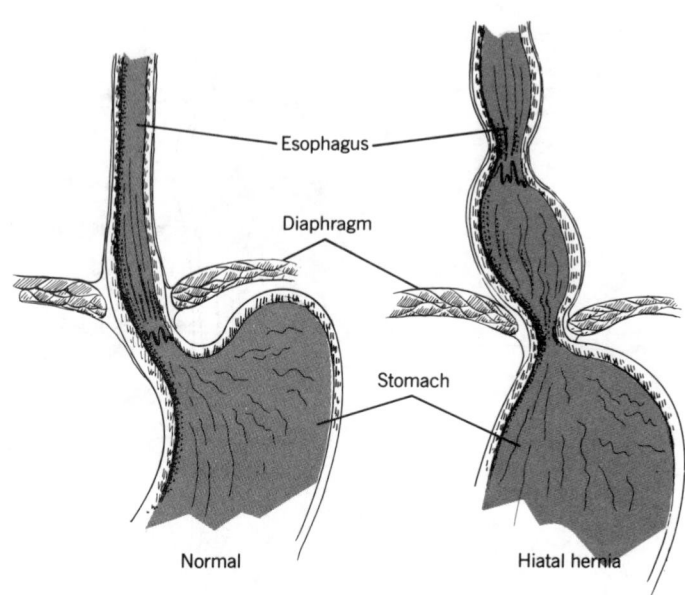

FIGURE 19-3 A hiatal hernia.

Mixing. Peristaltic contractions mix food thoroughly with gastric juices to form chyme.

Pyloric sphincter valve
A circular muscle that controls the movement of food from the pyloric region of the stomach into the duodenum.

Regulation of the flow of cyme. Chyme is released in small quantities into the duodenum through opening and closing of the **pyloric sphincter valve** (Fig. 19-4).

Facilitates absorption of vitamin B$_{12}$, iron, and calcium. The stomach secretes an intrinsic factor that aids the absorption of vitamin B$_{12}$ in

TABLE 19-1 RESTRICTED BLAND DIET

Purpose:	Designed to decrease peristalsis and avoid irritation of the gastrointestinal tract.
Use:	Used in treatment of hiatal hernia. Also used as a transitional diet in treatment of various diseases of the gastrointestinal tract in which inflammation or spasms are present.
Examples of foods:	Foods that are chemically, mechanically, or thermally irritating are removed from the diet. Some examples of foods that are eliminated are fried foods, most raw fruits and vegetables, caffeine, alcohol, coarse breads and cereals, and highly seasoned foods.
Adequacy:	Diet is adequate.

Source: Chicago Dietetic Association, *Manual of Clinical Dietetics,* second edition. Philadelphia, W.B. Saunders Company, 1981. Reprinted by permission.

TABLE 19-2 SUMMARY OF HIATAL HERNIA

Pathophysiology	Causes	Symptoms	Diet Therapy
Protrusion of part of stomach through esophagus opening in diaphragm	Congenital weakness of diaphragm Aging process Obesity Pregnancy Tight-fitting clothes	Pyrosis Reflux Dysphagia	Bland diet Small, frequent feedings No foods eaten 3–4 hours before bedtime Elevation of head of bed

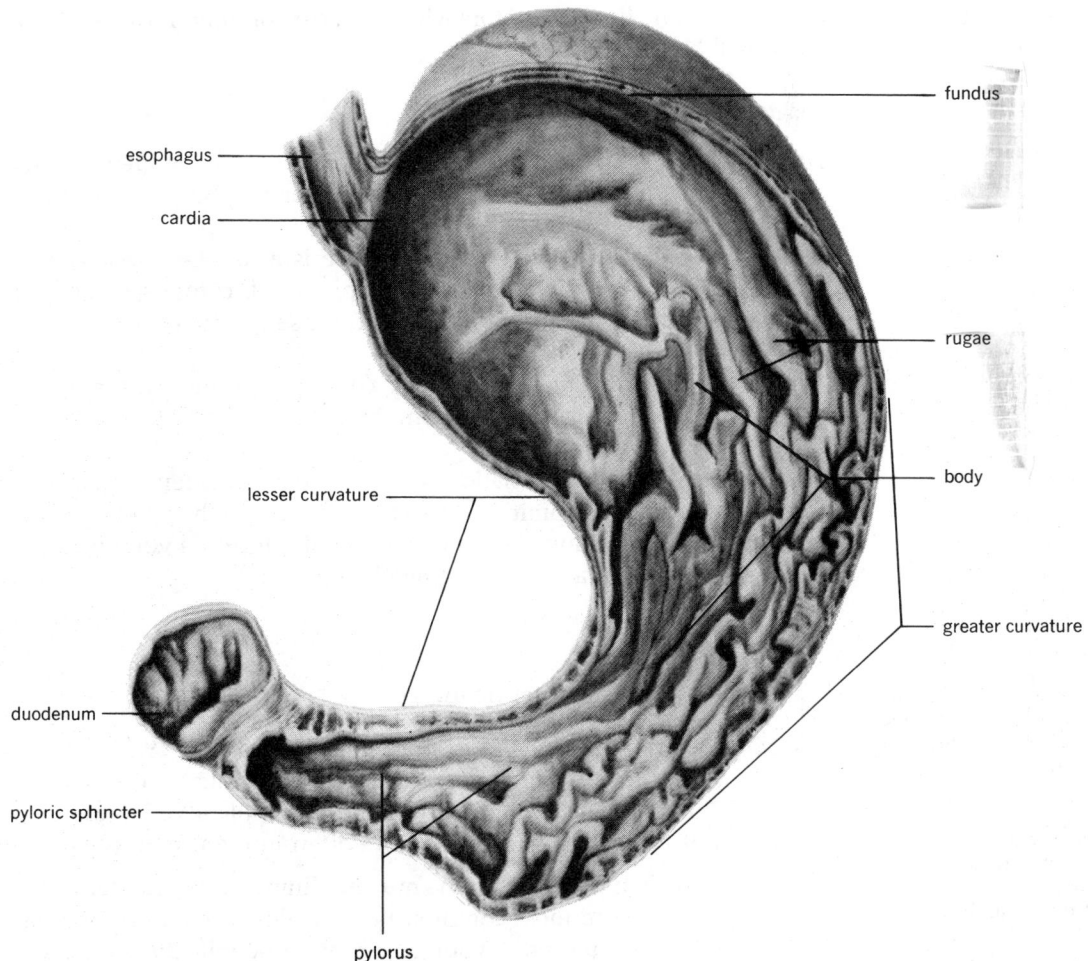

FIGURE 19-4 Anatomy of the stomach. (From J.R. McClintic, *Basic Anatomy and Physiology of the Human Body.* New York: John Wiley & Sons, Inc., © 1980. Reprinted by permission.)

the small intestine. Also, the hydrochloric acid (HCl) in the stomach helps to convert iron from a +3 charge to a +2 charge, which is more readily absorbed. HCl increases the solubility and thereby the absorption of calcium.

Any stomach disorder interferes with one or more of these functions.

DISORDERS

Gastritis

Gastritis A condition in which the gastric mucosa is inflamed.

Gastritis involves inflammation of the gastric mucosa, which is the mucous membrane lining the stomach. The most common form, acute gastritis, will be discussed.

Acute Gastritis

Edematous Refers to a condition of edema.

Acute gastritis is a common disorder characterized by a reddened, **edematous** mucosa, with small erosions and hemorrhages.

Cause. Probably the most common cause is alcohol, especially when consumed in combination with aspirin. Spicy foods composed of pepper, vinegar, and mustard are also known to cause gastritis.

Epigastric pain Same as epigastric distress.

Symptoms. An affected person may complain of anorexia, **epigastric pain,** and in some cases severe vomiting.

Diet Therapy. The inflammation subsides when the offending foods are witheld; therefore, if vomiting persists, no foods can be given by mouth and parenteral nutrition should be instituted. Once the vomiting stops, a bland diet and antacids should be given.

Peptic Ulcer

Peptic ulcer A deterioration or lesion in the mucosal lining of the stomach or duodenum.

Gastric ulcer A deterioration of the gastric mucosa generally located along the lesser curvature of the stomach.

Duodenal ulcer A deterioration of the mucosal lining of the duodenum.

There are two types of **peptic ulcers.**

Gastric. Deterioration of the gastric mucosa (see Fig. 19-5) along the lesser curvature of the stomach causes most gastric ulcers (see Fig. 19-6). This type occurs most frequently in people 40–55 years of age and about two and a half times more often in men than in women.

Duodenal. This type occurs in the mucosal lining of the duodenum (see Fig. 19-6). It is the most common type of ulcer accounting for about 80% of all peptic ulcers. A younger group of people, 25–50 years old, tend to develop this type.

Cause. The exact cause of ulcers is not known. However, ulcers seem to occur when there is an imbalance between the amount of hydrochloric

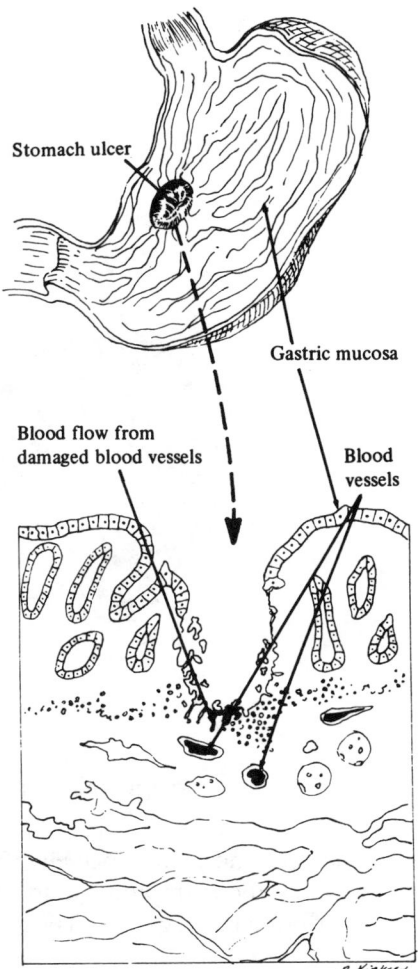

FIGURE 19-5 A gastric ulcer. (From T. Randall Lankford, *Integrated Science for Health Students*, 2nd ed., 1979. Reprinted by permission of Reston Publishing Company, a Prentice-Hall Company, 11480 Sunset Hills Road, Reston, VA 22090.)

acid (HCl), pepsin enzyme, and mucosal resistance. Normally, the gastric and duodenal mucosae are very effective in preventing deterioration of the stomach and duodenal walls. An imbalance can result from a variety of factors. Most often it occurs in people who are tense, hard-driving, and anxious. Research has also shown that alcohol, caffeine, and nicotine tend to predispose a person to the development of ulcers.

Symptoms. Epigastric pain, occurring 1–3 hours after eating or at night, is a common symptom. Apparently the pain results from HCl coming in contact with exposed nerve endings in the lesion. Eating a meal

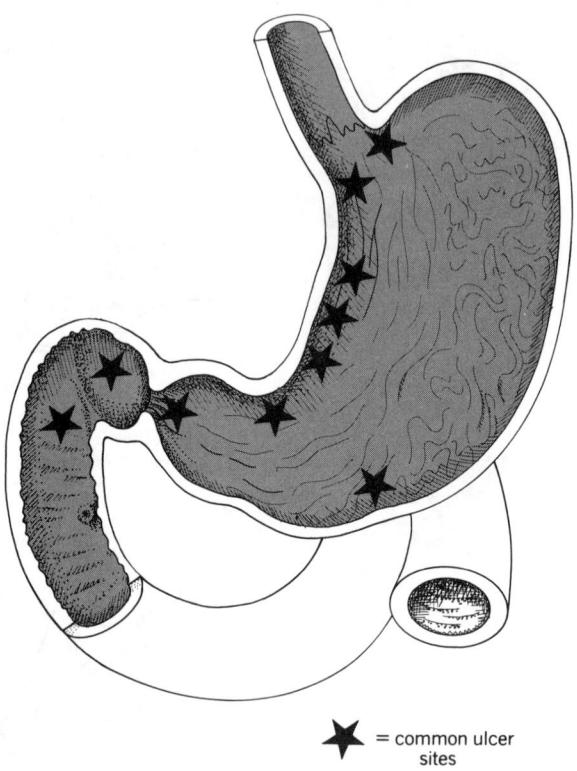

★ = common ulcer sites

FIGURE 19-6   Sites of gastric and duodenal ulcers.

relieves the pain, since chyme coats the nerve endings and blocks the HCl. Other symptoms tend to vary depending upon whether the ulcer is duodenal or gastric. These symptoms are as follows:

Gastric Ulcer	Duodenal Ulcer
Nausea	Heartburn
Anorexia	Good appetite
Vomiting	Weight gain
Weight loss	Constipation

Apparently the weight gain in duodenal ulcers results from the fact that the patient has a good appetite and consumes food to reduce pain.[2]

Diet Therapy. The primary goal of dietary management is to buffer or inhibit acid secretions. This goal is accomplished by eating small, frequent meals and avoiding alcohol and caffeine, which stimulate secretion of HCl.

Bland diet A diet that restricts the use of many spicy foods.

Sippy diet A diet that consists of hourly feedings of whole milk and cream.

Liberal diet A diet that allows a variety of foods.

Vagus nerve The tenth cranial nerve. It stimulates gastric glands in the stomach to secrete hydrochloric acid and pepsin enzyme.

There is disagreement among nutritionists as to whether the diet should be **bland**, **Sippy**, or **liberal**. Current literature favors a liberal diet, since a person cannot realistically follow a strict bland diet. Also, such a diet tends to create anxiety and demoralize the person. However, a 1977 survey of hospital dietitians revealed that a bland diet was used in 77% of hospitals in this country. It also showed that many patients believed that their diet should be bland.[3]

For a long time, a sippy diet was advocated as the best diet for healing an ulcer. The diet progresses to cooked cereals, soft-cooked eggs, custards, strained soups, and pureed fruits and vegetables. The theory behind this diet is that the protein in whole milk buffers the HCl and the fat helps to keep food in the stomach, since it delays gastric emptying, prolonging the buffering action. The diet lost favor with experts when the relationship of saturated fat to myocardial infarction and atherosclerosis was shown.

Today the sippy diet is not recommended except for acute bleeding ulcers. Then it is recommended that skim milk be substituted for whole milk and that cream plus polyunsaturated fats be used.

Antacid drugs are prescribed to neutralize activity up to about pH 5 (from a normal pH of 1–3), which significantly reduces pepsin enzyme activity.

Rest is prescribed, since it reduces vagus nerve activity. The **vagus nerve** stimulates the release of HCl from glands in the stomach.[4]

Current Dietary Treatment

The current dietary treatment for ulcers is a more liberal individualized diet than the traditional bland diet. The objectives of the diet are as follows:

- To decrease gastric acid secretion
- To neutralize gastric acidity
- To promote healing of the ulcer

Most nutritionists and research studies indicate that a strict bland diet is not necessary when the ulcer patient shows no symptoms. General guidelines for an ulcer diet for a symptom-free person are as follows:

Three meals should be eaten rather than six small feedings per day. Three meals per day cause less stimulation of gastric acid secretion than six small meals. In addition, the extra meals interfere with antacid therapy to reduce gastric acidity, and thus are more harmful than to three meals.

Bedtime snacks should be eliminated. The traditional approach was to include bedtime snacks in order to coat the ulcer while the person was sleeping. However, this practice is not now recommended, since the snacks actually stimulate gastric acid secretion.

Milk and cream feedings should not be used to reduce acidity. While milk should be included, it should not be used as a way to lower gastric acidity. Milk protein does initially neutralize HCl, but it also stimulates secretion of the acid. Cream is high in saturated fat, which can promote weight gain and increase the risk of atherosclerosis.

Completely eliminating certain foods is unwarranted. Research does not indicate that totally eliminating certain foods is beneficial. If a food causes repeated discomfort, it should be eliminated. Caffeine-containing beverages (coffee, tea, cola drinks) typically do increase gastric acid secretion but may be taken in moderation.

Omission of foods containing fiber has not been found to be beneficial to ulcer patients. Omission of gas-forming foods such as baked beans, cabbage, milk, nuts, and onions has not been found to aid the healing of ulcers. However, black pepper, chili powder, and nicotine may cause distress and need to be limited.

Excessive alcohol intake should be avoided. Alcohol can damage the gastric mucosa; therefore, excessive intake should be avoided in order to increase the healing of ulcers.

In reference to specific details, the diet should contain an adequate level of protein for healing. In addition, it should contain a moderate amount of fat for suppression of gastric secretions and peristaltic contractions. The principles of a chronic peptic ulcer diet are provided in Table 19-3.

Professionals disagree on the best dietary treatment when the ulcer is active and the person shows symptoms. Some prescribe a conservative bland diet. This diet is similar to the conservative Sippy diet. Essentially, foods from each of the exchange lists are chosen that are soft, bland,

TABLE 19-3 CHRONIC PEPTIC ULCER DIET

Purpose:	Decrease gastric irritation and excessive gastric acid irritation.
Use:	Treatment of chronic peptic ulcer disease.
Examples of modifications:	Three regular meals are recommended. Eliminate between meal and bedtime snacks, as they interfere with antacid therapy. Alcohol should be eliminated. Anatacids should be given 1 hour and 3 hours after meals and prior to bedtime in order to keep the acidity of the stomach within tolerable limits.
Adequacy:	Diet is adequate in all nutrients.

Source: Chicago Dietetic Association, *Manual of Clinical Dietetics,* second edition. Philadelphia, W.B. Saunders Company, 1981. Reprinted by permission.

TABLE 19-4 SUMMARY OF GASTRIC ULCER

Pathophysiology	Causes	Symptoms	Diet Therapy
Lesion in mucosal lining of stomach or duodenum	Not known, but results from imbalance of HCl, pepsin, and mucosal resistance	Epigastric pain 1–3 hours after eating Nausea Anorexia Heartburn Weight loss	Avoidance of alcohol, caffeine, and other mucosal irritants Liberal diet or one that allows wide variety of foods Bland or Sippy diet recommended only in bleeding ulcer cases

Hypercalcemia High blood calcium level.

and chemically nonirritating. Six small meals are given to aid the neutralization of gastric acidity. Milk is omitted in patients with lactose intolerance, milk allergy, or **hypercalcemia.** Table 19-4 provides a summary of the pathophysiology, causes, symptoms, and diet therapy for a gastric ulcer. See the sample menu for a liberal peptic ulcer diet.

Complications. Complications of peptic ulcers are as follows:

Hemorrhage. Approximately 25% of peptic ulcer patients lose blood at some time. Duodenal ulcers tend to bleed more often than gastric ulcers.

Perforation An opening through the gastric or duodenal wall.

Perforation. This is an opening through the gastric or duodenal wall.

Pyloric obstruction A condition in which the pyloric sphincter becomes scarred and stenosed (the opening is narrowed).

Pyloric obstruction. Sometimes the pyloric sphincter becomes scarred and stenosed (the opening becomes narrowed).

Patients who develop these complications generally are treated surgically, with a subtotal gastrectomy (see Fig. 19-7) being one example. This procedure removes the distal 50–75% of the stomach.[5]

Dumping Syndrome (Postgastrectomy Syndrome)

Tachycardia An abnormally rapid heartbeat.

After a gastrectomy, a person may experience a combination of symptoms: weakness, a desire to lie down, nausea, profound sweating, **tachycardia,** and dizziness. The changes in blood vessels and the small intestine related to the dumping syndrome are shown in Figure 19-8 and are as follows:

Rapid entrance of food into the duodenum. Chyme enters the duodenum rapidly as a result of the removal of the majority of the stomach

SAMPLE MENU FOR A LIBERAL PEPTIC ULCER DIET

Exchange

	Breakfast
1 fruit	½ cup orange juice
1 bread	½ cup oatmeal
½ milk	4 oz. milk (whole or low fat)
1 medium-fat meat	1 poached egg or egg substitute
2 fat	2 slices broiled bacon or bacon substitute
1 bread	1 slice toast
1 fat	1 tsp butter or margarine
	1 tbsp jelly
	2 tsp sugar
	1 cup coffee, if tolerated

	Lunch
1 ½ vegetable	6 oz vegetable soup
2 medium–fat meat	2 oz. beef patty on bun
1 vegetable	Sliced tomato and lettuce
1 fat	1 tbsp french dressing
1 fruit	4 apricot halves
	2 sugar cookies
1 milk	8 oz milk (whole or low fat)

	Dinner
1 vegetable	½ cup tomato juice
3 lean meat	3 oz broiled chicken
1 bread	½ cup mashed potatoes
1 vegetable	½ cup peas
1 fruit	½ cup fruited jello salad
	½ cup orange sherbet
1 bread	1 slice bread
1 fat	1 tsp butter or margarine
½ milk	4 oz milk (whole or low fat)

Analysis and Comments

- An analysis of this diet shows 2 milk, 4 ½ vegetable, 3 fruit, 4 bread, 6 meat, and 5 fat exchanges. This menu reinforces the point that a liberal diet should not exclude certain foods but rather should be an optimum diet with foods from all exchange groups.

- The number of milk exchanges is 2, which reinforces the point that a great deal of milk should not be used for antacid therapy.

- The 5 fat exchanges provide a moderate amount of fat for suppression of gastric secretions and peristaltic contractions.

Source: Menu adapted from Chicago Dietetic Association, *Manual of Clinical Dietetics,* 2nd ed. Philadelphia, W.B. Saunders Company, 1981. Reprinted by permission.

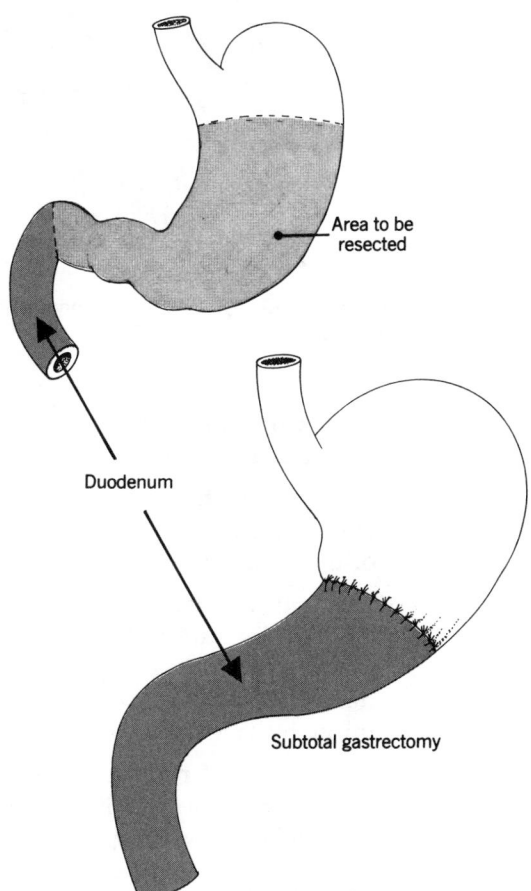

Area to be resected

Duodenum

Subtotal gastrectomy

FIGURE 19-7   A subtotal gastrectomy surgical procedure.

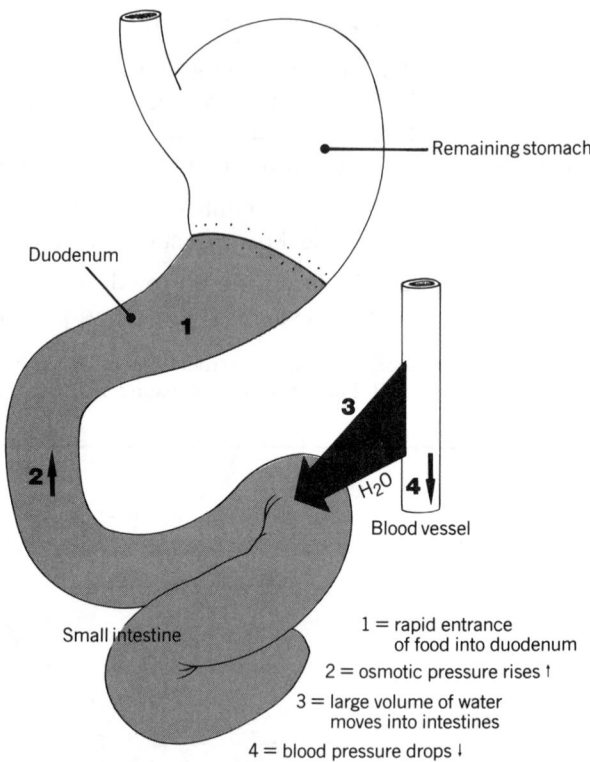

Remaining stomach

Duodenum

Blood vessel

Small intestine

1 = rapid entrance
    of food into duodenum
2 = osmotic pressure rises ↑
3 = large volume of water
    moves into intestines
4 = blood pressure drops ↓

FIGURE 19-8   Dumping syndrome and changes in blood vessels and the small intestine.

and pyloric sphincter. Normally, the stomach and pyloric sphincter store and gradually release food into the duodenum.

Increased osmotic pressure in the intestines. Osmotic pressure increases considerably in the duodenum and small intestine as a result of the rapid entrance of a large amount of food.

Movement of a large volume of water into the intestines. A higher osmotic pressure in the intestines compared to the blood results in the movement of a large volume of water into the intestines. This movement of water by osmosis results from the fact that water moves through all membranes from a low osmotic to a high osmotic pressure.

Decreased blood pressure. The movement of water out of the blood into the intestines results in a drop in blood pressure and is the cause of weakness, sweating, tachycardia, and dizziness.[6]

Dietary Treatment. Dumping syndrome can be best controlled by diet. Objectives of diet therapy and explanation of the dumping syndrome

TABLE 19-5 POSTGASTRECTOMY DIET

Purpose:	Designed to retard the rapid passage of food into the intestine and decrease the formation of a concentrated hyperosmolar solution. Adequate kilocalories are provided for tissue building and for prevention of weight loss.
Use:	Used for persons who have undergone surgical procedures that accelerate the normal emptying time of the stomach; total gastrectomy and Billroth I and II anastomoses are examples.
Examples of foods:	Simple sugars are kept to a minimum. Proteins and fats are increased. Meals are small and frequent. Liquids are generally served between meals rather than with meals, thus slowing the passage of food from stomach into the intestines.
Adequacy:	Adequacy of the diet depends upon the extent of surgery; vitamin B_{12} absorption is inadequate due to loss of intrinsic factor when the stomach is removed; therefore, vitamin B_{12} injections are required.

Source: Chicago Dietetic Association, *Manual of Clinical Dietetics*, second edition. Philadelphia, W.B. Saunders Company, 1981. Reprinted by permission.

are discussed below. The principles of a postgastrectomy diet are provided in Table 19-5.

Minimize the quantity of food eaten at meals and increase the number of meals. Eating small meals means that smaller amounts of food are released into the duodenum. Therefore, the osmotic pressure in the intestine will be lower. The number of meals should be increased to six per day.

Avoid simple sugars. Simple sugars in the intestines increase osmotic pressure more than fats and proteins, causing great movement of water out of blood into the intestines. Simple sugars that move into the blood also cause temporary hyperglycemia, with increased insulin secretion. This action is followed by hypoglycemia, with symptoms of weakness and dizziness, about 2–3 hours after rapid entrance of sugar into blood.

Avoid liquids 30 minutes before and 1 hour after meals. Liquid ingested during these times will move large amounts of food (chyme) out of the stomach and into the intestines faster than the food would move without liquid consumption.

Increase the ratio of calories from polyunsaturated fat and proteins. Since carbohydrates are reduced, calories come primarily from polyunsaturated fat and proteins. Fat also delays emptying of the stomach,

thereby reducing the chance of rapid movement of food into the duodenum and initiating dumping syndrome symptoms.

Increase caloric intake to 2,000–3,500 kcal.[7]

See the sample menu for the dumping syndrome diet.

Long-Range Nutritional Problems After a Subtotal Gastrectomy. The
nurse, as well as all members of the health team, needs to be aware of
and plan for possible long-term nutritional problems in a patient who
has undergone a subtotal gastrectomy. Some of the more common problems are discussed below (see Fig. 19-9).

Hypocalcemia. The previous discussion of stomach functions mentioned that the HCl in the stomach increases the absorption of calcium
by increasing its solubility. With the removal of a large portion of the
stomach, the ability to absorb calcium is reduced. This reduction can
result in the following problems:

Muscle tetany: abnormal skeletal muscle contraction.

Osteoporosis: a decline in bone mass. The reduction in calcium absorp-
    tion results in the removal of calcium from bones, causing their mass
    to decline.

Anemia. A patient may suffer from iron deficiency anemia as a result
of decreased iron absorption. The stomach aids in the absorption of iron,
as discussed at the beginning of this chapter, and this function is decreased as a result of a subtotal gastrectomy. Since iron is essential to
red blood cell (RBC) production, this surgery results in a decreased
production of RBCs or anemia.

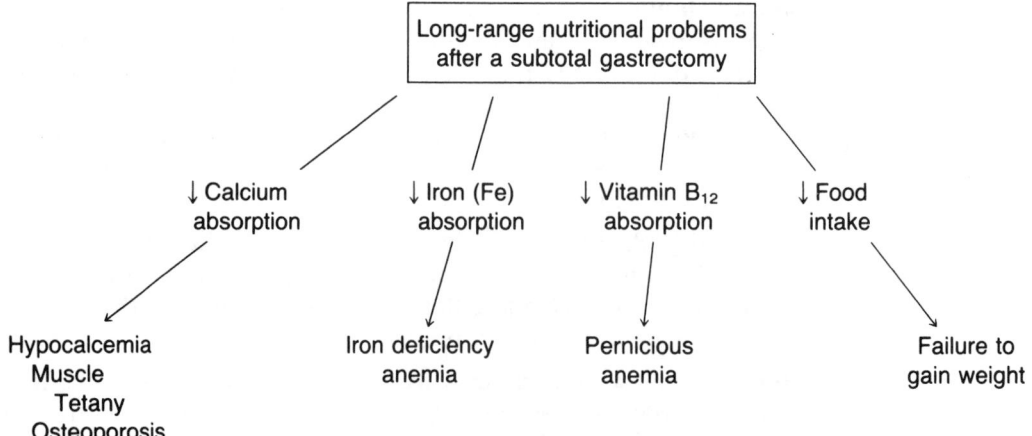

FIGURE 19-9 Long-range nutritional problems after a subtotal gastrectomy.

SAMPLE MENU FOR THE DUMPING SYNDROME
(POSTGASTRECTOMY SYNDROME)

Exchange	
	Breakfast
2 medium-fat meat	2 fried eggs
2 bread	2 slice toast
2 fat	2 tsp butter
	1 cup coffee
	(take 30–60 minutes after eating)
	Mid-Morning Snack
1 low-fat meat	$\frac{1}{4}$ cup cottage cheese
1 bread	2 graham crackers
	Lunch
3 medium-fat meat	3 oz hamburger patty
2 bread	1 cup mashed potatoes
1 fat	1 tsp margarine
1 fruit	$\frac{1}{4}$ cantaloupe
	iced tea with lemon and sugar substitute
	(take 30–60 minutes after eating)
	Mid-Afternoon Snack
1 medium-fat meat	2 tbsp peanut butter
1 bread	6 saltine crackers
	Supper
4 medium-fat meat	4 oz boiled ham
2 bread	1 cup rice
1 vegetable	$\frac{1}{2}$ cup carrots
2 fat	2 tsp butter
1 fruit	$\frac{1}{4}$ cup unsweetened peach slices
	iced tea with lemon and sugar substitute
	(take 30–60 minutes after eating)
	Evening Snack
1 high-fat meat	1 oz cheddar cheese
1 fat	1 strip bacon
1 bread	1 slice bread

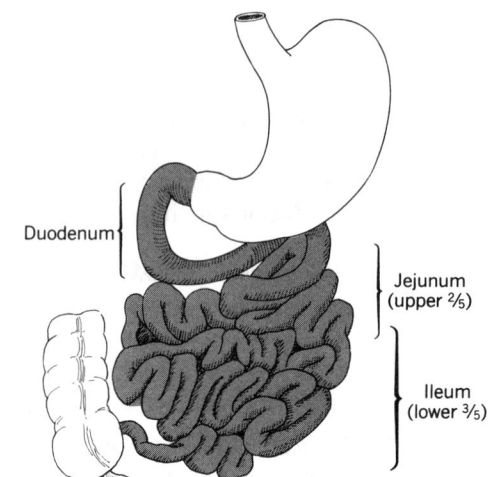

FIGURE 19-10 The regions of the small intestine.

sites (see Fig. 19-11) into blood and lymph. In addition, water, electrolytes, and vitamins are absorbed at specific sites. Knowledge of these absorption sites is necessary in order to understand how disease of the intestine may cause specific nutritional deficiencies.

Secretion of hormones. Various hormones (ex-gastrin and cholecystokinin) are secreted that affect the activity of stomach, pancreas, and gallbladder.

MALABSORPTION DISORDERS

Nontropical Sprue (Celiac Disease, Gluten-Sensitive Enteropathy)

Nontropical sprue affects both children and adults. It appears in children primarily between the ages of 1 and 5 years and in adults primarily between 30 to 40.

Celiac disease A disease characterized by the degeneration and atrophy of the intestinal villi, induced by the ingestion of foods containing gluten.

Gluten A water-soluble protein found in wheat, rye, barley, and oats.

Peptidase enzyme An enzyme that catalyzes the degradation of a harmful peptide.

Celiac disease is characterized by degeneration and atropy of intestinal villi induced by the ingestion of foods containing **gluten** (a water-insoluble protein found in wheat, rye, barley, and oats).

Cause. The exact cause is unknown, but two theories suggest an inborn error of metabolism and an immune reaction. The inborn error of metabolism is an inherited inability to produce a **peptidase** enzyme. Lack of the enzyme allows a buildup of a harmful peptide, resulting in damage to the villi. The immune reaction theory proposes that gluten causes a hypersensitive reaction to the intestinal mucosa.[9]

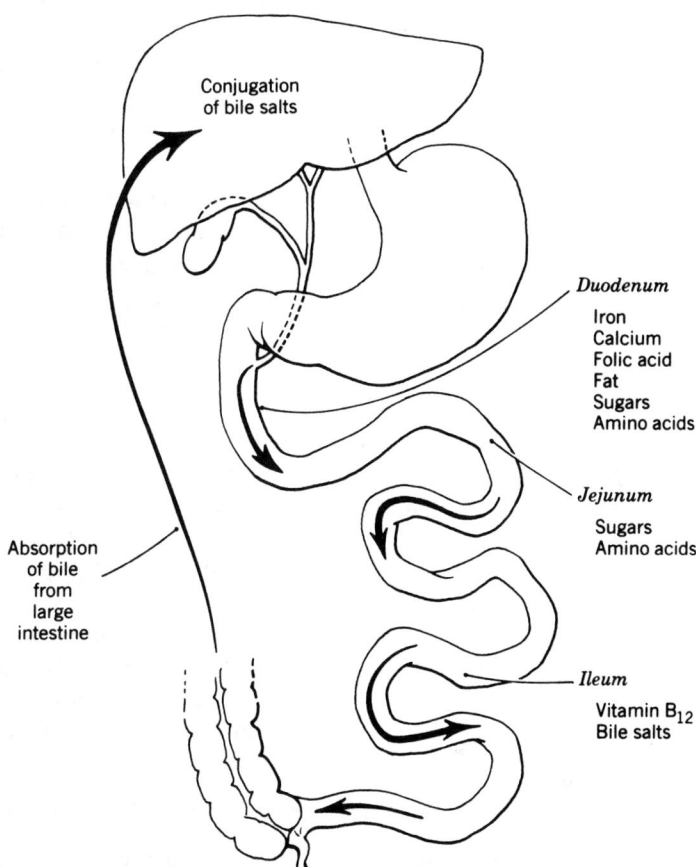

FIGURE 19-11 Specific sites along the small intestine where nutrients are absorbed. (Reproduced with permission from S.A. Price and L.M. Wilson, *Pathophysiology: Clinical Concept of Disease Processes*, 2nd ed. New York: McGraw-Hill Book Company, 1982.)

Pathophysiology. The intestinal mucosa reacts to gluten in ways that cause the intestinal villi to atrophy, shorten, become club-shaped, or fuse. The end result is that the absorption surface area is decreased; therefore, the afflicted individual does not absorb nutrients very efficiently.

Symptoms. Diarrhea is a common symptom, with the stools being fatty (steatorrhea), foul-smelling, greasy, and bulky. This symptom is common in both children and adults. Other symptoms in children are more subtle, such as irritability, failure to gain weight, and muscle wasting. A child may go into a **celiac crisis.** These problems can cause dehydration, acidosis, and even death.

Celiac crisis An attack of watery diarrhea and vomiting.

TABLE 19-6 GLUTEN-RESTRICTED DIET

Purpose:	Diet is designed to avoid foods that contain the protein gluten.
Use:	Used for patients who have nontropical sprue (celiac disease or gluten-induced enteropathy).
Examples of foods:	General diet with elimination of all foods containing the grains wheat, rye, oats, barley, and buckwheat.
Adequacy:	Diet is adequate.

Source: Chicago Dietetic Association, *Manual of Clinical Dietetics*, second edition. Philadelphia, W.B. Saunders Company, 1981. Reprinted by permission.

Diet Therapy. Diet therapy involves a low-gluten diet. The principles of a gluten-restricted diet are provided in Table 19-6. Ideally, the diet should exclude all foods that contain gluten. However, this plan is impossible to implement, so the best one can hope for is to reduce dietary gluten to a minimum. Table 19-7 lists foods containing gluten, as well as the by-products of gluten-containing foods. See the sample menu for a gluten-restricted diet.

Other aspects of diet therapy for celiac sprue are given in Table 19-8. The diet has to be supplemented with vitamins, minerals, and electrolytes, since they are not absorbed adequately. The diet should also be high in kilocalories, since food is not adequately absorbed.

Lactose Intolerance (lactase Deficiency)

Lactose (disaccharide) is hydrolyzed, or broken down, into glucose and galactose by the enzyme lactase. This enzyme normally is located in the

TABLE 19-7 GLUTEN-CONTAINING FOODS

Foods	
Wheat	Barley
Oats	Rye
By-Products	
Flours	Malted milk
Cereals	Beer and ale
Many commercial soups	Bread and crackers
Puddings (except cornstarch and tapioca ones)	Breaded meats
	Wheat germ
Macaroni, spaghetti, noodles, oatmeal, and granola	

SAMPLE MENU FOR A GLUTEN-RESTRICTED DIET

Exchange	
	Breakfast
1 fruit	½ cup orange juice
1 bread	¾ cup corn flakes
2 fat	2 strips bacon
1 bread	1 slice low-gluten bread
1 fat	margarine
1 milk	1 cup skim milk
	1 cup coffee with sugar
	Lunch
3 lean meat	3 oz baked fresh fish (halibut, trout, red snapper, etc.)
1 bread	1 small baked potato
1 vegetable	½ cup sliced tomatoes plus lettuce
1 bread + 1 fat	1 piece corn bread (2 × 2 × 1 in.) (made without flour)
1 fat	1 tsp margarine
1 fruit	4 apricot halves
	iced tea with lemon and sugar
	Dinner
	7 oz beef bouillon
3 lean meat	3 oz broiled chicken
1 vegetable	½ cup green beans
1 bread	1 slice low-gluten bread
1 fat	1 tsp margarine
	cherry gelatin (1 envelope)
1 milk	1 cup skim milk
	iced tea with lemon and sugar

Analysis and Comments

• An analysis of this menu shows that it contains 2 milk, 2 vegetable, 2 fruit, 5 bread, 6 meat, and 6 fat exchanges.

- In reference to the exchanges, the following foods should be eliminated:

  Milk: commercial chocolate milk and malted milk.

  Vegetables: creamed or breaded.

  Fruit: none.

  Bread: all breads made with wheat, rye, oats, barley, and buckwheat should be eliminated. Notice that this menu includes low-gluten bread and cornbread. Any breads or cereals that contain corn (cornbread, corn tortillas) or rice (rice wafers, Rice Krispies, and puffed rice) are allowed and should definitely be included, since they are the only grain sources that can be tolerated.

  Meat: meats excluded are prepared meats such as sausage, frankfurters, bologna, luncheon meat, and commercial hamburger, meat loaf, croquettes, gravy, cream sauce and processed cheese.

  Fat: cream substitutes, whipped toppings, and commercial salad dressings (typically contain gluten stabilizers) must be eliminated.

  Miscellaneous: puddings (except cornstarch and tapioca) must be eliminated. All beverages that contain wheat, rye, oats, or barley, such as beer and ale, must be eliminated. In addition, chili sauce, soy sauce, and bottled meat sauces contain these grains and must be eliminated.

- Sometimes the gluten-restricted menu initially decreases the number of fat exchanges and fiber to decrease diarrhea and steatorrhea.

- Between meals, bedtime snacks are given to achieve a high kilocalorie intake.

- This menu and similar ones are typically deficient in thiamin and iron, since wheat, barley, oats, and rye must be eliminated. Therefore, it is recommended that the diet be supplemented with daily vitamins and minerals.

Source: Menu adapted from Texas Dietetic Association, *Diet Manual*, 3rd ed. Austin: Texas Dietetic Association, 1981. Reprinted by permission.

---

brush border of the intestinal mucosa. Some people have a deficiency of lactase; therefore, the quantity of lactose builds up, resulting in increased osmotic pressure in the small intestine (see Fig. 19-12). This increased osmotic pressure causes a large amount of water to shift into the intestine, resulting in increased motility and diarrhea. Malabsorption of nutrients occurs due to the motility.

Congenital lactase deficiency A rare inherited intolerance of lactase throughout life.

Cause. There are three causes of lactase deficiency. **Congenital lactase deficiency** is a rare inherited condition. Persons who have it are intol-

TABLE 19-8 SUMMARY OF CELIAC DISEASE

Pathophysiology	Causes	Symptoms	Diet Therapy
Atrophy, shortening, and decrease in size of intestinal villi	Inborn error of metabolism Immune reaction	Diarrhea Irritability Muscle wasting	Eliminate gluten containing foods Diet prescription: high protein, high carbohydrate, low to moderate fat, and high calories Vitamin, mineral, and electrolyte supplementation

Secondary lactase deficiency A condition that may develop as a secondary problem in a person who has a disease of the small intestine such as celiac disease, Crohn's disease, or protein-calorie malnutrition.

Developmental lactase deficiency A condition that results from a gradual decrease in lactase during childhood and adolescence.

erant of lactose throughout their lives. **Secondary lactase deficiency** may develop as a secondary problem in a person who has a small intestine disease such as celiac disease, Crohn's disease, or protein-calorie malnutrition (PCM). **Developmental lactase deficiency** results from a gradual decrease in the lactase level during childhood and adolescence, until it is quite low in the adult. Approximately 70% of American blacks have

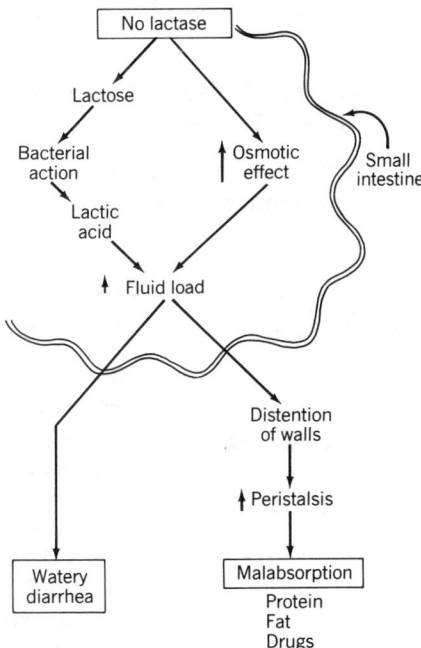

FIGURE 19-12 The effects on the small intestine caused by lactase deficiency. (Reproduced with permission from R.B. Howard and N.H. Herbold, *Nutrition in Clinical Care.* New York: McGraw-Hill Book Company, 1978.)

this condition, along with significant percentages of Orientals and American Indians.

The tolerance of milk by these groups varies considerably, and many are able to tolerate and benefit from inclusion of moderate amounts of milk and other dairy foods in their diet.

Symptoms. The increased osmotic pressure in the small intestine from ingestion of milk results in a bloated feeling, flatulence, belching, cramps, or diarrhea.

Diet Therapy. An infant who has a congenital lactase deficiency can obtain the necessary nutrients from soybean formulas that contain low levels of lactose. Adults with secondary and developmental deficiencies can frequently tolerate partially fermented diary products (which have reduced or absent lactose) such as cottage cheese, buttermilk, sour cream, yogurt, and hard cheese. The principles of a lactose-restricted diet are provided in Table 19-9.

A lactase enzyme powder (Lact-Acid) can be added to milk, thereby hydrolyzing lactose to galactose and glucose. This makes it possible for lactase-deficient individuals to drink milk without experiencing the previously mentioned symptoms.[10] Table 19-10 summarizes important information about lactase deficiency.

Crohn's disease An inflammatory disease that is located primarily in the ileum region of the small intestine and may extend into the large intestine.

Crohn's Disease (Inflammatory Bowel Disease)

Crohn's disease is an inflammatory disease that is located primarily in the ileum region of the small intestine but may extend into the large

TABLE 19-9 LACTOSE-RESTRICTED DIET

Purpose:	Provide foods that contain a minimum of lactose.
Use:	Used to reduce symptoms in people who do not tolerate lactose well due to a deficiency of the enzyme lactase.
Examples of foods:	General diet, with a reduction of milk and milk products that contain lactose. Most people can tolerate about 4 to 8 oz of milk if consumed with meals. Yogurt and other fermented foods are generally tolerated, since lactose is altered by fermentation. Breast milk contains more lactose than cow's milk, so breast feeding is not recommended for infants born with congenital lactose intolerance.
Adequacy:	Diet will lack calcium but will be adequate in all other nutrients; calcium supplements or the use of milk substitute is recommended.

Source: Chicago Dietetic Association, *Manual of Clinical Dietetics*, second edition. Philadelphia, W.B. Saunders Company, 1981. Reprinted by permission.

TABLE 19-10 SUMMARY OF LACTOSE INTOLERANCE

Pathophysiology	Causes	Symptoms	Dietary Treatment
Lack of lactase enzyme activity	Congenital Secondary Developmental	Bloated feeling Flatulence Belching Cramps Diarrhea	Lactose-free formula for infants Partially fermented dairy products—cottage cheese, buttermilk, sour cream yogurt— generally can be pretty well tolerated.

Granuloma A tumor-like mass of granulation tissue.

Serosa The outer layer of the intestine.

intestine. The intestinal wall may also have **granulomas** extending through all layers, including the **serosa** (see Fig. 19-13). The disease occurs frequently in young adults and is seen in mild, moderate and severe forms.

Cause. The exact cause is unknown. Some theories focus on infectious agents, autoimmune disase, and possibly a genetic link.

Symptoms. The symptoms tend to vary depending on the severity of the condition and the area of the gastrointestinal tract affected. Mild intermittent bloody diarrhea, two to five stools per day, and pain in the lower abdomen are common symptoms. Some patients also develop steatorrhea, weight loss, and anemia. Other malabsorption symptoms may be present. Young children may experience growth retardation.[11]

Diet Therapy. The general dietary goals are to rest the small intestine so that healing can occur and to avoid nutritional deficiency states. These goals are best achieved by excluding foods that are high in fiber (raw fruits and vegetables) and residue. See the sample menu for a minimum-

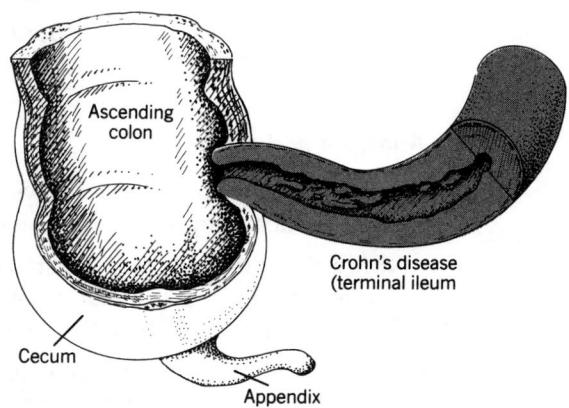

FIGURE 19-13   Internal view of the ileum showing Crohn's disease.

SAMPLE MENU FOR A MINIMUM-RESIDUE DIET

Exchange	
	Breakfast
1 fruit	½ cup strained orange juice
1 bread	½ cup cream of wheat
2 medium-fat meat	2 poached eggs
2 bread	2 slices of white toast
2 fat	2 tsp margarine
	Lunch
2 low-fat meat	2 oz tender, lean roast beef
1 vegetable	½ cup buttered rice
1 vegetable	½ cup tomato juice
1 bread	1 slice white bread
1 fat	1 tsp margarine
	angel food cake
	iced tea
	Dinner
	1 cup beef broth
1 bread	½ cup macaroni
1 fruit	¼ cup grape juice
1 bread	slice white bread
1 fat	1 tsp margarine
	plain orange gelatin
	iced tea

Analysis and comments

- An analysis of this menu shows 0 milk, 2 vegetable, 2 fruit, 6 bread, 4 meat, and 4 fat exchanges.
- Notice that the fruits and vegetables are either juices or soft vegetables as opposed to fresh whole fruits and fibrous vegetables. These adaptations reduce the level of residue.
- Foods from the meat exchange list are either soft foods (eggs) or tender beef, which are low in fiber and will form little residue.

- Notice that there are no milk exchanges. The reason is that milk can be fermented by bacteria in the large intestine, thereby forming a large amount of residue.

- Due to its adaptations and exclusions, this menu is deficient in the RDA levels of calcium, iron, vitamin A, riboflavin, and vitamin D. If it is to be followed for a long period, these vitamins and minerals should be supplemented.

Source: Menu adapted from Texas Dietetic Association, *Diet Manual*, 3rd ed. Austin: Texas Dietetic Association, 1981. Reprinted by permission.

residue diet. Table 19-11 provides the pathophysiology, cause, symptoms, and diet therapy for Crohn's disease.

Medium chain triglycerides (MCTs) should be used to replace the fats that are not being absorbed.

To promote healing of the intestinal wall, the diet should be high in protein and carbohydrate and low in fat. Supplementation with vitamin B_{12} may be necessary due to malabsorption (see Fig. 19–11 for site of vitamin B_{12} absorption). Supplementation with iron and folic acid may be necessary due to blood loss from tissue destruction. Patients with severe Crohn's disease respond very favorably to total parenteral nutrition (hyperalimentation), especially when they are to undergo surgery.[12]

LARGE INTESTINE (COLON)

The large intestine is a continuation of the alimentary canal from the small intestine. It is a muscular tube about 5 ft in length and is noticeably

TABLE 19-11 SUMMARY OF CROHN'S DISEASE (INFLAMMATORY BOWEL DISEASE)

Pathophysiology	Etiology	Symptoms	Diet Therapy
Inflammation of intestinal mucosa in ileum region Granulomas extending through wall of intestine	Exact cause unknown Possibly due to infectious agents, autoimmune, or genetic component	Mild diarrhea Lower abdominal pain Steatorrhea Weight loss Anemia	Rest the small intestine Low-fiber, low-residue diet High protein and carbohydrate levels Supplementation with iron, folate, and vitamin B_{12}

Cecum The first portion of the large intestine to which the small intestine attaches and from which the appendix extends.

Ileocecal valve A valve that is located between the ileum and the cecum.

Ascending colon The portion of the large intestine that ascends upward on the right side of the body from the cecum to the liver.

Transverse colon The portion of the large intestine that extends across the abdomen from the right to the left.

Descending colon The portion of the large intestine that extends downward along the left side of the abdomen.

Sigmoid colon The S-shaped portion of the large intestine between the descending colon and the rectum.

larger in diameter than the small intestine. It extends from the **cecum** to the anal canal and is divided into the cecum, colon, and rectum (see Fig. 19–14). The **ileocecal** valve guards the entrance into the cecum. The colon is subdivided into the **ascending, transverse, descending,** and **sigmoid** colons. The last major region of the large intestine is the rectum. The final inch of the rectum is called the *anal canal* and is guarded by internal and external sphincter muscles.

The functions of the large intestine are related to the final processing of materials that enter from the small intestine:

Reabsorption of water and electrolytes. About 600 ml of water with electrolytes are absorbed through the colon wall into the blood, compared with about 8,000 ml absorbed by the small intestine.

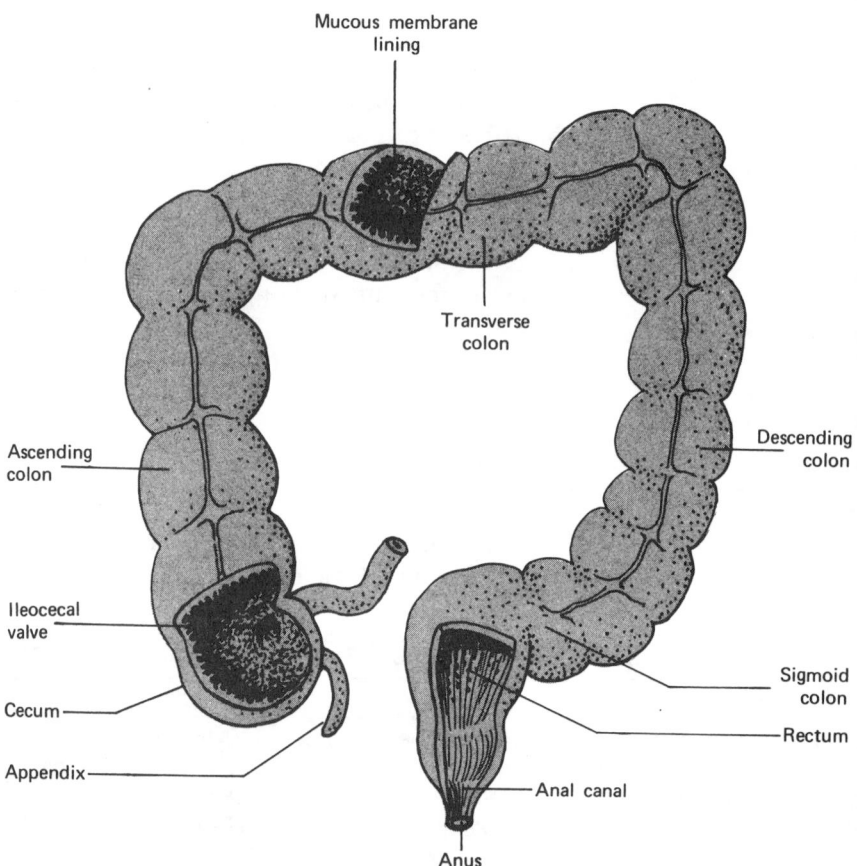

FIGURE 19-14 The large intestine and its subdivisions. (From S.R. Burke, *Human Anatomy and Physiology for the Health Sciences.* New York: John Wiley & Sons, Inc., © 1980. Reprinted by permission.)

Elimination of wastes (feces). Nonabsorbed residue, bacteria, nonabsorbed water, and electrolytes are excreted as feces by the anal canal.

Intestinal flora Bacteria in the large intestine.

Synthesis of vitamins. **Intestinal flora** synthesize several vitamins, including vitamin K and some of the B complex group.

DISORDERS

Colonic diverticulosis A condition characterized by small, sac-like herniations of the colon mucosa called *diverticula*.

Colonic Diverticulosis and Diverticulitis

Colonic diverticulosis is a condition characterized by small, sac-like herniations of the colon mucosa (see Fig. 19–15) called *divertculae*. The

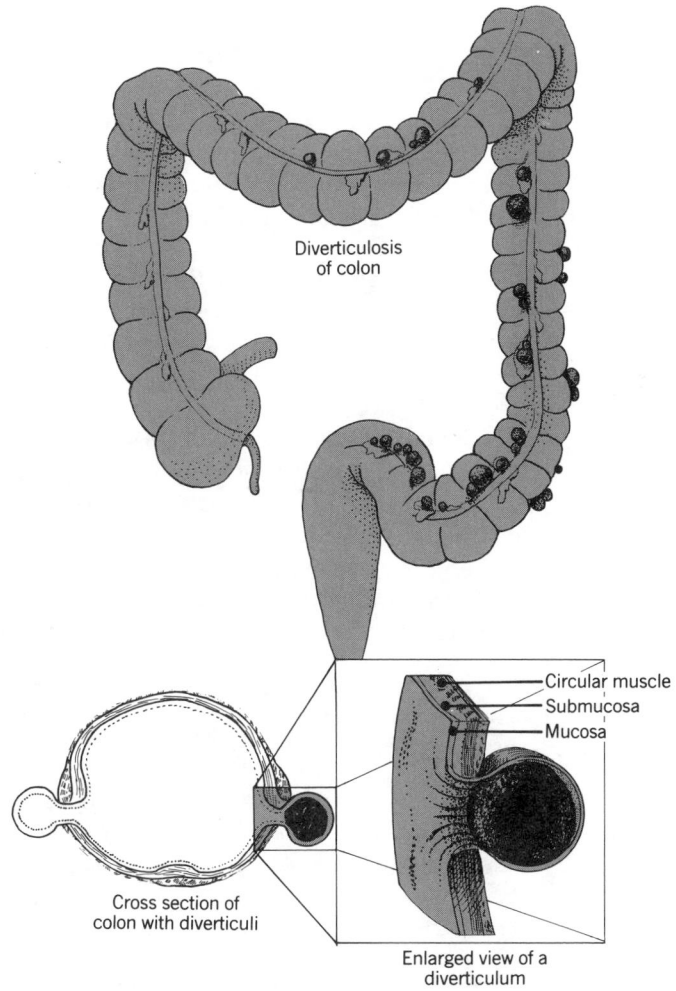

FIGURE 19-15 Diverticulosis of the large intestine.

most common initial site of diverticula formation is the sigmoid colon. The incidence of diverticulosis is higher in people over 40 years of age than in younger people. Between 15 and 30% of diverticulosis cases develop into the inflammatory condition called **diverticulitis**.

Diverticulitis Inflammatory condition of diverticula caused by bacterial growth and action arising from food residues and fecal matter.

Cause. One basic cause of this disease is a low-fiber diet. The mechanism by which a low-fiber diet results in the formation of diverticula is as follows:

Low-fiber foods	→ increased segmentation of colon to move residue along	→ increased intraluminal pressure within intestine	→ protrusion of intestinal mucosa through intestinal wall

A high-fiber diet basically prevents diverticulosis, since the feces occupy a greater volume and are heavier. This condition results in less segmentation of the colon in moving the feces along, thereby generating less intraluminal pressure.[13]

Symptoms of Colonic Diverticulosis. Symptoms are minimal, with occasional abdominal discomfort. Constipation is not a symptom of diverticulosis but rather an indication that conditions are right for its development.

Diet Therapy of Colonic Diverticulosis. The treatment consists of prevention, which is accomplished by increasing the amount of fiber and bulk in the diet. This diet decreases intraluminal pressure and reduces the possible development of diverticula. If diverticula are already present, they may revert to a normal state if a high-fiber diet is consumed and intraluminal pressure remains lowered over a period of time. The principles of a high-fiber diet are provided in Table 19–12.

TABLE 19-12 HIGH-FIBER DIET

Purpose:	Promotes regular elimination and increases fecal excretion.
Use:	Used in treatment of diverticular disease, atonic constipation, and irritable bowel syndrome.
Examples of foods:	Almost all foods on a general diet are included; includes three to four servings of food high in indigestible carbohydrates (fiber).
Adequacy:	The diet is adequate.

Source: Chicago Dietetic Association, *Manual of Clinical Dietetics*, second edition. Philadelphia, W.B. Saunders Company, 1981. Reprinted by permission.

Symptoms of Diverticulitis. If diverticulosis develops into diverticulitis, the symptoms are an increase in the total white blood cell count, fever, left lower quadrant abdominal pain, abdominal distention, flatulence, slight nausea, and constipation. Occasionally, bloody stools and/or intestinal obstructions may occur.

Diet Therapy for Diverticulitis. The initial treatment of an acute attack of diverticulitis is bed rest, antibiotics, stool softeners, and a liquid diet. If there is no evidence of obstruction, **fistulas, abscesses,** or perforation, the diet may progress to normal. Bulk agents such as Metamucil or bran may be gradually included, but large quantities should be avoided. After the inflammation has subsided, a high-fiber diet may be followed.[14]

Fistulas Abnormal tube-like passages within the body tissue, usually between two internal organs.

Abscesses Localized collections of pus in cavities formed by the disintegration of tissues.

Ulcerative Colitis (Inflammatory Bowel Disease)

Ulcerative colitis is similar to Crohn's disease in that it is an inflammatory disease with other features in common. It is common in adults between the ages of 20 and 40 years. Ulcerative colitis is about five times more common than Crohn's disease.

The ulcers are located in the mucosa (see Fig. 19-16) and submucosa of the large intestine, as opposed to the granulomas in Crohn's disease extending through all layers of the small intestine wall. The initial ulcers

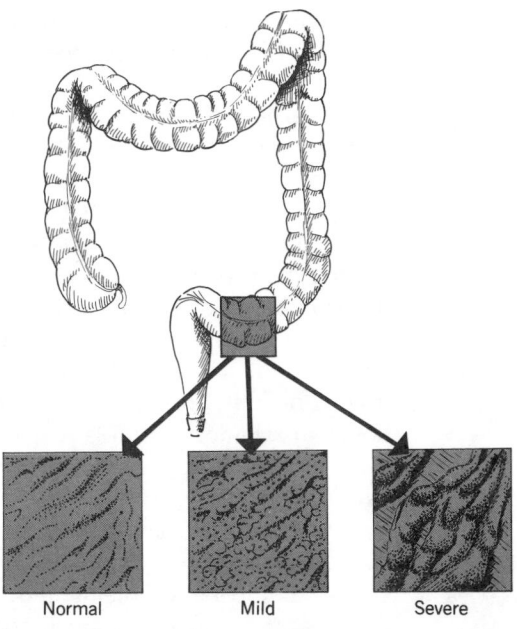

Normal   Mild   Severe

FIGURE 19-16 Ulcerative colitis of the large intestine.

are located in the rectum and sigmoid colon regions, from which they tend to spread upward.

Cause. As with Crohn's disease, the exact cause is unknown. Some theories are as follows:

- Genetic. There is a strong familial relationship in colitis.
- Autoimmunity. Antibodies from the colon and the diseased region have been found in the serum of ulcerative colitis patients.
- Psychological stress. Much controversy has been generated over this theory. It is now considered to play a secondary role.

Acute fulminating A condition that occurs suddenly with great intensity.

Chronic intermittent (recurrent) colitis A type of ulcerative colitis that is characterized by mild diarrhea and intermittent, slight bleeding.

Chronic continuous A condition that persists for a long time and shows either little change or an extremely slow progression over a long period.

Exacerbations Increased severity and complications.

Symptoms. The symptoms vary depending on whether the patient has **acute fulminating, chronic intermittent (recurrent),** or **chronic continuous** colitis. Most ulcerative colitis patients have the chronic intermittent (recurrent) type. The attacks are short and may occur at intervals ranging from months to years. There may be little or no fever. It is common for the patient to suffer frequent **exacerbations** and repeated hospitalizations.

The chronic loss of blood and mucus may result in anemia, dehydration, and hypoproteinemia. Chronic poor protein intake may also contribute to hypoproteinemia. Crampy abdominal pain and weight loss are common symptoms. Patients may be deficient in vitamin B_{12} if the ileum region of the small intestine is affected.

Ulcerative colitis patients frequently exhibit an intolerance to milk, since lactase depletion is secondary to the disease.

Osmotic overload A condition that results in the movement of large amounts of water into the intestines from the blood.

Diet Therapy. The principal goals of diet therapy are to control inflammation, maintain the patient's nutritional status, give symptomatic relief, and prevent infection.

A bland, low-residue diet may be helpful during attacks but is not believed to help prevent the symptoms. A new and quite successful approach to treating acute attacks of this chronic disease is 4–6 weeks of total parenteral nutritional therapy with simultaneous drug therapy.

The protein in the diet should be high, 1.5 g per kilogram of desired body weight per day. The caloric level should be 2,400–3,600 kcal/day. If eggs or milk are not well tolerated, manufactured (packaged) nutritional supplement formulas are excellent for providing kilocalories and protein, provided they do not present the intestine with an **osmotic overload.**

Any foods that may irritate the mucosa, such as raw fruits and vegetables, are eliminated.

Iron should be supplemented, due to loss of blood, but because of diarrhea and malabsorption it should be administered parenterally or intramuscularly. Vitamin B_{12} should also be administered parenterally.[14]

TABLE 19-13 SUMMARY OF ULCERATIVE COLITIS

Pathophysiology	Etiology	Symptoms	Diet Therapy
Ulcers in mucosa and submucosa of large intestine	Exact cause unknown Theories Genetic Autoimmunity Stress	Diarrhea Crampy abdominal pain Anemia Hyproteinemia	Low-residue diet Bland diet Total parenteral nutrition High protein level High calorie level Eliminate milk if patient is intolerant Supplement iron and vitamin B_{12}

Anticholinergic drugs Drugs that block the passage of impulses through the parasympathetic nerves.

Total colectomy Removal of the colon.

Ileostomy An opening into the ileum for drainage of fecal matter.

Anticholinergic drugs help to relieve cramps and diarrhea. Emotional support from the health team is very important to successful treatment.

If dietary, drug, and emotional help fail, surgical intervention is indicated. The most common procedure is a **total colectomy** and the creation of a permanent **ileostomy**.[15]

Table 19-13 summarizes information about ulcerative colitis.

CASE STUDY: PEPTIC ULCER AND THE DUMPING SYNDROME

John is a 45-year-old Spanish-American who is admitted to a hospital with complaints of epigastric fullness, nausea, dizziness, tachycardia, and generalized malaise 2–3 hours after eating.

Family History. Father died of a heart attack last year. Mother, age 63, alive and well. Five brothers and three sisters.

Personal History. Frequent alcohol but no tobacco use. No medications. Subtotal gastrectomy 6 years ago. Has not been taking vitamin and mineral supplements or following the prescribed diet.

Laboratory Findings		Normal Values
Serum iron	40 μg/dl	65–150 μg/dl
Serum calcium	7.3 mg/dl	9–11 mg/dl
Serum glucose	40 mg/dl	70–120 mg/dl
	at 2 hours of oral glucose tolerance test	
Bone biopsy indicated Osteoporosis		
Hemoglobin	8 g/dl	13–16 g/dl
Hematocrit	33%	42–50%

Present illness. A diagnosis of early postprandial (after-meal) dumping syndrome, anemia, and osteoporosis.

Using the above information plus material in this chapter, answer the following questions.

1. John's subtotal gastrectomy probably was for a _____ ulcer.

   A. gastric
   B. duodenal

2. The basis for the low serum iron and calcium values is _____ .

   1. partial stomach removal.   3. decreased amount of HCl
   2. decreased amount of   4. decreased pepsin enzyme
      mucus.

       A. 1, 2, 3 B. 1, 3 C. 2, 4 D. 4 E. all of these

3. John's laboratory values indicate that he is probably suffering from _____ anemia.

   A. pernicious
   B. iron deficiency
   C. folic acid
   D. none of these

4. The following dumping syndrome diet has been planned for John. Using the exchange lists (Appendix A), calculate the protein, fat, and carbohydrate values in grams; then choose from the answers below:

	Exchanges	Protein (g)	Fat (g)	Carbohydrate (g)
Meat (all medium fat)	15			
Fat	18			
Fruit	2			
Vegetables	2			
Bread	3			
Total				

   A. protein, 115 g; fat, 165 g; carbohydrate, 75 g
   B. protein, 105 g; fat, 90 g; carbohydrate, 185 g
   C. protein, 185 g; fat, 75 g; carbohydrate, 150 g
   D. none of these

5. The total kilocalories for this diet are:
   A. 3,510
   B. 1,985
   C. 2,245
   D. none of these

6. The caloric ratio is protein, 1.5; fat, 5; and carbohydrate, 1. The reason(s) why the fat and protein ratios are high and the carbohydrate ratio low is (are):
   1. fat and protein supply needed calories
   2. fat delays gastric emptying
   3. carbohydrate leaves the stomach first and may produce symptoms of the dumping syndrome
   4. none of these
      A. 1, 2, 3   B. 1, 3   C. 2, 4   D. 4

7. Food from one exchange list is intentionally omitted from the diet, which is _____ and the reason is due to its _____ content.
   A. cereal—carbohydrate
   B. milk—fat
   C. liquid—water
   D. milk—carbohydrate (lactose)

8. In reference to question 7, which important mineral (contained in an omitted food) is lacking and therefore must be given as an oral supplement?
   A. sodium
   B. cobalt
   C. potassium
   D. calcium

9. The basis for some of John's dumping syndrome symptoms is rapid movement of water from the blood into the intestines, thereby lowering blood pressure.
   A. true   B. false

10. John has not been following his prescribed diet, and an increased intake of simple sugars is probably a major reason for the symptoms and activity mentioned in question 9.
    A. true   B. false

Discussion Questions

1. Explain the reason for low serum glucose levels, or hypoglycemia, at the end of 2 hours after initiation of the oral glucose tolerance test.

2. Explain the reason for John's osteoporosis.

3. In reference to question 4, show how these exchanges could be distributed to provide six meals per day.

4. Write a 1-day menu for John that can be used with the exchanges in the previous question. (Refer to Table 1-2 for specific foods for the Spanish-American culture).

OUTLINE

ESOPHAGUS

This is a muscular collapsible tube about 250 cm (10 in.) in length. It begins at the base of the pharynx and extends through the diaphragm, joining the stomach. Its function is to move a bolus (round mass) of food from the pharynx to the stomach.

Disorders of the Esophagus
Hiatal Hernia
The stomach protrudes through an opening in the diaphragm.

Causes: causes include congenital weakness of the diaphragm, aging, obesity, pregnancy, and tight-fitting clothes.

Symptoms: symptoms include heartburn (pyrosis), dyphagia, substernal pain, and vomiting.

Diet therapy: bland diet and small, frequent feedings; antacids help neutralize stomach acidity; no foods should be eaten 3 to 4 hours before bedtime; the head of the bed should be elevated to avoid reflux.

STOMACH

The stomach has four basic functions:

- Storage: temporarily stores partially digested food (chyme).
- Mixing: peristaltic contractions mix food to form chyme.
- Regulation of the flow of chyme: the pyloric sphincter value gradually releases chyme into the duodenum.
- Aids in absorption of vitamin B_{12}, iron and calcium

Disorders
Gastritis
Gastritis is the inflammation of the gastric mucosa; acute gastritis is the most common form. The mucosa is reddened and edematous, and hemorrhages are present.

Causes: alcohol consumed with aspirin, spicy foods containing pepper, vinegar, and mustard.

Symptoms: are anoxeria, epigastric pain, and vomiting.

Diet therapy consists of removing offending foods, causing inflammation to subside. Total parenteral nutrition, along with a bland diet, has been successful.

Peptic Ulcer
Gastric: ulcer consists of deterioration of the gastric mucosa along the lesser curvature.

Duodenal: ulcer consists of deterioration of the mucosa in the duodenum. It is the more common peptic ulcer; about 80% of ulcers are duodenal.

The cause is an imbalance between the amount of HCl, pepsin enzyme, and mucosal resistance.

Symptoms include epigastric pain 1–3 hours after eating, heartburn, anorexia, vomiting, weight loss, and constipation.

Diet Therapy
The Sippy diet was advocated as the best diet for many years. It consists of hourly feedings of whole milk and cream and progresses to cooked cereals, soft-cooked eggs, custards, strained soups, and pureed fruits and vegetables.

The theory behind the diet is that protein in whole milk buffers the HCl and fat helps to keep food in the stomach, thereby prolonging the buffering action of food.

This diet lost favor with experts when the relationship of saturated fat to myocardial infarction and atherosclerosis was identified.

The Sippy diet is not recommended today except in bleeding ulcers; then skim milk should be substituted for whole milk and cream.

Antacid drugs are prescribed to neutralize acidity.

Rest is prescribed, since it reduces vagus nerve activity and therefore the release of HCl.

Current Dietary Therapy for Peptic Ulcer
The current treatment is a more liberal individualized diet than the Sippy diet.

General guidelines for an ulcer diet for a symptom-free person are as follows:

- Three meals rather than six small feedings per day should be eaten.
- Bedtime snacks should be eliminated.
- Milk and cream feedings should not be used to reduce acidity.
- Completely eliminating certain foods is unwarranted.
- Excessive alcohol intake should be avoided.

The diet should contain an adequate level of protein for healing and a moderate amount of fat for suppression of gastric secretions and peristaltic contractions.

Professionals disagree on the best dietary treatment when the ulcer is active and the person is showing symptoms; a conservative bland diet is prescribed by some professionals.

Complications

Hemorrhage: loss of blood, which is more frequent with duodenal than gastric ulcer.
Perforation: a hole or opening in the gastric or duodenal wall.

Pyloric obstruction: scarring or narrowing of the pyloric valve.

Dumping Syndrome (Postgastrectomy Syndrome)
Symptoms
Symptoms may occur after a gastrectomy operation; they include weakness, nausea, sweating, tachycardia, and dizziness. The changes that result in these symptoms are presented in the sequence in which they occur:

Rapid entrance of food into the duodenum
Increased osmotic pressure in the intestines
Movement of a large volume of water into the intestines
Decreased blood pressure

Dietary Treatment

- Minimize the quantity of food and increase the number of meals
- Avoid simple sugars
- Avoid liquids 30 minutes before and 1 hour after meals
- Increase the ratio of calories from polyunsaturated fat and proteins
- Increase caloric intake to 2,000–3,500 kcal.

Long-Range Nutritional Problems After a Subtotal Gastrectomy

- Hypercalcemia
- Anemia
- Reduced food intake and absorption

Dietary Counseling

- Small, frequent feedings
- Emphasis on protein, fat, and limited carbohydrate
- Gradual additions of foods
- No fluids at meals
- Vitamin and mineral supplements.

SMALL INTESTINE

This organ is 6–7 m (19–23 ft) long and is composed of the duodenum, jejunum and ileum. It has three functions: complete digestion of food, absorption of nutrients, and secretion of hormones.

Malabsorption Disorders
Nontropical Sprue (Celiac disease),
Gluten-sensitive Enteropathy
This is degeneration and atrophy of intestinal villi induced by foods that contain *gluten*.

Cause: there are two theories: an inborn error of metabolism, with an inability to produce peptidase, or an immune reaction to gluten.

Pathophysiology: intestinal villi atrophy and shorten, decreasing the surface area.

Symptoms. there is diarrhea and steatorrhea in adults. Children have irritability, failure to gain weight, and muscle wasting.

Diet therapy: a low-gluten diet; vitamin, mineral, and electrolyte supplements; and 3,000–3,500 kcal.

Lactose Intolerance (Lactase Deficiency)
The person lacks the lactase enzyme, which results in lactose buildup and osmotic pressure in the intestines, a shift of fluids into the intestines, increased motility, and malabsorption.

Causes: congenital, secondary, and developmental.

Symptoms: a bloated feeling, flatulence, belching, cramps, and diarrhea.

Diet therapy: a lactase-free formula for infants and partially fermented dairy products for adults.

Crohn's Disease (Inflammatory Bowel Disease)
This disease is located primarily in the ileum region and may extend into the large intestine; *granulomas* (nodular clumps) extending through all layers of the intestinal wall are common. The disease is common in young adults.

Cause: theories concern infectious agents, an autoimmune disease, and a genetic factor.

Symptoms: diarrhea, pain in the lower abdomen, steatorrhea, weight loss, and anemia.

Diet therapy: a low-fiber (low-residue) diet, high protein and carbohydrate and low fat levels; the diet should be supplemented with iron, folate, and vitamin B_{12}. Total parental nutrition is needed for severe cases.

LARGE INTESTINE (COLON)

This organ, which is 5 ft in length, is divided into the cecum, colon, and rectum. The ileocecal valve guards the entrance to the cecum. External and internal sphincter muscles guard the exit. Its functions are reabsorption of water and electrolytes, elimination of wastes (feces), and synthesis of vitamins.

Disorders of the Large Intestine
Colonic Diverticulosis and Diverticulitis
There are small sac-like herniations of the colon mucosa called *diverticula;* a common site is the sigmoid colon. Diverticulitis is inflammation of diverticula.

Cause: low-fiber foods cause increased intraluminal pressure in the intestine.

Symptoms of colonic diverticulosis: minimal constipation indicates the possible development of the condition.

Diet therapy for colonic diverticulosis: high fiber and bulk in diet.

Symptoms of diverticulitis: increase in total white blood cell count, fever, left lower quadrant pain, flatulence, slight nausea, and constipation.

Diet therapy of diverticulitis: antibiotics, stool softeners and liquid diet initially, gradual progression to a normal diet. After inflammation subsides, a high-fiber diet may be followed.

Ulcerative Colitis (Inflammatory Bowel Disease)

Ulcers are located in the mucosa and submucosa of the large intestine; initial ulcers are located in the rectum and sigmoid colon regions.

Cause: theories concern a genetic component, autoimmunity, and psychological stress.

Symptoms: chronic intermittent (recurrent) colitis is characterized by mild diarrhea and intermittent colitis by slight bleeding, anemia, dehydration and hypoproteinemia, and vitamin B_{12} deficiency.

Diet therapy: a bland low-residue diet is needed during attacks. Total parenteral nutrition with drug therapy is a new, effective treatment. A high-calorie diet is needed. Iron should be supplemented parenterally due to the loss of blood. Surgical intervention is indicated in many cases.

REVIEW QUESTIONS

TRUE (A) OR FALSE (B)

Questions 1–27

1. The primary goal of the diet in hiatal hernia is to prevent reflux by a bland diet and small frequent feedings.
2. A person who is receiving a hiatal hernia diet should not eat food 3–4 hours before bedtime.
3. A gastric ulcer is the most common type of peptic ulcer.
4. The exact cause of peptic ulcers is known to be the result of being tense, hard-driving, and anxious.
5. A constant state of epigastric pain is a common symptom of a gastric or duodenal ulcer.
6. The primary goal of peptic ulcer dietary management is to buffer or inhibit acid secretions in the stomach.
7. The Sippy diet is the recommended diet for peptic ulcers, since it has been proven to be superior to the liberal diet.
8. General guidelines for an ulcer diet for a symptom-free person are three meals rather than six small meals per day, elimination of bedtime snacks, avoidance of milk and cream feedings

to reduce acidity, and avoidance of excessive alcohol.

9. The dumping syndrome is a combination of symptoms—weakness, a desire to lie down, nausea, profound sweating, tachycardia, and dizziness—that often develop after a subtotal gastrectomy.
10. Dietary treatment of the dumping syndrome includes increased consumption of simple sugars and decreased consumption of fats.
11. Some of the long-term problems related to a subtotal gastrectomy are hypercalcemia and constipation.
12. One theory about the cause of nontropical sprue is that the protein gluten, found in wheat, causes an immune reaction to the intestinal mucosa.
13. Some of the common symptoms of nontropical sprue are diarrhea, fatty stools (steatorrhea), and muscle wasting.
14. All products that may contain wheat, and thus gluten, must be eliminated from the diet, with breaded vegetables, chicken fried steak, and gravy being examples.
15. All breads and cereals that contain wheat, corn, and rice must be eliminated from a gluten-restricted diet. (For the answer, consult the analysis and comments on the sample menu for the gluten-restricted diet.)
16. A gluten-restricted diet involves merely increasing the amount of food consumed to achieve adequacy in the intake of certain nutrients such as thiamine and iron. (The comments for question 15 are applicable here.)
17. Congenital lactase deficiency is the most common type of lactase deficiency and is very prevalent in American blacks and Orientals.
18. Lactase deficiency can result in malabsorption of nutrients due to increased motility and diarrhea.
19. A lactose-intolerant individual must avoid all dairy products, including cottage cheese, buttermilk, sour cream, yogurt, and hard cheese.
20. Symptoms of Crohn's disease include bloody diarrhea, pain in the lower abdomen, and possibly steatorrhea.
21. The dietary goal of Crohn's disease is to rest the small intestine, which is best accomplished by excluding foods high in fiber and residue.
22. A person who has diverticulitis has herniations of the small intestine mucosa, constipation, and few other minimal symptoms.
23. The treatment of diverticulosis is a liquid diet, bed rest, antibiotics, and stool softeners.
24. A high-fiber diet is recommended for diverticulitis after inflammation has subsided, since it decreases intraluminal pressure, thereby decreasing the chance of diverticuli formation.

25. Ulcerative colitis is characterized by ulcers in the mucosa of the rectum and sigmoid colon, with diarrhea, crampy abdominal pain, and weight loss being common symptoms.
26. The principal goals of diet therapy for ulcerative colitis are to control inflammation, maintain the patient's nutritional status, give symptomatic relief, and prevent infection.
27. An ulcerative colitis diet should consist of high levels of protein and decreased amounts of raw fruits and vegetables, plus iron and vitamin B_{12} supplements.

MULTIPLE CHOICE

Questions 28–40

28. Hiatal hernia is characterized by:
   1. possibly being caused by aging and obesity
   2. complaints of heartburn, reflux, and difficulty in swallowing
   3. diet therapy consisting of a bland diet and small, frequent feedings
   4. no food being eaten 3–4 hours before bedtime
      A. 1, 2, 3   B. 1, 3   C. 2, 4   D. 4
      E. all of these
29. The exact cause of peptic ulcers is not known; however, the condition can result from:
   1. an imbalance in the amount of HCl
   2. an imbalance in the amount of pepsin enzyme
   3. an imbalance in mucosal resistance of the gastric mucosa
   4. eating a chronic low-fiber diet
      A. 1, 2, 3   B. 1, 3   C. 2, 4   D. 4
      E. all of these
30. Current dietary therapy for peptic ulcer includes
   1. six small meals per day
   2. inclusion of a bedtime snack
   3. consumption of whole milk as opposed to skim milk
   4. limitation of black pepper, chili powder, and nicotine
      A. 1, 2, 3   B. 1, 3   C. 2, 4   D. 4
      E. all of these
31. The symptoms or changes in blood vessels and the small intestine that may result from a subtotal gastrectomy are _____ and the reason(s) is (are) _____.
   1. increased osmotic pressure in the intestines—rapid entrance of food into the duodenum
   2. increase in blood pressure—large volume of water moving out of the intestines

3. weakness, sweating, and tachycardia—drop in blood pressure due to movement of water out of the blood
4. slow entrance of food into the duodenum—removal of the majority of the stomach and pyloric sphincter
   A. 1, 2, 3   B. 1, 3   C. 2, 4   D. 4
   E. all of these
32. The dietary treatment for control of dumping syndrome is (are)
   1. an increased quantity of food at three meals
   2. avoidance of simple sugars
   3. drinking liquids with meals
   4. increasing the number of kilocalories from polyunsaturated fat and proteins
      A. 1, 2, 3   B. 1, 3   C. 2, 4   D. 4
33. Long-range nutritional problems that are possible following a subtotal gastrectomy are
   1. hypocalcemia and osteoporosis
   2. iron deficiency and pernicious anemia
   3. fear of eating
   4. high blood cholesterol level
      A. 1, 2, 3   B. 1, 3   C. 2, 4   D. 4
      E. all of these
34. The immune theory of the cause of celiac disease is that _____ causes the intestinal villi to _____, thereby decreasing absorption.
   A. simple sugars—be destroyed
   B. corn and rice—enlarge and become distorted in shape
   C. gluten—atrophy, shorten, and fuse
   D. fats—become ulcerated
35. Infants who have congenital lactose intolerance can obtain necessary nutrients from ___ _____ and adults with secondary lactose intolerance can tolerate partially fermented dairy products such as _____.
   A. fat formulas—skim milk and skim cheese
   B. soybean—cottage cheese and buttermilk formulas
   C. sucrose—low-fat butter and ice cream formulas
   D. none of these
36. A menu for a minimum-residue diet, such as for Crohn's disease, has the following characteristics and adaptions:
   1. numerous servings of fresh fruits and fibrous vegetables
   2. two servings of skim milk
   3. six servings of high-fiber bread
   4. supplements of calcium, iron, vitamin A, riboflavin, and vitamin D
      A. 1, 2, 3   B. 1, 3   C. 2, 4   D. 4
      E. all of these
37. A chronic low-fiber diet may cause diverticu-

losis, and the mechanism that results in the formation of diverticula is

A. low-fiber foods → increased segmentation → of colon

→ increased intra-luminal pressure within intestine → protrusion of intestinal mucosa through intestinal wall

B. high-fiber foods → decreased segmentation → of colon

→ decreased intra-luminal pressure within intestine → protrusion of intestinal mucosa through intestinal wall

38. Initial treatment of an acute attack of diverticulitis consists of:
1. a high-fiber diet   2. stool softeners
3. a high-residue diet   4. a liquid diet
    A. 1, 2, 3   B. 1, 3   C. 2, 4   D. 4
    E. all of these

39. Chronic intermittent ulcerative colitis typically occurs in the mucosa and submucosa layers of the _____ regions of the large intestine and is characterized by _____.
A. ascending and transverse—severe diarrhea and bleeding
B. cecum and ascending—steatorrhea and constipation
C. rectum and sigmoid—mild diarrhea and slight bleeding
D. none of these

40. Dietary and drug therapy for ulcerative colitis includes
1. total parenteral nutrition
2. decreased amounts of raw fruit and vegetables
3. iron and vitamin B_{12} supplements
4. administration of anticholinergic drugs
    A. 1, 2, 3   B. 1, 3   C. 2, 4   D. 4
    E. all of these

DISCUSSION QUESTIONS

1. Discuss the general guidelines of a liberal individualized diet for peptic ulcer.
2. Describe the long-range nutritional problems that are possible following a subtotal gastrectomy.
3. Discuss the cause, symptoms and diet therapy for lactose intolerance.
4. Describe the mechanism by which a low-fiber diet may cause diverticulosis.

5. Discuss the causes, symptoms, and diet therapy for ulcerative colitis.

REFERENCES

1. D.P. Burkitt. "Hiatus hernia: Is it preventable?" *American Journal of Clinical Nutrition*, 34(3), 428–431 (1981).
2. K.G. Wormsley: "Duodenal ulcer: An update." *Mount Sinai Journal of Medicine*, 48(5), 391–396 (1981).
3. T. Beaudette. "Nutritional problems and controversies in gastrointestinal diseases." *Nutrition in Practice*, 2(1), 18 (1982).
4. D.J. Shearman and D. Hetzel. "The medical management of peptic ulcer." *Annual Review of Medicine*, 30, 61–79 (1979).
5. S.A. Price and L.M. Wilson. *Pathophysiology: Clinical Concepts of Disease Processes*, 2nd ed. New York: McGraw-Hill Book Co., 1982, pp. 224–225.
6. R.B. Howard and N.H. Herbold. *Nutrition in Clinical Care*, 2nd ed. New York: McGraw-Hill Book Co., 1981, pp. 362–363.
7. E.R. Woodward. "The late postprandial syndrome." *Major Problems in Clinical Surgery*, 20, 159 (1976).
8. M.L. Green and M.L. Harry. *Nutrition in Contemporary Nursing Practice*, New York: John Wiley and Sons, 1981, pp. 649–656.
9. R.K. Chandra and S. Sahni. "Immunological aspects of gluten intolerance." *Nutrition Reviews*, 39, 117–120 (1981).
10. T. Gilat. "Carbohydrate and milk intolerance." *Practical Gastroenterology*, 4, 32–5 (1980).
11. H.L. Segal and L.N. Chessin. "Etiology of granulomatous disease of the gut (Crohn's disease)." *Journal of Clinical Gastroenterology*, 3, 321–325 (1981).
12. L. Descas and J. Vignal. "Total parenteral nutrition in the management of Crohn's disease." *World Journal Surgery*, 4, 161–162 (1980).
13. J.L.A. Roth. "Medical management of diverticular disease of the colon." *Current Concepts in Gastroenterology*, 2, 19 (1977).
14. G.M. Levine. "Nutritional support in gastrointestinal disease." *Surgical Clinic of North America*, 61, 701 (1981).
15. V.W. Fazio and R.B. Turnbull. "Ulcerative colitis and Crohn's disease of the colon: Review of surgical options." *Medical Clinic of North America*, 34, 1135–1159 (1980).

20 DISORDERS OF THE LIVER, GALLBLADDER, AND PANCREAS

OBJECTIVES

Upon completion of this chapter, you should be able to:

1. Name and give examples of the four liver functions.

2. Give the cause and symptoms of hepatitis.

3. Name the most common cause of cirrhosis and describe the underlying causes of portal hypertension, esophageal varices, and ascites.

4. Describe the dietary treatment of hepatitis and cirrhosis in terms of the amounts of kilocalories, protein, carbohydrate, fat, vitamin supplements, and sodium.

5. Discuss the drug treatments of hepatitis and cirrhosis and their possible side effects.

6. Name the precipating factor that results in hepatic coma, as well as the symptoms.

7. Discuss how the dietary treatment of hepatic coma is different from that of hepatitis and cirrhosis.

8. Discuss the roles of antibiotics and lactulose in the treatment of hepatic coma.

9. Discuss the theories of what causes formation of gallstones.

10. Describe the dietary treatment of gallstones.

11. Describe the location and functions of the pancreas.

12. Name the symptoms of pancreatitis.

13. Discuss the dietary and drug treatments of pancreatitis.

14. Explain how mucus produced in cystic fibrosis affects the pancreas and lungs.

15. Describe the dietary and drug treatments of cystic fibrosis.

INTRODUCTION

The gallbladder, pancreas, and liver attach to the intestinal portion of the gastrointestinal tract (see Fig. 20-1). These accessory digestive organs contribute important chemical compounds to the small intestine. In addition, the pancreas and liver play important roles in metabolic reactions.

LIVER

FUNCTIONS

The liver (see Fig. 20-1) is the largest organ in the body and carries on many metabolic reactions. These functions can be grouped into four areas: synthesis, decomposition, storage, and detoxification.

Bile A fluid secreted by the liver that emulsifies fat molecules in the small intestine.

Fibrinogen A blood protein that contributes to blood clotting.

Albumin A blood protein that regulates the osmotic pressure of the blood.

Synthesis

Production of bile. The liver produces approximately 600–800 ml bile per day.

Production of blood proteins. **Fibrinogen** and prothrombin proteins are vital to blood clotting. A third protein is **albumin,** which is the primary contributor to the osmotic pressure of the blood.

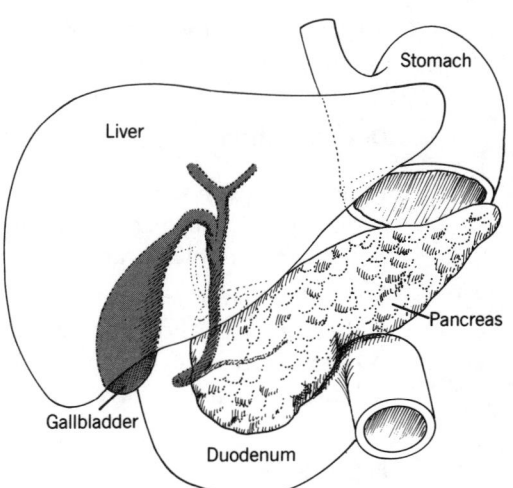

FIGURE 20-1 The liver, gallbladder, and pancreas. (Courtesy of the National Institute of Public Health.)

Glycogenesis. Insulin promotes the synthesis of glycogen by combining many glucose molecules.

Cholesterol. Liver cells synthesize cholesterol, some of which become a component of bile.

Synthesis of lipoproteins. Very-low-density lipoproteins (VLDL) and low-density lipoproteins (LDL) are synthesized and transport cholesterol and other lipids to the tissues.

Urea. Urea is synthesized from ammonia molecules, which result from deamination of amino acids.

Decomposition

Phagocytic cells Cells that carry on phagocytosis, such as some white blood cells.

Bilirubin A pigment produced by the breakdown of heme and secreted into bile.

Destruction of red blood cells (RBCs). Phagocytic cells decompose worn-out RBCs. **Bilirubin** is a product of this decomposition and is incorporated into bile.

Glycogenolysis. Decomposition of glycogen and release of glucose is stimulated by glucagon when the blood glucose level drops below 70 mg/dl.

Hydrolysis of lipids. The liver hydrolyzes cholesterol, phospholipids, and lipoproteins to fatty acids and glycerol.

Steroid hormone inactivation. Several steroid hormones (aldosterone, glucocorticoids, estrogen, progesterone, and estrogen) are inactivated.

Storage

Vitamin and mineral storage. Fat-soluble vitamins, vitamin B_{12}, copper, and iron are stored in the liver.

Detoxification

Hepatic coma A coma that results from the buildup of ammonia, which increases as a result of the liver's inability to convert ammonia to urea.

Hepatitis A viral infection that results in inflammation of the liver tissue.

Drug and alcohol detoxification. Liver cells can decompose, thereby detoxifying most drugs and alcohol. This function is one reason why chronic alcoholism can result in cirrhosis (discussed later).

Detoxification of ammonia to urea. As mentioned above, the liver synthesizes urea; however, another way of describing this function is detoxification of ammonia. When this function fails, ammonia can build up to a toxic level, resulting in **hepatic coma.**[1]

DISEASES

Three common liver diseases are **hepatitis,** cirrhosis, and hepatic coma. These conditions are discussed in an increasing order of severity.

SGOT Serum glutamic oxaloacetic transaminase, an enzyme found especially in the heart and

Hepatitis

Hepatitis A and B are the two most common forms. A comparison of the two is as follows:

	Hepatitis A	Hepatitis B
Synonyms	Infectious hepatitis	Serum hepatitis
Groups with highest incidence	Young children, especially in institutions	All age groups; common in drug addicts and hemodialysis patients
Transmission	Fecal-oral route; shellfish	Blood transfusion is most common
Symptoms	Fatigue, anorexia, jaundice, light stools, dark urine, elevated enzyme levels (**SGOT and SGPT**), enlargement of the liver, and abnormal liver function test	

liver. An elevated level in the blood is indicative of liver damage.

SGPT Serum glutamic pyruvic transaminase, an enzyme found in several tissues including the liver. An elevated level in the blood is indicative of liver disease.

Chronic persistent hepatitis An inflammation of the liver that may last for 4–8 months.

Interstitial Between-parts. Interstitial fluid, which is located between cells, is an example.

Laennec's cirrhosis Cirrhosis caused by chronic alcoholism.

Biliary atresia Congenital destruction or closure of one or more bile ducts in the liver.

Hemochromatosis An inherited disease in which a person absorbs and deposits excessive amounts of iron in the liver.

The majority of hepatitis A and B infections are mild, with complete recovery. In hepatitis A, the symptoms are sometimes so mild that the person may think he or she simply has the flu.

Treatment of viral hepatitis is nonspecific, but bed rest and a nutritious diet (discussed below) are essential. Most hepatitis cases show signs of recovery 1–2 weeks after the onset of jaundice. Stools regaining their abnormal color, jaundice lessening, and lightening of the urine color are examples of normal recovery signs.

From 5 to 10% of hepatitis patients experience **chronic persistent hepatitis,** which lasts for 4–8 months. Approximately the same percentage experience a relapse as a result of alcohol ingestion or excessive physical activity. A small number of hepatitis patients experience destruction of liver tissue and cirrhosis.[2]

Cirrhosis of the Liver

The term cirrhosis means inflammation and scarring of **interstitial** (between parts) tissue. Cirrhosis of the liver results in destruction of liver cells, which are replaced by scar tissue. Destruction of liver cells and replacement by scar tissue result in decreased functioning of the liver. (See Case Study: Liver disease, at end of chapter, for reinforcement and application of information about cirrhosis of the liver.)

Causes. In the United States, chronic alcoholism is the most common cause and is called **Laennec's cirrhosis.** Chronic severe hepatitis can also cause cirrhosis. Other causes of cirrhosis include obstruction and absence of or injury to bile ducts. For example, **biliary atresia** and **hemochromatosis** can also result in cirrhosis.

Palmar erythema Bright red palms.

Spider angioma Spider-shaped blood vessels.

Symptoms. The early onset of cirrhosis is subtle, including symptoms such as, anorexia, weight loss, and fatigue. Other examples of early symptoms are **palmar erythema** and **spider angioma.** Decreased inactivation of the steroid hormone estrogen results in the formation of spider-shaped blood vessels. These are seen in the skin, especially in the neck, shoulder, and chest regions. Intense itching is often reported; it results from deposits of bile in the skin. This condition and jaundice occur because pigments are not being processed normally by the liver. A later symptom is the accumulation of triglycerides or the development of fatty liver. These problems result from the inability to synthesize enough lipoproteins to transport fats out of the liver. All of these symptoms result from the loss of various liver functions.

A second group of symptoms results from scar tissues altering the normal flow of blood through the liver. Normally, the liver receives about one-third of the blood the heart pumps each minute. The major blood supply is from the portal vein (see Fig. 20-2), through which the

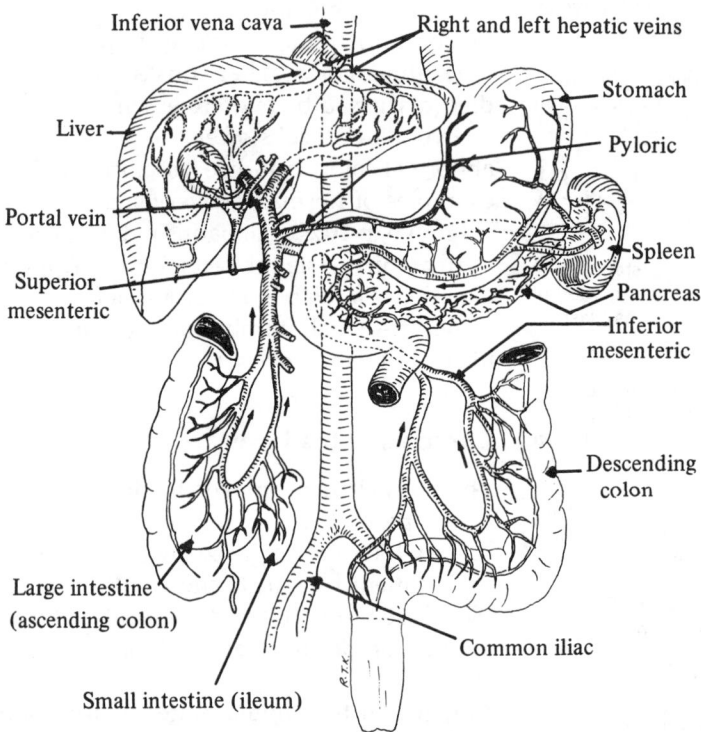

FIGURE 20-2 The portal vein, which supplies most of the blood to the liver, and the hepatic veins, which drain blood from the liver into the inferior vena cava. (From T. Randall Lankford, *Integrated Science for Health Students,* 3rd edition, 1984. Reprinted by permission of Reston Publishing Company, a Prentice-Hall Company, 11480 Sunset Hills Road, Reston, VA 22090.)

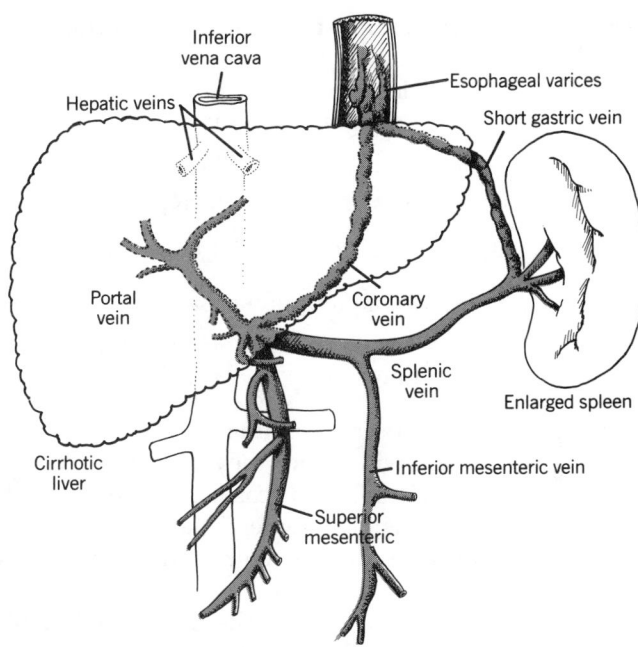

FIGURE 20-3 Collateral venous channels that drain blood around the liver in cirrhosis. (Courtesy of the National Institute of Public Health.)

Inferior vena cava The vein that drains the blood from the lower part of the body to the right atrium of the heart.

Hepatic veins Veins that drain the blood from the liver into the inferior vena cava.

Portal hypertension Abnormally increased pressure in the portal circulation.

Collateral channels Veins that are used as detour routes from the liver connecting to veins from the lower esophagus.

Esophageal varices Dilation of esophageal veins.

Ascites The accumulation of fluids in the abdominal cavity.

liver receives products of digestion from the gastrointestinal tract. After the blood flows through the liver, it empties into the **inferior vena cava** through the **hepatic veins.** Scar tissue decreases blood flow into the liver through the portal vein. This decreased flow results in **portal hypertension** and the development of detour routes around the liver. These detour routes are called **collateral channels** and involve veins from the liver connecting to veins from the lower esophagus (see Fig. 20-3). Portal hypertension often results in **esophageal varices.** About 70% of advanced cirrhosis patients experience these varices, and bleeding from them is a common cause of death.

A major symptom or complication of scar tissue in the liver is **ascites.** Many of the dietary modifications for cirrhotic patients are based on preventing or reducing ascites; therefore, it is important to understand the three major changes that lead to ascites:

Decreased albumin. The development of scar tissue results in gradual loss of liver functions such as synthesis of albumin. Decreased albumin in the blood results in a lowering of blood osmotic pressure. This low osmotic pressure in the veins of the gastrointestinal tract prevents the normal pulling of fluids into veins. Instead, the fluid is pulled into the abdominal cavity, where the osmotic pressure is higher.

Portal hypertension. Increased pressure in the portal vein helps to force fluids out of the blood into the abdominal cavity.

Hyperaldosteronism An increased level of the hormone aldosterone.

Hyperaldosteronism. This hormone stimulates the absorption of sodium by the kidneys and normally is degraded by the liver. Hyperaldosteronism causes increased retention of sodium, which further aggravates the ascites.[3]

Dietary Treatment of Hepatitis and Cirrhosis

The two goals of diet therapy in hepatitis and cirrhosis are:

- To maintain homeostasis by providing kilocalories and nutrients
- To enhance the functions of the liver and allow for healing and cellular renewal

Nausea, vomiting, and anorexia are the most difficult symptoms to deal with, since they directly affect food intake and malnutrition complicates liver disease. When the symptoms are severe, intravenous solutions or parenteral fluids of 5–10% glucose and 3.5% protein hydrolysates should be given until the symptoms subside.

Diet Treatment. The diet prescription for hepatitis and cirrhosis is the same: high kilocalories, high protein, high carbohydrate, and moderate fat.

The caloric content should be 35–50 kcal per kilogram of recommended body weight, or approximately 2,000–3,000 kcal for an adult. The increase in kilocalories over the normal amount a sedentary person needs (about 30 kcal/kg) is important for regeneration of liver tissue. See the sample menu for a high-protein, moderate-fat, high-carbohydrate diet.

A high protein intake should provide 1.5–2.0 g of protein per kilogram of desired body weight. This protein intake is two to almost three times the Recommended Dietary Allowance (RDA) for protein for adults with 0.8 g per kilogram of body weight. The increased protein is important for several reasons:

- To protect the liver from further degeneration
- To repair and restore liver tissue
- To form bile acids
- To replenish plasma proteins
- To provide lipotropic factors

Liptropic factors Compounds that contribute to the formation of lipoproteins that transport fats out of the liver.

Protein sources should be of high biological value and especially high in foods that contain **lipotropic factors.** Foods especially rich in lipotropic factors are egg yolks, meat, fish, and cereals. If the condition progresses to hepatic coma, protein must be restricted (discussed below).

Carbohydrate intake should be 300–400 g/day, or approximately 60%

SAMPLE MENU FOR A HIGH-PROTEIN, MODERATE-FAT, HIGH-CARBOHYDRATE DIET

Exchange		P (g)	F (g)	C (g)
	Breakfast			
1 fruit	½ grapefruit	—	—	10
1 bread	½ cup bran flakes	2	—	15
1 medium-fat meat	1 scrambled egg	7	5	—
2 bread	2 slices whole wheat toast	4	—	30
2 fat	2 tsp margarine	—	10	—
	1 tbsp jelly* (3 tsp)	—	—	15
	1 cup coffee	—	—	—
	Lunch			
4 lean meat	4 oz broiled fish	28	12	—
1 bread	1 small baked potato	2	—	15
1 fat	1 tsp margarine	—	5	—
1 vegetable	½ cup asparagus	2	—	5
2 bread	2 slices whole wheat bread	4	—	30
2 fat	2 tsp margarine	—	10	—
	1 tbsp jelly* (3 tsp)	—	—	15
2 fruit	1 banana	—		20
1 milk	1 cup skim milk	8	—	12
	Mid-Afternoon Snack			
1 milk	1 cup skim milk	8	—	12
1 bread	2 graham crackers	2	—	15
	Dinner			
4 lean meat	4 oz broiled chicken (skin removed)	28	12	—
1 bread	1 small baked potato	2	—	15
2 fat	2 tsp margarine	—	10	—
1 vegetable	½ cup string beans	2	—	5
2 bread	2 plain rolls	4	—	30

1 fat	1 tsp margarine	—	5	—
	1 tbsp apple jelly* (3 tsp)	—	—	15
1 milk	1 cup skim milk	8	—	12
Evening Snack				
1 milk	1 cup skim milk	8	—	12
2 bread	2 slices whole wheat bread	4	—	30
	2 tbsp jelly* (6 tsp)	—	—	30
	Totals	123	69	353

Key: Protein (P), Fat (F), Carbohydrate (C)

Calculations of Nutrient Levels

$$
\begin{array}{rl}
\text{Protein: } 123 \text{ g} \times 4 \text{ kcal/g} = & 492 \text{ kcal} \\
\text{Fat: } 69 \text{ g} \times 9 \text{ kcal/g} = & 621 \text{ kcal} \\
\text{Carbohydrate: } 353 \text{ g} \times 4 \text{ kcal/g} = & 1,412 \text{ kcal} \\
\text{Total} & 2,525 \text{ kcal}
\end{array}
$$

Percentage of total kilocalories due to protein:

$$\frac{492 \text{ kcal}}{2,525 \text{ kcal}} \times 100 = 19\%$$

fat:

$$\frac{621 \text{ kcal}}{2,525 \text{ kcal}} \times 100 = 25\%$$

carbohydrate:

$$\frac{1,412 \text{ kcal}}{2,525 \text{ kcal}} \times 100 = 56\%$$

Analysis of Menu and Calculations

- An analysis of this menu shows that there are 4 milk, 2 vegetable, 3 fruit, 12 bread, 9 meat, and 8 fat exchanges.

- In order to achieve a high-protein diet while achieving a moderate-fat diet, there are eight servings of lean meat, one serving of medium-fat meat, and no servings of high-fat meat.

- Notice that much of the carbohydrate in the menu is from the sugar group, which is not one of the exchanges. The amount of carbohydrate in each tablespoon and teaspoon is given.

- Fat is kept to a moderate level by including skim milk rather than whole milk. The 8 fat exchanges should be polyunsaturated rather than saturated fat. This is especially important, since the fat in the 9 meat exchanges is all saturated.

The asterisk (*) in the menu indicates foods that are not part of an exchange list. Rather, these foods are members of the sugar group. The amount of carbohydrate in a tablespoon (3 tsp) of jelly is 5 g/tsp or 15 g/tbsp.

of the total kilocalories. Carbohydrate intake is important so that protein can be spared from being used as an energy source.[4]

Moderate fat consumption of 25–40% of the kilocalories is recommended. Whole dairy products and eggs should be the main source of fat, as opposed to greasy foods. Medium chain triglyceride (MCT) oils may help to reduce fat infiltration in the liver, since they do not use the chylomicron transport system. However, since MCTs are metabolized in the liver, some authorities recommend that they not be given to cirrhosis patients. Fat is important for absorption of fat-soluble vitamins and energy, and to increase the palatibility of the meals. The principles of a low-fat diet are provided in Table 20-1.

Vitamin supplements include thiamin, which is important for the metabolism of carbohydrates, proteins, fats, and vitamin B_{12}. Vitamin K is given to counteract the bleeding tendency that results from decreased synthesis of prothrombin. Vitamin C helps to provide collagen, which is important for tissue regeneration.

If a person has ascites, this condition can be helped by restricting sodium in the diet, with 22–40 mEq/day (500–920 mg/day) being a common amount. A major problem with this restriction is that protein may also be restricted, since many foods high in protein are also high in sodium (see Appendix I for the sodium content of foods). Powdered

TABLE 20-1 LOW-FAT DIET (40–45 g)

Purpose:	The diet is designed to limit the total amount of fat to 40–45 g.
Use:	Used in diseases of the liver, gallbladder, or pancreas in which there is an impairment of fat digestion and absorption.
Examples of foods:	Foods with a high fat content are omitted and those that cause gaseous distention may be omitted.
Adequacy:	Diet is adequate.

Source: Chicago Dietetic Association, *Manual of Clinical Dietetics,* 2nd ed. Philadelphia, W.B. Saunders Company, 1981. Reprinted by permission.

protein supplements can be used to help offset this problem. In addition, low-sodium milk (Lonalac) is a good source of protein and allows the use of other foods with a higher sodium content. Water intake often has to be limited to 1,000–1,500 ml/day.

Drug Treatment. Frequently, diuretics have to be administered in order to decrease the ascites condition. Spironolactone (Aldactone) is a diuretic that blocks the activity of aldosterone, thereby decreasing absorption of sodium while potassium is reabsorbed. It is important that diuresis not result in too rapid a fluid loss in order to prevent disastrous changes in plasma volume. A general goal is a loss of no more than 0.5 kg/day if person has ascites only and not more than 1 kg/day if he or she also has peripheral edema.[5]

Potential complications of diuretics are numerous, with hypokalemia being an example. Hypokalemia can cause a cirrhotic condition to degenerate into a hepatic coma (discussed next).

A drug that helps give relief from itching is cholestyramine (Questran), which binds with bile in the intestine and prevents its reabsorption. However, it can reduce absorption of vitamin B_{12}, MCT, iron, and calcium. See Chapter 16 for details about effects of diuretics and cholestyramine (Questran).

Hepatic Coma

Hepatic coma occurs when cirrhosis progresses to the point where the liver cannot adequately detoxify ammonia to urea. A person experiencing this condition usually is not in a comatose state but rather exhibits mental disturbances such as disorientation and behavioral changes. Sleep patterns may be altered and a flapping tremor of the hands may occur when the arms are extended.

Ammonia results from the deamination of amino acids, with the gastrointestinal tract being the main source. Intestinal bacteria produce ammonia by interacting with cells from the intestinal mucosa and blood cells that result from esophageal varices. Ammonia levels increase in the blood to the point where they cause malfunction of the brain tissue; therefore, the name **hepatic encephalopathy** is often used to describe this condition.

Hepatic encephalopathy
A condition caused by increased levels of ammonia in the blood, which leads to a malfunction of brain tissue.

Dietary Treatment. Regulating protein intake is the key to treating hepatic coma. Since ammonia can also be formed by bacterial action, antibiotic therapy is used to destroy intestinal bacteria.

Low protein, low fat, high carbohydrate levels and high kilocalories are the diet prescription for hepatic coma. Elimination of foods that contain preformed ammonia (certain cheeses, chicken, salami, peanut butter, and potatoes) is essential. See the following boxed material concerning the treatment of hepatic coma with branched chain amino acids.

One somewhat controversial approach to treating hepatic coma is the use of special solutions containing branched chain amino acids (leucine, isoleucine, and valine) rather than nonbranched aromatic amino acids (phenylalanine, tyrosine, and tryptophan). Branched chain amino acids are not metabolized in the liver; therefore, they do not increase ammonia levels, but they do help to maintain a positive nitrogen balance. Some studies on hepatic coma patients have shown recovery when they received a special total parenteral nutrition (TPN) solution containing 35% branched chain amino acids, as opposed to the 22% found in most commercial mixtures. An oral supplement that is high in branched chain amino acids is Hepatic Aid (McGaw Laboratories).

The use of branched chain amino acids is controversial, since some studies have not achieved positive results in the patient awakening sooner from a coma compared to the results achieved with a more traditional diet with low levels of nonbranched amino acids. In addition, studies have not proven that the nonbranched amino acids tryptophan and phenylalanine definitely cause hepatic coma.[6]

Dietary protein intake should be decreased to 0.5 g per kilogram of body weight, or 20–40 g of protein per day. See the sample menu for a 20-g protein diet. A diet containing less than 40 g of protein is deficient in many nutrients, such as protein, niacin, riboflavin, thiamin, calcium, phosphorus, and iron. If a person is in a coma, he or she must be placed on a zero protein diet for a few days until the ammonia decreases to a safe level. This diet involves complete elimination of some exchanges, such as milk, vegetables, and meat. Other exchanges, such as bread, allow some foods, such as low-protein bread and pasta only. Also, only certain fruits are allowed, such as cranberry juice and apple juice. The diet is high in carbohydrates and fat and should supply 1,500–2,000 kcal to prevent breakdown of tissue proteins.[7]

As the person's condition improves, protein intake can be increased gradually by 10–15 g/week to 40–50 g/day.

Drug Treatment. Neomycin sulfate (Mycifradin) is an antibiotic that destroys bacteria that can break down protein and urea into ammonia. Possible nutritional side effects include reduced absorption of calcium, iron, and vitamin B_{12}. In addition, this antibiotic can increase fecal excretion of sodium and potassium.

Lactulose (Cephulac) reduces the amount of ammonia absorbed from the large intestine into the blood. This drug causes acidification of the

SAMPLE MENU FOR A 20-G PROTEIN DIET

Exchange	
	Breakfast
1 fruit	½ cup orange juice
1 bread	½ cup oatmeal
1 milk	1 cup skim milk
3 fat	3 strips of bacon
1 bread	1 slice low-protein bread
2 fat	2 tsp margarine
	1 tbsp jelly
	1 cup coffee
	4 tsp sugar
	Mid-Morning Snack
	8 oz Kool-Aid with ¼ cup high-calorie, low protein powder (e.g., Contra-lyte) added
	Lunch
1 vegetable	½ cup sliced tomatoes
1 fat	1 tbsp french dressing
1 fruit	½ cup peaches
1 fruit	½ cup applesauce
	½ cup fruit cocktail
1 bread	1 slice low-protein bread
3 fat	3 tsp margarine
	1 tbsp jelly
	8 oz gingerale
	Mid-Afternoon Snack
	8 pieces candy
	8 oz Seven-Up
	Dinner
1 medium fat meat	1 poached egg
1 bread	1 slice low-protein bread
1 vegetable	½ cup spinach
1 vegetable	½ cup asparagus

1 fat	1 tbsp french dressing
	1 cup Italian water ice
3 fat	3 tsp margarine
	1 cup tea
	2 tsp sugar

Bedtime Snack

8 oz Kool-Aid with $\frac{1}{4}$ cup high-calorie, low-protein powder (e.g., Contro-lyte) added

Analysis and Comments

- An analysis of this diet shows that it contains 1 milk, 3 vegetable, 3 fruit, 4 bread, 1 meat, and 13 fat exchanges.

- In order to keep the protein level at 20 g, the menu includes only 1 meat and 1 milk exchange. The four bread exchanges are low-protein bread, which contains 0.5 g protein or less, compared to 2 g per slice in normal bread.

- The high number of fat exchanges is important to provide kilocalories. In addition, kilocalories are provided by the foods from the sugar group (e.g., jelly, Kool-Aid) and the high-kilocalories, low-protein powder.

- Due to the restriction in protein, the menu is deficient in protein, niacin, riboflavin, thiamin, and calcium.

Source: Menu adapted from Chicago Dietetic Association, *Manual of Clinical Dietetics,* 2nd ed. Philadelphia: W.B. Saunders Company, 1981. Reprinted by permission.

large intestine, with the end result being that ammonia is converted to ammonium ions, which cannot be absorbed. Some side effects of lactulose are diarrhea, flatulence, and abdominal discomfort.[8]

GALLBLADDER

FUNCTION

The gallbladder is a sac whose walls consist of smooth muscle and have a mucosal lining. It is located on the inferior surface of the liver (see Fig. 20-1). Storage and concentration of bile from the liver are the functions of the gallbladder. Concentrated bile is released into the duodenum through the common bile duct when the gallbladder is stimulated to contract. The hormone **cholecystokinin** stimulates the gallbladder to contract when it is secreted from the duodenum on the entrance of fat from the stomach.

Cholecystokinin A hormone that stimulates the gallbladder to contract and release bile.

Bile is composed of bile salts, cholesterol, bilirubin, and lecithin. The liver secretes about 700 ml of bile per day, which is important in emulsification and digestion of fats (see Chapter 4 for details).

DISORDERS

Cholecystitis An inflammation of the gallbladder that results from bacterial infection or gallstones.

Cholecystitis is inflammation of the gallbladder and frequently results from bacterial infection or **gallstones. Cholelithiasis** is the formation of stones in the gallbladder. About 80% of all gallstones are composed chiefly of cholesterol.

Gallstones Stone-like masses that form in the gallbladder.

Cholelithiasis The formation of stones in the gallbladder.

Gallstone Formation and Symptoms

It is believed that gallstones develop when cholesterol in bile becomes too concentrated. Two reasons for the increased cholesterol level are increased cholesterol synthesis and a decrease in the amount of bile. Cholesterol gradually precipitates out of solution, with the end result being the formation of gallstones (see Fig. 20-4).

Many persons have gallstones but no symptoms, that is, they have "silent gallstones." Others may experience severe, steady pain in the epigastric area that lasts for at least 20 minutes and usually up to 2–4 hours. There may be pain between the shoulder blades or in the right

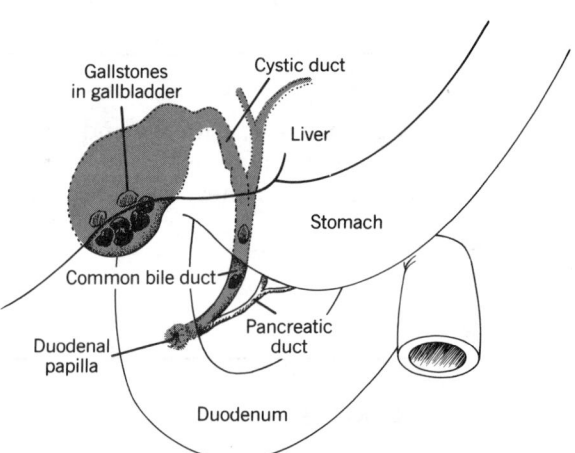

FIGURE 20-4 Gallstones in the gallbladder and common bile duct. (Courtesy of the National Institute of Public Health.)

Cystic duct A duct that drains bile from the gallbladder to the common bile duct.

shoulder. There may be nausea or vomiting. Frequently, gallstones move into the **cystic duct** (see Fig. 20-4), which causes cholecystitis. The symptoms appear after a person eats fatty foods. When fat enters the duodenum, it causes secretion of the hormone cholecystokinin, which stimulates the gallbladder to contract and release bile into the duodenum.

Women are three times more likely than men to develop gallstones. Both men and women who are obese and eat many dairy products plus animal fats are likely to form gallstones.

Dietary Treatment

The goal of diet therapy is to avoid foods that produce painful symptoms or cause the gallbladder to contract. Persons with cholecystitis or cholelithiasis may experience bloating and belching after eating greasy or rich foods or specific foods such as garlic, onions, bell peppers, apples, or other gas formers. Individual food intolerances should be avoided, and a low-fat diet of about 40 g/day will bring relief. See Table 20-2 for foods on each exchange list that are allowed and disallowed.

Protein intake should be normal, but carbohydrate and total kilocalorie intake generally should be decreased, since most people who have gallbladder problems are obese. Restriction of dietary cholesterol has not been shown to reduce the amount of cholesterol synthesized by the liver. The reason is that the liver synthesizes about 60% of the total cholesterol in the body, despite the amount in the diet.

Cholecystectomy Surgical removal of the gallbladder.

If a **cholecystectomy** is performed, a low-fat diet should be continued for a few months. Since bile is synthesized by the liver, after a few months fat can be gradually increased to the amount tolerated by the person.[9]

Drug Treatment

Chenodeoxycholic acid (Chenix) can be administered to dissolve gallstones. This drug is a naturally occurring bile acid that decreases the synthesis of cholesterol. However, the potential side effects (diarrhea and possible liver damage) can be quite severe in some people.[8]

PANCREAS

FUNCTIONS

The pancreas, a rather large gland, extends from the duodenum behind the stomach to the spleen (see Fig. 20-1). Its functions are to secrete digestive enzymes and sodium bicarbonate into the duodenum. See

TABLE 20-2 40-g FAT DIET

Food Group	Foods Allowed	Foods Not Allowed
Milk group (2 cups daily): Milk	Skim milk, nonfat dry milk, buttermilk made from skim milk, condensed skim milk, cocoa made from skim milk, yogurt made from skim milk.	All other milk, including whole milk and low-fat milk (2%), low-fat yogurt.
Meat group (two servings daily) Meat, poultry and fish	Limited to 5 oz daily: lean beef, lamb, ham, veal, or poultry; lean fish such as cod, flounder, haddock, bluefish, perch, bass, whitefish; water-packed salmon and tuna. All meats prepared without fat and served without sauces or gravies.	Fatty meats, bacon, sausage, luncheon meats, frankfurters, corned beef; processed meats, fish, or poultry; fatty fish or fish canned in oil; fried meats; poultry skin.
Eggs	Egg whites as desired; one egg yolk per day may be substituted for 1 oz of meat, if tolerated.	Egg yolks in excess of one per day.
Meat substitutes	Low-fat cheese and uncreamed cottage cheese; dried beans and peas if they do not cause gaseous distress.	All cheese other than those allowed, peanut butter, nuts.
Vegetable and fruit group Potato and substitute	White and sweet potatoes; macaroni, noodles, spaghetti and rice.	Fried potatoes, potato chips, potatoes prepared with cream sauce or butter.
Vegetables	All fresh, frozen, or canned vegetables except those on the avoid list.	All buttered, creamed, or fried vegetables. Omit the following if they cause distress: broccoli, brussel sprouts, cabbage, cauliflower, chives, corn, cucumber, garlic, onion, green pepper, radishes, rutabagas, turnips, sauerkraut.
Fruit	All except those on the avoid list.	Avocado, olives, coconut. If the following cause gaseous distress, they should be omitted: raw apple, melon, and banana.
Bread and cereal group (four servings daily) Bread and crackers	Whole grain and enriched breads except those on the avoid list; graham crackers, soda or saltine crackers.	Hot breads such as muffins, biscuits, pastries, sweet rolls, doughnuts, pancakes, waffles, french toast; high-fat snack crackers.

TABLE 20-2 *(Continued)*

Food Group	Foods Allowed	Foods Not Allowed
Cereals	All except those on the avoid list.	Cereals prepared with chocolate, fat, coconut, or nuts.
Miscellaneous foods		
Fats	3 level tsp daily: butter, margarine or oil, which may be used on bread or in cooking. One strip of crisp bacon may be substituted for 1 tsp of fat if well tolerated.	Any fat in excess of the amount allowed; all fried foods, cream, salt pork, lard, visible fat on meat, gravies, and salad dressings.
Soups	Fat-free broth and bouillon, homemade soup made with skim milk and allowed vegetables.	Commercial soups, cream soups prepared with whole milk.
Desserts and Sweets	Gelatin desserts, sherbet, fruit ices, angle food cake, meringue cookies, pudding made with skim milk; sugar, syrup, honey, jam, jelly, gum drops, plain sugar candy.	Ice cream, rich pastries, pie, cake, cookies. Any prepared with chocolate, coconut, or nuts.
Beverages	Coffee, tea, carbonated beverages	None.
Miscellaneous	Salt, pepper, herbs and spices in moderation, catsup, mustard, vinegar, cocoa, lemon juice, flavoring extracts, nonstick cooking pan spray.	Garlic, barbeque sauce, chili sauce, steak sauce, cream sauce, gravy, nuts, olives, pickles, chocolate, popcorn.

Source: A Diet Manual for Hospitals and Nursing Homes, 3rd ed. Austin: Texas Dietetic Association, 1979. Reprinted by permission.

Chapters 3, 4, and 5 for the specific roles of the enzymes. The sodium bicarbonate neutralizes the acidic chyme that enters the duodenum from the stomach. In addition, the pancreas secretes insulin and glucagon, as described in Chapter 18.

DISORDERS

Pancreatitis

Autodigestion Self-digestion

Pancreatitis is inflammation of the pancreas and may be acute or chronic. This inflammation is an example of **autodigestion**. Normally, the pancreatic enzymes are secreted in an inactive form into the duodenum, where they are activated. Autodigestion is initiated when these inactive enzymes accumulate in the pancreas and become activated. The protein-digesting enzyme trypsin is especially responsible for degradation of the pancreas tissue. The normal endocrine functions (secretion of insulin and glucagon) and exocrine functions (secretion of enzymes) are lost as the pancreatic tissue is degraded and replaced by fibrous tissue.

Cystic fibrosis A genetic disorder characterized by the production of very thick mucus by mucus-producing glands and increased concentration of sodium in sweat.

Pleurisy Inflammation of the pleura membrane that lines and covers the lungs in the thoracic cavity.

Causes and Symptoms. Exactly how the enzymes become activated is not understood. Their blockage and accumulation have been found to result from blockage of the pancreatic duct by gallstones, alcohol abuse, certain drugs (corticosteroids and thiazide diuretics), and **cystic fibrosis**. It is not understood how these factors produce the attacks.

The symptoms usually begin with a mild, steady pain in the upper abdomen, which usually increases in severity and may last for several days. Other symptoms include nausea, vomiting, low-grade fever, increased pulse rate, jaundice, **pleurisy,** and shortness of breath. In the most severe cases, bleeding can occur in the pancreas, leading to shock and often death.

Frequently, acute pancreatitis can result in elevated blood glucose levels due to decreased secretion of insulin and elevated blood lipid levels. Characteristically, amylase (a carbohydrate-splitting enzyme) is found in elevated amounts in the blood

Dietary Treatment. The goal of treatment is to relieve pain by reducing the stimulation of the pancreas and to prevent additional damage to the pancreas.

To reduce stimulation of the pancreas, no food is given by mouth for 24–48 hours. Intravenuos fluids or tube feedings of elemental formulas are administered during this time. Also, to help relieve pain, a nasogastric tube may be inserted and the stomach contents suctioned out.

Once the pain subsides, the diet should consist of clear liquids (see Table 25-1 for details of this diet) followed by progression to a low-fat, high-carbohydrate, high-protein diet. The low-fat diet basically is the same as the one prescribed for gallbladder problems—a 40-g low-fat diet (see Table 20-2).

The low-fat diet is important because pancreatitis is almost always accompanied by steatorrhea as a result of a decreased level of pancreatic lipase. In addition to low-fat foods, the diet should include MCT oils (which are readily absorbed without requiring digestion), MCT margarines, or preparations that combine sugar, vitamins, essential fatty acids, and minerals with MCT oils such as Portagen or Pregestimil. Approximately 3 tbsp of MCT oil can be added each day to foods such as skim milk, homemade salad dressing, and milkshakes made of whole milk, sugar, and vanilla. The MCTs should reduce the steatorrhea as well as enhance the absorption of fat-soluble vitamins, which should be increased.[10]

Alcohol, as well as any other gastric irritants, must be totally eliminated. Gradually the person progresses to six small, bland meals. As mentioned above, it is not uncommon for pancreatitis to result in decreased insulin secretion; therefore, if the blood glucose level begins to rise, the amount of carbohydrates should be lowered and complex carbohydrates should be generally used.

Drug Treatment. Antacids shoulds be given to help neutralize the acidic bile that enters the duodenum, since the secretion of bicarbonate from the pancreas is hindered. The antacids also enhance the activity of pancreatic enzymes (Cotazym, Cotazym-s) that can be given in tablet or capsule form with or before meals.[8]

Cystic Fibrosis

Cystic fibrosis is a genetic disorder that is usually evident in early infancy, with the diagnosis being often made before 6 months of age. This disorder is characterized by production of very thick mucus by the mucus-producing glands and an increased concentration of sodium in sweat. Cystic fibrosis can affect many organs, but the lungs and pancreas are affected most severely, as described:

Pancreas. The thick mucus blocks the entrance of pancreatic enzymes into the duodenum. As a result, the digestion of carbohydrates, proteins, and especially fats is impaired. The buildup of enzymes gradually results in destruction, atrophy, and replacement of pancreatic tissue with fibrous tissue.

Lungs. Mucus clogs the bronchi and bronchioles (cartilaginous air tubes in the lungs), which can result in overinflation, emphysema, and **atelectasis.** In addition, the mucus leads to recurrent pulmonary infections such as pneumonia and even respiratory failure. Management of pulmonary complications is critical in determining the survival of a cystic fibrosis patient.[11]

Atelectasis A collapsed state of the lungs, which may involve all or part of the lungs.

The impairment of digestion and absorption in cystic fibrosis often cause the child to be malnourished or fail to gain weight. As a result, many young patients experience growth failure, and are short and very thin for their age. Fat malabsorption in cystic fibrosis is especially serious, with steatorrhea, osteoporosis, and low levels of fat-soluble vitamins being the result.

Dietary Treatment. The goals of dietary treatment of cystic fibrosis are as follows:

• To provide adequate protein for growth and immunity

• To provide adequate kilocalories for growth and development

• To prevent or control pulmonary infections

• To maintain electrolyte balance (especially sodium)

In reality, providing adequate nutrients and kilocalories requires increases in most of them, since a cystic fibrosis patients does not absorb nutrients very effeciently.

Hydrolysates Solutions
with amino acids.

Protein intake should be 6–8 g per kilogram of ideal body weight, or about twice the normal amount for growth, to compensate for the amount that is not absorbed. Infants with cystic fibrosis are usually given high-protein formulas (e.g., Pregestimil and Albumaid) with protein **hydrolysates** that do not equire digestion. For noninfant CF patients, the best protein foods are those that provide the most protein, vitamins, and minerals while keeping dietary fats to a minimumm. Broiled, stewed, or roasted lean meats, fish, and fowl are best.

Kilocalorie intake should be increased by 50–100% over the child's RDA, or to about 150 kcal/per kilogram of ideal body weight per day. This increased amount is required to offset malabsorption and to help fight the frequent infections that occur. In addition, the increased kilocalories are required for the patient's laborious breathing.

Simple carbohydrate intake should be high in order to help supply the increased level of kilocalories. However, complex carbohydrates should be decreased, since they require the enzyme amylase to be digested.

If the person experiences steatorrhea and abdominal pain, fat intake may have to be reduced to 25–30 g/day. If there is no steatorrhea, the level of fat tolerated can be individualized. MCT oils are recommended especially for those who do not tolerate fat well.

An increase in salt to 2–4 g/day may be needed to offset that lost through perspiration, especially during periods of fever, diarrhea, and increased sweating. Iron must also be increased, since pancreatic enzymes (discussed under the heading "Drug Treatment") decrease its absorption.

Water- and fat-soluble vitamin supplements are usually given, with riboflavin being especially important due to the high level of kilocalories. Vitamin A is very important since it maintains the integrity of the respiratory and digestive mucosae. Another fat-soluble vitamin that must be increased is vitamin K, since antibiotic therapy destroy many intestinal bacteria. Fat-soluble vitamins should be given in a water-miscible form, since they can be absorbed in water or in the absence of fat.

Drug Treatment. Pancreatic enzyme supplements are an important part of successful treatments, with Cotazym and Cotazym-s being examples. A pancreatic powder (Viokase) may be used in carbohydrate foods. Pancreatic supplements should never be mixed with the formula of an infant.

Other drugs that are given are antibiotics to help fight or reduce infections. Expectorants or mucolytic drugs are used to thin bronchial mucous secretions, factilitating their removal. Bronchodilator drugs are also given to dilate bronchial tubes and increase the passage of air into the lungs. The nutritional side effects of these drugs vary, depending on the specific drug, but include nausea, anorexia, vomiting, and diarrhea. While these drugs will reduce the respiratory problems of a cystic fibrosis patient, they may interfere with the person's digestion and absorption.

CASE STUDY: LIVER DISEASE

Mr. E. is an alcoholic who has been drinking heavily for the past 8 years. Recently, he has been experiencing abdominal pain, fatigue, and anorexia and has noticed jaundice in his eyes. In addition, he complains of frequent itching of his skin. The physical and laboratory findings are as follows:

Physical Findings:	
2+ peripheral edema	Palmar erythema
Jaundice	Weight loss (156 lb), with
Spider angiomas	usual weight being 166 lb

Laboratory Findings:		*Normal Values*
Serum albumin	2.8 g/dl	3.5–5.0 g/dl
Serum potassium	3.0 mEq/liter	3.2–4.6 mEq/liter
Total bilirubin	1.6 mg/dl	0.15–1.0 mg/dl
Prothrombin time	14 seconds	12 seconds
Hemoglobin	9.7 g/dl	13–16 g/dl
Hematocrit	27.6%	42–50%
Serum triglycerides	453 mg/dl	10–200 mg/dl

An upper gastrointestinal tract series reveals esophageal varices.

Diet Prescription:	*Medications:*
High protein	Aldactone
High carbohydrate	Folic acid
Moderate fat	Iron
Low sodium	Cholestyramine
Fluid restriction 1,000 ml/day	
Smooth diet	

1. Some of Mr. E's symptoms and their causes are:
    1. jaundice—bile secretion prevented by liver cell destruction and bile absorbed into the blood.
    2. high blood triglyceride level—inability of the liver to synthesize lipoproteins
    3. ascites—drop in blood osmotic pressure due to decreased albumin
    4. spider angiomas—dilation of blood vessels due to portal hypertension

   A. 1, 2, 3   B. 1, 3   C. 2, 4   D. 4   E. all of these

2. Which of the following nutrient values are appropriate for Mr. E?

    1. 10–15 g protein   3. 25–30 g fat
    2. 400 g carbohydrate   4. 3,000 kcal

   A. 1, 2, 3   B. 1, 3   C. 2, 4   D. 4   E. all of these

3. Mr. E was placed on a 250-mg (11-mEq) sodium diet, the purpose of which is to _____.
   A. reduce deposition of sodium in the liver
   B. reduce ascites and peripheral edema
   C. decrease the load on the kidneys
   D. none of these

4. Based on Mr. E's weight (156 lb or 71 kg) and the normal allowance of protein on a high-protein intake, Mr. E's protein intake should be _____ g.
   A. 100–142
   B. 55–85
   C. 23–32
   D. none of these

5. If Mr. E's condition worsened to prehepatic coma, which of the protein values in question 4 would be appropriate for this condition?
   A. 100–142 g
   B. 55–85 g
   C. 23–32 g
   D. none of these

6. Which of the following foods are the best sources of protein and lipotropic factors?
   A. sardines, liver, egg yolks, cereals
   B. milk, pinto beans, peanuts, soybeans
   C. hard cheese, legumes, peanut butter
   D. none of these

7. A moderate amount of fat is prescribed to _____.
   A. absorb fat-soluble vitamins
   B. increase the palatibility of meals
   C. provide kilocalories
   D. all of these

8. The smooth diet will help relieve which of Mr. E's problems?
   A. portal hypertension
   B. low albumin levels
   C. esophageal varices
   D. none of these

9. To facilitate the metabolism of carbohydrates, help correct the decreased prothrombin level, and provide collagen for tissue regeneration, his diet should include which of the following vitamin supplements?
   A. thiamin, vitamin A, vitamin E, and vitamin B_{12}
   B. thiamin, vitamin K, vitamin C
   C. vitamin A, vitamin D, vitamin E
   D. none of these

10. The role of the medications that Mr. E is taking is:
    1. spironolactone—a diuretic that blocks the activity of sodium
    2. folic acid—increases the level of prothrombin
    3. cholestyramine—decreases itching by decreasing the absorption of bile
    4. iron—increases hematocrit and hemoglobin
       A. 1, 2, 3   B. 1, 3, 4   C. 2, 3   D. 2   E. all of these

11. Some of the nutritional side effects of cholestyramine are reductions in _____?
    A. vitamin K, folic acid, iron, and fat
    B. vitamin B_{12}, MCTs, iron, and calcium
    C. thimain, protein, fat, vitamin C, and vitamin A
    D. none of these

OUTLINE

LIVER

Functions
Synthesis, decomposition, storage, and detoxification.

Diseases

Hepatitis
Viral infection.

Symptoms: fatigue, anorexia, jaundice, light stools, elevated enzyme levels (SGOT and SGPT), enlargement of the liver, and abnormal liver function test.

Cirrhosis of the Liver
Inflammation and scarring of liver tissue followed by replacement with fibrous tissue.

Causes: chronic alcoholism, obstruction, absence of or injury to bile ducts, chronic severe hepatitis, and hemochromatosis.

Symptoms: anorexia, weight loss, fatigue, palmar erythema, spider angioma, jaundice, portal hypertension, esophageal varices, and ascites.

Dietary Treatment of Hepatitis and Cirrhosis
High kilocalories: 35–50 kcal per kilogram of ideal body weight or 2,000–3,000 kcal/day.

High protein: 1.5–2.0 g protein per kilogram of ideal body weight; foods high in lipotropic factors (egg yolks, meat, fish, and cereals) should be increased.

High carbohydrate: 300–400 g/day.

Moderate fat: 25–40% of total kilocalories per day; use of medium-chain triglycerides (MCTs) may help to reduce fatty infiltration of the liver.

Vitamin supplements: thiamin, vitamin K, and vitamin C.

Restriction of sodium: if the person has ascites, intake of sodium has to be restricted to about 22–40 mEq/day (500–920 mg/day).

Drug Treatment of Hepatitis and Cirrhosis
Diuretics: used to decrease ascites; spironolactone (Aldactone) blocks the activity of aldosterone, decreasing the absorption of sodium; a potential complication is hypokalemia.

Cholestyramine (Questran): relieves itching by binding with bile and preventing reabsorption; side effects include reduced absorption of vitamin B_{12}.

Hepatic Coma
This occurs when cirrhosis progresses to the point where the liver cannot adequately detoxify ammonia to urea.

Dietary Treatment
The dietary treatment of cirrhosis and hepatic coma is basically the same, except that treating hepatic coma involves decreasing the amount of dietary protein to 20–40 g/day. If the person is in a coma, a zero protein diet is necessary.

Drug Treatment
Neomycin sulfate (Mycifradin): an antibiotic that destroys bacteria that produce ammonia; possible side effects are reduced absorption of calcium, iron, and vitamin B_{12}.

Lactulose (Cephulac): reduces the amount of ammonia absorbed from the large intestine; possible side effects are diarrhea, flatulence, and abdominal discomfort.

GALLBLADDER

Function
Located on the inferior surface of the liver; stores and concentrates bile and then secretes it into the duodenum when stimulated by the hormone cholecystokinin.

Disorders
Cholecystitis: inflammation of the gallbladder from bacterial infection or gallstones.

Cholelithiasis: formation of gallstones, which are composed primarily of cholesterol.

Gallstone Formation and Symptoms
Theorized to result when cholesterol in bile becomes too concentrated due to increased cholesterol synthesis and a decrease in the amount of bile.

Symptoms: severe, steady pain in the epigastric area; pain between the shoulder blades or in the right shoulder; nausea and vomiting.

Dietary Treatment
Low fat: about 40 g/day.

Protein: normal intake.

Carbohydrate: generally should be decreased, since most people with gallbladder problems are obese.

Drug Treatment
Chenodeoxycholic acid (Chenix), a naturally occurring bile acid, will dissolve gallstones; possible side effects are diarrhea and liver damage.

PANCREAS

Functions
Gland that extends from the duodenum behind the stomach to the spleen.

Functions: Secretes digestive enzymes and sodium bicarbonate into the duodenum; secretes insulin and glucagon.

Disorders
Pancreatitis
Inflammation of pancreatic tissue; accumulation of enzymes that digest tissue; an example of auto-digestion (self-digestion).

Causes: blockage of enzymes entering the duodenum results from gallstones, alcohol abuse, certain drugs (corticosteroids and thiazide diuretics), and cystic fibrosis.

Symptoms: pain in the upper abdomen, nausea, vomiting, low-grade fever, increased pulse rate, jaundice, pleurisy, and shortness of breath.

Dietary Treatment
Main goal is to reduce stimulation to the pancreas and prevent additional damage.

No food by mouth for 24–48 hours; tube or intravenous feeding during this time.

Once pain subsides, there is progression to clear liquid diet and then to a low-fat, high-carbohydrate, high-protein diet. The low-fat diet contains about 40 g, or the same as a gallbladder diet.

To reduce steatorrhea the diet should include MCTs.

Drug Treatment
Antacids neutralize acidic bile from stomach; pancreatic enzymes (Cotazym, Cotazym-s).

Cystic Fibrosis
Genetic disorder that results in excessive amount of very thick mucous; mucous blocks secretion of pancreatic enzymes and clogs respiratory passageways; results in pulmonary infections and respiratory failure.

Dietary Treatment
High protein: 6–8 g per kilogram of body weight; infants should be given high-protein formulas (Pregestimil and Albumaid).

High kilocalories: kilocalories should be increased by 50–100% or about 150 kcal per kilogram of ideal body weight.

High carbohydrate: simple carbohydrates should be increased but complex carbohydrates should be reduced, since they require the enzyme amylase to be digested.

Low fat: if the person experiences steatorrhea and abdominal pain, fat intake has to be decreased to 25–30 g/day.

Increased salt: to 2–4 g/day to offset that lost through perspiration.

Increased amounts of fat- and water-soluble vitamins: riboflavin is especially important due to the high kilocalorie intake; vitamin A is important for the respiratory and intestinal mucosae; vitamin K is increased because of destruction of intestinal bacteria by antibiotics.

Drug Treatment
Pancreatic enzymes (Cotazym and Cotazym-s) are given to help digest food.

Antibiotics: fight or reduce infections.

Expectorants or mucolytic drugs: thin bronchial mucous secretions.

Bronchiodilator drugs: dilate bronchial tubes to allow more air into lungs.

REVIEW QUESTIONS

TRUE (A) OR FALSE (B)
Questions 1–27

1. The metabolic functions of the liver can be grouped into synthesis, decomposition, storage and detoxification.
2. The most common cause of cirrhosis is hepatitis.
3. Development of fatty liver in cirrhosis results from the inability of the liver to synthesize enough lipoproteins to transport fats out of the liver.
4. Portal hypertension followed by the development of collateral blood channels and esophageal varices results from the inability of the liver to detoxify urea.
5. Many of the dietary modifications for cirrhotic patients are based on preventing or reducing ascites.
6. Three major changes that lead to the development of ascites are decreases in the following—hydrolysis of lipids, vitamin and mineral storage, and synthesis of cholesterol.
7. The diet prescription for hepatitis and cirrhosis is high kilocalories (30 kcal/kg), high protein (0.8 g/kg), high carbohydrate (150 g/day) and moderate fat.
8. Three important roles of protein in hepatitis and cirrhosis are to repair and restore liver tissue, to form bile acids, and to provide lipotropic factors.
9. Restricting sodium in cases of ascites is common but may also restrict sources of protein, since foods high in sodium frequently are also high in protein.
10. Two drugs that are frequently administered to cirrhosis patients are diuretics (spironolactone) to reduce itching and cholestyramine to help reduce ascites.

11. Spironolactone can decrease the level of blood potassium and cholestyramine can reduce the absorption of vitamin B_{12}, MCTs, iron, and calcium.

12. A person showing signs of hepatic coma (disorientation and behavioral changes) should be on a diet that includes 60–80 g protein per day.

13. Two drugs and their effects in improving hepatic coma are lactulose, which destroys ammonia-producing bacteria in the intestines, and neomycin sulfate, which reduces the amount of ammonia absorbed.

14. Possible nutritional side effects of lactulose are diarrhea, flatulence, and abdominal discomfort.

15. Two possible reasons for the formation of gallstones are increased cholesterol synthesis and a decreased amount of bile synthesized by the liver.

16. The persons most likely to develop gallstones are men and women who are obese and eat many dairy products and animal fats.

17. The diet for patients with cholecystitis or cholelithiasis is very low in fat (20 g or less), high in protein (1.5 g/kg) and high in carbohydrates (300–400 g).

18. A person who has had the gallbladder surgically removed (cholecystectomy) has to be on a low-fat diet, due to decreased bile production, for the rest of his or her life.

19. Pancreatitis is an example of autodigestion, in which pancreatic enzymes are not secreted and their accumulation results in digestion of pancreatic tissues.

20. The dietary goals of treatment of pancreatitis are to relieve pain by reducing stimulation of and prevent additional damage to the pancreas.

21. Steatorrhea may be a problem with cirrhosis but not with pancreatitis.

22. MCTs are important in a pancreatic diet because they enhance the absorption of proteins.

23. Drug treatment of pancreatitis includes antacids to help neutralize acidic bile and pancreatic enzymes (Cotazym).

24. Cystic fibrosis is a genetic disorder that severely affects the liver and intestines.

25. Cystic fibrosis results in little digestion of nutrients, especially fats, since mucous blocks the secretion of pancreatic enzymes.

26. A cystic fibrosis diet might include 6–8 g of protein per kilogram of body weight for growth and to compensate for the amount that is not absorbed.

27. Vitamins A and K are increased in cystic fibrosis diets, with K being important to maintain the integrity of respiratory and digestive mucosa.

MULTIPLE CHOICE

Questions 28–38.

28. Hepatic coma can result from which liver malfunction?
    A. hydrolysis of lipids
    B. synthesis of cholesterol
    C. detoxification of ammonia to urea
    D. production of bile

29. Major changes in a cirrhosis patient that leads to the development of ascites are:
    1. decreased albumin
    3. hyperaldosteronism
    2. portal hypertension
    4. decreased bile production
    A. 1, 2, 3   B. 1, 3   C. 2, 4   D. 4
    E. all of these

30. Which of the following are a correct diet prescription for hepatitis and cirrhosis?
    1. high kilocalories (35–60 kcal/kg)
    3. high protein (1.5–2.0 g/kg)
    2. high fat (60–80 g)
    4. high sodium (2–4 g/day)
    A. 1, 2, 3   B. 1, 3   C. 2, 4   D. 4
    E. all of these

31. A potential complication of diuretics like spironolactone to treat ascites is _____.
    A. too rapid of fluid loss
    B. increased level of blood sodium
    C. low level of blood potassium
    D. B, C
    E. A, C

32. Two sources of ammonia that can result in hepatic coma are _____ and _____.
    A. deamination of amino acids—intestinal bacteria from the gastrointestinal tract
    B. conversion of urea in the liver—preformed ammonia in foods
    C. portal vein—liver
    D. none of these

33. Cholelithiasis and cholecystitis patients may receive relief from a diet that consists of:
    A. low fat (60–80 g/day)
       high protein (1.5 g/kg/day)
       high carbohydrate (300–400 g/day)
    B. low fat (40 g/day)
       normal protein (0.8 g/kg)
       decreased kilocalories for weight loss
    C. moderate fat (90–120 g/day)
       low protein (0.4 g/kg)
       normal carbohydrate (50% of total kilocalories)
    D. none of these

34. Symptoms of gallstones are:
    1. epigastric pain   2. nausea and vomiting

3. pain in the right shoulder
4. appearance of symptoms after eating fatty foods
   A. 1, 2, 3   B. 1, 3   C. 2, 4   D. 4
   E. all of these

35. Pancreatitis can result in loss of _____ and _____, which are the normal pancreatic functions.
   A. insulin and glucagon secretion—secretion of cholecystokinin
   B. bile secretion—cholesterol synthesis
   C. insulin and glucagon secretion—of enzymes secretion
   D. none of these

36. Cystic fibrosis patients experience great difficulty in digesting and absorbing nutrients, especially fats; the reason is _____.
   A. damage to the liver
   B. thick mucus blocks the secretion of enzymes from the pancreas
   C. there is no bile from the gallbladder
   D. an acidic condition in the stomach destroys enzymes

37. Dietary treatment for cystic fibrosis includes:
   1. high protein (6–8 g/kg) for growth
   2. low kilocalories for weight loss
   3. high carbohydrate intake but a decrease in complex carbohydrates, since they require the enzyme amylase for digestion
   4. low salt level due to the presence of edema
   A. 1, 2, 3   B. 1, 3   C. 2, 4   D. 4
   E. all of these

38. Drug treatment for cystic fibrosis includes:
   A. pancreatic enzyme supplements
   B. antibiotics to fight infections
   C. expectorants or mucolytic agents to thin mucus secretions
   D. bronchodilator drugs to dilate the bronchi
   E. all of these

DISCUSSION QUESTIONS

1. Describe the dietary treatment of hepatitis and cirrhosis in relation to the amounts of kilocalories, protein, carbohydrate, fat, vitamin supplements, and sodium.

2. Discuss the differences in the dietary treatment of hepatic coma compared to hepatitis and cirrhosis.

3. Discuss the roles of antibiotics and lactulose in the treatment of hepatic coma.

4. Discuss the dietary and drug treatments of cystic fibrosis.

REFERENCES

1. T.R. Lankford *Integrated Science for Health Students*. Reston, Va.: Reston Publishing Co., 1983, pp. 392–393.
2. L.S. Brunner and D.S. Suddarth. *Textbook of Medical-Surgical Nursing*, 5th ed. Philadelphia: J.B. Lippincott Co., 1984, pp. 862–869.
3. D.H. Van Thiel et al. "Gastrointestinal and hepatic manifestations of chronic alcoholism." *Gastroenterology, 81,* 594–615 (1981).
4. J. Smith et al. "Enteral hyperalimentation in undernourished patients with cirrhosis and ascites. "*American Journal of Clinical Nutrition, 35,* 56–72 (1982).
5. R.P. Dodd. "Ascites: When the liver can't Cope." *RN, 47*(10), 26–30 (1984).
6. "Dietary treatment of Hepatic Encephalopathy." *Nutrition and the M.D., 8* (8), 4 (1982).
7. P.S. Johnson and T.G. Jensen. *The Diet and Nutrition Reference of Hermann Hospital and the University of Texas Medical School at Houston.* Houston: Hermann Hospital, 1980, pp. 44–45.
8. *Drugs: Nurse's Reference Library.* Springhouse, Pennsylvania: Intermed Communications, Inc., 1982.
9. C.J. Thorpe and J.A. Caprini. "Gallbladder disease: Current trends and treatments. "*American Journal of Nursing, 80,* 2181 (1980).
10. B.G. Morrissey. *Therapeutic Nutrition.* Philadelphia: J.B. Lippincott Co., 1984, pp. 305–308.
11. S.A. Price and L.M. Wilson. *Pathophysiology: Clinical Concepts of Disease Processes*, 2nd ed. New York: McGraw-Hill Book Co., 1982, p. 440.

21

DISEASES OF THE CARDIOVASCULAR SYSTEM

OBJECTIVES

Upon completion of this chapter, you should be able to:

1. Describe atherosclerosis in terms of the modifications of blood vessels.

2. Name the nonmodifiable and modifiable risk factors of atherosclerosis.

3. Discuss how dietary modifications of cholesterol, polyunsaturated versus saturated fats, and fiber can influence the development of atherosclerosis.

4. Distinguish between type II and type IV hyperlipoproteinemia in terms of lipid elevation, age range and frequency, and characteristics.

5. Distinguish between dietary and drug treatment of type II and type IV hyperlipidemia.

6. Discuss the role of kilocalories, sodium intake, calcium and magnesium, and potassium on essential hypertension.

7. Name the components of a stepped care approach in the treatment of hypertension.

8. Discuss specific details of a moderate sodium-restricted diet in treating hypertension.

9. Give two examples of diuretics, sympatholytics, and vasodilator drugs and their effects in controlling hypertension.

10. Describe three nutritional ways in which the workload on the heart can be reduced in a myocardial infarct patient.

11. Discuss the effects of two antiarrhythmic drugs and their side effects on the heart.

12. Give two examples of cardiotonic glycoside drugs in terms of their effects and nutritional side effects in treating congestive heart failure.

INTRODUCTION

Cardiovascular diseases are diseases of the blood vessels and the heart. In 1979, over 50% of all deaths in the United States were due to cardiovascular diseases.[1] Approximately one-fourth of these people were under age 65, with an average life expectancy of 69 for men and 77 for women. In addition to the high number of premature deaths, the cost of cardiovascular disease was $26.7 billion in 1977.[2]

ATHEROSCLEROSIS

Atherosclerosis The thickening and loss of elasticity of the walls of arteries.

Atheroma An abnormal mass of fatty or lipid material with a fibrous covering often found in the inner lining of arteries.

Lumen Inner open space in a tube such as blood vessel or the intestine.

A major cardiovascular disease is **atherosclerosis.** "Hardening of the arteries," the lay term for atherosclerosis, occurs in the walls of medium- and large-sized arteries. There are several causes of atherosclerosis, but the only one that is treatable by nutrition is the accumulation of fatty plaques. The thickening of the arterial walls results from **atheroma** (see Fig. 21-1). The plaques initially are composed primarily of cholesterol and later may become encapsulated by fibrous tissue. As the plaques enlarge, they decrease the **lumen** and elasticity of the arteries. These changes decrease the amount of blood flowing through the arteries, as well their ability to dilate and contract. The amount of blood reaching the tissues decreases and the heart has to work harder to pump blood through the narrowed arteries.

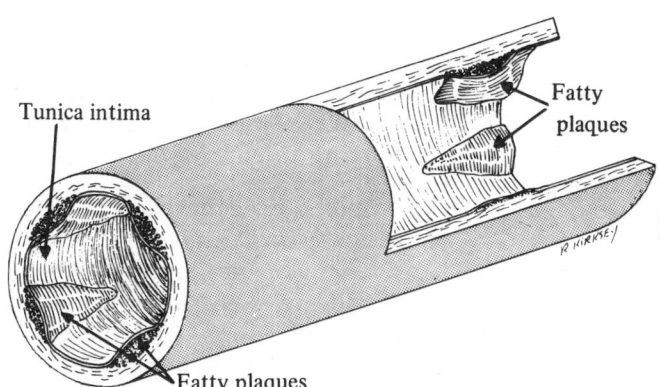

FIGURE 21-1 Fatty plaques inside arteries. (From T. Randall Lankford, *Integrated Science for Health Students*, 3rd ed., 1984. Reprinted by permission of Reston Publishing Company, a Prentice-Hall Company, 11480 Sunset Hills Road, Reston , Va. 22090)

Coronary arteries Arteries that supply blood to the myocardium (heart tissue).

Ischemia The lack of blood flow and oxygen to a body part that is often due to an obstruction of an artery, as in atherosclerosis.

Angina pectoris Acute pain in the chest resulting from ischemia of the heart muscle.

Necrosis Death of tissue.

Myocardial infarction A condition in which a portion of the heart tissue becomes necrotic. Commonly referred to as a *heart attack*.

Atherosclerosis of the **coronary arteries** initially results in **ischemia,** which is indicated by **angina pectoris** pain. Prolonged ischemia heart disease can result in **necrosis.** The lay term for this condition is *heart attack* and the medical term is **myocardial infarction.**

CAUSATIVE FACTORS

It is believed that many factors interact to cause atherosclerosis. They are referred to as *risk factors* and are classified as nonmodifiable and modifiable factors.

Nonmodifiable Biologic Risk Factors

Age, sex, and family history are examples of nonomidifiable factors.

Age. Research and statistics show that cases of coronary atherosclerosis increases with age, especially after age 40.

Sex. Women before menopause are less susceptible to atherosclerosis than men. After menopause, women are equally susceptible. Estrogen has been theorized as the possible reason why women have greater immunity than men.

Family history. The chances of developing atherosclerosis appear to be higher if it has been detected in close relatives (parents, brothers, and sisters). It is not known how genetic inheritance predisposes a person to atherosclerosis; however, it is theorized that it may be linked to familial disorders (type III and type V hyperlipidemia) or obesity.

Modifiable Risk Factors

Major risk factors in the development of atherosclerosis are elevated blood lipid level, hypertension, cigarette smoking, diabetes mellitus, and a high-fat diet. All these factors can be altered, decreasing the chances of developing atherosclerosis.

Elevated blood lipids levels. An elevation of the level of blood lipids (cholesterol, triglycerides, and phospholipids) is called *hyperlipidemia* and is a potent indicator of the severity and prematurity of the disease. The blood cholesterol level relates most directly to the risk of developing atherosclerosis. The American Heart Association states that a person whose blood cholesterol level is consistenly above 250 mg/dl has a threefold increased risk of developing atherosclerosis. The optimal cholesterol level is under 200 mg/dl.

Hypertension. High blood pressure, or hypertension, exists when the systolic pressure is over 140 mm Hg and the diastolic pressure is 90 mm Hg. Increased blood pressure pushes lipids into the arterial wall with great force; therefore, a greater risk of plaque development exists. A person with a systolic blood pressure above 150 mm Hg has twice as great a risk of developing atherosclerosis as a person with a systolic pressure under 120 mm Hg.

Cigarette smoking. Smoking is apparently related to atherosclerosis in that the nicotine in cigarettes is a vasoconstrictor, which decreases blood flow through arteries.

Diabetes mellitus. Research has shown that diabetics experience a greater number and more severe cases of atherosclerosis than nondiabetics. The exact reason is unknown, but it may result from their high level of blood lipids.

High-fat diet. A diet that has a high concentration of cholesterol and saturated fat contributes to hyperlipidemia and obesity. Both of these conditions increase the stress or workload on the heart.[2]

Three other risks that contribute to coronary heart disease are sedentary life-style, psychological stress, and personality type. Stress always results in the release of large amounts of epinephrine and norepinephrine, which can result in an increase in blood pressure and pumping by the heart. Research shows that psychological stress is handled by some people in such a way as to increase their risk of developing atherosclerosis. These people have a personality characterized by intense competitiveness, ambition, aggressiveness, and a sense of time urgency.

As mentioned at the beginning of the discussion of atherosclerosis, various factors interact to cause the disease. This statement is reinforced by the fact that in the presence of two or more factors, the risk of developing atherosclerosis is not additive but rather **synergistic.** As an example, if a person has a high blood cholesterol level and elevated diastolic blood pressure and smokes, his or her chances of having a coronary heart attack are eight times greater than those of someone who does not have any of these risk factors. However, if an individual has only two of these risk factors, his or her chances of having an attack are four times greater than someones who does not have any of them.

Synergistic The combined effect is greater than the sum of the parts.

Diet as a Modifiable Risk Factor

Nutritional experts do not all agree that diet alone can lower the risk of atherosclerosis. However, groups such as the American Heart Association do believe that certain modifications in the diet can reduce the level of cholesterol and triglycerides.

Cholesterol. Chapter 4 discussed the chemical structure, functions, and endogenous and exogenous sources of cholesterol. It was indicated that cholesterol is definitely important in the body. However, an excessive level of cholesterol in the blood is one of the major risk factors in atherosclerosis.

Cholesterol absorption is directly proportional to cholesterol intake. About 40% of dietary cholesterol is absorbed. Therefore, lowering the intake of cholesterol should lower the amount absorbed into the blood. Cholesterol from dietary sources does not have as powerful an effect on serum cholesterol as saturated fat does. Consuming a diet that is low in saturated fat, high in polyunsaturated fat, and low in cholesterol will decrease serum cholesterol levels from 8 to 18%. If cholesterol intakes are reduced to less than 300 mg/day, serum cholesterol levels will decrease regardless of endogenous cholesterol production. Appendix C lists the cholesterol and saturated fat content of some common foods. The principles of a fat-controlled diet are provided in Table 21-1.

It was noted in Chapter 4 that cholesterol and other lipids are transported in the blood as lipoproteins [chylomicrons, very-low-density lipoprotein (VLDL), low-density lipoprotein (LDL), and high-density lipoprotein (HDL)], with VLDL and LDL transporting the majority of cholesterol from the liver to the tissues. HDL transports cholesterol from the tissues or plaques to the liver, where it is decomposed into bile. Research shows that the higher the level of LDL, the greater the risk of atherosclerosis. However, the higher the level of HDL, the lower the risk of atherosclerosis, since this lipoprotein actually lowers the level of serum cholesterol. Dietary LDL is lowered when the saturated fat intake is reduced. Serum HDL levels apparently cannot be increased by diet but rather by increasing exercise. Sustained aerobic exercise for 20 minutes at least four times a week is necessary to raise the serum HDL level.[3]

TABLE 21-1 FAT-CONTROLLED DIET

Purpose:	To reduce serum lipid levels.
Use:	Used for persons with elevated serum cholesterol levels or people who are high-risk candidates for atherosclerosis and coronary heart disease.
Examples of foods:	Based on a general diet with the following adjustments: • Fat is limited to 30% of total kilocalories. • Dietary cholesterol should be limited to 250–300 mg. • Simple sugars and alcohol may be limited, since they can cause elevation of serum triglyceride levels, which is a causative factor in atherosclerosis.
Adequacy:	Diet is adequate.

Source: Chicago Dietetic Association, *Manual of Clinical Dietetics*, 2nd edition. Philadelphia, W.B. Saunders Company, 1981. Reprinted by permission.

Polyunsaturated versus Saturated Fats. Research shows that an increase in polyunsaturated fats (review the discussion of saturated and unsaturated fats in Chapter 4) can reduce the serum cholesterol level. The desirable ratio of polyunsaturated to saturated fats (P:S) is 1:1 and may be achieved in three ways. One way is to add polyunsaturated fat to the diet. The second way is to consume less saturated fat. Table 21-2 presents some suggestions on how to decrease the amount of saturated fat in the diet. The third way is to decrease saturated fat and increase unsaturated fat until a ratio of 1:1 is achieved. Table 21-3 ranks fats and oils from most polyunsaturated to most saturated.

TABLE 21-2 HOW TO DECREASE FAT, ESPECIALLY SATURATED FAT

1. Limit beef, pork, lamb and whole milk cheese consumption to a combined total of 20 ounces per week. (Each ounce contains approximately 1 teaspoon of saturated fat.)
2. When you do eat meat, select the leanest cuts and remove all visible fat before eating.
3. Use poultry, fish and legumes to replace red meat several times a week.
4. Avoid luncheon meats, frankfurters and sausage because they are so high in fat.
5. Skim the fat off broths, soups and gravies.
6. Bake, broil and boil meats. Avoid frying whenever possible.
7. Switch to nonfat or lowfat milk.
   a. Whole milk contains the equivalent of 2 teaspoons of butter per cup.
   b. Lowfat milk contains only about 1 teaspoon of butter per cup.
   c. Nonfat or skim milk contains no butter.
   d. If you prefer whole milk, you can reduce your intake of fats from other sources.
8. Use cheeses made with part skim milk rather than those made with whole milk. Recommended cheeses include:
   a. Cottage, Farmer, Sapsago, Edam, Gouda.
   b. Ricotta, Parmesan, Mozzarella, Gruyere, Jarlesberg Swiss.
9. Decrease your intake of rich dishes made with butter, cream, palm oil, coconut oil and/or cocoa butter.
10. Avoid food products bearing the terms *hardened* or *hydrogenated* vegetable oil.
11. Use only small portions of fresh butter, margarine (listing liquid oil as the first ingredient) and mayonnaise as spreads.
12. Use salad dressings sparingly. (One ladleful can contain as much as 200 calories of fat!)

Source: High Level Health: A Proven Health Promotion Program. Green Bay, WI: Sun Valley Health Institute, 1982. Reprinted with permission.

TABLE 21-3
POLYUNSATURATED OILS

Safflower	Most
Sunflower	polyunsaturated
Corn	
Walnut	
Soybean	
Wesson	
Crisco	
Sesame	least
Cottonseed	polyunsaturated

Source: High Level Health: A Proven
Health Promotion Program. Green Bay,
Wisc.: Sun Valley Health Institute, 1982.
Reprinted with permission.

Fiber. The dietary fiber types lignin, pectin, and guargum (from fruits and oatbran) have been shown to help lower LDL cholesterol levels by approximately 15%. It is suggested that the dietary fiber reduces the absorption of bile acids from the intestinal tract. This reduction causes more cholesterol from the liver to be degraded to bile acids, thereby reducing the serum cholesterol level.

ELEVATED BLOOD LIPID LEVELS

Hyperlipoproteinemia
Elevated blood lipoprotein level.

Persons who have atherosclerosis often have elevated levels of blood lipids, with chylomicrons, triglycerides, and cholesterol being the most common. Hyperlipidemia refers to elevated blood lipid levels and **hyperlipoproteinemia** refers to elevated blood lipoprotein levels. It is not unusual for these two terms to be used inerchangeably.

Types of Hyperlipoproteinemia

There are six basic types of hyperlipoproteinemia: types I, IIa, IIb, III, IV, and V. Types II and IV are the most common, and types I and V are not associated with an increased incidence of atherosclerotic disease. The types of hyperlipoproteinemia are based on which of the classes of lipoproteins (see Chapter 4 for details of the five classes of lipoproteins) are elevated; LDL and VLDL are the ones most commonly elevated.

LDL transport more cholesterol than any other lipoproteins, and VLDL transport primarily triglycerides. Therefore, the two lipids that are primarily elevated are cholesterol and triglycerides. Table 21-4 presents information on which lipids are elevated, as well as the age range, frequency, and characteristics of the four types of hyperlipoproteinemia that are associated with atherosclerosis.

TABLE 21-4 SUMMARY OF HYPERLIPOPROTEINEMIAS

Hyperlipoproteinemia Type	Cholesterol[a] (Normal, 150–250 mg/dl)	Triglycerides (Normal 10–200 mg/dl)	Age Range and Frequency	Characteristics
IIa (autosomal dominant)	300–600	Normal	All ages; severe cases occur in early childhood	Xanthoma (yellowish lesion) in tendons; corneal arcus (whitish line around edge of cornea); premature atherosclerosis
IIb	300–600	150–400	Usually adult; common	Xanthoma (palmar) premature atherosclerosis
III	350–800	400–800	Adult	Xanthoma (palmar) premature atherosclerosis
IV (familial)	Normal or slightly elevated	200–1,000	Adult; very common	Obesity; often develops as a secondary problem with diabetes mellitus

[a]The upper normal value for cholesterol of 250 mg/dl is for people up to age 29. After age 29 the upper normal value rises until at age 50+ the upper normal value is 330 mg/dl.

Autosomal dominant trait A dominant gene that is present on one of the 22 pairs of genes known as *autosomes*.

Nephrosis Kidney disease that is characterized by a large loss of proteins in the urine and edema (see Chapter 23).

Type IIa is a relatively common type of hyperlipoproteinemia, since it can be inherited as an **autosomal dominant trait.** It is not unusual for the problem to be detected in infants by 1 year of age. Premature atherosclerosis occurs rapidly, often resulting in death by age 30. This type of lipoproteinemia, as well as the others, can result from either primary causes (inherited disorders) or secondary causes (conditions such as diabetes, **nephrosis,** or obesity). Secondary causes of type IIa include nephrosis, **hypothyroidism,** and biliary obstruction. Once elevated blood lipid levels are detected, secondary causes must be ruled out before the appropriate treatment can be determined.

Type IV is probably the most common form of hyperliproproteinemia. While it can be genetically inherited, most causes result from the diet. Secondary causes include uncontrolled diabetes, alcohol abuse, renal dialysis, pregnancy, and pancreatitis. It is very common to find type IV hyperlipoproteinemia associated with diabetes and obesity.[4]

DIETARY AND DRUG TREATMENT OF LIPOPROTEIN DISORDERS

A summary of the dietary treatment of types II–IV hyperlipoproteinemia is presented in Table 21-5. Diet is the basic treatment of hyperlipoproteinemia. In some cases, diet alone is not effective and drugs must also be used. The following discussion presents the goals of dietary and drug treatment of hyperlipoproteinemia. In addition, details of dietary and drug treatment of type II will be compared with those of type IV.

TABLE 21-5 SUMMARY OF TYPES II–IV HYPERLIPOPROTEINEMIA

	Type IIa	Type IIb and Type III	Type IV
Diet prescription	Low cholesterol polyunsaturated fat increased	Low cholesterol Approximately: 20% Cal. Protein 40% Cal. Fat 40% Cal. CHO	Controlled CHO (approx. 45% calories) Moderately restricted cholesterol
Calories	Not restricted	Achieve and maintain "ideal" weight, i.e. reduction diet if necessary	Achieve and maintain "ideal" weight, i.e., reduction diet if necessary
Protein	Not restricted	High protein	Not restricted except to limit weight
Fat	Saturated fat intake limited Polyunsaturated fat intake increased	Controlled to 40% of calories (polyunsaturated fats recommended in preference to saturated fats)	Not limited other than control of pts. wt. (polyunsaturated fats recommended in preference to saturated fats)
Cholesterol	As low as possible; only source of chol. is meat in diet	Less than 300 mg. only source of chol. is meat in diet	Moderately restricted to 300–500 mg.
Carbohydrate	Not limited	Controlled; concentrated sweets are restricted	Controlled concentrated sweets are restricted
Alcohol	May be used with discretion	Limited to 2 servings (subst. for CHO)	Limited to 2 servings (subst. for CHO)

The Dietary Management of Hyperlipoproteinemia. A Handbook for Physicians and Dietitians. National Heart and Lung Institute, Bethesda, Md. Revised 1974.

Goals and Principles of Diet and Drug Therapy

The goals of the therapy are to reduce cholesterol and triglycerides to desirable levels. Its achievement requires permanent changes in eating habits that must be followed for life. Generally, drugs are not used to treat hyperlipoproteinemia unless diet therapy has been unsuccessful for at least 3 months.

Lowering the cholesterol level with diet therapy generally can be achieved by:

• Restricting cholesterol intake to less than 300 mg/day

• Reducing saturated fat intake

• Increasing polyunsaturted fat intake

An elevated level of cholesterol is the basic problem with type II hyperlipoproteinemia; therefore, the following comments are applicable to lowering cholesterol levels. (*See Case Study: Hyperlipoproteinemia, at end of chapter, for reinforcement and application of hyperlipoproteinemia information.*)

The P:S ratio is more important than the amount of fat in the diet. A P:S ratio of 2:1 is most beneficial in reducing blood cholesterol level. In order to restrict cholesterol, the diet must exclude egg yolks and liver. In addition, beef and pork intakes should be limited. (See Appendix C for cholesterol values of specific foods.)

The P:S ratio can be accomplished by increasing the intake of polyunsaturated foods such as tub margarines and liquid oils and increasing the intake of vegetables. Saturated fats can be reduced by restricting the

---

SAMPLE MENU FOR TYPE IIa HYPERLIPOPROTEINEMIA

Exchange	
	Breakfast
1 fruit	½ cup orange juice
1 bread	¾ cup corn flakes
1 medium-fat meat	1 omelet made with egg substitute
1 bread	1 slice whole wheat toast
1 fat	1 tsp margarine
	1 tsp jelly
1 milk	1 cup skim milk
	1 cup coffee
	Lunch
3 lean meat	3 oz fish (halibut, trout, red snapper, etc.)
1 bread	1 small potato
1 vegetable	½ cup sliced tomatoes
	½ cup shredded lettuce
1 fat	1 tsp french dressing
1 bread	1 slice french bread
1 fat	1 tsp low-fat margarine
	4 oz angel food cake
	iced tea with lemon and sugar

	Dinner
	1 cup beef bouillon
3 lean meat	3 oz broiled chicken (no skin)
1 vegetable	½ cup green beans
1 bread	1 slice whole wheat bread
1 fat	1 tsp low-fat margarine
1 fruit	1 medium peach
1 milk	1 cup skim milk
	iced tea with lemon and sugar

Analysis and Comments

- An analysis of the menu shows that it contains 2 milk, 2 vegetable, 2 fruit, 5 bread, 7 meat, and 4 fat exchanges.
- The cholesterol level is kept to less than 300 mg/day by modifications in certain exchanges:

    Milk: skim milk is used as opposed to whole milk, thereby reducing the saturated fat intake.

    Meat: three modifications are used to reduce fat and cholesterol intake. First, 6 of 7 meat exchanges are from the lean group. Second, the 1 medium-fat exchange is an egg substitute as opposed to a whole egg or even an egg yolk. Third, the number of ounces of meat exchanges is 7. In order to reduce cholesterol intake, it is best to keep the total number of meat exchanges to 9 or fewer.

    Bread: no sweet rolls or other breads with added fat should be used.

    Vegetables: vegetables should not be prepared with butter or cream sauces and should not be fried.

    Fat: margarines should be low in fat.

    Miscellaneous: beef bouillon helps to provide some nutrients without adding much cholesterol. Angel food cake is an example of a dessert that is low in cholesterol. Some examples of desserts that are high in cholesterol and should be excluded are commercial cakes, pies, cookies, ice cream, and desserts, which contain whole milk or egg yolks.

Source: Menu adapted from Texas Dietetic Association, *Diet Manual*, 3rd ed. Austin: Texas Dietetic Association, 1981. Reprinted by permission.

consumption of butter, whole milk, coconut oil (used in popping corn commercially), palm oil (found in nondairy creamers), and animal fat as on steaks, chops, and bacon. See the sample menu for type IIa hyperlipoproteinemia.

Persons who follow this diet and increase their physical activity should be able to lower their LDL level and thereby their cholesterol. Increased physical activity will also increase their HDL level, which will lower their cholesterol level.

Lowering triglyceride levels by diet therapy generally can be achieved by:

- Weight reduction
- Carbohydrate restriction
- Elimination of concentrated sweets
- Reduction of alcohol intake

Elevated triglyceride levels is the common lipid disorder in type IV hyperlipoproteinemia. As mentioned above, this disorder is frequently a complication of obesity and diabetes. Therefore, a reduction in daily kilocalories to lose weight will reduce triglyceride levels as well as help reduce obesity and diabetes.

Carbohydrate intake should be almost exclusively from complex carbohydrate sources. Concentrated sweets should be restricted. A major difference in the type IV diet compared to the type II diet is the recommended reduction in alcohol. Alcohol has been found to increase triglyceride levels, whereas it does not affect cholesterol levels. See the sample menu for type IV hyperlipoproteinemia.

Drug Treatment for Types II and IV Hyperlipoproteinemia

As mentioned earlier, if dietary treatment after approximately 3 months has not been successful in lowering cholesterol and triglyceride levels, drugs may be used in conjunction with the diet. Long-term use of a particular antilipemic drug should not continue unless it produces at least a 15% drop in lipid levels within 4–6 weeks or reduction of xanthomas occurs.

Cholestyramine (Questran) and colestipol (Colestid) are two commonly used drugs for type IIa hyperlipoproteinemia. They both lower levels of blood cholesterol by preventing its absorption from the intestines. This mechanism can result in some side effects such as constipation, nausea, vomiting, abdominal discomfort, and vitamin A, D, and K deficiencies from decreased fat absorption.[5] Table 21-6 summarizes information about these drugs.

SAMPLE MENU FOR TYPE IV HYPERLIPOPROTEINEMIA (1,200 KCAL)

Exchange	
	Breakfast
1 fruit	½ cup orange juice
1 bread	¾ cup corn flakes
1 fat	1 tsp margarine
1 milk	1 cup skim milk
	coffee with sugar substitute
	Lunch
3 lean meat	3 oz broiled chicken (no skin)
1 bread	½ cup rice
1 vegetable	½ cup green beans
1 vegetable	½ cup sliced tomatoes
1 fruit	1 small apple
2 fat	2 tsp margarine
1 milk	1 cup skim milk
	iced tea with sugar substitute
	Dinner
3 lean meat	3 oz baked fish (e.g., halibut, trout, red snapper)
1 bread	½ cup mashed potatoes
1 vegetable	½ cup cooked cabbage
1 fruit	12 fresh grapes
1 fat	1 tsp margarine
	iced tea with sugar substitute

Analysis and Comments

- An analysis of this menu shows that it contains 2 milk, 3 vegetable, 3 fruit, 3 bread, 6 meat, and 4 fat exchanges.

- The bread and fruit exchanges are few in order to reduce the amount of carbohydrates.

- Foods from the miscellaneous and other group are limited to those that are low in carbohydrate.

> • The intake of saturated fat is reduced, while the total fat intake is not limited.
>
> *Source:* Menu adapted from Texas Dietetic Association, *Diet Manual,* 3rd ed. Austin: Texas Dietetic Association, 1981. Reprinted by permission.

In addition, cholestyramine and colestipol can reduce the absorption of acidic compounds such as digitalis, warfarin, iron, and tetracyclines. Therefore, these compounds should be given 1 hour before administration of cholestyramine and colestipol.

Clofibrate (Atromid-S) is used in treating types IIb and IV hyperlipoproteinemia. The exact mechanism by which it lowers triglyceride levels is not known. It lowers cholesterol levels mildly by decreasing its synthesis in the liver. Some of the nutritional side effects of the drug are nausea, diarrhea, vomiting, and weight gain.

Nicotinic acid, or niacin, can be used for types II and IV hyperlipoproteinemia, but it is never the first drug of choice. Apparently, it functions to lower the level of cholesterol by reducing the synthesis of LDL. Nicotinic acid can result in severe gastrointestinal upset, headaches, itching, flushing, and hyperglycemia. Table 21-6 summarizes information about clofibrate and nicotinic acid.

Some research groups have found that administering a combination of colestipol (30 g/day) and nicotinic acid (increasing doses up to 6–7.5 g/day) significantly reduces LDL cholesterol levels and the size of xanthomas. The side effects can be prominent and include constipation, gastrointestinal irritation, and **systemic flushing.**

Systemic flushing Redness throughout the body as a whole.

HYPERTENSION

Hypertension is a symptom that is manifested as an elevated **systolic** and/or **diastolic** blood pressure. The major effect of hypertension is on

TABLE 21-6 DRUGS USED IN TYPES II AND IV HYPERLIPOPROTEINEMIA

Type of Hyperlipoproteinemia	Drugs	Lipid Lowered	Nutrition-Related Side Effects
IIa	Cholestyramine (Questran)	Cholesterol	Constipation; abdominal discomfort; vitamin A, D, and K deficiencies;
	Colestipol (Colestid)	Cholesterol	reduced absorption of digitalis, warfarin, iron, and tetracyclines
IV	Clofibrate (Atromid-S)	Triglyceride	Nausea, diarrhea, vomiting, and weight gain
II and IV	Nicotinic acid	Cholesterol and triglyceride	Nausea, vomiting, hyperglycemia

the blood vessels. The increased tension and pressure cause the lining of the blood vessels to become thickened and the lumen narrowed. This thickening and narrowing change the flow of blood to the heart and kidneys and can eventually cause damage to these organs. Hypertension is a major risk factor for heart disease, stroke, and renal disease and affects approximately 18% of adult Americans.

DIAGNOSIS

The diagnosis of hypertension is based on three consecutive readings that are elevated by two or more standard deviations above the norm for the age group. The upper limit of normal blood pressure for the 18- to 44-year-old age group is:

$$\frac{140 \text{ mm Hg (systolic)}}{90 \text{ mm Hg (diastolic)}}$$

Hypertension and degrees of severity are as follows:

Mild hypertension: diastolic pressure 90–104 mm Hg

Moderate hypertension: diastolic pressure 105–114 mm Hg

Severe hypertension: diastolic pressure 115–129 mm Hg

Malignant hypertension: diastolic pressure greater than 130 mm Hg[6]

TYPES AND CAUSES

Essential Hypertension

Essential hypertension A type of hypertension for which there is no known cause.

About 90% of all cases of hypertension are essential. While there is no known cause of essential hypertension, factors that can influence it are genetic predisposition (approximately 20% of the population is so predisposed), race (approximately twice as many blacks as whites), body weight, level of exercise, cigarette smoking, psychological stress, and diet. The following discussion concerns the role of various dietary factors on blood pressure.

Kilocalorie intake. Research shows that weight reduction in overweight hypertensives can reduce their blood pressure.

Sodium intake. Many researchers believe that some of the genetically predisposed individuals are sensitive enough to their current levels of sodium intake to cause hypertension. However, other researchers disagree. Currently, scientific and medical research has not shown that there is a causal relationship between hypertension and sodium consumption at the present levels.[7]

While dietary sodium may not cause hypertension, various groups such as the U.S. Department of Agriculture (USDA) and the Department of Health and Human Services (DHHS) believe that a reduction in the sodium intake of healthy adults would not adversely affect their health.[8] (Details on sodium reduction are presented later)

Calcium and magnesium. Calcium and magnesium are closely inter-related, and some studies have shown that when they are reduced, an increase in blood pressure can occur.[9]

Potassium. The ratio of sodium to potassium may be more important in causing hypertension than the level of sodium alone. The relationship between sodium and potassium is normally inverse. In other words, when there is a high level of potassium there is a low level of sodium. Research indicates that this is the best relationship for preventing hypertension.[10] Current diets tend to be high in sodium and low in potassium; this may be the reason for hypertension in genetically predisposed individuals.

Secondary Hypertension

Secondary hypertension can be traced to a specific disease or disorder such as kidney disease, **primary aldosteronism**, and **Cushing's disease**.

Primary aldosteronism An excessive secretion of the hormone aldosterone from the adrenal gland. It is characterized by hypertension, hypokalemia, muscular weakness, and polydipsia.

Cushing's disease A condition caused by an excessive secretion of hormones from the cortex region of the adrenal glands.

STEPPED CARE TREATMENT PROGRAM FOR HYPERTENSION

People who have at least mild, essential hypertension (basically those with a diastolic pressure between 90 and 104 mm Hg) have recently been helped by a stepped care approach. This approach involves the following:

- Dietary sodium restriction
- Weight control measures
- Moderate exercise
- Drug therapy

Essentially, in this approach the mild hypertensive implements the first three steps (weight control only if necessary) simultaneously. If these steps are not successful in lowering blood pressure to 90 mm Hg or below, drug therapy is also implemented.[11] Only dietary sodium restriction and drug therapy will be discussed at this point, since weight control and exercise have been adequately covered in previous chapters.

Dietary Sodium Restriction

Sodium Level in the Normal Diet. It is estimated that Americans consume about 3 g (1 tsp) to 12 g (5 tsp) of salt (NaCl) per day.[7] However, the amount of sodium (Na) in these same diets varies from 1.2 to 4.8 g. The reason for the difference in the amount of salt (NaCl) and sodium (Na) is that salt is composed of 40% Na and 60% chloride (Cl).

As mentioned in Chapter 7, animal foods generally contain more sodium than plant foods. Therefore, exchange lists that, on the average, contain more sodium are list 1 (milk) and list 5 (meat), but only cured meats such as ham and bacon and some cheeses such as cheddar. One exception to the statement that list 2 (vegetables) is lower in sodium is canned vegetables that do not state "no salt added," since canning normally involves addition of salt. Table 21-7 lists the sodium values for each exchange list.

Sodium Measurement. Sodium may be measured in grams (g), milligrams (mg), and milliequivalents (mEq). The relationships between the three are as follows:

1 g sodium = 1000 mg sodium

1 tsp salt = 2,300 mg sodium = 100 mEq

1 mEq sodium = 23 mg sodium

TABLE 21–7 SODIUM VALUES FOR FOODS ON THE SIX EXCHANGE LISTS

Exchange List	Food Group	Amount	Na+ (mg)	Na+ (mEq)
1	Milk			
	Whole	1 cup	120	5
	Skim	1cup	120	5
	Milk, low sodium	1 cup	7	—
	Buttermilk, salted	1 cup	280	13
2	Vegetables			
	Cooked, raw, fresh, frozen	½ cup	9	—
	Canned	½ cup	230	10
3	Fruits	1 serving	2	—
4	Bread or cereal			
	Low sodium or made without salt	1 slice	5	—
	Salted yeast bread	1 slice	150	7
5	Meat, poultry, fresh fish cooked without salt	1 oz	25	1
	Cheese, cottage (dry)	¼ cup	5	—
	cheddar	1 oz	207	9
	Egg	1	70	3
6	Fat			
	Unsalted	1 tsp	—	—
	Salted		50	2

Levels of Sodium-Restricted Diets. Physicians often use a variety of terms for ordering a sodium-restricted diet. Diet orders should specify the level of sodium in either milligrams or milliequivalents. The following terms are nonspecific, open to a wide range of interpretation, and should not be used without specific *sodium* levels being given: *low salt, no salt, salt free, salt poor, sodium restricted,* and *low sodium.*

The following are standard sodium levels for sodium-restricted diets:[12]

Mild (2,000–3,000 mg; 87–130 mEq sodium) (Approximately 1 to 1¼ tsp of sodium.)

- No more than ½ tsp (1,150 mg sodium) of salt added in cooking.
- No salt added to food at the table.
- No salty foods (crackers, pretzels, potato chips, corn chips, etc.).
- Frequently used as a maintenance diet for hypertension, renal, and heart patients at home.
- See sample menu for 2,000 to 3,000-mg diet.

Moderate (1,000 mg; 44 mEq sodium) (Slightly less than ½ tsp of sodium).

- No salt used in cooking.
- No salt added to food at the table.
- No salty foods.
- Replacement of some natural-sodium foods with foods processed without salt (e.g., salt-free canned vegetables, bread).
- Foods containing moderate amounts of sodium may be limited, such as milk, eggs, and desserts.
- This level is very difficult to achieve as a maintenance diet at home.
- See Sample menu for 1,000 mg; 44 mEg sodium diet.

Strict (500 mg; 22 mEq sodium) (Approximately ¼ of a tsp of sodium)

- First three comments for the above restriction applicable here.
- Meat limited to 5–6 oz total per day
- Replacement of all natural-sodium foods with foods processed without salt.
- Milk is limited to 2 cups or servings per day.

Unsalted margarine is used.

- This level of restriction is extremely difficult to achieve and should be used for only short term or tests in a hospital.

Severe (250 mg; 11 mEq sodium) (Approximately 1/10 of a tsp of sodium)

- Identical to the 500-mg sodium diet except that 2 cups of regular milk must be replaced by low-sodium milk.

SAMPLE MENU FOR A 2,000- to 3,000-mg DIET

Exchange	
	Breakfast
1 fruit	½ cup orange juice
1 bread	½ cup oatmeal
1 milk	1 cup skim milk
1 medium-fat meat	1 poached egg
1 bread	1 slice toast
1 fat	1 tsp margarine
	1 tsp jelly
	1 cup coffee
	4 tsp sugar
	Lunch
	6 oz unsalted vegetable soup
2 medium-fat meat	2 oz beef patty
1 vegetable	½ cup sliced tomatoes
	1 tbsp oil and vinegar dressing
1 fruit	4 halves of dried apricots
	2 sugar cookies
1 milk	1 cup skim milk
	Dinner
1 vegetable	½ cup low-sodium tomato juice
3 lean meat	3 oz broiled chicken
1 bread	½ cup mashed potatoes
1 vegetable	½ cup peas (frozen)
	½ cup fruited jello salad
1 bread	1 slice bread
1 fat	1 tsp margarine
	½ cup orange sherbert
	1 cup coffee

Analysis and Comments

- An analysis of this menu shows that it consists of 2 milk, 3 vegetable, 2 fruit, 4 bread, 6 meat, and 2 fat exchanges.

• The menu does not limit any exchanges. The main restrictions are in foods from the miscellaneous or other group. Notice that the soups are unsalted and that an oil and vinegar dressing is used as opposed to other dressings that are higher in sodium. Also notice that no salty foods (crackers, pretzels, potato chips, or corn chips) are included.

Source: Menu adapted from Chicago Dietetic Association, *Manual of Clinical Dietetics,* 2nd ed. Philadelphia: W.B. Saunders Company, 1981. Reprinted by permission.

• This diet should be used only in cases of extreme edema or for hospital tests.

The principles of sodium-controlled diets are provided in Table 21–8.

Another source of sodium that needs to be considered is the public water supply. The sodium standard for public water should be about 20 mg/liter, as recommended by the American Heart Association, to help protect heart and kidney patients. However, public water supplies may contain more or less sodium, depending on the geographic location. Water containing over 100 mg/liter of sodium probably should be avoided by hypertensives, who instead should use bottled, distilled water for drinking and cooking.[13]

Specific Details of Dietary Restriction. Moderate sodium restriction (to approximately 1,000 mg sodium) in two recent controlled trials has been found to be successful in lowering blood pressure.[11]

In addition to lowering sodium, increasing potassium in the diet is important. These two dietary changes helps to achieve a low-sodium, high-potassium diet, which, as discussed earlier, is beneficial in lowering blood pressure. Foods naturally high in potassium are those on the fruit exchange, 4, list with oranges, bananas, and dried fruits. Foods from the meat exchange list, 5, and the vegetable exchange list, 2, contain smaller amounts.

SAMPLE MENU FOR A 1,000-mg DIET

Exchange	
	Breakfast
1 fruit	½ cup orange juice
1 bread	½ cup unsalted oatmeal

1 milk	1 cup skim milk
1 medium-fat meat	1 unsalted poached egg
1 bread	1 slice regular toast
1 fat	1 tsp unsalted margarine
	1 tbsp jelly
	1 cup coffee
	4 tsp sugar

Lunch	
	6 oz unsalted vegetable soup
3 medium-fat meat	3 oz unsalted beef patty
1 vegetable	½ cup sliced tomatoes
	1 tbsp vinegar and oil dressing
1 fruit	4 dried apricot halves
1 milk	1 cup skim milk

Dinner	
1 vegetable	½ cup low-sodium tomato juice
3 lean meat	3 oz unsalted broiled chicken
1 bread	½ cup unsalted mashed potatoes
1 vegetable	½ cup low-sodium canned peas
	½ cup fruited jello salad
1 bread	1 slice regular bread
1 fat	1 tsp unsalted margarine
	½ cup orange sherbert
	1 cup coffee
	2 tsp sugar

Analysis and Comments

- An analysis of this menu shows that it contains 2 milk, 3 vegetable, 2 fruit, 4 bread, 7 meat, and 2 fat exchanges.
- Notice that the only major difference between this menu and the 2,000- to 3,000-mg menu is the use of salt-free or low-salt foods.

Source: Menu adapted from Chicago Dietetic Association, *Manual of Clinical Dietetics,* 2nd ed. Philadelphia: W.B. Saunders Company, 1981. Reprinted by permission.

TABLE 21-8 SODIUM-CONTROLLED DIETS

Purpose:	Sodium-controlled diets are designed to avoid excessive retention of sodium.
Use:	Used for persons with fluid retention caused by cardiovascular, renal, or hepatic diseases.
Sodium restriction:	Examples of specific sodium-controlled diets:
	No added salt (approximately 4 g sodium or 174 mEq)
	All foods on the general diet are used, but salt is not used at the table.
	2,000–3,000 mg sodium (87–130 mEq)
	$\frac{1}{2}$ tsp regular table salt may be used, either in the preparation of food or at the table.
	Foods with high salt content are omitted but can be calculated into the diet in place of the $\frac{1}{2}$ tsp table salt.
	1000 mg (43 mEq). *This level is not recommended for home use.*
	No salt is used in the preparation of food or at the table. Canned or processed foods containing sodium are omitted. Four servings of regular bread are allowed daily.
	500 mg sodium (22 mEq). *This level should be used for the short term or tests only.*
	No salt is used in the preparation of food or at the table. Canned or processed foods containing sodium are omitted. Certain vegetables containing high levels of natural sodium are omitted.
	250 mg sodium (11 mEq). *This diet is not recommended, but could be used for the short term or tests only.*
	No salt is used in the preparation of food or at the table. Canned or processed foods containing sodium are omitted. Certain vegetables containing high natural sodium are omitted. Low-sodium milk is used instead of regular milk.
Adequacy:	All the sodium modifications are adequate, with the possible exceptions of the 250-mg and 500-mg sodium diets. Unless carefully planned, these two diets can be inadequate in some nutrients.

Source: Chicago Dietetic Association, *Manual of Clinical Dietetics,* 2nd ed. Philadelphia, W.B. Saunders Company, 1981. Reprinted by permission.

Mechanism of the Low-Sodium Diet in Lowering Blood Pressure.
Essentially, a low-sodium diet functions as a natural diuretic to reduce
the volume of extracellular fluid. As a result, the work on the heart is
reduced, as is **peripheral resistance** in the arterioles and capillaries.
Reduction in peripheral resistance is apparently the main factor responsible for the long-term effect of salt restriction on blood pressure. It may
take a few weeks to a couple of months for a hypertensive person to
benefit from a low-sodium diet. The more successful the person is in
restricting the sodium intake, the less likely will be the need for drug
therapy.

Peripheral resistance
Resistance to the passage
of blood through small
blood vessels, especially
the arterioles.

Suggestions to Help Reduce Sodium Intake. Hypertensives often find
it difficult to reduce their sodium intake drastically, primarily because
the food tastes unpalatable. One way to increase compliance with the
diet is to introduce the person to spices that add flavor to food but do
not contain sodium. Some sodium-free spices are the following:

Allspice	Paprika
Bay leaves	Pepper
Curry powder	Sage
Lemon juice	Thyme
Nutmeg	Vanilla extract

Learning to read labels for sources of sodium is important. Some substances in foods that contain sodium are the following:

Baking powder	Monosodium glutamate
Baking soda	Sodium alginate
Disodium phosphate	Sodium benzoate
Sodium propionate	

In general, processed foods, milk, and dairy products are high in sodium. Some medications, such as antacids, antibiotics, cough medicines,
laxatives, pain relievers, and sedatives, may contain sodium. Even some
toothpastes and mouthwashes contain sodium.

Drug Therapy

People who have diastolic blood pressures above 100 mm Hg and mild
hypertensives who do not respond adequately to dietary therapy often
need drug therapy as a part of the stepped care approach to treatment.
Essentially, there are three types of antihypertensive drugs:

Diuretics. Diuretics reduce blood volume by causing excretion of fluid
through the kidneys. The end result is a reduction in extracellular

fluid volume, less work on the heart, and less peripheral resistance of the blood vessels.

Many diuretics are known as thiazide diuretics, hydrochlorothiazide (HydroDiuril) being an example. They cause a loss of sodium but also of potassium. Therefore, when these diuretics are administered, foods high in potassium or supplements must be consumed to avoid hypokalemia. Symptoms of hypokalemia are general muscle weakness, muscle cramps, vomiting, anorexia, rapid heart rate, listlessness, and lethargy.

Some diuretics, such as spironolactone (Aldactone) and triamterene (Dyrenium), lower sodium and water but conserve potassium. If foods high in potassium or supplements are given with this type of diuretic, there is a chance that hyperkalemia will develop. Symptoms of hyperkalemia are a slow heart rate, nausea, diarrhea, irritability, and mental confusion.

However, spironolactone and triamterene are less potent than the thiazide diuretics that cause loss of potassium. Table 21-9 summarizes information about the diuretics and their side effects.

TABLE 21-9 SUMMARY OF ANTIHYPERTENSIVE DRUGS

Type of Antihypertensive Drug	Name of Drug	Nutritional Side Effects
Thiazide diuretic		
	Hydrochlorothiazide (HydroDiuril)	Anorexia, nausea, hypokalemia, and hyperglycemia
	Chlorothiazide (Diuril)	Same as above
Non-potassium-wasting diuretic		
	Spironolactone (Aldactone), Triamterene (Dyrenium)	Anorexia, nausea, and hyperkalemia
Sympatholytics		
	Propranolol (Inderal)	Nausea, vomiting, diarrhea, and hypoglycemia
	Methyldopa (Aldomet)	Diarrhea, dry mouth
	Guanethidine (Ismelin)	Diarrhea, dry mouth, and edema
Vasodilators		
	Hydralazine (Apresoline)	Nausea, vomiting, diarrhea, and anorexia
	Prazosin (Minipress)	Vomiting, diarrhea, and nausea
	Minioxidil (Loniten)	Edema

Sympatholytics. These drugs dampen the effects of the sympathetic nervous system on the heart and blood vessels. The end result is decreased cardiac output and decreased peripheral resistance.

Propranolol (Inderal) and methyldopa (Aldomet) are two examples of sympatholytic drugs. A more potent drug is guanethidine (Ismelin). Table 21-9 summarizes information about the sympatholytic drugs.

Vasodilators. This group of drugs decreases peripheral resistance, as do the sympatholytics, but in a different manner. Vasodilators act directly on the blood vessel walls to increase their diameter, thereby reducing blood pressure.

Hydralazine (Apresoline) and prazosin (Minipress) are two examples of vasodilator drugs. A more potent drug is minoxidil (Loniten).[5] Table 21-9 summarizes information about these drugs.

MYOCARDIAL INFARCTION

A myocardial infarction (also known as *heart attack, coronary occlusion,* or *coronary*) is a condition in which a portion of the heart tissue is necrotic. As discussed earlier in the chapter, the main contributor is atherosclerosis of the coronary arteries.

DIET THERAPY

The basic dietary principle for a heart attack patient is to reduce the workload on the heart and improve cardiac output. This can be accomplished nutritionally in three ways:

• Keep the size of the meals small
• Reduce to ideal body weight if necessary
• Eliminate excess body fluid

In addition, the following foods are avoided, since they can cause stress on the heart: foods that cause gaseous discomfort or distention, very hot or cold foods, and foods containing stimulants.

A diet progression for a myocardial infarct patient may be as follows:

First 24–48 hours

• Nothing is given by mouth; an intravenous line is established for intravenous fluids and drugs.

After 1–2 days

• Usually the first oral meals are clear liquids and skim milk (the possibility of distention due to lactose intolerance should be monitored).

- No caffeine is given.
- Fluids are usually limited to 1,000–1,500 ml.
- Sodium restriction is necessary if edema is present.

After about 3 or 4 days

- A soft, low-kilocalorie, mildly restricted-sodium diet (2,000 kcal) is given.
- Fat and cholesterol are restricted.
- Six small meals are given to avoid distention.

Rehabilitation phase

- A moderate-fat and cholesterol-controlled diet (depending on blood lipid levels) is given.
- There is mild sodium restriction (2,000–3,000 mg).
- Caffeine is restricted.

DRUG THERAPY

Antiarrhythmics Agents that prevent variations of the normal heart rhythm.

Calcium antagonists Antiarrhythmic drugs that are effective in managing some types of arrhythmias.

A cardiac-depressant or **antiarrhythmic** is a type of drug frequently administered to a myocardial infarction patient. These drugs are used to treat or prevent atrial and ventricular arrhythmias.

A new class of antiarrhythmic drugs called **calcium antagonists,** or slow channel blockers, has been found effective in managing some types of arrhythmias, with few side effects. Verapamil (Calan) is an example of a drug in this category. A nutritional side effect is constipation.

Quinidine, procainamide (Pronestyl), and lidocaine (Xylocaine) are examples of conventional antiarrhythmics. Anorexia, nausea, vomiting, and abdominal pain are common side effects of these drugs. Quinidine may also cause visual disturbances, confusion, and fever. In addition, an alkaline urine decreases excretion of quinidine and can lead to **quinidine intoxication.**[5] Therefore, when a patient is receiving quinidine, the diet needs to be low in alkaline ash foods (milk, vegetables, and fruits except cranberries, prunes, and plums).

Qunidine intoxication A poisoned state due to a buildup of the drug quinidine.

CONGESTIVE HEART FAILURE

Congestive heart failure A condition in which the heart is damaged to the point where it is unable to pump blood adequately to the tissues.

Congestive heart failure is a condition in which the heart is damaged to the point where it is unable to pump blood adequately to the tissues. This condition is often called **decompensation.** The term *congestion* comes from the fact that this condition often results in pulmonary edema. Since the kidneys, like all body tissues, do not receive enough blood, they set into motion a mechanism to conserve sodium and water throughout the body. The end result is peripheral edema and ascites. The excess fluid increases the load on the heart and can further weaken it.

DIET THERAPY

The diet principle in congestive heart failure is basically like that of a myocardial infarction patient: to reduce the workload of the heart. Therefore, a low-kilocalorie (if the patient is overweight or obese), sodium-restricted, and sometimes fluid-restricted diet is common for congestive heart failure. Also, a soft diet with avoidance of gaseous food and foods containing stimulants is common in diet therapy.

DRUG THERAPY

Cardiotonic glycosides
A group of drugs that increase the strength of heart contractions.

Two basic groups of drugs used to treat congestive heart failure are diuretics and drugs that increase the strength of heart muscle contractions. **Cardiotonic glycosides** is the general name for the group of drugs that increase the strenth of heart contractions.

Three common examples of cardiotonic drugs are digitalis, digitoxin (Crystodigin), and digoxin (Lanoxin). All three are potent drugs, and signs of drug toxicity can occur even when normal doses are administered. Some of the common nutritional side effects of these drugs are nausea, vomiting, diarrhea, and anorexia.[5] These drugs should not be administered with milk or high-calcium foods, since their effects are diminished. High-fiber meals also reduce their absorption. In addition, they tend to cause hypokalemia; therefore, foods high in potassium or supplements should be consumed when a person is taking any of these cardiotonic drugs.

CASE STUDY: HYPERLIPOPROTEINEMIA

Mr. T is a 52-year-old ex-vice president of a bank. He has come into a clinic for a yearly health checkup. Below are the assessment findings for this person.

Physical Findings	*Normal Values*
Height: 5 ft 9 in. (69 in.)	
Weight: 191 lb.	148–160 lb
Blood pressure: $\frac{145 \text{ mm Hg}}{95 \text{ mm Hg}}$	Upper limit $\frac{140 \text{ mm Hg}}{90 \text{ mm Hg}}$

Laboratory Findings

Serum cholesterol: 480 mg/dl	Upper limit for age 50+ is 330 mg/dl
Serum triglycerides: 100 mg/dl	10–190 mg/dl
LDL: 200 mg/dl	60–120 mg/dl
HDL: 56 mg/dl	57–80 mg/dl

Other Information

Occupation: retired early because of disability

Activity: minimal physical activity; spends days reading and watching TV.

Nutrition: eats three meals per day and an evening snack; three or four beers per day.

Other: no known present or previous disorders; smokes two packs of cigarettes per day.

Using the above information and material in Chapter 21 answer the following questions.

1. What type of hyperlipoproteinemia does Mr. T have?
   A. type IIa   C. type III
   B. type IIb   D. type IV

2. The modifiable risk factors that Mr. T has for the development of atherosclerosis are

   1. overweight   3. elevated cholesterol level

   2. sex   4. age

   A. 1, 2, 3   B. 1, 3   C. 2, 4   D. 4   E. all of these

3. The basic diet for Mr. T should be one of _____.
   A. low saturated fat, restricted carbohydrates, no alcohol consumption
   B. weight reduction, restricted carbohydrate, salt restriction
   C. decreased saturated fat and increased polyunsaturated fat, increased HDL, weight loss, exercise
   D. none of these

For the fats listed below, choices 4 through 12, mark an A or a B based on the following key:
   A = polyunsaturated fat and should be increased in Mr. T's diet
   B = saturated fat and should be decreased in Mr. T's diet

___ 4. coconut oil   ___ 6. corn oil

___ 5. safflower oil   ___ 7. butter

___ 8. tub margarines   ___ 11. bacon drippings

___ 9. Crisco   ___ 12. skim milk

___ 10. soybean oil

13. The following meal represents a typical breakfast for Mr. T before being put on a low-cholesterol diet. Use information in Appendix C to calculate the total amount of cholesterol in this meal.

    2 scrambled eggs, 4 slices bacon
    swiss cheese (1 cu in) on an english muffin
    6 oz orange juice
    coffee with nondiary creamer, 2 tsp sugar

The total amount of cholesterol for this meal is _____ mg.

    A. 330
    B. 780
    C. 540
    D. none of these

14. The major source of cholesterol in Mr. T's breakfast is _____ and a suggestion for decreasing the cholesterol from this source but still retaining some of its nutrients is _____.

    A. bacon—to substitute beef bacon for pork
    B. cheese on muffin—to substitute low-kilocalorie bread and cheese
    C. eggs—to eat the egg whites only or Egg Beaters.
    D. nondairy creamer—to eliminate cream from his coffee
    E. none of these

15. For his other meals, Mr. T can increase his P:S ratio by increasing his consumption of _____ and decreasing his consumption of _____.

    A. tub margarines, liquid oils, and vegetables—butter, whole milk, coconut oil, and animal fat
    B. skim milk, butter, and animal fat—liquid oils, vegetables, and animal fats
    C. egg whites, whole milk, and animal fat—skim milk, sweets, and low-kilocalorie bread
    D. none of these

16. According to Table 21-5, how much total cholesterol should Mr. T be consuming per day?

    A. moderately restricted to 300–500 mg
    B. severely restricted to as little as possible, with meat being the only source
    C. not restricted
    D. none of these

17. Part of Mr. T's dietary advice is to increase his intake of fiber, like the kind he might get naturally from fruits and oatbran, and to increase his exercise level. The increase in fiber is to _____ and the increase in exercise is designed to _____.

    A. increase HDL—decrease Mr. T's weight

    B. decrease LDL—increased HDL

    C. decreased synthesis of cholesterol—increase degradation of cholesterol in the liver

    D. none of these

18. If Mr. T's diet does not lower his cholesterol adequately, he may need to take medication, with _____ being example(s) and possible side effects being _____.

    A. spironolactone—anorexia, nausea, and hyperkalemia (Aldactone)

    B. chlorothiazide—same as above (Diuril)

    C. hydralazine—diarrhea and vomiting (Apresoline)

    D. cholestyramine—constipation, vitamin A, D, and K deficiencies

OUTLINE

ATHEROSCLEROSIS

Atherosclerosis is thickening and loss of elasticity of arterial walls.

Accumulation of lipid plaques (atheromas) is the cause.

It can result in ischemia, necrosis, and myocardial infarction.

Causative Factors
Nonmodifiable Biologic Risk Factors
Age, sex, and family history.

Modifiable Risk Factors
Elevated blood lipid levels, hypertension, cigarette smoking, diabetes mellitus, and high fat intake.

The presence of two or more factors increases the risk of atherosclerosis in a synergistic way as opposed to an additive way.

Diet as a Modifiable Risk Factor
The cholesterol level in the blood can be reduced by decreasing the amount in the diet.

Saturated fat in the diet has a greater influence on serum cholesterol than does dietary cholesterol.

Consuming a diet that is low in saturated fat, high in polyunsaturated fat, and low in cholesterol will decrease the serum cholesterol level 8–18%.

Decreasing the LDL in the diet can reduce the serum cholesterol level, which can be done by reducing the intake of saturated fat.

Increasing the HDL reduces the serum cholesterol level, which can be done by increasing exercise.

Increasing polyunsaturated fats and decreasing saturated fats to a 1:1 ratio can reduce the serum cholesterol level.

Elevated Blood Lipid Levels
Atherosclerosis is often accompanied by elevated levels of blood lipids—chylomicrons, triglycerides, and cholesterol being the most common.

Types of Hyperlipoproteinemia
There are six types of hyperlipoproteinemia or conditions in which lipoproteins are elevated.

Type IIa: common, since it can be inherited as an autosomal dominant trait; elevated LDL and cholesterol are the basic problems. It is detected in people of all ages, even in infants by 1 year of age. Premature atherosclerosis occurs rapidly, often resulting in death by age 30. Secondary causes are nephrosis, hypothroidism, and biliary obstruction.

Type IV: probably the most common type of hyperlipoproteinemia. The basic problem is elevated triglycerides. Most cases result from diet. Secondary cause include diabetes, alchohol abuse, renal dialysis, pregnancy, and pancreatitis. It is commonly associated with diabetes and obesity.

Dietary and Drug Treatment of Lipoprotein Disorders
Goals and Principles of Diet and Drug Therapy
Type IIa: increase the P:S ratio to about 2:1. Egg yolks and liver should be excluded; beef and pork should be limited.

Drug treatment should not be started until after 3 months of unsuccessful dietary treatment.

Cholestyramine (Questran) and colestipol (Colestid) are commonly used drugs for type IIa hyperlipoproteinemia or to reduce cholesterol. They lower the level of cholesterol by decreasing its absorption from the intestine.

Side effects of cholestyramine and colestipol include constipation, abdominal discomfort, and vitamin A, D, and K deficiencies from decreased fat absorption.

Type IV: reduce daily kilocalorie intake to achieve weight loss. Carbohydrate intake should be almost exclusively from complex carbohydrates. Concentrated sweets should be restricted; a reduction in alcohol is recommended, since it can raise triglyceride levels.

Clofibrate (Atromid-S) is a drug used to treat types IIb and IV hyperlipoproteinemia. Side effects of clofibrate are nausea, diarrhea, vomiting, and weight gain.

Nicotinic acid, or niacin, can be used to treat types II and IV but is never the first drug of choice.

Some groups have found that administering a combination of colestipol and nicotinic acid can significantly reduce LDL cholesterol levels and the size of xanthomas.

HYPERTENSION

Diagnosis
Hypertension is elevated diastolic or systolic pressure on three different occasions.

Types and Causes
Essential Hypertension
There is no known cause; 90% of hypertension is essential. Factors that can influence essential hypertension are genetic predisposition, race, body weight, level of exercise, cigarette smoking, psychological stress, and diet.

Effects of Dietary Factors on Blood Pressure

Kilocalorie intake: weight reduction in overweight hypertensives can reduce blood pressure.

Sodium intake: research is inconclusive as to whether reducing the sodium intake will definitely reduce blood pressure. However, many groups believe that a reduction might reduce blood pressure and will not hurt the individual.

Calcium and magnesium: reduction of both can increase blood pressure.

Potassium: the ratio of sodium to potassium is very important in reducing blood pressure. The ratio that is most beneficial is low sodium and high potassium.

Secondary Hypertension

Caused by diseases or disorders such as aldosterone and Cushing's disease.

Stepped Care Treatment Program for Hypertension

Mild, essential hypertensive people have recently been helped by a stepped care approach;—dietary sodium restriction, weight control, moderate exercise, and drug therapy.

Dietary Sodium Restriction

Sodium Level in the Normal Diet

Americans consume 3 g (1 tsp) to 12 g (5 tsp) of salt (NaCl) per day. However, this is only 1.2–4.8 g of sodium (Na) per day, since salt is composed of 40% Na and 60% chloride.

Sodium Measurement

1 g sodium = 1,000 mg sodium

1 tsp of salt = 2,300 mg sodium = 100 mEq

1 mEq sodium = 23 mg sodium

Levels of Sodium-Restricted Diets

Mild (2,000–3,000 mg; 87–130 mEq sodium) (1 to $1\frac{1}{4}$ tsp of sodium)

Moderate (1,000 mg; 44 mEq sodium) (slightly less than $\frac{1}{2}$ tsp of sodium)

Strict (500 mg; 22 mEq sodium) ($\frac{1}{4}$ of a tsp of sodium)

Severe (250 mg; 11 mEq sodium) ($\frac{1}{10}$ of a tsp of sodium)

Specific Details of Dietary Restriction

Moderate sodium restriction (1,000 mg) is required.

Potassium intake should be increased, with foods from the fruit exchange being the best source. Foods from the meat and vegetable exchanges contain smaller amounts.

Mechanism of the Low-Sodium Diet in Lowering Blood Pressure

A low-sodium diet functions as a natural diuretic to reduce the volume of extracellular fluid. This reduces both the work on the heart and peripheral resistance.

It may take a few weeks to a couple of months for the diet to lower the blood pressure of a hypertensive person.

Drug Therapy

Diuretics

The thiazide type cause a loss of sodium but also of potassium. Hydrochlorothiazide (HydroDiuril) is an example. There is a potential side effect of hypokalemia.

Nonpotassium-wasting diuretics. Spironolactone (Aldactone) and triamterene (Dyrenium) lower sodium levels but conserve potassium. There is a potential side effect of hyperkalemia (high blood pressure).

Sympatholytics

These drugs dampen the effects of the sympathetic nervous system on the heart and blood vessels. Propranolol (Inderal) and methyldopa (Aldomet) are examples.

Vasodilators

These drugs decrease peripheral resistance by causing vasodilation of blood vessels. Hydralazine (Apresoline) and prazosin (Minipress) are examples.

MYOCARDIAL INFARCTION—HEART ATTACK

This is a condition in which heart tissue is necrotic or dead.

Diet Therapy

The basic dietary principle for a heart attack patient is to reduce the workload on the heart. This is done in three ways: keeping meals small, reducing body weight to ideal weight if necessary, and eliminating excess body fluid.

The diet progression for a myocardial infarct patient may be: nothing by mouth and IV fluids > clear liquid diet > soft, low-kilocalorie, mildly restricted sodium diet > moderate-fat, cholesterol-controlled diet.

Drug Therapy

Cardiac depressants, or antiarrhythmics, are a common class of drugs used in treating myocardial infarction.

Calcium antagonists such as verapamil (Calan) are a new class of antiarrhytmic drugs. Constipation appears to be the only nutritional side effect.

Quinidine, procainamide (Pronestyl), are lidocaine (Xylocaine) are examples of conventional antiarrhythmic drugs. Side effects of quinidine include visual disturbances, confusion, and fever. Alkaline urine decreases excretion of quinidine and leads to quinidine intoxication.

CONGESTIVE HEART FAILURE

This occurs when the heart is unable to pump blood to the tissues adequately. Congestion occurs in the lungs and other tissues as a result of the failure of blood to circulate adequately from the capillary beds back to the heart. Also, congestion results from compensatory mechanisms set into motion by the kidneys.

Diet Therapy

Diet is essentially the same as that for a myocardial infarction patient.

Drug Therapy

Two basic groups of drugs used in treating congestive heart failure are diuretics and drugs that increase the strength of heart contractions, cardiotonic glycosides. Digitalis, digitoxin (Crystodigin), and digoxin (Lanoxin) are three examples of cardiotonic drugs. Side effects are nausea, vomiting, diarrhea, and anorexia. Calcium diminishes their effects. They can also cause hypokalemia.

REVIEW QUESTIONS

TRUE (A) OR FALSE (B)

Questions 1–25

1. Atherosclerosis is a weakening of arterial walls with the formation of outer extending sacs.
2. Atherosclerosis can decrease the lumen of coronary arteries, resulting in angina pectoris.
3. The risk of developing atherosclerosis, for anyone who has two or more modifiable risk factors, is not additive but rather synergistic.
4. Cholesterol from dietary sources has a more powerful effect on serum cholesterol levels than does saturated fat.
5. If cholesterol intake is reduced to less than 300 mg/day, serum cholesterol level will decrease regardless of endogenous cholesterol production.
6. Increasing the blood level of high-density lipoproteins (HDLs) will lower the level of blood cholesterol.
7. Increasing the blood level of low-density lipoproteins (LDLs) will lower the level of blood cholesterol
8. Blood LDL levels will increase when the intake of saturated fats is reduced.
9. Type IIa hyperlipoproteinemia can occur at any

age, since it is inherited and is characterized by a high level of cholesterol.
10. Type IV hyperlipoproteinemia is characterized by a high level of triglycerides and is often associated with diabetes and obesity.
11. The diet for a person with type IIa hyperlipoproteinemia is one in which P:S level is 1:2.
12. The amount of polyunsaturated fat in the diet could be increased by increasing the consumption of butter, whole milk, coconut oil (popping corn oil), and palm oil (found in nondiary creamers).
13. Cholestyramine (Questran) and colestipol (Colestid) help lower cholesterol levels in type IIa people by increasing its degradation in the liver.
14. Scientific and medical research has proven that there is a definite causal relationship between sodium consumption and hypertension.
15. A decrease in both sodium and potassium levels in the diet is beneficial in reducing hypertension.
16. Low dietary calcium intake can cause an increase in blood pressure.
17. In general, animal foods contain more sodium than plant foods; therefore, the milk and meat exchange lists contain more sodium than the other lists.
18. A strict sodium (500 mg, 22 mEq) diet has been found easy to achieve for people who have mild essential hypertension.
19. A person on a moderate (1,000 mg, 44 mEq) sodium-restricted diet cannot add salt to food and needs to limit the intake of milk and eggs.
20. Reduction in peripheral resistance is apparently the main factor responsible for the long-term effect of salt restriction.
21. If thiazide diuretics like hydrochlorothiazide (HydroDiuril) are used in treating hypertension, foods such as bananas and oranges should be limited in the diet.
22. The basic dietary principle for a heart attack patient is to increase foods and drugs that will increase the strength of heart muscle contractions.
23. A person who has suffered a myocardial infarct should be kept on total parenteral nutrition for a lengthy period of time to allow maximum relaxation and healing of the heart.
24. A heart attack patient who is receiving the drug quinidine should also have a diet that is low in alkaline ash foods (milk, vegetables, and fruits except cranberries, prunes, and plums).
25. The cardiotonic drugs such as digitalis, digitoxin (Crystodigin), and digoxin (Lanoxin) should not be administered with milk or high-calcium foods, since they can diminish the effects of the drugs.

26. Modifiable risk factors in developing atherosclerosis include:
    1. elevated blood lipid levels
    2. cigarette smoking
    3. diabetes mellitus
    4. age
       A. 1, 2, 3   B. 1, 3   C. 2, 4   D. 4
       E. all of these

27. Which of the following comments about cholesterol and atherosclerosis is not true?
    A. Cholesterol absorption is inversely proportional to intake
    B. Cholesterol from dietary sources has a more powerful effect on blood cholesterol levels than saturated fat
    C. Consuming a diet that is high in saturated fat and low in polyunsaturated fat will decrease serum cholesterol levels
    D. A, B
    E. A, B, C

28. Type IIa hyperlipoproteinemia can be described as:
    1. an elevated level of triglycerides
    2. an elevated level of cholesterol
    3. a problem that can be helped by weight loss
    4. a problem that can be helped by increasing the P:S ratio
       A. 1, 2, 3   B. 1, 3   C. 2, 4   D. 4
       E. all of these

29. Type IV hyperlipoproteinemia is characterized as:
    1. an elevated level of triglycerides
    2. a frequent complication of obesity and diabetes
    3. being helped by reducing the consumption of alcohol
    4. a problem that is helped more by restricting total kilocalories than fat intake
       A. 1, 2, 3   B. 1, 3   C 2, 4   D. 4
       E. all of these

Questions 30–34. Choose either A, B, or C.

A = reduction in this factor can reduce blood pressure

B = increase in this factor can reduce blood pressure

C = this factor cannot be altered but can influence blood pressure

___ 30. kilocalorie intake
___ 31. genetic predisposition to hypertension
___ 32. calcium and magnesium
___ 33. potassium
___ 34. sodium

35. Which of the following presents the steps, in the proper sequence, for a stepped care treatment program for hypertension?
    A. dietary sodium restriction, drug therapy, weight control measures, and moderate exercise
    B. drug therapy, moderate exercise, weight control measures, and dietary sodium restriction
    C. dietary sodium restriction, weight control measures, moderate exercise, and drug therapy
    D. none of these

36. The mechanism of a low-sodium diet in lowering blood pressure is initial reduction of _____, which is followed by reduction of _____.
    A. blood cholesterol—body weight and blood pressure
    B. the volume of extracellular fluid—work on the heart and peripheral resistance
    C. edema—sodium and calcium
    D. none of these

37. After a heart attack, which of the following help to reduce the workload of the heart?
    1. keep size of meals small
    2. increase fiber in diet
    3. eliminate excess body fluid
    4. increase foods like ice cream, which contain many kilocalories in small portions
       A. 1, 2, 3   B 1, 3   C 2, 4   D. 4
       E. all of these

MATCHING

Questions 38–41

Match each drug in column A with the dietary modifications or dietary problems that are appropriate for that drug in column B.

	A	B
___ 33.	hydrochlorothiazide (HydroDiuril)	A. need foods low in potassium to avoid hyperkalemia
___ 39.	quinidine	B. need foods high in potassium to avoid hypokalemia
___ 40.	spironolactone (Aldactone)	C. diet low in alkaline ash foods
___ 41.	digitalis	D. diet low in calcium

DISCUSSION QUESTIONS

1. Describe atherosclerosis in terms of modifications of blood vessels and possible end results with atherosclerosis of the coronary arteries.
2. Discuss specific dietary modifications of cholesterol, polyunsaturated versus saturated fats, and fiber on decreasing the development of atherosclerosis.
3. Distinguish between type II and type IV hyperlipoproteinemia in terms of elevated lipid level, age range and frequency, and characteristics.
4. Discuss specific details of a moderate sodium-restricted diet in treating hypertension.
5. Describe three nutritional ways in which the workload on the heart can be reduced for a myocardial infarct patient.

REFERENCES

1. U.S. Department of Health and Human Services. *Ninth Report of the National Heart, Lung, and Blood Advisory Council*, NIH Publication No. 81-2334. Bethesda, Md.: National Heart and Lung Institute, 1981.
2. *Heart Facts*. Dallas: American Heart Association, 1976.
3. R.I. Levy and B.M. Rifkind. "The structure, function, and metabolism of high-density lipoproteins: A status report." *Circulation* (*Supplement IV*) 62, 7, Table 4 (1982).
4. U.S. Department of Health, Education, and Welfare. *The Dietary Management of Hyperlipoproteinemia*. Bethesda, MD. Publication No. (NIH) 78-110, 1978.
5. *Drugs: Nurse's Reference Library*. Springhouse, PA: Intermed Communications, Inc., 1982.
6. R. Stamler, J. Stamler, WF Riedlinger, et al. "Weight and blood pressure. Findings in hypertension screening of 1 million Americans." *Journal of the American Medical Association, 240*, 1607 (1978).
7. Federation of American Societies for Experimental Biology. *Evaluation of the Health Aspects of Sodium Chloride and Potassium Chloride as Food Ingredients*. Prepared for the Bureau of Foods, Food and Drug Administration, U.S. Department of Health, Education and Welfare, Washington, DC, 1979.
8. The National Research Council, *Toward Healthful Diets*. Washington, D.C.: National Academy of Sciences, 1980.
9. H. Kesteloot and J. Geboers. "Calcium and blood pressure." *Lancet 1*, 813 (1982).
10. R.L. Tannen. "Effects of potassium on blood pressure control." *Annals of Internal Medicine.* 98(Pt. 2), 773 (1983).
11. "Five-Year Findings of the Hypertension Detection and Follow-Up Program. I. Reduction in mortality of persons with high blood pressure, including mild hypertension." *Journal of the American Medical Association, 242*, 2562 (1979).
12. Committee on Sodium-Restricted Diets, Food and Nutrition Board, National Research Council. *Sodium-Restricted Diets and the Use of Diuretics. Rationale, Complications, and Practical Aspects of Their Use*. Washington, D.C.: National Academy of Sciences, 1979.
13. E.J. Calabrese and R.W. Tuthill. "A review of literature to support a sodium drinking water standard." *Journal of Environmental Health, 40*, 80–83 (1977).

22 DISEASES OF THE RESPIRATORY SYSTEM

OBJECTIVES

Upon completion of this chapter, you should be able to:

1. Describe bronchitis in terms of tissue changes, characteristic problems exhibited by bronchitis patients, and underlying causes.

2. Describe emphysema in terms of tissue changes, characteristic problems exhibited by emphysema patients, and underlying causes.

3. Discuss diet therapy for bronchitis and emphysema.

4. Discuss two reasons why malnutrition is common in respiratory insufficiency and respiratory failure.

5. Give the formula for calculating basal energy expenditure (BEE) for men and women.

6. Describe pneumonia in terms of changes in the lungs, symptoms, and diet therapy.

7. Give the causative organism of tuberculosis, tissue changes, and diet therapy.

8. Discuss lung cancer (bronchiogenic cancer) in terms of symptoms, nutritionally related side effects of therapy, and dietary treatment.

9. Give some of the respiratory problems associated with cystic fibrosis.

10. Discuss optimal nutrition, antibiotics, and expectorants in the treatment of respiratory problems related to cystic fibrosis.

INTRODUCTION

Nutrition is important in regard to respiratory diseases. Poor nutrition in children has been associated with increased frequency of respiratory infections. In some studies, starving children and adults have been found to have emphysema-like changes. Recovery from pulmonary diseases can be affected by the type of nutritional care the person receives.[1]

This chapter discusses some of the more common respiratory disorders and the role that nutrition may play in recovering from them.

CHRONIC OBSTRUCTIVE PULMONARY DISEASE

Chronic obstructive pulmonary disease (COPD) A group of disorders that obstruct the air flow into and out of the lungs.

Chronic obstructive pulmonary disease (COPD) refers to a group of disorders that obstruct air flow into and out of the lungs. COPD includes bronchitis, emphysema, and asthma.

The severity of COPD is significant. The death rate is more than 40,000 per year, making it the sixth leading cause of death. In addition, more than 13 million Americans suffer from emphysema and chronic bronchitis.[2] COPD is found primarily in men over 45 years of age; however, the incidence in women is now steadily increasing.

BRONCHITIS

Ventilation The ability to move air into and out of the lungs.

Dyspnea Labored breathing.

Cyanotic Bluish color of the skin due to reduced level of oxygen.

Emphysema A disease characterized by the gradual destruction of alveoli, enlargement of distal air spaces, and trapping of air.

Cor pulmonale Hypertrophy of the right side of the heart.

Bronchitis is a chronic infection of the lower respiratory tract or the bronchial tree (see Fig. 22-1). The condition is characterized by a regularly returning cough due to excessive mucus secretion and an inability to expel it. In addition, the bronchioles become constricted, resulting in decreased **ventilation** and **dyspnea.** Decreased ventilation often results in a **cyanotic** condition. The body build of chronic bronchitis sufferers often tends toward obesity, and because of their persistent bluish color, clinicians often refer to them as "blue boaters".[3]

The underlying cause of bronchitis is frequent respiratory infections. The condition can progress to **emphysema,** discussed below, and can result in **cor pulmonale.** Cor pulmonale results from increased difficulty of the right side of the heart in pumping blood to the lungs. As the bronchioles become constricted, thereby decreasing blood flow to them, the right side of the heart has to work harder to pump blood to the lungs.

PULMONARY EMPHYSEMA

Emphysema is characterized by gradual destruction of alveoli, enlargement of distal air spaces, and trapping of air (see Fig. 22-2). Loss of

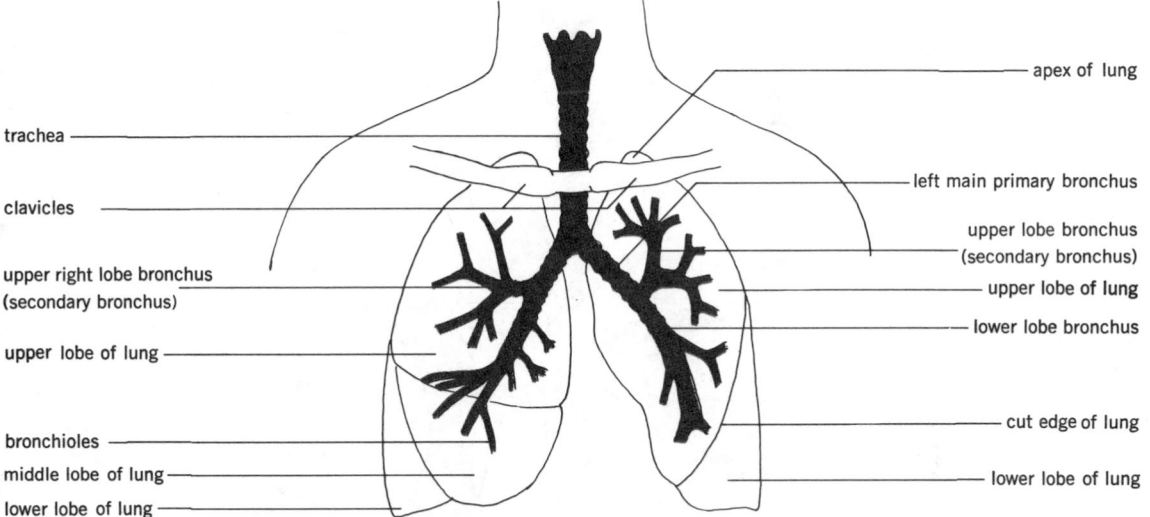

FIGURE 22-1 The bronchial tree. (J.R. McClintic, *Basic Anatomy and Physiology of the Human Body.* New York: John Wiley & Sons, Inc., © 1980. Reprinted by permission.)

Barrel chest An appearance of the chest often seen in people who suffer from chronic asthma attacks.

Pulmonary therapy Treatment of lung diseases.

Intermittent positive-pressure breathing The use of a ventilator for treatment of patients with inadequate breathing.

elasticity allows the bronchi to collapse during expiration, making it very difficult for them to expire. There is progressive loss of lung tissue and destruction of alveolar blood capillaries. Mucus secretions are increased and accumulate due to ineffectual coughing. As more and more alveoli are hyperextended, the lungs become overdistended, causing the diaphragm to flatten. As a result, it becomes more and more difficult to breathe with the diaphragm. Instead, the person becomes more of a chest breather, relying on the intercostal muscles. These changes result in the formation of a **barrel chest.**

Unlike bronchitis, there is adequate oxygenation of tissues and no cyanosis develops; therefore, clinicians frequently refer to these patients as "pink puffers." People suffering from emphysema characteristically are thin, with muscle wasting and recent weight loss. There are three basic reasons for these changes:

- Extra energy is required to eat

- Increased physical effort is required to eat

- The full stomach presses on the diaphragm and causes dyspnea[3]

The basic cause of emphysema is chronic irritation of the lungs. Cigarette smoking and inhaled irritants are the two most common sources.

Drugs are used to liquefy secretions, dilate the bronchi, and treat infections. In addition, **pulmonary therapy, intermittent positive-pressure breathing,** aerosol treatments, and oxygen in low concentrations are used in treating emphysema.

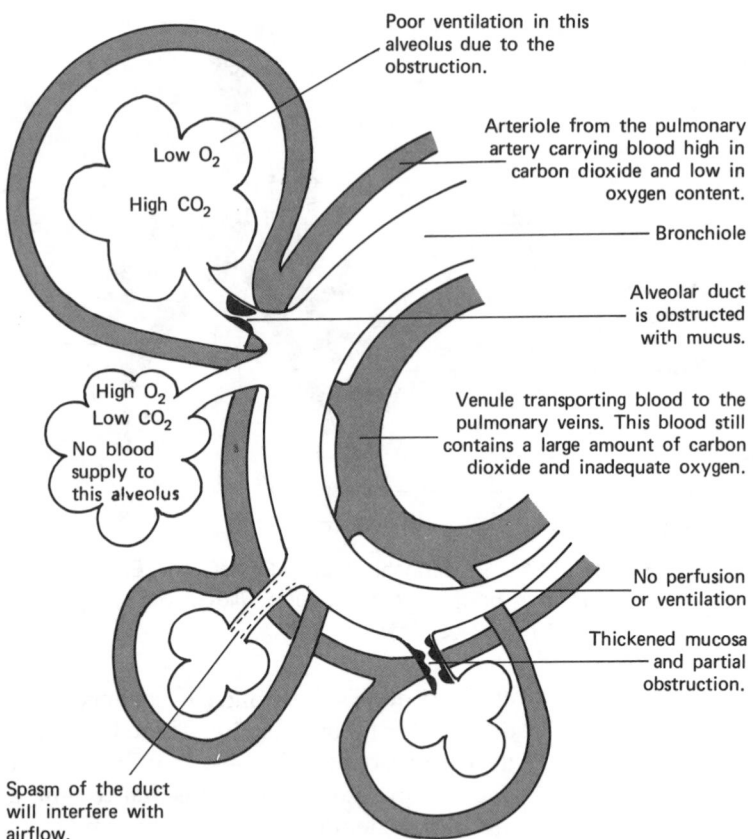

Poor ventilation in this alveolus due to the obstruction.

Arteriole from the pulmonary artery carrying blood high in carbon dioxide and low in oxygen content.

Bronchiole

Alveolar duct is obstructed with mucus.

Venule transporting blood to the pulmonary veins. This blood still contains a large amount of carbon dioxide and inadequate oxygen.

No perfusion or ventilation

Thickened mucosa and partial obstruction.

Low O_2

High CO_2

High O_2 Low CO_2 No blood supply to this alveolus

Spasm of the duct will interfere with airflow.

FIGURE 22-2 Emphysema is characterized by gradual destruction of alveoli, enlargement of distal air spaces, and trapping of air. (Reproduced by permission from S.R. Burke, *The Composition and Function of Body Fluids*, 3rd ed. St. Louis, 1980, The C.V. Mosby Co.)

DIET THERAPY

Eating is often very difficult for chronic bronchitis and emphysema patients. Dyspnea accompanied by air swallowing, coughing, persistent mucus production, and side effects of medications often result in anorexia and weight loss. In addition, when they do eat a large meal, the resulting full stomach pushes up on the diaphragm, decreasing the ability of the lungs to inflate.

The general diet plan is a high-kilocalorie diet with five to six small meals per day. Small meals require less energy to consume and decrease the fear that eating will bring on coughing spells and increase breathing difficulties.

In addition to high kilocalories, high protein and especially high levels of vitamins A and C are important in a COPD diet. The possibility of protein-calorie malnutrition (PCM) of the marasmic type should be as-

Acute respiratory failure (ARF) Inadequacy of the respiratory function in maintaining the body's need for an oxygen supply and for carbon dioxide removal while at rest.

Bronchial pneumonia Inflammation of the bronchi in the lungs.

Liquefaction Conversion into a liquid form.

Respiratory insufficiency A condition that results when the exchange of oxygen and carbon dioxide is insufficient for the body's needs during normal activities.

Respiratory failure A condition that develops when the blood pH becomes too acidic, the pCO_2 increases, and the PO_2 decreases.

Adult respiratory distress syndrome (ARDS) A variety of acute lung lesions that cause deficient oxygenation of the blood.

Endotracheal tube An airway catheter inserted into the trachea that removes secretions and maintains an adequate air passageway.

Alveolar surfactant A protein compound that is important in inflating the lungs.

Basal Energy Expenditure (BEE) The amount of energy expended by a person is at rest.

sessed in patients with COPD, especially those with emphysema. It is important to include enough protein in the diet to prevent a negative nitrogen balance. A negative nitrogen balance will result in the catabolism of the intercostal and diaphragm muscles, predisposing the person to **acute respiratory failure,** discussed below.

Vitamin A is important for maintenance and restoration of respiratory epithelial tissues. Without maintenance and restoration of this tissue, the person is strongly predisposed to respiratory infection and **bronchial pneumonia,** which could be fatal. Vitamin C is important for synthesis of collagen for the respiratory mucosa and blood vessels. Liquid blenderized or commercial formulas may be beneficial. Administering oxygen while the person is eating may be helpful. High-kilocalorie between-meal snacks should be offered to help achieve a high kilocalorie intake.

A COPD patient should be encouraged to consume an adequate level of fluids for hydration and **liquefaction** of mucus secretions. Gas-producing foods should be avoided, since they can cause upward pressure on the diaphragm, increasing dyspnea. (See Case Study: COPD in a 45-Year-Old Man, at end of Chapter for reinforcement and application of COPD information.)

NUTRITION IN RESPIRATORY INSUFFICIENCY AND RESPIRATORY FAILURE

COPD can worsen into **respiratory insufficiency** failure. **Respiratory failure** can develop if the blood pH becomes too acidic, the pCO_2 increases, and the pO_2 decreases. Patients who go into **acute respiratory failure (ARF),** including **adult respiratory distress syndrome (ARDS),** require special mechanical ventilatory techniques and are very susceptible to malnutrition. There are two reasons why malnutrition may develop. First, an **endotracheal tube,** required for mechanical ventilation, decreases oral intake of food. Second, it is more difficult for the patient to communicate a feeling of hunger.[4]

As discussed above, a negative nitrogen balance can result in catabolism of the diaphragm and intercostal muscles, as well as decreasing the ability to produce the **alveolar surfactant.** Some studies of mechanically ventilated patients showed that their average kilocalorie intake was only 1,050 per day, whereas their actual need was 1,440. In addition, their protein intake was only 26 g/day and they were receiving no vitamin supplementation.

The patient's fat stores can be assessed by measuring skinfold thickness and muscle mass by measuring midarm muscle circumference. As mentioned above, it is important to make sure that the total kilocalorie intake is adequate for the patient's metabolic needs. One formula that can be used to estimate the **Basal Energy Expenditure** (BEE) of resting individuals who are not under stress is as follows:

Men:

$$BEE = 66 + (13.7 \times wt) + (5 \times ht) - (6.8 \times age)$$

Example: A 47-year-old, 5 ft 9 in. (69 in.) man who weighs 145 lb.

$$BEE = 66 + (13.7 \times 145\ lb) + (5 \times 69\ in.) - (6.8 \times 47)$$
$$66 + (1,987) + (345) - (320) = 2,078\ kcal$$

Women:

$$BEE = 655 + (9.6 \times wt) + (1.7 \times ht) - (4.7 \times age)$$

Example: A 35-year-old, 5 ft 2 in. (62 in.) woman who weighs 115 lb

$$BEE = 655 + (9.6 \times 115) + (1.7 \times 62) - (4.7 \times 35)$$
$$655 + (1,104) + (105) - (165) = 1,699\ kcal$$

As stated above, these calculations are for resting people who are not under stress. However, people who are experiencing respiratory insufficiency or respiratory failure are under stress. Therefore, for these people who are under stress, 1.2 to 1.5 times the BEE is usually adequate to meet their current nutritional needs.[5]

If possible, the enteral route is best for providing nutrients. However, aspiration is a complication of feeding by the enteral route, especially with the already-compromised respiratory system (see Chapter 17 for other complications of enteral nutrition). Total parental nutrition (TPN) by a central vein is the best alternative after enteral nutrition (see Chapter 17 for details of TPN). See the following boxed material on respiratory-dependent COPD patients.

A new formula for respiratory-dependent COPD patients is PULMOCARE (Ross Laboratories). This formula is designed to minimize CO_2 production by supplying high fats and low carbohydrates. Carbon dioxide retention is a problem with patients who are suffering from respiratory insufficiency or failure. Cachexia often complicates this condition due to to the fact that malnutrition and weight loss increase the catabolism of the diaphragm and intercostal muscles.

Fats supply concentrated energy but reduce the production of CO_2. PULMOCARE provides 55% of kilocalories as fat, 28% as carbohydrates, and 17% as protein. Lowering CO_2 production results in less respiratory effort, thereby decreasing stress to the respiratory system.[6]

PNEUMONIA

Pneumonia An acute infection of the lung tissue.

Bacterial pneumonia A type of pneumonia in which the alveoli become filled with exudate that interferes with the exchange of gases.

Exudate Fluid with a high content of protein and cellular debris.

Unproductive No expulsion of sputum.

Sputum Mucous secretion from the lungs, bronchi, and trachea.

There are many factors that predispose a person to **pneumonia**. Malnutrition, chronic lung disease, bacteria, and virus infections some of the more common causative agents.

In **bacterial pneumonia,** the alveoli become filled with **exudate,** which interferes with exchange of gases. Respiration is rapid and shallow. Symptoms include coughing, which at first may be dry and **unproductive,** chest pain, and fever. As the inflammation spreads, the cough becomes productive, and the **sputum** has a rusty color due to the presence of blood.[4]

A person suffering from pneumonia loses a great deal of fluid as a result of high fever, profuse perspiration, and dyspnea.

DIET THERAPY

A high fluid and electrolyte intake of approximately 3000 ml/day is important to replace the large losses. In addition, the fluids act to thin mucus, which makes expulsion easier. Often the patient is vomiting and so ill that parenteral infusion of fluids is the only option.

At least 1,500 kcal/day should be administered in order to meet the patient's increased metabolic needs. Generally a liquid blenderized or commercial formula diet is tolerated better than solid food if administered orally.[3]

TUBERCULOSIS

Tuberculosis A bacterial infectious disease caused by the bacterium *Mycobacterium tuberculosis*.

Tubercle A small, rounded nodule produced by the bacterium *Mycobacterium tuberculosis*.

Caseous necrosis Necrosis of the tubules in which the dead tissue assumes a cheesy appearance.

Tuberculosis is a bacterial infectious disease caused by the bacterium *Mycobacterium tuberculosis*. It is usually confined to the lungs but can involve the kidneys, bones, and lymph nodes.

In the lungs, the bacteria form **tubercles** that may heal, leaving scar tissue, or they may be reactivated (see Fig. 22-3). If the condition becomes reactivated, the tubercles undergo necrosis; the dead tissue have a cheesy appearance, and the condition is called **caseous necrosis.** Healing occurs with calcification of the caseous tissue. The treatment of tuberculosis is chemotherapy.

DIET THERAPY

An optimum diet with large quantities of proteins, minerals, and vitamins is recommended. Protein is important for healing of the tubercles. Calcium is especially important for calcification of the tubercles, with at

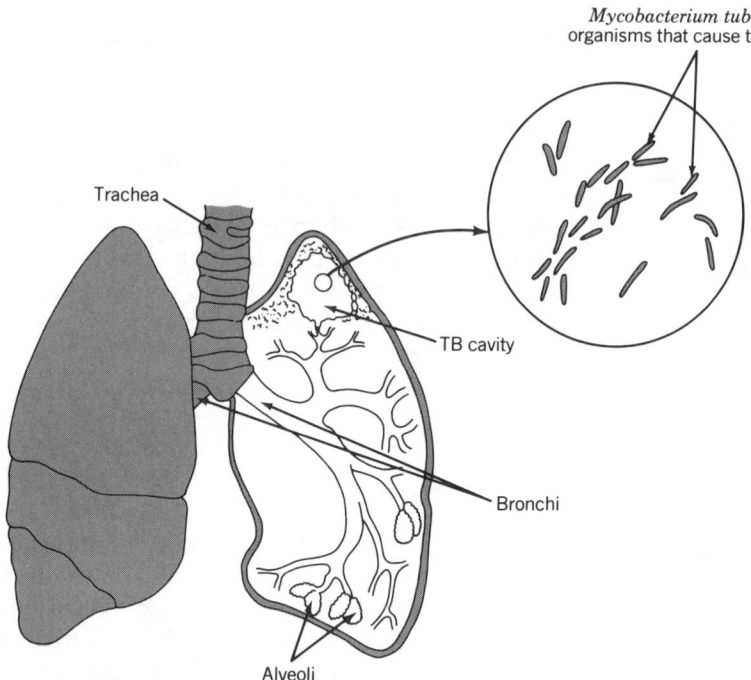

FIGURE 22-3 Tuberculosis. (From T. Randall Lankford, *Integrated Science for Health Students*, 2nd ed., 1979. Reprinted by permission of Reston Publishing Company, a Prentice-Hall Company, 11480 Sunset Hills Road, Reston, Va. 22090.)

least one quart of milk per day being recommended. In addition to milk, the diet may include cheeses, yogurt, and the addition of nonfat dry milk to beverages, casseroles, soups, and desserts.[7]

LUNG CANCER (Bronchiogenic Cancer)

Bronchiogenic cancer A malignant tumor of the lung that originates in the epithelial lining of the bronchi.

Metastasis The transfer of a cancerous tumor.

Bronchiogenic cancer is a malignant tumor of the lung that originates in the epithelial lining of the bronchi. Lung cancer is the most common type found in men, and the incidence in women has been increasing in the last several years. The most common cause is cigarette smoking, with persons who smoke one pack per day or more being at greatest risk.[8] Another possible cause of lung cancer is preexisting pulmonary diseases such as tuberculosis and COPD.

    Metastasis frequently occurs from the lungs to other regions of the body by the blood and lymph. Some of the symptoms are a persistent cough that may be productive of sputum, dyspnea, wheezing, chest pain, and repeated infections of the upper respiratory tract. Later symptoms are weight loss, fatigue, anorexia, nausea, and vomiting.

Medical management involves surgical therapy, radiation therapy, chemotherapy, and immunotherapy. Surgical therapy offers the only type of cure and is usually successful only in the early stages of the disease. Radiation therapy and chemotherapy may be helpful in slowing the metastasis of cancer and providing symptomatic relief.

Dysphagia Difficulty in swallowing.

When the lungs and chest are treated by radiation therapy, the esophagus may be irritated, resulting in **dysphagia.** As a result, tube feedings may be necessary. The drugs used in chemotherapy are among the most powerful and destructive of tissues that are available. They often cause nausea, vomiting, and anorexia, as well as tissue destruction and diarrhea. Some drugs prevent absorption of folic acid and cause iron deficiency through blood loss. As a result of these problems, hyperalimentation is the only alternative.

DIET THERAPY

Patients suffering from lung cancer, as well as other cancers, often experience PCM. This results from many factors such as internal metabolic changes, anorexia, vomiting, nausea, and malabsorption of nutrients.

To avoid or correct PCM, a cancer patient needs approximately 1.2–1.5 g protein per kilogram of body weight daily. To be sure that the protein is used properly, 2,000 kcal/day are required for patients who are not malnourished. A malnourished patient may need as many as 4,000 kcal/day.

In addition to having protein deficits, cancer patients frequently are low in vitamins and minerals, requiring therapeutic doses.

Due to anorexia, an altered sense of taste, and vomiting, oral feeding will not meet the nutritional needs of the cancer patient. As a result, tube feeding and TPN are required. TPN is especially important if the patient has lost 7% of his or her body weight within 2 months or has been unable to eat for 5 days and is unlikely to eat for another week.[9] Some practical dietary suggestions for lung cancer and other cancer patients are as follows:

- Encourage small, high-calorie, high-protein snacks such as yogurt, peanut butter, cream soups, eggs, and fresh fruits.

- Additional kilocalories at meals or snacks can be provided by milkshakes, eggnog, pudding, custard, ice cream, butter, and gravy.

- Pain and nausea interfere with eating; therefore, pain and antinausea medications could be timed to be given 30 minutes before meals.

- For dry mouth problems, foods can be moistened with butter, gravy, cheese sauce, and cream.

- Nausea can be helped by giving the patient dry crackers, toast, and carbonated drinks.

CYSTIC FIBROSIS

Cystic fibrosis is a disorder that is characterized by the production of very thick mucus by the mucous-producing glands and increased concentration of sodium in sweat. As described in Chapter 20, the thick mucus can block the pancreatic and hepatic ducts, leading to digestive disorders. The mucus can also cause respiratory disorders, which constitute the most serious threat to life.

The respiratory disorders result from the fact that the abnormally thick mucus accumulates and clogs the bronchi and bronchioles (see Fig. 22-4). It is quite difficult for the child to expel the mucus, which serves as an excellent medium for bacterial growth. As a result, the child has recurrent episodes of pneumonia. In addition to the infections, accumulation of mucus can lead to overinflation, emphysema, and collapse of alveoli. These structural changes cause a reduction in oxygen-carbon dioxide exchange, resulting in hypoxia, hypercapnia (excess carbon dioxide in blood), and acidosis.

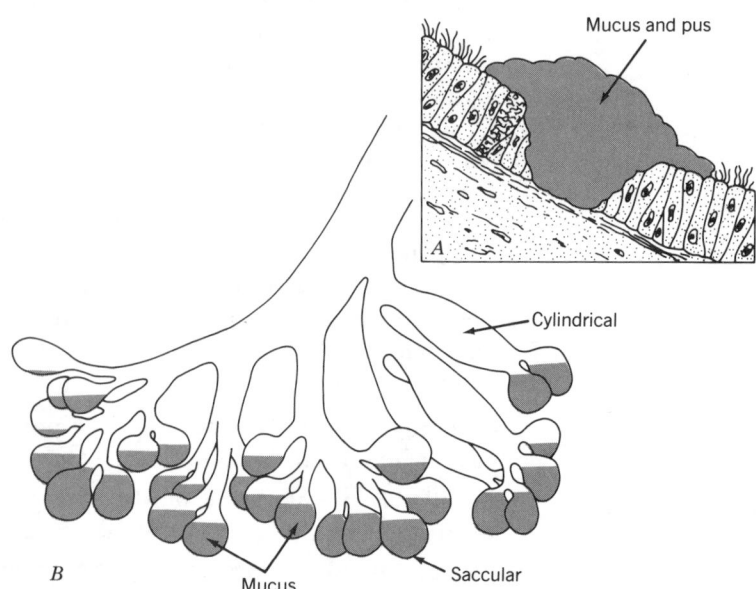

FIGURE 22-4 Bronchiectasis. (*a*) Longitudinal section of a bronchial wall damaged by chronic infection. (*b*) A collection of purulent material in the bronchioles leading to persistent infection. (Reproduced with permission from S.A. Price and L.M. Wilson, *Pathophysiology: Clinical Concepts of Disease Processes*, 2nd ed. New York: McGraw-Hill Book Company, 1982.)

DRUG THERAPY

Management of the respiratory problems involves intermittent aerosol therapy, a mist tent (a controversial approach that is frequently not used with newly diagnosed patients), postural drainage, expectorants (particularly iodides), antibiotics, and optimal nutrition. The details of optimal nutrition are presented in Chapter 20. The various drugs used often have the following nutritional side effects:

Antibiotics. Antibiotics are administered to fight and reduce infections. Tetracyclines, novobiocin, and chlamphenical are common examples. Tetracyclines frequently cause vomiting, diarrhea, anorexia, and nausea. They should not be administered with milk, since calcium forms insoluble tetracycline complexes that cannot be absorbed. Two tetracyclines, doxycycline (Doxychel and Vibramycin) and minocycline (Minocin and Vectrin), are two exceptions to this rule. In addition to a need for large amounts of vitamins in cystic fibrosis due to malabsorption, tetracyclines decrease absorption of some vitamins, such as folic acid and vitamin B_{12}. They also decrease the synthesis of vitamin K.

Chloramphenicol and novobiocin can result in nausea, vomiting, anorexia, diarrhea, and intestinal hemorrhage.

Expectorants or mucolytic drugs. These drugs decrease the viscosity of sputum, loosening the secretions and making them easier to expel.

Several of the popularly used drugs contain iodine (e.g., potassium iodide), and long-term use can lead to goiter and hypothyroidism. These medications have a strong metallic taste and are more acceptable when administered in grape juice or other fruit juices.[10]

CASE STUDY: COPD IN A 45-YEAR-OLD MAN

Mr. L is a 45-year-old man who has a long history of COPD. He has had many previous hospitalizations for congestive heart failure.

Four days before his admission, he noticed increasing shortness of breath and generally felt ill. On admission, he was described as a thin, middle-aged man who was experiencing adult respiratory distress syndrome (ARDS) and appeared chronically ill. It was decided to place Mr. L on a respirator.

Physical Findings	Normal Values
Height: 5 ft 11 in. (71 in.)	
Weight: 142 lb	154–166 lb (medium frame)

Blood pressure: $\dfrac{160 \text{ mm Hg}}{90 \text{ mm Hg}}$ Upper limits: $\dfrac{140 \text{ mm Hg}}{90 \text{ mm Hg}}$

Laboratory Findings	
Blood gases	
$PaO_2 = 40$ mm Hg	75–100 mm Hg
$PaCO_2 = 62$ mm Hg	35–45 mm Hg
pH = 7.28	7.35–7.45
Bicarbonate = 21 mEq/liter (HCO_3^-)	20–30 mEq/liter
Protein in urine	Negative

Using the information above and the material in this chapter, including the discussion of a new formula for respiratory-dependent COPD patients, answer the following questions.

1. A major nutritional factor that health professionals need to monitor in Mr. L's case is _____ .
   A. weight gain
   B. dehydration
   C. malnutrition
   D. metabolic alkalosis

2. Mr. L's diet should prevent a negative nitrogen balance, since this condition can result in catabolism of which respiratory muscles?
   A. triceps and biceps
   B. diaphragm and intercostals
   C. pectoralis major and rectus abdominis
   D. sternocleidomastoid and deltoid

3. The metabolic needs of Mr. L using the BEE formula multiplied by 1.5 are
   A. 2,060 kcal
   B. 2,360 kcal
   C. 3,158 kcal
   D. 3,090 kcal

4. If possible, the best route to administer the kilocalories to Mr. L is _____ but a complication is _____ .
   A. parenteral—edema
   B. enteral—osmotic overload
   C. parenteral—hyperglycemia
   D. enteral—aspiration

5. Since Mr. L, when admitted, was experiencing retention of CO_2, which was contributing to his acidotic condition, which nutrient should contribute the majority of kilocalories to his diet?

   A. carbohydrate   B. protein   C. fat

6. The diet for Mr. L, in addition to the previous comments, should contain adequate to increased amounts of

   1. vitamin A   3. vitamin C

   2. liquids   4. gas-producing foods

       A. 1, 2, 3 B. 1, 3 C. 2, 4 D. 4 E. all of these

7. If Mr. L were not experiencing CO_2 retention and were not receiving artificial respiration, his diet might consist of

   1. six small meals per day

   2. high calories

   3. high protein

   4. liquid blenderized formulas

       A. 1, 2, 3 B. 1, 3 C. 2, 4 D.   E. all of these

OUTLINE

CHRONIC OBSTRUCTIVE PULMONARY DISEASE (COPD)

COPD is a group of disorders that obstruct air flow into and out of lungs; they include bronchitis, emphysema, and asthma. COPD is the sixth leading cause of death, and more than 13 million Americans suffer from emphysema and chronic bronchitis.

Bronchitis

Bronchitis is a chronic infection of the lungs characterized by a regularly returning cough due to excess mucus production and an inability to remove it, dyspnea, and cyanosis. The basic cause is frequent respiratory infections. It can progress to emphysema, with cor pulmonale being a possible complication.

Pulmonary Emphysema

Pulmonary emphysema is characterized by destruction of alveoli, enlargement of distal air spaces, and trapping of air. Loss of elasticity results in collapse of alveoli, causing great difficulty in expiration. Progressive loss of lung tissue and destruction of alveolar blood vessels result in hyperextension of lungs and difficulty in breathing with the diaphragm. The person breathes more with the intercostal muscles, with the end result being a "barrel chest" appearance.

Emphysema patients are usually very thin for three reasons: (1) extra energy is required for eating; (2) increased physical effort is required to eat; and (3) a full stomach presses on the diaphragm and causes dyspnea.

Diet Therapy

The general diet plan requires high levels of kilocalories and five to six small meals per day; high protein and high levels of vitamins A and C are also needed.

It is important to assess the COPD patient for PCM of the marasmic type. It is also important to prevent a negative nitrogen balance, which could result in catabolism of the diaphragm and intercostal muscles, predisposing the person to acute respiratory failure.

Vitamin A: important for maintenance and restoration of respiratory epithelial tissue.

Vitamin C: important for synthesis of collagen for respiratory tissue and blood vessels.

Liquid blenderized or commercial formulas can be very beneficial. Intake of adequate levels of fluids is very important for hydration and liquefaction of mucus.

Nutrition in Respiratory Insufficiency and Respiratory Failure

Acute respiratory failure (ARF) and adult respiratory distress syndrome (ARDS) require special mechanical ventilatory techniques. There are two reasons why malnutrition may develop: (1) the endotracheal tube decreases oral food intake; (2) it is more difficult for the patient to communicate a feeling of hunger.

It is important to assess the patient's protein and fat stores, as well as the basal energy expenditure (BEE) requirements to prevent malnutrition.

PNEUMONIA

Pneumonia is an acute infection of the lung tissue; infection often results in accumulation of exudate in the lungs, interfering with the exchange of gases. The person loses large amounts of fluids as a result of high fever, profuse perspiration, and dyspnea.

Diet Therapy

High fluid and electrolyte levels of approximately 3,000 ml are needed to replace the large losses. At least 1,500 kcal should be consumed daily to meet the increased metabolic needs of the patient.

TUBERCULOSIS

Tuberculosis is a bacterial infection that involves the bacterium *Mycobacterium tuberculosis*. Bacteria cause the formation of tubercles (lesions), which either heal or can reactivate. If reactivation occurs, the lesions undergo necrosis, with the formation of caseous necrosis.

Diet Therapy

An optimum diet with high quantities of proteins, minerals, and vitamins is recommended. Calcium is especially important for calcification of the tubercles, which is needed for healing; at least one quart of milk per day is important. In addition, calcium can be increased by eating cheeses and yogurt and by adding nonfat dry milk to beverages, casseroles, soups, and desserts.

LUNG CANCER (Bronchiogenic Cancer)

Lung cancer is a malignant tumor of the lung that originates in the epithelial lining of the bronchi. The most common cause is smoking, with those who smoke one pack per day or more being at greatest risk. Early symptoms are a persistent cough, dyspnea, wheezing, chest pain, and repeated infections of the upper respiratory tract; later symptoms are weight loss, fatigue, anorexia, nausea, and vomiting.

Diet Therapy

PCM is a common complication of lung cancer as well as other cancers; to avoid this problem, it is recommended that the diet contain 1.2–1.5 g protein per kilogram of body weight daily. In addition, 2,000 kcal/day are required for patients who are not malnourished, and 4,000 kcal/day for malnourished patients.

Cancer patients frequently are deficient in minerals and vitamins, as well as protein; therefore, therapeutic doses are needed.

TPN is required when the patient cannot consume enough food orally and if the patient has lost 7% of body weight within 2 months or has been unable to eat for 5 days and is unlikely to eat for another week.

See the text for a list of practical dietary suggestions for lung cancer.

CYSTIC FIBROSIS

Cystic fibrosis produces large amounts of thick mucus, which accumulates and clogs the bronchi and bronchioles. The cystic fibrosis child is very susceptible to pneumonia and other respiratory problems such as emphysema, collapse of alveoli, hypoxia, hypercapnia, and acidosis.

Drug Therapy

Treatment involves optimal nutrition (described in Chapter 19). In addition, drugs play a major role in treatment. Some of the drugs and their nutritional side effects are as follows:

- Antibiotics: used to treat infections. Tetracyclines can cause vomiting, diarrhea, anorexia, and nausea. They should not be administered with milk, since calcium combines with them to form insoluble complexes. Also, they can cause decreased absorption of folic acid and vitamin B_{12} and decreased synthesis of vitamin K.
- Expectorants or mucolytic drugs: loosen secretions and make expulsion easier. Possible side effects of drugs that contain iodide (e.g., potassium iodide) are goiter and hypothyroidism.

REVIEW QUESTIONS

TRUE (A) OR FALSE (B)

Questions 1–17

1. Chronic obstructive pulmonary disease (COPD) includes problems like tuberculosis, pneumonia, and lung cancer.
2. Bronchitis involves collapse of alveoli and trapping of air.
3. People suffering from emphysema frequently are thin, with muscle wasting and recent weight loss.
4. Emphysema patients are thin and wasted because extra energy is required to eat, increased physical effort is required to eat, and a full stomach presses on the diaphragm and causes dyspnea.
5. The general diet plan for COPD is low kilocalories, high protein, and high levels of vitamins D and K.
6. Adequate to high levels of fluids are important in COPD to lower temperature and aid dysphagia (difficult swallowing).
7. It is common for people who are in respiratory insufficiency or respiratory failure to be susceptible to malnutrition.
8. The energy needs of a patient in respiratory insufficiency or respiratory failure are less than those when the patient is not in this condition.
9. TPN is always the best method for feeding respiratory patients.
10. The general diet plan for pneumonia is a low-fluid, low-protein, high-carbohydrate diet.
11. Exchange of gases in tuberculosis is hampered by tubercles (lesions) that destroy epithelial and blood tissues.
12. Diet therapy for tuberculosis includes high levels of calcium for calcification and healing of tubercles.
13. Radiation therapy and chemotherapy for cancer often alter the patient's metabolism such that less kilocalories, protein, and vitamins are needed.
14. Management of respiratory problems related to cystic fibrosis involves optimal nutrition, intermittent aerosol therapy, mist tent, postural drainage, expectorants, and antibiotics.
15. Tetracyclines should be administered with milk to reduce irritation to the gastrointestinal tract.
16. One reason for increasing the vitamin content in the diet of cystic fibrosis patients is to compensate for losses caused by some tetracycline antibiotics.
17. Some of the more popular expectorants or mucolytic drugs used to treat cystic fibrosis contain a large amount of sodium, leading to a high level of sodium in the blood.

MULTIPLE CHOICE

Questions 18–26

18. Common characteristics of emphysema patients are:

| 1. overweight | 3. recent weight gain |
| 2. thinness | 4. muscle wasting |

A. 1, 2, 3   B. 1, 3   C. 2, 4   D. 4
E. all of these

19. Some of the common nutritional problems of COPD patients are:
   1. increased metabolism and voracious appetite
   2. negative nitrogen balance
   3. decreased absorption of nutrients
   4. large meals causing dyspnea
   A. 1, 2, 3   B. 1, 3   C. 2, 4   D. 4
   E. all of these

20. A negative nitrogen balance or malnutrition in a COPD patient can result in:
   1. catabolism of intercostal muscles
   2. catabolism of the diaphragm
   3. decreased synthesis of epithelial tissue in the respiratory mucosa
   4. increased predisposition to acute respiratory failure
   A. 1, 2, 3   B. 1, 3   C. 2, 4   D. 4
   E. all of these

21. Which of the following two meals is appropriate for a COPD patient who needs high kilocalories, high protein, and high levels of vitamins A and C?
   A. cheeseburger on a bun with mayonnaise, ½ tomato with lettuce, french fries, and 1 cup whole milk
   B. ½ cup cream of wheat, lettuce salad, ½ cup peas, 1 cup skim milk, 1 banana

22. An adequate to high level of fluid intake in COPD patients is important for:
   A. reducing temperature
   B. replacing fluids lost due to diarrhea
   C. replacing fluids lost because of increased perspiration
   D. liquefaction of mucus secretions

23. The basal energy expenditure (BEE) for patients who are in acute respiratory failure (ARF) or adult respiratory distress syndrome (ARDS) is _____ .
   A. lower than when patients are not in this condition.
   B. 1.2–1.5 times the BEE if the patients are stressed.
   C. 0.5–1.0 times the BEE if the patients are stressed.
   D. none of these

24. The diet therapy for a person suffering from pneumonia is:
   1. an intake of 3,000 ml or more of fluids per day
   2. strictly parenteral intake of fluids and nutrients
   3. intake of at least 1,500 kcal/day to compensate for increased metabolism

4. low protein intake to reduce exudate in lungs
   A. 1, 2, 3   B. 1, 3   C. 2, 4   D. 4
   E. all of these

25. Diet therapy for tuberculosis includes _____
   _____ .
   A. low protein, moderate fat, and low carbohydrate in order to relax the lungs
   B. high iron, high folacin, vitamin B_{12}, and a normal amount of protein
   C. high protein, minerals (especially calcium), and vitamins
   D. parenteral infusion of high-kilocalorie, low-protein formulas

26. Dietary treatment for lung cancer includes:
   A. a low-kilocalorie, low-fat, low-protein diet to reduce the work of the lungs
   B. 0.8 g of protein per kilogram of ideal body weight, 1,200 kcal, and low fat
   C. high calcium, high levels of vitamin D, E, and K, and normal protein intake
   D. 1.2–1.5 g protein per kilogram of body weight per day, 4,000 kcal, and high vitamins plus minerals

DISCUSSION QUESTIONS

1. Discuss the diet therapy for bronchitis and emphysema.
2. Discuss two reasons why malnutrition is common in respiratory insufficiency and respiratory failure.
3. Calculate the BEE for a man who is experiencing respiratory failure. He is 49 years old, 5 ft 10 in., and weighs 147 lb.
4. Discuss lung cancer (bronchiogenic cancer) in terms of symptoms, nutritionally related side effects of therapy, and dietary treatment.

REFERENCES

1. T. Beaudette. "Nutrition and pulmonary disorders." *Seminars in Nutrition*, 3 (3) 1–15 (1983–1984).
2. T.E. Petty. *Chronic Obstructive Pulmonary Disease*, New York: Dekker, Marcel, Inc., 1978.
3. S.M. Lewis and I.C. Collier. *Medical-Surgical Nursing: Assessment and Management of Clinical Problems*. New York: McGraw-Hill Book Co., 1983, pp. 523–524.
4. L.S. Brunner and D.S. Suddarth. *The Lippincott Manual of Nursing Practice*, 3rd ed. Philadelphia: J.B. Lippincott Co., 1982.
5. A.G. Driver and M. Lebrun. "Iatrogenic malnutrition in patients receiving ventilatory sup-

port." *Journal of the American Medical Association*, 244, 2195 (1980).

6. Communique. Columbus, OH: Ross Laboratories, March 29, 1985.

7. L.H. Bodinski. *The Nurse's Guide to Diet Therapy*. New York: John Wiley and Sons, 1980, pp. 203–204.

8. *Cancer 1981 Facts and Figures.* New York: American Cancer Society, 1980.

9. M.A. Crosley. "Watch out for nutritional complications of cancer." *RN*, 48(3), 22–27 (1985).

10. *Drugs. Nurse's Reference Library.* Nursing 82 Books. Springhouse, PA.: Intermed Communications, Inc., 1982.

557

Erythropoietin A hormone, secreted by the
kidneys, that stimulates
erythropoiesis.

Erythropoietin. Stimulation of erythropoiesis (maturation of red blood
cells in the red bone marrow) is the role of this hormone.

Renin. This hormone causes formation of the compound angiotensin,
which ultimately raises blood pressure by vasoconstriction.

Renin A hormone that
causes the formation of
the compound angio-
tensin.

Active form of vitamin D. Vitamin D enters the kidneys in an inactive
form and is secreted in the active form 1,25-dihydroxycholecaciferol
(calcitriol), which increases the absorption of calcium and phosphorus
from the intestine, from the bones, and in the kidneys.

These functions show that the kidneys play a major role in regulating
the internal environment of the body.

NEPHRON: FUNCTIONAL UNIT OF THE KIDNEY

Nephron The structural
and functional unit of the
kidney.

The functional unit of the kidney is the **nephron** (see Fig. 23-1). Since
renal diseases affect different regions and functions of the nephron, it
is important to have some knowledge of them. The nephron has three
major functions: filtration, reabsorption, and secretion. These functions
and the locations where they occur in the nephron will be discussed
next.

Glomerulus A capillary
tuft within the Bowman's
capsule of a nephron.

Bowman's capsule A
proximal portion of a
renal tubule that encloses
the glomerulus of a
nephron.

GLOMERULAR FILTRATION

Blood enters the **glomerulus** of each **Bowman's capsule** under high
pressure, which causes large amounts of **filtrate** to be filtered from the
blood. The filtration process is not selective; therefore, both nutrients
and wastes are filtered from the blood.

Filtrate A fluid present
in Bowman's capsule. It
is formed by filtration of
blood in the glomeruli.

The **glomerular filtration rate (GFR)** averages about 125 ml/min, or
about 180 liters/day. **Creatinine clearance** (normal values = 95–135 ml/min)
is used as a measure of the GFR. Kidney disease frequently decreases
the creatinine clearance rate, resulting in decreased filtration of the wastes
out of the blood. When the filtration decreases to a certain level, dialysis
is required. This topic will be discussed later.

**Glomerular filtration rate
(GFR)** The amount of filtrate formed.

Creatinine clearance The
rate at which the nitrogen
compound creatinine is
filtered out of the blood
by the kidneys.

REABSORPTION

Threshold level The
amount of nutrients that
will be reabsorbed into
the blood of the neph-
rons. When this level is
reached, no more reab-
sorption of the nutrients
will occur.

The tubular system of the kidney reabsorbs the important nutrients that
were filtered out according to the **threshold level** of each substance. In
other words, most of the nutrients are found in the blood at a certain
threshold level, and when the absorption of each nutrient has been
reached, the excess will be excreted in the urine.

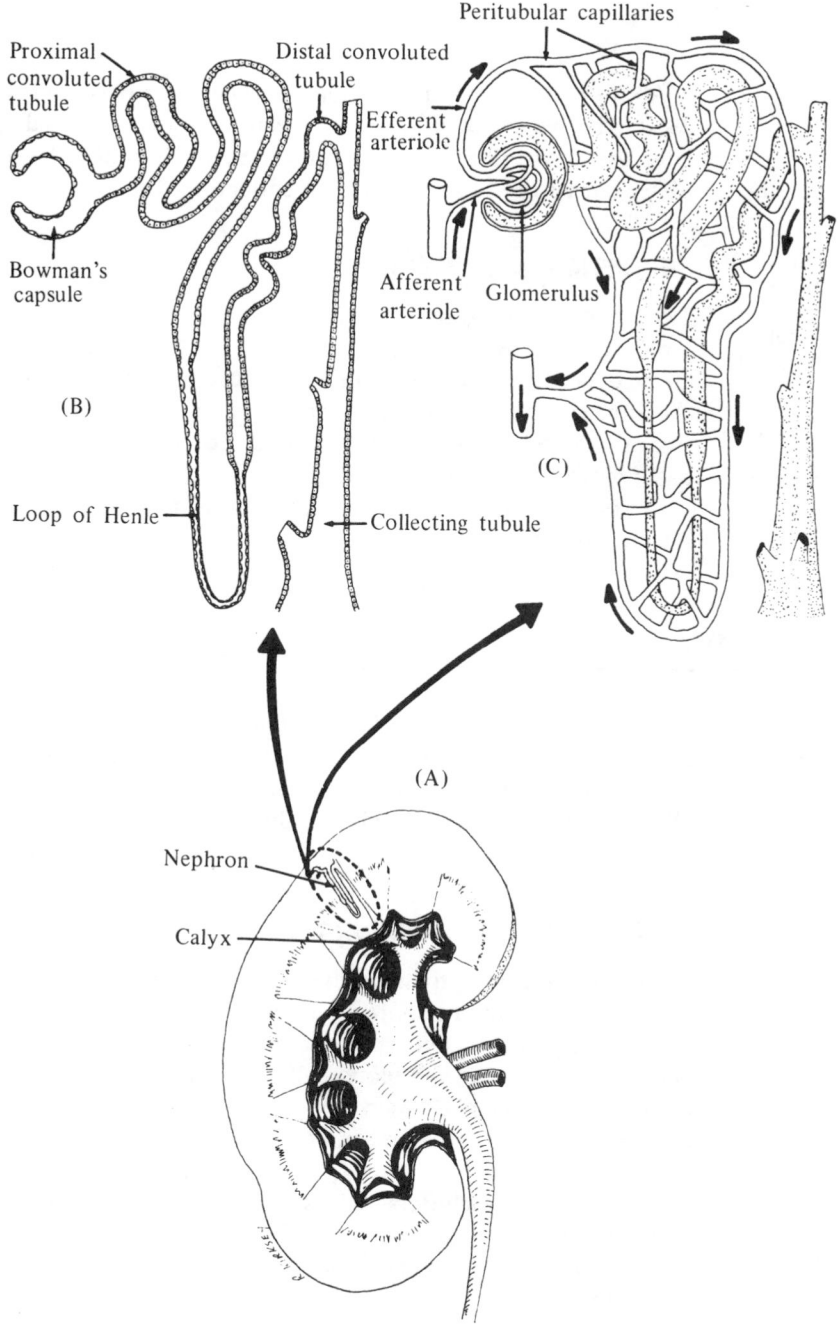

FIGURE 23-1 Parts of the kidney. (*a*) The sagittal section of a kidney shows a nephron. (*b*) The sagittal section of a nephron shows the regions. (*c*) A glomerulus within a Bowman's capsule and peritubular capillaries surrounding the regions of a nephron. (From T. Randall Lankford, *Integrated Science for Health Students*, 3rd ed., 1984. Reprinted by permission of Reston Publishing Company, a Prentice-Hall Company, 11480 Sunset Hills Road, Reston, Va. 22090.)

Proximal tubule The portion of the renal tubule attached to Bowman's capsule. Most reabsorption of nutrients occurs here.

About 80% of the reabsorption occurs in the **proximal tubule** (see Fig. 23-1). The hormone aldosterone (secreted by the adrenal gland) stimulates the absorption of sodium and the excretion of potassium from the **distal convoluted tubule** and the **collecting duct.**

Distal convoluted tubule The portion of the renal tubule that is farthest from Bowman's tubule. Some water reabsorption and secretion occur here.

SECRETION AND BLOOD pH

The kidneys help to regulate the pH of the blood by secreting hydrogen ions and reabsorbing basic bicarbonate ions. Metabolic reactions produce an excess of hydrogen ions; therefore, to keep the pH of the blood within the normal range (7.35–7.45), the kidneys secrete the hydrogen ions from the blood in the distal convoluted tubule into the urine. In addition, basic bicarbonate ions are reabsorbed into the blood.

Collecting duct A duct that carries urine from the distal convoluted tubule of the nephron to the pelvic region.

In addition, many different medications are secreted from the blood into the urine.

KIDNEY DISEASES

Acute renal disease Sudden onset of kidney disease.

Kidney diseases may result from temporary or permanent damage to the nephrons and may occur as either **acute renal disease** or **chronic renal disease.** In acute renal disease, there is usually recovery; however, with chronic disease, there is usually little if any recovery, and dialysis or transplantation are generally the only ways to avoid death.

Chronic renal disease Gradual onset of kidney disease.

Acute glomerulonephritis A form of kidney disease that involves inflammation of the glomeruli.

ACUTE GLOMERULONEPHRITIS

Acute glomerulonephritis involves inflammation of the glomeruli, frequently as a result of streptococci infections. The inflammation increases the **porosity** of the glomerular membrane to the point where large molecules (proteins and red blood cells) are filtered out of the blood. However, other substances such as urea and creatinine are not filtered out adequately, since the glomeruli are damaged from the infection.

Porosity The state of being porous.

Besides streptococcal infections other possible causes of acute glomerulonephritis include shock, **septic abortion,** surgery in other areas of the body, and drugs.

Septic abortion An abortion in which a uterine infection is spread to the general circulation.

Symptoms and their causes associated with acute glomerulonephritis are as follows:

Hematuria Blood in the urine.

Hematuria. Blood in the urine results from the increased porosity of the glomeruli, as well as from damage to them.

Proteinuria Protein in the urine.

Proteinuria. Protein in the urine also results from the increased porosity of the glomerular membranes. Frequently the protein is albumin; therefore, the symptom is often called **albuminuria.**

Albuminuria Albumin in the urine.

Edema. Loss of protein causes a reduction in the osmotic pressure of the blood therefore, an imbalance occurs in the exchange of fluids in the capillaries (see Chapter 7 for details on this fluid exchange).

Oliguria Diminished urine output.

Oliguria. This is diminished urine output to about 500 ml/day, or about a 50% drop from a normal of about 1,000–1,500 ml/day. This decrease results from increased damage to the nephrons.

The following symptoms may occur with acute glomerulonephritis but are not always present.

Increase in blood urea nitrogen (BUN). Diminished urine output frequently results in an increase in the waste compound urea.

Hypertension. Damage to the glomeruli results in reduced blood flow through the nephrons. This activates the renin-angiotensin mechanism in a compensatory step to increase blood flow to the kidneys. The end result is an increase in blood pressure.

In addition, frequently the person with acute glomerulonephritis exhibits nausea and anorexia.[1]

Dietary and Drug Treatment

The basic dietary treatment for acute glomerulonephritis is as follows:

- During oliguria, fluid intake needs to be limited to the amount lost during the previous day. This involves not only restricting the amount of fluid consumed orally but also knowing the amount in the foods consumed. See Table 23-1 for the approximate amount of water in exchange groups.

- Fruit juices are given orally to supply carbohydrates and to help maintain energy needs and spare protein breakdown, but the total amount should be within the prescribed fluid limits. The person needs to be monitored for hyperkalemia, which is a potential problem with oliguria and consumption of fruit juices. See Table 23-2 for approximate amounts of potassium per exchange list.

- Protein needs to be limited to about 40 g/day during a period of oliguria. Once oliguria has ended, protein intake is increased to compensate for urinary losses and to restore lost serum protein.

- Sodium restriction is necessary with edema. See Table 23-2 for approximate amounts of sodium per exchange list.

Drug treatment includes antibiotics for residual group A beta-streptococcal infection, antihypertensive drugs, and diuretics for edema.[2]

TABLE 23-1 WATER CONTENT OF EXCHANGE GROUPS

Exchange	Approximate % of Water	Approximate Amount of Water Per Exchange Serving
Milk	85	1 cup = 204 ml
Vegetables	70–95	½ cup = 70-95% × wt. of vegetables (See Appendix G for weights of specific vegetables)
Fruit	70–95	½ cup = 70-95% × wt. of fruit (See Appendix G for weights of specific fruits
Bread	35	1 slice = 11 ml
Cooked cereals	80–90	½ cup = 98–110 ml
Dry cereal	3	¾ cup = 0.5–1.0 ml
Meat		
Cooked rare	75	1 oz = 23 ml
Cooked well done	40	1 oz = 12 ml

Comments

Fluid restriction in oliguria frequently is limited to the amount lost in urine plus 400–600 ml, which represents the approximate amount of fluid lost per day through the skin, lungs, and feces. For example, a urinary excretion of 250 ml/day would permit a fluid intake of about 750 ml.

Using the approximate values for water content in exchanges (given above), a diet can be designed that includes the water consumed orally plus the amount present in the exchange groups.

Source: Adapted from D.F. Tver, *Nutrition and Health Encyclopedia.* New York: Van Nostrand Reinhold Co., 1981. All rights reserved.

CHRONIC GLOMERULONEPHRITIS

Repeated episodes of glomerulonephritis lead to loss of nephrons and of kidney function, especially filtration. The problem is characterized by increased loss of protein and by accumulation of urea and creatinine.

Dietary treatment of chronic glomerulonephritis is identical to that of acute glomerulonephritis unless the condition worsens to a stage termed **nephrotic syndrome.**

Nephrotic syndrome A stage of kidney disease that is characterized by large losses of protein in the urine, severe edema, low serum protein levels, elevated levels of cholesterol and other serum lipids, and anemia.

NEPHROTIC SYNDROME

Nephrotic syndrome is characterized by large losses of protein in the urine, severe edema, low serum protein levels, elevated levels of cholesterol and other serum lipids, and anemia. The massive losses of protein can result in tissue wasting, which is often masked by edema. The elevated cholesterol level is a result of increased lipoprotein production

TABLE 23-2 SODIUM AND POTASSIUM VALUES OF EXCHANGE LISTS

Exchange	Serving Size	Sodium (mg)	Potassium (mg)
Milk			
Whole or skim	1 cup	120	335
Low sodium	1 cup	7	600
Vegetables	½ cup	9	110–245
Starchy vegetables	Varies	2–10	110–190
Fruits	Varies	2	135–200
Bread			
Regular	1 slice	60	30
Low sodium	1 slice	5	30
Meat	1 oz or equivalent	25	100
Fat	1 tsp or equivalent	—	—

Comments

The values above are average values for each exchange list.
Specific comments about each exchange list

- Milk. Foods to be avoided due to their high sodium and potassium levels are chocolate milk, condensed milk, ice cream, malted milk, milkshake, milk mixes, and sherbet.

- Vegetable. Vegetables to be avoided due to their high potassium levels are baked beans, dried beans, lima beans, fresh broccoli, brussels sprouts, raw carrots, raw celery, peas, spinach (fresh or frozen), and potatoes (in skin or frozen). Vegetables to be avoided due to their high sodium levels are carrots, spinach, canned beets, turnips, dandelion greens, collards, and mixed vegetables.

- Fruit. For potassium- and sodium-restricted diets, the following fruits should be avoided: all dried and frozen fruits with sodium sulfite added, fresh apricots, avocado, bananas, glazed fruits, maraschino cherries, nectarines, prunes, and raisins.

- Bread. The following foods on the bread exchange list should be avoided on sodium- and potassium-restricted diets: yeast breads or rolls made from commercial mixes, quick breads made with baking powder, commercial baked products, graham crackers (except low-sodium dietetic ones), self-rising flour, salted popcorn, potato chips, pretzels, and waffles.

- Meat. Meats to avoid are all canned, salted, or smoked meats (e.g., bacon, bologna, corned beef, ham, sausage, kosher meats, and luncheon meats); all canned, salted, or smoked fish (e.g., anchovies, caviar, cod, herring, halibut, sardines, salmon, and tuna); cheddar, cottage, American, and Swiss cheeses should be avoided on sodium-restricted diets.

Source: Reprinted with permission of Macmillan Publishing Company from *Normal and Therapeutic Nutrition,* 16th edition, by Corinne H. Robinson and Marilyn R. Lawler. Copyright © 1982 by Macmillan Publishing Co. Reprinted by permission.

(especially low-density lipoproteins) by the liver. Anemia results from decreased secretion of erythropoietin.

The goal of dietary and drug treatment of nephrotic syndrome is to alleviate the symptoms of edema, protein malnutrition, and hyperlipidemia. The most effective means of preventing edema and initiating **diuresis** is severe sodium restriction. Nephrotic syndrome results in very little sodium excretion or about 230 mg/day (10 mEq/day). Therefore, dietary sodium intake must be equally low and must not exceed 10 mEq/day.

Protein malnutrition can be helped by high protein intake (65–200 g/day or, more accurately, 1.5 g per kilogram of ideal body weight). As with any high-protein diet, it needs to be accompanied by a high kilocalorie intake (35–50 kcal per kilogram of ideal body weight). When necessary, high-protein supplements and tube feeding may be used.

The hyperlipidemia problem that accompanies nephrotic syndrome is often type IIa and IIb, with type V being the most common. The diet should be appropriate for the type of hyperlipoproteinemia.

Losses of calcium, potassium, and vitamin D may occur with nephrotic syndrome. The symptom of bone pain may indicate calcium deficiency and muscular pain indicates potassium deficiency. Diets should contain adequate amounts of these minerals and iron in order to prevent deficiency symptoms.[3]

RENAL FAILURE

Renal failure results when enough damage to the kidneys has occurred so that they no longer adequately excrete nitrogenous wastes (urea, uric acid, and creatinine) and maintain the composition of the various electrolytes in the blood. Diagnosis is generally based on azotemia. The volume of urine decreases to the point of oliguria and even to **anuria.** If renal failure progresses to a severe stage, the person may develop **uremic syndrome,** which is a complex of symptoms caused by azotemia. The symptoms and their sources are discussed later.

Like the other renal diseases, renal failure can be sudden or **acute renal failure** and the person can regain normal function of the kidney tissue. Alternatively, the failure may occur gradually and is referred to as **chronic renal failure.**

Acute Renal Failure

A rapid drop in the urine volume to about 500 ml can result from dehydration, fever, allergic reactions, immunologic reactions, shock, and glomerulonephritis. When the urine volume drops below 600 ml/day, the excretion of urea, uric acid, and creatinine is not adequate and these waste products may increase to toxic levels.

Diuresis Increased urine flow.

Renal failure A condition in which kidney damage is severe enough that the kidneys no longer excrete the nitrogenous wastes or maintain the electrolytes in the blood.

Anuria Execretion of less than 50 ml of urine per day.

Uremic syndrome A complex of symptoms that result from an extremely high level of nitrogenous wastes in the blood.

Acute renal failure Sudden onset of renal failure.

Chronic renal failure Gradual onset of renal failure.

Dietary and Drug Treatment. Dietary treatment of acute renal failure is as follows:

Discover and treat the cause. Since acute renal failure is an abrupt problem that results from a cause other than damage to the kidneys, it is important to determine the cause and treat it before permanent damage to the kidneys occurs.

Maintain fluid homeostasis. Fluid intakes should replace urine output plus **insensible water loss,** with about 400 ml/day allowed for this loss. During the oliguric phase, fluid intake will be low, but during the diuretic phase, it must be increased in order to prevent **hypovolemic shock** and dehydration. Diuretics may be necessary during the oliguric phase to prevent uremic syndrome and edema.

Maintain mineral homeostasis. Potassium is not excreted in acute renal failure and may build up in the blood, since it is a by-product of tissue destruction. Potassium intake should be restricted to 30–50 mEq/day (1,200–2,000 mg/day). Dialysis may be used when there is an urgent need to reduce serum potassium levels. It is possible to lose large amounts of potassium during the diuretic phase, which may result in hypokalemia. When this occurs, potassium chloride may be added to the diet.

Prevent malnutrition. Prevention of possible malnutrition may hasten recovery and improve survival. Protein catabolism in cases of vomiting and diarrhea is prevented by administering amino acids and glucose in parenteral solutions. The majority of the kilocalorie intake should come from carbohydrates and fat, since their waste products are not excreted through the impaired kidneys. Kilocalorie intake should be high (50 kcal per kilogram of ideal body weight) to prevent tissue breakdown and promote synthesis of new tissue.

Prevent uremic syndrome. If the levels of urea and other wastes are high, **peritoneal dialysis** or **hemodialysis** may have to be used to diminish their toxic effects.

Chronic Renal Failure

Chronic renal failure occurs over a long period of time and is usually secondary to other diseases such as diabetes mellitus, chronic glomerulonephritis, atherosclerosis, and malignant hypertension.

Chronic renal failure can progress through four stages. Stage 1 is characterized by loss of 50 to almost 70% of the kidney tissue. This stage is frequently not distinguishable, since the kidneys can continue to function normally even with this amount of damage. Stage 2 is characterized by damage to more than 75% of the kidney tissue. At this stage, the ability of the kidneys to filter out nitrogenous wastes is decreased to the

---

Insensible water loss Fluid lost through the skin, vomiting, diarrhea, and fever (averages about 400–600 ml per day).

Hypovolemic shock Shock caused by low blood volume.

Peritoneal dialysis Infusion of dialysate fluid through a tube into the abdominal cavity. Nitrogenous wastes, excess fluids, and electrolytes are exchanged from the blood through the peritoneum into the dialysate fluid. The fluid is then drained out.

Hemodialysis Circulation of arterial blood from the body into a machine called a *dialyzer.* Through diffusion and osmosis, nitrogenous wastes, excess fluid, and electrolytes are exchanged from the blood into the dialysate. The cleansed blood is then returned to the body.

End-stage renal disease (ESRD) The stage of chronic renal failure in which 90% of the kidney tissue is damaged.

Uremia (uremic syndrome) A complex of symptoms that result from an extremely high level of nitrogenous wastes in the blood.

Renal osteodystrophy A complication of end-stage renal disease that is characterized by the loss of calcium from the bones and bone mass.

Giordano-Giovannetti (G-G) diet A diet used to treat chronic renal failure.

point where mild azotemia occurs. Stage 3 is characterized by moderate to severe azotemia. Stage 4 occurs when 90% of the kidney tissue is damaged. This stage is often called **end-stage renal disease (ESRD).** At this point, the GFR has decreased to about 10–12 ml/min (normal, 95–135 ml/min), with the end result being **uremia (uremic syndrome).**

Some of the symptoms of uremic syndrome are fatigue, weakness, decreased mental alertness, hyperglycemia, hyperlipidemia, hypertension, anorexia, nausea, and vomiting. In later stages, pH and metabolic imbalances result in gastrointestinal ulcers and bleeding. A major complication of ESRD is **renal osteodystrophy.** Renal failure results in retention of phosphorus and loss of calcium (refer to Chapter 7 for information on the reciprocal relationship of calcium and phosphorus).

Dietary and Drug Treatment. The basic goals of nutritional care in chronic renal failure include the following:

Regulation of protein intake. As renal function and the GFR decrease, so does dietary protein intake. Table 23-3 presents the amount of protein intake in relation to creatinine clearance. The **Giordano-Giovannetti (G-G) diet** is frequently used to supply protein, kilocalories, sugar, and fats. The diet (Table 23-4) provides about 20 g of high-quality protein with almost all the essential amino acids. The low level of protein intake causes the body to use some of the urea to make the nonessential amino acids. The end result is a positive nitrogen balance and a reduction in urea levels.

Fluid intake to balance urinary output and insensible losses. Fluid intake should not exceed urinary output and the amount from the insensible losses. Allowing about 400–600 ml for insensible losses, plus the amount excreted in the urine, is usually adequate.

Regulation of sodium intake to balance output. Sodium intake is dependent on urinary sodium excretion, the presence of edema, the serum sodium level, and blood pressure. When hypertension, edema, and oliguria are present, sodium intake must be restricted to equal urinary sodium output. When vomiting and diarrhea are present, sodium intake needs to be increased.

TABLE 23-3 PROTEIN INTAKE IN RELATION TO CREATININE CLEARANCE

Creatinine Clearance (ml/min)	Protein Allowance (g/day)
30–20	50
20–15	40
15–10	30
10–5	25

TABLE 23-4 GIORDANO-GIOVANNETTI DIET

20 g protein per day	Amount of protein per exchange
1 egg	(7 g)
¾ cup milk or 1 oz meat	(7 g)
½ lb low-protein bread	(1.5 g)
or	
1 piece of regular bread	
2–4 vegetable exchanges	(2 g per exchange)
Fats and sweets as desired to supply adequate kilocalorie intake	

Determination of potassium balance. Hyperkalemia may occur when the volume of urine formed is very low or anuric. Potassium restriction depends on serum potassium levels and urinary potassium loss.

Control phosphorus intake. As mentioned earlier, ESRD results in retention of phosphorus; therefore, the amount in the diet depends on the degree of renal function. Generally, a low-protein diet is low in phosphorus. However, foods that are high in phosphorus and therefore may need to be restricted are dried beans and peas, dried fruit, milk, nuts, whole grain breads, whole grain cereals, and peanut butter. Another method used to control the phosphorus level is to administer aluminum hydroxide medications such as Amphojel, Basaljel, and Alu-Caps. These compounds bind with phosphorus in the intestines and prevent its absorption. The advantage of these compounds is that they do not require restriction of foods that are high in phosphorus. However, some people find them unpalatable, and they can cause constipation.

Control energy requirements. Kilocalorie requirements range from 1,800 to 3,500 per day, based on the individuals height, age, weight, sex, and activity level. Since individuals suffering from ESRD frequently do not have much desire to eat, it is difficult to get them to consume this level of kilocalories. Therefore, their diet frequently must include concentrated caloric sources such as honey, heavy cream, sugar, hard candy, butter, jam, and jelly. This high kilocalorie intake is very important to avoid protein degradation and therefore, an elevation of the urea level.

Provide vitamin and mineral supplementation. A diet that is low in protein is also low in various vitamins such as thiamin, riboflavin, niacin, pyridoxine, ascorbic acid, and vitamin D. It is also deficient in iron and calcium. Ironically, renal failure results in iron and calcium deficiencies, with iron deficiency resulting from gastrointestinal tract ulcers. Calcium deficiency results from the inability of the kidneys to

TABLE 23-5 PROTEIN-SODIUM-POTASSIUM-CONTROLLED DIET FOR RENAL DISEASE

Purpose:	Designed to minimize complications frequently associated with acute and chronic renal failure and to maintain ideal body weight (IBW).
Use:	A guide for planning diets for persons with acute or chronic renal failure.
Examples of foods:	Diet provides specific amounts of protein, electrolytes, and fluid, depending on the individual's needs.
Adequacy:	Diets containing less than 40 g protein are deficient in the following nutrients: protein, niacin, riboflavin, thiamin, calcium, phosphorus, and iron for both men and women. Levels of protein between 40 and 60 g are deficient in niacin, riboflavin, thiamin, and calcium for men and calcium and iron for women.

Source: Chicago Dietetic Association, *Manual of Clinical Dietetics*, 2nd ed. Philadelphia, W.B. Saunders Company, 1981. Reprinted by permission.

activate vitamin D or secrete calcitriol (dihydroxycholecalciferol). Calcium should be supplied from supplements, with 1,200–1,600 mg/day being necessary to prevent loss of bone mass. A multivitamin preparation can provide iron and the above-mentioned vitamins.[4] The principles of a protein-sodium-potassium controlled diet for renal disease are provided in Table 23-5. (*See Case Study: Chronic Renal Failure, at end of Chapter, for reinforcement and application of chronic renal failure information.*)

DIALYSIS TREATMENT

Diet alone is not always successful in preventing uremia. At this point, the nitrogenous wastes have to be removed by dialysis, or else the person will die from complications of ESRD. The determination of when dialysis is required is based on the GFR. A commonly used figure is a GFR of 5–10 ml/min compared to a normal level of 125 ml/min. There are two types of dialysis: hemodialysis and peritoneal dialysis.

HEMODIALYSIS

In hemodialysis (see Fig. 23-2), the person's arterial blood, rich in nitrogenous wastes, is circulated from the body into a machine called a *dialyzer*. The blood circulates through semipermeable dialysis membranes that are bathed by a **dialysate** fluid. This fluid is similar in com-

Dialysate A fluid that bathes semipermeable dialysis membranes in dialyzer.

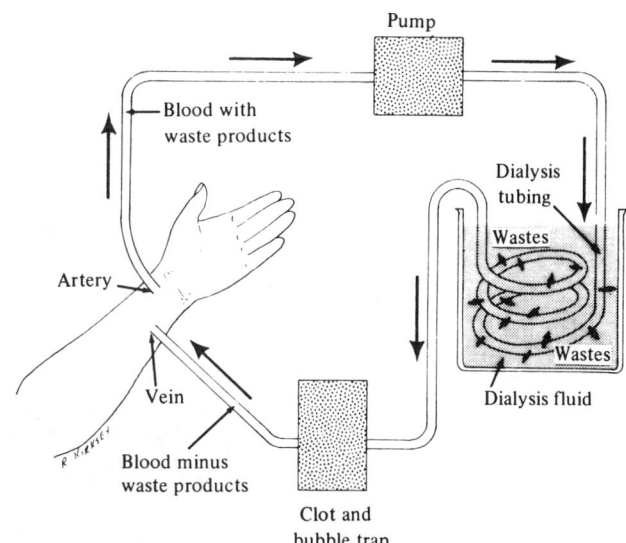

FIGURE 23-2 A dialysis kidney machine removes wastes from blood through dialysis tubing. (From T. Randall Lankford, *Integrated Science for Health Students*, 3rd ed., 1984. Reprinted by permission of Reston Publishing Company, a Prentice-Hall Company, 11480 Sunset Hills Road, Reston, Va. 22090.)

position to normal plasma. By diffusion and osmosis, the nitrogenous wastes, excess fluid, and electrolytes are exchanged from the person's blood into the dialysate. The cleansed blood is returned to the patient by a vein. The entire process takes about 4–6 hours and is repeated about three times per week.

One disadvantage of hemodialysis is loss of about 9–12 g of amino acids per 6-hour treatment. Hepatitis is a potential complication with nutritional implications. Another disadvantage is the cost; hospital-based hemodialysis is estimated to cost about $25,000 per year and home hemodialysis about $18,000 per year.

PERITONEAL DIALYSIS

Peritoneum membrane A membrane that covers most of the abdominal pelvic organs and through which exchange of nutrients and wastes occurs in peritoneal dialysis.

Peritoneal dialysis utilizes the **peritoneum membrane.** Dialysate fluid is infused through a tube into the person's abdominal cavity (see Fig. 23-3). The nitrogenous wastes, excess fluids, and electrolytes are exchanged from the person's blood through the peritoneum into the dialysate fluid. After about 20–40 minutes, the dialysate fluid with the wastes is drained out. For chronic but not acute cases, the procedure is repeated over 8–12 hours, three to five times a week. For acute conditions, the procedure is repeated over 36–72 hours.

Intact proteins can be lost (about 6–8 g/day) with peritoneal dialysis.

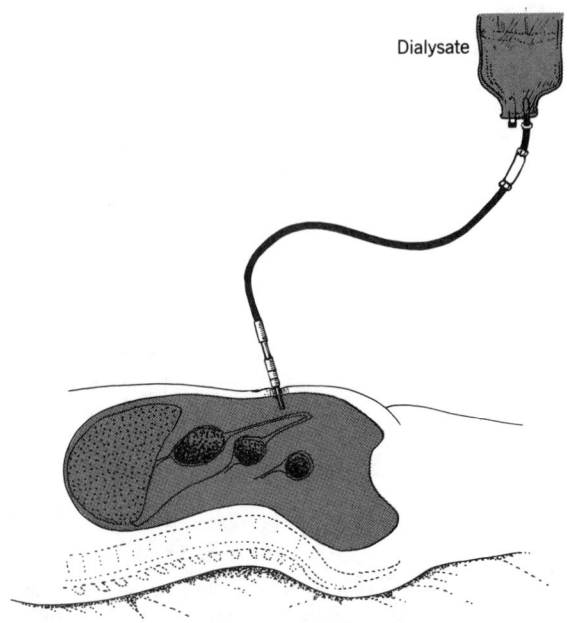

FIGURE 23-3 Peritoneal dialysis.

Another disadvantage of peritoneal dialysis is the potential for hyperglycemia due to the diffusion of large amounts of glucose into the blood.[5]

Diet Therapy for Dialysis Treatments

The diet therapy for hemodialysis and peritoneal dialysis is basically the
same as for predialysis for most nutrients, with the exception of proteins
and fluids.

	Hemodialysis	*Peritoneal Dialysis*	*Comments*
Proteins	Higher than for predialysis	Higher than for predialysis	Increased protein is required for both, due to loss of amino acids by hemodialysis and loss of intact proteins by peritoneal dialysis.
Fluids (ml/day)	Lower than for predialysis	Lower than for predialysis	With 90% of the nephrons destroyed and a GFR of 5–10 ml/min, the amount of fluid removed is very low compared to that of a predialysis person; if fluid intake is not restricted, the person experiences edema and weight gain.

RENAL CALCULI (KIDNEY STONES)

Kidney stones (renal calculi) Material that is composed of calcium phosphate, calcium oxalate, or a mixture of both.

Hyperparathyroidism An excessive secretion of the parathyroid hormone from the gland.

Kidney stones (renal calculi) are composed primarily of calcium phosphate, calcium oxalate, or a mixture of both. Various problems can cause these salts to precipitate out of urine, such as **hyperparathyroidism,** bone disease, and ingestion of excessive amounts of antacids (as is common in peptic ulcer treatment). Kidney stones may develop either in the kidney or the bladder, where they can obstruct the urinary system, resulting in infection and pain.

DIETARY AND DRUG TREATMENT

Many physicians do not consider diet to be important in treating kidney stones. Others use diet along with medications.

A high fluid intake of about 2,400–4,000 ml (at least 10–12 glasses) per day is very important to dilute the concentration of calcium in the urine. A reduction in the calcium level to about 400–600 mg/day is commonly recommended. This restriction is usually achieved by the removal of milk and dairy products. (See the sample menu for a calcium-restricted diet.) Increasing the acidity of urine helps to prevent the formation of calcium stones; this is accomplished by giving medications along with an acid ash diet. An **acid ash diet** includes foods that form an acid urine, such as cereals, meat, bread, fish, and eggs; foods high in protein tend to be good acid formers.

Acid ash diet A diet that includes foods that will form an acid urine.

If tests indicate that a person is forming calcium oxalate stones, foods high in oxalic acid should be restricted. Foods high in oxalic acid include asparagus, spinach, cranberries, plums, tea, cocoa, coffee, green beans, tomatoes, almonds, and cashews.

Thiazide diuretics such as chlorothiazide (Diuril) are often used, since they reduce renal excretion of calcium. A potential problem with this drug is hypercalcemia. Cholestyramine (Questran) can be administered to lower oxalate absorption; however, it also impairs absorption of iron and vitamin B_{12}.[2]

CASE STUDY: CHRONIC RENAL FAILURE

Ms. White, age 78, is admitted to the emergency room in a semicomatose state with severe nausea, vomiting, lack of coordination, and a complaint of weakness. She has been a diabetic for several years.

SAMPLE MENU OF A CALCIUM-RESTRICTED DIET

Exchange

Breakfast

1 fruit	½ cup raspberries
1 bread	¾ cup corn flakes
1 milk	1 cup skim milk
1 medium-fat meat	1 soft-cooked egg
1 bread	1 slice Italian bread
1 fat	1 tsp margarine
	1 tsp jelly
	1 cup coffee

Lunch

3 lean meat	3 oz cold sliced turkey
2 bread	2 slices Italian bread
1 bread	1 small potato
2 fat	2 tsp margarine
	4 oz angel food cake
1 fruit	¾ cup strawberries

Dinner

3 medium-fat meat	3 oz pork loin
1 bread	½ cup noodles
1 fat	1 tsp margarine
1 vegetable	½ cup zucchini squash
1 bread	1 hard roll made without milk
1 fat	1 tsp margarine
	½ cup fruit salad
	iced tea with lemon

Analysis and Comments

- An analysis of this menu shows the following exchanges, with the approximate amount of calcium in parentheses: 1 milk (290 mg), 1 vegetable (25 mg), 2 fruit (25 mg), 7 bread (35 mg), 7 meat (25 mg), and 5 fat (0 mg). The total amount of calcium is 400 mg.
- In order to achieve a calcium-restricted diet of 400–600 mg, the following exchanges and comments are important:

Milk. This is the most important exchange group that has to be limited, since 1 cup contains 290 mg. In addition, since it is important that an acid ash diet be followed for the treatment of calcium stones, it is important to restrict milk, since it causes an alkaline ash diet.

Vegetables. This exchange group does not provide much calcium; however, there are some vegetables that should be avoided due to their higher calcium levels: dried beans, broccoli, green cabbage, greens, and okra. In addition to avoiding these vegetables, this exchange group in general does not help provide an acid ash diet, but rather an alkaline ash.

Fruit. Fresh, canned, or cooked fruits are low in calcium. Cranberries and plums are also good acid formers. Dried fruits should be avoided.

Bread. Many breads have to be avoided, since they are prepared with milk. Examples of breads that can be readily consumed are French or Italian breads (without added milk), pretzels, saltines, matzoh, and water rolls.

Meat. Beef, lamb, veal, pork, and poultry all contain little calcium. However, seafood such as crabs, lobster, oysters, salmon, and sardines should be avoided.

Fat. All fats are low in calcium, except for mayonnaise, sweet cream, and sour cream.

Source: Menu adapted from C.H. Robinson and M.R. Lawler, *Normal and Therapeutic Nutrition,* 16th ed. New York: Macmillan, 1982. Reprinted by permission.

Physical Findings	Normal Values
Height 62 in.	
Weight 150 lb	118–132 lb
Blood pressure 220/98 mm Hg	Upper limit, 140/90 mm Hg
Edema in lower extremities	
Laboratory Values	
Blood urea nitrogen (BUN) 52 mg/dl	10–20 mg/dl
Creatinine clearance 15 ml/min	95–135 ml/min
Serum phosphorus 5.9 mg/dl	3–6 mg/dl
Serum calcium 7.1 mg/dl	8.5–10.5 mg/dl

Laboratory Values	Normal Values
Hemoglobin 8.6 g and hematocrit 27.0%	12–14 g/dl 40–48%
Serum potassium 6.3 mEq/liter	3.5–5.0 mEq/liter

Ms. White is diagnosed as having ESRD with severe chronic renal failure, severe fluid overload, hypertension, uremia, and anemia.

1. Ms. White's diagnosis of severe chronic renal failure and uremia are based primarily on which laboratory values?
   A. hemoglobin and hematocrit
   B. blood pressure values
   C. BUN, creatinine, and phosphorus
   D. calcium and blood pressure values

2. Ms. White's high BUN values indicate
   1. that she has been eating too much protein
   2. a significant decrease in filtration by nephrons
   3. a probable need for dialysis
   4. decreased absorption by nephrons
       A. 1, 2, 3   B. 1, 3   C. 2, 4   D. 4   E. all of these

3. Ms. White could suffer cardiac arrhythmias as a result of which substance that is present in an abnormal amount, according to the laboratory values?
   A. calcium
   B. iron
   C. phosphorus
   D. potassium

In order to reduce Ms. White's BUN level but still provide an adequate amount of proteins to avoid tissue breakdown, she is placed on the G-G (Giordano-Giovannetti) diet.

Using the key below and information in Table 23-4, determine which meals would provide 20 g of high-quality protein, and kilocalorie from sugars and fats.
   Key:
   a = meal allowed
   b = meal not allowed

___ 4. 2 eggs

> 6 oz meat
> $\frac{1}{2}$ lb normal bread (approximately 8 slices)
> 1 cup green beans
> 2 tbsp of jelly
> 2 tsp of butter

5. 1 egg
   1 oz meat
   $\frac{1}{2}$ cup asparagus
   $\frac{1}{2}$ cup carrots
   1 slice of bread + 1 teaspoon of butter + 2 tbsp jelly

6. Ms. White's fluid intake–urine output is: fluid intake per 24 hours, 3,500 ml; urine output per 24 hours, 900 ml. This record indicates that Ms. White is experiencing
   A. normal fluid output with intake
   B. fluid retention
   C. edema
   D. A, C
   E. B, C

7. In reference to the fluid figures given in question 6, what could be done to improve this condition?
   A. limit fluid intake to 3,500 ml
   B. limit fluid intake to 900 + 400 to 600 ml
   C. place Ms. White on dialysis
   D. A, C
   E. B, C

8. If Ms. White is placed on periodic peritoneal dialysis, her diet should be higher in _____ than a nondialysis diet.
   A. kilocalories
   B. carbohydrates
   C. fats
   D. proteins
   E. none of these

9. Ms. White is taking Basaljel tablets, which help her condition by _____ .
   A. decreasing her edema
   B. increasing her serum calcium level
   C. decreasing her serum phosphorus level
   D. decreasing her urea level

10. Ms. White is also taking the medication ferrous gluconate, which will help her _____ condition.

    A. potassium

    B. phosphorus

    C. anemic

    D. creatinine

FUNCTIONS OF THE KIDNEYS

Excretory Function
This is the most important function. The substances excreted are urea, uric acid, creatinine, excess water, electrolytes, and foreign substances.

Endocrine Function
The hormones secreted are erythropoietin, renin, and the active form of vitamin D (calcitriolor 1,25-dihyroxycholecalciferol).

NEPHRON: FUNCTIONAL UNIT OF THE KIDNEY

Glomerular Filtration
This occurs in the glomerulus of Bowman's capsule; both nutrients and wastes are filtered out; the glomerular filtration rate (GFR) averages about 125 ml/min; creatinine clearance is a measure of the GFR (95–135 ml/min is normal).

Reabsorption. Substances are reabsorbed up to their threshold level; about 80% of reabsorption occurs in the proximal tubule. Aldosterone stimulates the absorption of sodium and the excretion of potassium in the distal tubule and the collecting duct.

Secretion and Blood pH. The kidneys help regulate the pH of the blood by secreting hydrogen ions from blood into urine and reabsorbing bicarbonate ions.

KIDNEY DISEASES

Acute Glomerulonephritis
This condition is an inflammation of glomeruli, frequently caused by streptococci bacteria. Increased porosity of the membranes results in a loss of large molecules like proteins and red blood cells.

Symptoms
Hematuria, proteinuria, edema, oliguria, increase in BUN, and hypertension.

Dietary and Drug Treatment
- Fluid intake limited to the amount lost the previous day during oliguria.
- Increased carbohydrate intake primarily from fruit juices.
- Limited protein intake to about 40 g/day during oliguria.
- Sodium restriction during edema.

Chronic Glomerulonephritis
It can be caused by repeated episodes of glomerulonephritis.

Symptoms
Increased loss of protein, accumulation of urea and creatinine.

Dietary and Drug Treatment
Same as that of chronic glomerulonephritis.

Nephrotic Syndrome
Symptoms
Large losses of protein in urine, severe edema, low serum protein level, elevated blood cholesterol level, and anemia.

Dietary Treatment
- Severe sodium restriction to about 230 mg/day (10 mEq/day).
- High protein intake (about 1.5 g per kilogram of ideal body weight).
- High kilocalorie intake (35–50 kcal per kilogram of ideal body weight).
- Diet appropriate for the type of hyperlipidemia (type V is most common).
- Increased intake of calcium, potassium, and vitamin D.

Renal Failure
This condition is diagnosed when the kidneys cannot filter out nitrogenous wastes adequately, leading to azotemia, oliguria, and even anuria.

Acute Renal Failure
This condition can be caused by dehydration, fever, allergic reactions, immunologic reactions, shock, and glomerulonephritis.

Dietary and Drug Treatment
- Discover and treat the cause
- Maintain fluid homeostasis
- Maintain mineral homeostasis
- Prevent malnutrition
- Prevent uremic syndrome

Chronic Renal Failure
This condition occurs over a long period of time. It is usually secondary to diseases such as diabetes mellitus, chronic glomerulonephritis, atherosclerosis, and malignant hypertension.

It can progress through four stages, with stage 4 occurring when 90% of the kidney tissue is damaged. Uremia and uremic syndrome occur, and if the GFR decreases to 5–10 ml/min, dialysis must be administered.

Symptoms

Fatigue, weakness, decreased mental alertness, hyperglycemia, hyperlipidemia, hypertension, anorexia, nausea, and vomiting. Renal osteodystrophy is a major complication.

Dietary and Drug Treatment

- Regulation of protein intake
- Fluid intake to balance urinary output and insensible losses
- Regulation of sodium intake to balance output
- Potassium restriction
- Control of phosphorus intake
- Increased energy level from concentrated carbohydrates and fats
- Vitamin and mineral supplementation

DIALYSIS TREATMENT

Dialysis is required when the GFR decreases to 5–10 ml/min; the waste level and uremia are so high that the patient will die without dialysis.

Hemodialysis

Blood from the patient is circulated into the dialyzer through dialysis membranes that are bathed by dialysate fluid. Wastes, fluids, and water are exchanged from blood with dialysate. Cleansed blood is returned to the patient through a vein.

The disadvantage of this process is a loss of 9–12 g of amino acids per 6-hour treatment.

Peritoneal Dialysis

The peritoneum membrane in the abdominal cavity is used to exchange wastes from the blood to the dialysate fluid in the abdominal cavity. The disadvantage of this process is a loss of 6–8 g of intact proteins per day of treatment.

Diet Therapy for Dialysis Treatments

It is the same as for predialysis except for proteins and fluids. There is increased intake of protein for both types of dialysis to replace the losses. Fluid intake is lower than during predialysis due to the inability of the kidneys to carry on filtration adequately.

RENAL CALCULI (KIDNEY STONES)

Kidney stones are composed mainly of calcium phosphate, calcium oxalate, or a mixture of both.

They can be caused by hyperparathyroidism, bone disease, or ingestion of excessive amounts of antacids.

Dietary and Drug Treatment

- High fluid intake (2,400–4,000 ml of water, or 10 to 12 glasses)
- Reduction in calcium level to 400–600 mg. The restriction of milk and dairy products usually is adequate.
- Increased consumption of acid-forming (high-protein) foods
- Reduced consumption of foods high in oxalic acid if the person is forming calcium oxalate stones.
- Use of thiazide diuretics to increase urination and decrease excretion of calcium.
- Cholestyramine can lower oxalate absorption.

REVIEW QUESTIONS

TRUE (A) OR FALSE (B)

Questions 1–17

1. A major function of the kidneys is excretion of aldosterone, renin, and erythropoietin.
2. A person who has damaged kidneys may have anemia due to decreased secretion of erythropoietin.
3. Filtration is a major function of the kidneys and can be determined by measuring the creatinine clearance.
4. Reabsorption of sodium and potassium occurs in the proximal tubule of the nephron.
5. Nephrons help regulate the normal pH of the blood by typically secreting bicarbonate and absorbing hydrogen ions.
6. Dietary treatment of acute glomerulonephritis includes high fluid intake to flush out the wastes plus high protein intake during oliguria to restore damaged tissues.
7. The diet for nephrotic syndrome is high protein (1.5 g per kilogram of ideal body weight) and high kilocalories (35–50 kcal per kilogram of ideal body weight).
8. Renal failure occurs when the kidneys no longer adequately excrete the nitrogenous wastes (urea, uric acid, and creatinine) and the volume of urine produced drops to 50% of normal.
9. Two components of dietary treatment of acute renal failure are restriction of potassium and intake and provision of kilocalories primarily from carbohydrates and fat.
10. Stage 4 of chronic renal failure is called *end-stage renal failure,* and the GFR is decreased to about 10–12 ml/min.
11. As renal function and GFR decrease in chronic renal failure, protein intake is increased to restore damaged tissue.

12. The Giordano-Giovannetti (G-G) diet supplies only about 20 g of protein, with almost all the essential amino acids and urea used to synthesize nonessential amino acids.
13. A major complication of ESRD is renal osteodystrophy, which is retention of too much calcium.
14. ESRD diets frequently have a restriction on foods high in phosphorus, such as dried beans and peas, dried fruit, milk, nuts, and whole grain cereals.
15. Hemodialysis has the disadvantage of causing amino acids to be lost (about 9–12 g per 6-hour treatment).
16. Peritoneal dialysis does not involve any nutrient losses and can be completed in a shorter period of time than hemodialysis.
17. Dietary treatment of calcium phosphate or calcium oxalate renal stones is an alkaline ash diet and reduction of foods high in protein.

MULTIPLE CHOICE

Questions 18–26

18. Substances that the kidneys excrete are:
    1. urea, uric acid, and creatinine
    2. renin
    3. excess amounts of sodium, potassium, and hydrogen ions
    4. active form of vitamin D

    A. 1, 2, 3   B. 1, 3   C. 2, 4   D. 4
    E. all of these

19. Kidney diseases can affect the functions of the nephrons, which are:
    1. filtration
    2. reabsorption
    3. secretion
    4. synthesis of fats

    A. 1, 2, 3   B. 1, 3   C. 2, 4   D. 4
    E. all of these

20. Symptoms associated with glomerulonephritis and the reasons for them are:
    1. hematuria—protein in the urine results from decreased porosity of the glomeruli.
    2. edema—retention of protein results in increased osmotic pressure
    3. proteinuria—blood in the urine results from damage to glomeruli.
    4. oliguria—diminished urine output to about 500 ml/day results from increased damage to nephrons

    A. 1, 2, 3   B. 1, 3   C. 2, 4   D. 4
    E. all of these

21. The anemia of ESRD results from
    A. decreased synthesis of renin
    B. decreased synthesis of erythropoietin
    C. bleeding from gastrointestinal ulcers
    D. A, B
    E. B, C

22. Uremia and uremic syndrome associated with ESRD results from a buildup of _____ due to decreased _____ in the nephrons.
    A. hydrogen ions—secretion
    B. nitrogenous wastes—reabsorption
    C. sodium and potassium—filtration
    D. nitrogenous wastes—filtration

23. Increased intake of calcium in renal failure is necessary to reduce _____ .
    A. loss of bone mass, or renal osteodystrophy
    B. potential for cardiac arrhythmias
    C. edema
    D. anemia

24. A renal failure diet may include the restriction of milk, nuts, whole grain breads, and peanut butter and the administration of Amphojel, Basaljel, or Alu-Caps to control the level of _____ .
    A. potassium
    B. phosphorus
    C. sodium
    D. calcium

25. Concentrated sugars and fats such as honey, sugar, heavy cream, butter, and jam are included in a renal failure diet is to achieve a _____ without producing nitrogenous wastes.
    A. high level of protein
    B. low level of calcium
    C. high energy intake
    D. none of these

26. Dietary and drug treatments of calcium phosphate and calcium oxalate kidney stones include:
    1. restricted fluid intake
    2. high fluid intake (2,400–4,000 ml) per day
    3. drugs that cause urine to become more alkaline
    4. increased intake of high-protein foods

    A. 1, 2, 3   B. 1, 3   C. 2, 4   D. 4
    E. all of these

DISCUSSION QUESTIONS

1. Discuss the dietary and drug treatment of acute glomerulonephritis.
2. Describe the dietary modifications necessary to alleviate the edema, protein malnutrition, and hyperlipidemia associated with nephrotic syndrome.

3. Describe the causes of chronic renal failure and the dietary treatment to alleviate the symptoms.

4. Discuss the dietary and drug treatments of calcium phosphate and calcium oxalate kidney stones.

REFERENCES

1. L.S. Brunner and D.S. Suddarth. *Textbook of Medical Surgical Nursing*, 5th ed. Philadelphia: J.B. Lippincott Co., 1984, pp. 1000–1002.

2. B.G. Morrissey. *Therapeutic Nutrition*. Philadelphia: J.B. Lippincott Co., 1984, pp. 323–327.

3. B.T. Burton and G.H. Hirschman. "Current concepts of nutritional therapy in chronic renal failure: An update." *Journal of the American Dietetic Association*, 82 359 (1983).

4. T. Beaudette. "Nutritional aspects of chronic renal disease." *Nutrition in Practice*. 1(5), 5–18 (1982).

5. B. Luke. *Principles of Nutrition and Diet Therapy*. Boston: Little, Brown, and Co., 1984, pp. 717–719.

24 NUTRITION AND CANCER

OBJECTIVES

Upon completion of this chapter, you should be able to:

1. Define cancer and compare its rate of occurrence in younger and older people.

2. Describe the relationship of diet to the possible causes of breast and colon cancers.

3. Give six dietary recommendations that may reduce the risk of cancer.

4. List four possible reasons for anorexia in cancer patients.

5. Describe cachexia in terms of its characteristics, major problems resulting from it, and two complications.

6. Describe diet therapy for cancer patients in terms of protein, kilocalories, and vitamin intake.

7. Give three ways in which diet can be modified to alleviate nausea and vomiting.

8. Discuss the advantages of tube feeding and parenteral nutrition in treating cancer.

INTRODUCTION

Neoplasm Tumor.

Cancer is an abnormal growth or **neoplasm** of the body cells. It tends to grow without control and can spread to secondary sites. It is the second leading cause of death in the United States. Cancer is primarily a disease of older people rather than younger ones, with the death rate being over 10 times greater at age 50 and 100 times greater at age 65 than it is at age 25.[1] The leading types of cancer in the United States, in decreasing order, are lung, colon, and breast cancer. Apparently, there is no relationship between diet and lung cancer, as there is with breast and colon cancer.

DIET AND POSSIBLE CAUSES OF BREAST AND COLON CANCERS

Current research suggests a link between diet and both breast cancer and colon cancer. It should be emphasized that the research has not proven that certain dietary deficiencies and excesses definitely cause cancer. Rather, it has shown certain relationships, as discussed below.

DIET AND BREAST CANCER

Research shows that breast cancer is related to a diet that is high in animal fat. One theory about how this relationship may induce the development of cancer is that high fat causes increased release of the hormones estrogen and prolactin. These hormones may alter the immune resistance of the breasts, making it prone to the development of tumors.[2]

DIET AND COLON CANCER

Most researchers believe that there is a close correlation between a high animal fat diet and colon cancer. A high-fat diet may cause colon cancer for the following reasons:

Carcinogenic A cancer-causing substance.

- A high-fat diet results in increased secretion of bile, which possibly is changed by intestinal bacteria into a **carcinogenic** form.
- Bile salts might be carcinogenic in large quantities.
- Fats themselves may be carcinogenic.[3]

    As mentioned in Chapter 3, one possible advantage of a high-fiber diet is prevention of colon cancer. Fiber may reduce the incidence of colon cancer by increasing the rate at which fats are moved through the colon, thereby decreasing the length of time the possible carcinogenic products are in contact with the colon walls. There are two other possible cancer-reducing factors of fiber: first, fiber dilutes the intestinal contents, which are therefore less irritating; second, certain fibers (lignin and pectin) may bind with bile and decrease its absorption.

DIETARY RECOMMENDATIONS TO REDUCE THE RISK OF CANCER

Despite the lack of definitive data that some nutrients can definitely cause cancer, a 1982 report by the National Academy of Sciences gave some dietary suggestions that may reduce the risk of common cancers. The committee offered the following dietary suggestions:[1]

- Reduce the intake of both saturated and unsaturated fats so that they compose approximately 30% of the daily kilocalories.
- Consume more fruits and vegetables, especially those high in vitamins A and C.
- Eat whole grain cereals (a good source of fiber) daily.
- Restrict the intake of salt-cured, salt-pickled, and smoked foods.
- Use alcohol in moderation.
- Avoid high-dose supplements of individual nutrients.

NUTRITIONAL PROBLEMS AND DIET THERAPY FOR CANCER PATIENTS

Two common nutritional problems associated with common cancers are anorexia and **cachexia.**

Cachexia A problem characterized by extreme weight loss, weakness, and severe wasting of tissues.

ANOREXIA

Anorexia, or decreased appetite, is the primary nutritional problem in cancer and is a major cause of cachexia. No one knows exactly what causes anorexia, but some of the possible reasons are altered tastes, a feeling of fullness, altered metabolism, and nausea or vomiting. The side effects of cancer therapy often result in anorexia.

CACHEXIA

Cachexia and malnutrition are synonymous. Loss of tissue protein is the major problem in cachexia, and one reason for the loss is that cancer results in increased metabolism. This is coupled with anorexia (decreased appetite and reduced protein intake) and the fact that tumors have a tendency to retain nitrogen. In addition, serum albumin tends to leak out of the blood into the tissue fluids. The end result of anorexia, retention of nitrogen in tumors and loss of albumin is less synthesis of proteins in the tissues.

In addition to protein deficiencies, cachexia typically results in anemia and vitamin A and vitamin C deficiencies (see Table 24-1). Anemia typically results from decreased availability of iron. The reasons for the vitamin A and C deficiencies are not known.

The major complications of cachexia are increased susceptibility to infections (due to decreased synthesis of protein antibodies) and decreased tolerance of cancer therapies (surgery, chemotherapy, and radiation therapy).[4]

DIET THERAPY

Two objectives of diet therapy for cancer patients are to meet the increased metabolic needs of the body and to alleviate the symptoms of

TABLE 24-1 HOW THE CANCER PATIENT WASTES AWAY

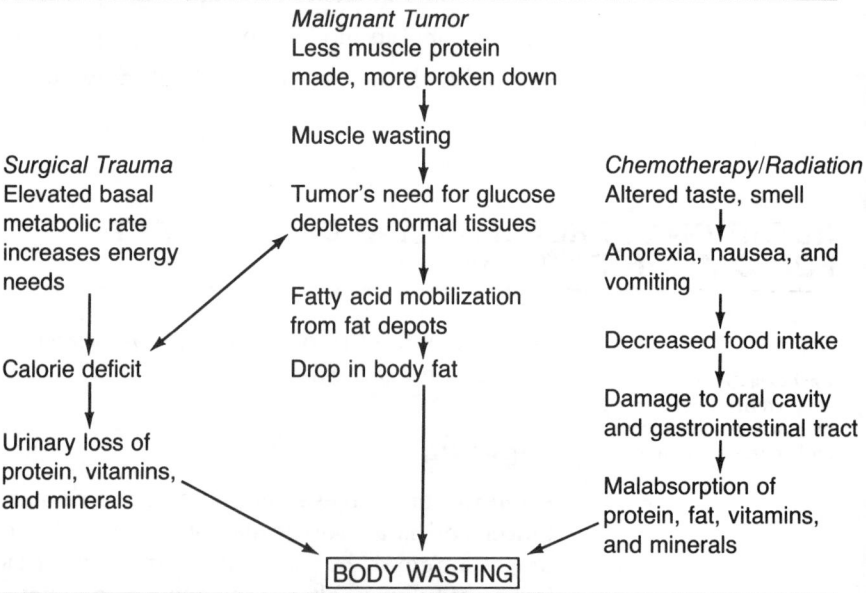

Source: Published in *RN*, a full-service nursing journal. Copyright © 1985 Medical Economics Company Inc., Oradell, N.J. March 1985, vol. 48. pp. 22–27. Reprinted by permission.

the disease or the side effects of the treatment. Specific details of diet therapy are as follows:

High protein. Increased protein intake is important to replace the tissue losses and increase the body's resistance to infection. Approximately 1 g protein per kilogram of ideal body weight is often adequate for a well-nourished patient and 2–3 g/kg for a malnourished patient.

High kilocalories. Due to the hypermetabolic condition that accompanies cancer, the diet should contain 2,000–4,000 kcal. Most of these kilocalories should be from nonprotein sources so that proteins can be spared for tissue synthesis. Since most cancer patients exhibit anorexia, getting them to increase their intake of kilocalories and proteins is not always easy. Some examples of how to accomplish this goal are as follows:

- Add milk powder to milk, cereals, soups, gravies, and ground meat.
- Add groud meat and cheese to dishes like soups and sauces.
- Increase the consumption of foods like eggs and peanut butter by adding them to other dishes.

Vitamin intake. Vitamins A and C typically need to be increased for most cancer patients, since they are usually deficient in these nutrients. Thiamin is usually increased to metabolize the high kilocalorie intake. Increased amounts of vitamin B_{12} and folacin help to alleviate anemia.

Nausea and vomiting are common side effects of chemotherapy. Antinausea medications can be given 30 minutes before meals to help alleviate this problem. However, they are frequently ineffective in cancer patients. These people can benefit by eating smaller meals, sipping clear beverages slowly, and eating foods cold rather than hot, since hot foods give off more aromas, which often cause nausea.

The taste alterations that often result from cancer frequently decrease the ability to taste salt and sugar; patients also often complain that meat smells rotten. In these cases, substitutions of milk, eggs, and cheeses provides sources of protein.

Oral feeding is always the method of choice. However, due to persistent anorexia, malnutrition, and the side effects of therapy, tube feeding and parenteral nutrition may have to be used. Until recently, parenteral nutrition was not used extensively for treating cancer. The reason was the fear that this aggressive nutritional support would cause increased growth of the tumor. However, studies show that tube feedings and parenteral nutrition enable a cancer patient to tolerate larger doses of chemotherapy and radiation therapy.[5]

CASE STUDY: CANCER PATIENT

Mr. S is a 50-year-old-man who has lung cancer. He has been receiving chemotherapy once a week. Currently, he is hospitalized for the management of anemia, which is often a side effect of chemotherapy.

Physical Findings	Normal Values
Height: 5 ft 10 in.	
Body weight: 141 lb (64 kg)	151–163 lb (medium frame)
Laboratory Findings	
Blood albumin: 2.5 g/dl	3.5–5.0 g/dl
Hemoglobin: 11.5 g/dl	13.5–18.0 g/dl
Hematocrit: 35%	40–54%
Ascorbic acid: 0.1 mg/dl	0.4–2.0 mg/dl
Vitamin A: 10 μg/dl	15–60 μg/dl

Using the above data and the information in this chapter, answer the following questions.

1. The above data indicate that Mr. S may be suffering from the nutritional problem called _____.
   A. neoplasm
   B. carcinoma
   C. cachexia
   D. myeloma

2. Mr. S is probably in a negative nitrogen balance, which is indicated by _____.
   A. the low ascorbic acid value
   B. the low blood albumin value
   C. the low vitamin A value
   D. none of these

3 Mr. S's condition and body weight indicate that the amount of protein he should be consuming is _____ g.
   A. 128–192
   B. 64
   C. 51
   D. 35–50

4. Mr. S's diet should contain approximately _____ kcal.
   A. 800–1,200
   B. 1,200–1,500
   C. 1,500–1,800
   D. 2,000–4,000

5. According to the data, Mr. S is anemic; therefore, increased amounts of _____ should be given to alleviate this problem.
   A. vitamins A and C
   B. vitamin B_{12} and folacin
   C. vitamins E and K
   D. none of these

6. Mr. S is anorexic; to help him increase his intake of kilocalories and protein, the following might be tried:
   1. add milk powder to milk, cereals, soups, gravies, and ground meat
   2. add ground meat and cheese to dishes like soups and sauces
   3. increase the consumption of foods like eggs and peanut butter by adding to them other dishes
   4. increase the consumption of citrus fruits
      A. 1, 2, 3   B. 1, 3   C. 2, 4   D. 4   E. all of these

7. Since Mr. S is undergoing chemotherapy, _____ and _____ might enable him to tolerate larger doses.
   A. weight loss—exercise
   B. enteral feedings—larger doses of vitamins
   C. weight gain—overnutrition
   D. tube feedings—parenteral nutrition

OUTLINE

Cancer is a neoplasm of body cells; it grows out of control and can spread. It is more prevalent in older people than in younger ones. The leading types of cancer in the United States are lung, colon, and breast cancer.

Diet and Possible Causes of Breast and Colon Cancers

Diet and Breast Cancer
Breast cancer is related to a diet high in animal fat; high fat possibly causes increased release of the hormones estrogen and prolactin, which possibly decrease the immunity of the breasts to cancer.

Diet and Colon Cancer
Colon cancer is related to a diet high in animal fat; possible reasons are:

- Conversion of increased bile to a carcinogenic form
- Bile salts might be carcinogenic in large quantities.
- Fats may be carcinogenic.

Dietary Recommendations to Reduce the Risk of Cancer

- Reduce saturated and unsaturated fats so that they compose 30% of the daily kilocalories.
- Consume more fruits and vegetables, especially those high in vitamins A and C.
- Eat whole grain cereals daily.
- Restrict the intake of salt-cured, salt-pickled, and smoked foods.
- Use alcohol in moderation.
- Avoid high-dose supplements of individual nutrients.

Nutritional Problems and Diet Therapy for Cancer Patients

Two common nutritional problems associated with cancers are anorexia and cachexia.

Anorexia
Possible causes are altered tastes, a feeling of fullness, altered metabolism, and nausea or vomiting.

Cachexia
It is characterized by extreme weight loss, weakness, and severe wasting of tissues. Loss of tissue protein is a major problem that results partially from increased metabolism. It may also be caused by anorexia, retention of nitrogen by tumors, and leakage of serum albumin into tissues.

Two complications are increased susceptibility to infections and decreased tolerance of cancer therapies.

Diet Therapy

- High protein. Approximately 1 g protein per kilogram of ideal body weight for a well-nourished patient and 2–3 g protein/kg for a malnourished patient.
- High kilocalories. From 2,000 to 4,000 kcal/day for tissue synthesis; most should come from nonprotein sources.
- Vitamin intake. Typically, increases in vitamins A and C, since they are usually deficient.
  Increased levels of thiamin for metabolism of nutrients.
  Increased amounts of vitamin B_{12} and folacin for anemia.
- Ways to reduce nausea and vomiting. Use of antinausea medications, eating smaller meals, slowly sipping clear beverages, eating foods cold rather than hot.
  Substitution of milk, eggs, and cheese for meats.
  If oral feeding is not possible or needs to be supplemented, tube feeding and parenteral nutrition are employed.

REVIEW QUESTIONS

TRUE (A) OR FALSE (B)
Questions 1–13

1. Cancer is as prevalent in younger people as it is in older ones.
2. Breast cancer is related to a low-fiber diet.
3. Research shows that there are certain links between diet and cancer, as opposed to definite proof that diet causes it.
4. Colon cancer is related to a low-fat diet.
5. Fiber may reduce the risk of colon cancer by increasing the rate at which food moves through the colon and binds with bile, thereby decreasing its absorption.
6. Dietary recommendations that might reduce cancer are reduction of fats to no more than 30% of total kilocalories and consumption of whole grain cereals daily.
7. Anorexia is the primary nutritional problem in cancer and is a major cause of cachexia.
8. Cachexia is characterized by weight gain and decreased metabolism.

9. The major complications of cachexia are weight loss and edema.
10. Diet therapy for cancer includes low levels of protein in order to reduce stress on the kidneys.
11. The diet for a cancer patient should be high in fat as a source of kilocalories.
12. Foods served cold are tolerated by anorexic and nauseated patients better than they are when served warm.
13. A major advantage of tube feeding and parenteral nutrition is the intake of a large amount nutrients despite anorexia or nausea.

DISCUSSION QUESTIONS

1. Give six dietary recommendations that may reduce the risk of cancer.
2. Describe cachexia in terms of characteristics, major problems resulting from it, and two complications.
3. Describe diet therapy for cancer patients in terms of protein, kilocalorie, and vitamin intake.
4. Discuss the advantages of tube feeding and parenteral nutrition in treating cancer.

REFERENCES

1. D.A. Wenck, M. Baren, and S.P. Dewan, *Nutrition: The Challenge of Being Well Nourished*, 2nd ed. Reston, Va.: Reston Publishing Co., Inc., 1983, pp. 438–446.
2. M.B. Lipsett, "Drugs and hormones." *Nutrition Today*, 13(5), 9 (1978).
3. E.L. Wynder, "Dietary habits in cancer." *Nutrition Today*, 13(5), 8 (1978).
4. T. Beaudette. "Diet, nutrition, and cancer." *Nutrition in Practice*, 1(2), 4–17 (1981).
5. M.E. Shils, "How to nourish the cancer patient." *Nutrition Today*, 16, 4–15 (1981).

25 PRE- AND POSTOPERATIVE NUTRITION

OBJECTIVES

Upon completion of this chapter, you should be able to:

1. State three ways in which preoperative nutrition is important.

2. Describe how kilocalories, proteins, vitamins, and minerals are important in the preoperative nutrition of an undernourished person.

3. Compare the difference in the preoperative diet 24 hours and 8 hours before surgery.

4. Describe a postoperative diet progression.

5. Give four ways in which a postoperative regular diet is beneficial to a person.

6. Describe the nutritional support for stages 1, 2, and 3 of burn care.

INTRODUCTION

Patients benefit from optimal nutrition preoperatively and postoperatively. A patient who is well nourished before surgery faces less of a chance of complications during and after surgery. A patient who is well nourished following surgery heals more quickly, fights infection better, loses less muscle tissue, and has a more positive attitude than a poorly nourished one.

PREOPERATIVE NUTRITION

Preoperative nutrition is important to meet the metabolic stress of surgery, improve wound healing, and increase resistance to infection. Two major nutritional problems in the preoperative period are undernutrition and obesity. The nutrients most needed by an undernourished patient are kilocalories, proteins, vitamins, and minerals. The importance of these nutrients for an undernourished patient before surgery are discussed next.

KILOCALORIES

Surgery is very stressful to the organ systems; an undernourished patient cannot compensate for the stress as effectively as a well-nourished one. There may not always be enough time to provide a high-kilocalorie diet orally before surgery. However, central vein total parenteral nutrition (TPN) is a way of providing a large amount of nutrients in a short period of time.

PROTEIN

During surgery, a patient who is deficient in protein (hypoproteinemia) is more susceptible to shock than one who is not, especially with great loss of blood. The liver is more threatened by anesthesia toxicity, and more edema occurs at the site of incision, all as a result of a low protein level. In contrast, adequate protein intake fortifies the patient for blood losses during surgery and for tissue catabolism.

In addition to these problems during surgery, a low protein level decreases the person's resistance to infection due to decreased synthesis of antibodies.

VITAMINS AND MINERALS

A deficiency of water-soluble vitamins hinders carbohydrate metabolism, which is increased during surgery. A deficiency of potassium may cause malfunction of the heart. Calcium and sodium are important for muscle and nerve activity. Vitamin K is important for blood clotting.

Obesity, the second major preoperative nutritional problem, presents a variety of potential problems:

- Fat tissue decreases the effects of some anesthetic agents.

- Greater strain on the heart is caused by increased fat.

- There is an increased chance of infection due to decreased resistance of fat tissue.[1]

PREOPERATIVE DIET

If there is enough time before surgery, an undernourished patient should be provided with a high-kilocalorie, high-protein, high-carbohydrate diet. Even a week of this type of diet can be valuable to the undernourished patient. Tube feeding and TPN may be required for some people who cannot consume food orally (see Chapter 17 for details on enteral-parenteral nutrition). An obese person should be placed on a weight loss diet.

Twenty-four hours before surgery, the diet should provide nutrients that cannot be stored by the body. These nutrients include glucose (the body has only about a 24-hour supply in the form of glycogen), B complex vitamins, and vitamin C. A high fluid intake is valuable during this time until fluids are withheld. If the person is iron deficient, iron supplementation is required.

Eight hours before surgery, all fluids and food are withheld. The reason is to help decrease regurgitation and aspiration of food, which can occur during anesthesia. If surgery is to be performed on the gastrointestinal tract, a restricted-residue diet is given for 2 or 3 days before surgery. The purpose of the diet is to reduce the amount of feces, which could interfere with surgery and lead to distention after surgery. A restricted-residue diet limits the amount of milk, fruits, and vegetables and allows only white bread. Many hospitals are now using synthetic low-residue and residue-free diets, since they contain simple carbohydrates, amino acids, essential fatty acids, minerals, and vitamins. They provide the important nutrients but are readily absorbed, with no remaining residue.

POSTOPERATIVE DIET

During surgery there is a loss of fluids and electrolytes; therefore, the immediate concern after surgery is to replace these losses. More fluids may be lost after surgery from vomiting, draining wounds, and diarrhea. Initially, fluids and electrolytes are replaced parenterally or enterally, since the person is usually nauseated and may be vomiting.

Once peristaltic contractions resume, the person can start receiving food orally. Frequently, a physician will order a diet progression from clear liquid to full liquid to a soft diet to a regular diet. See the sample menus for clear liquid and full liquid diets. Whether a progression through all of these diets is necessary, and at what rate, depends on the patient and on the severity and type of surgery. The faster the person can progress to a regular diet, the better. A regular diet, with its level of nutrients, enables the person to achieve a positive nitrogen balance, prevent weight loss, resist infection, and increase healing. Tables 25-1 through 25-4 present the principles of these diets.

TABLE 25-1 CLEAR (SURGICAL) LIQUID DIET

Purpose:	To minimize the amount of undigested material in the gastrointestinal tract.
Use:	Patients who have experienced surgery, vomiting, diarrhea, infections, and gastrointestinal problems will receive these diets.
Examples of foods:	Clear broth, plain Jello, water ice, all clear and strained fruit-juices of fruit drinks, tea, decaffeinated coffee, commercial low-residue, high-protein, high-calorie oral supplements; *no milk products are used, since they are high in residue.*
Adequacy:	Inadequate in all nutrients except vitamin C and should not be used for more than 1 or 2 days.

Source: Chicago Dietetic Association, *Manual of Clinical Dietetics*, 2nd ed. Philadelphia, W.B. Saunders Company, 1981. Reprinted by permission.

TABLE 25-2 FULL LIQUID DIET

Purpose:	To provide more nourishing fluids as the patient's gastrointestinal functions return to normal.
Use:	Transitional diet between the Clear Liquid Diet and the Soft Diet.
Examples of foods:	Milk and dairy products, fruit juices, strained vegetable juice, cooked or refined cereals, plain gelatin, and smooth pudding; the major difference between Full Liquid and Clear Liquid diets is the inclusion of milk and dairy products.
Adequacy:	May be low in protein, calories, iron, thiamin; vitamin and mineral supplements should be ordered if the diet continues for more than 3 to 4 days.

Source: Chicago Dietetic Association, *Manual of Clinical Dietetics*, 2nd ed. Philadelphia, W.B. Saunders Company, 1981. Reprinted by permission.

SAMPLE MENU FOR A CLEAR LIQUID DIET

Exchange	
	Breakfast
1 fruit	⅓ cup apple juice
	1 cup beef broth
	1 cup coffee
	1 tsp sugar
	Mid-morning Snack
	8 oz (1 cup) gingerale
	Lunch
	1 cup chicken broth
1 fruit	½ cup strained orange juice
	½ cup grape-flavored gelatin
	1 cup hot tea plus sugar
	Mid-Afternoon Snack
	8 oz grape juice
	Dinner
	1 cup beef broth
1 fruit	4 oz sweetened cranberry juice
	½ cup lime-flavored gelatin
	1 cup coffee or tea with sugar
	Bedtime Snack
	½ cup lime gelatin

Analysis and Comments

- An analysis of this diet shows that it contains 3 fruit exchanges. The miscellaneous foods contain various amounts of nutrients. Milk is not given since it is high in residue.

- Gelatin provides protein and the soups provide both protein and carbohydrate. Gingerale supplies carbohydrates and the fruit juices (orange and apple) supply carbohydrates along with some vitamin C and potassium.

- The amount of fluid given in a feeding is usually restricted to 30–60 ml/hour until the patient's tolerance improves.

> • If the diet is given after gastric surgery or myocardial infarction, the coffee and other caffeine beverages should be eliminated, since they stimulate hydrochloric acid secretion and increased heart rate.
>
> *Source:* Menu adapted from American Dietetic Association, *Handbook of Clinical Dietetics.* New Haven, Conn.: Yale University Press, 1981. Reprinted by permission.

Depending on the surgery and on whether the person is undernourished, TPN or tube feeding may be required. These diets are high in kilocalories and especially in proteins. In addition, it is important that the diets be high in the B complex vitamins, vitamin C, and vitamin K.[2]

TABLE 25-3 SOFT DIET

Purpose:	For patients who are physically or psychologically unable to tolerate a general diet.
Use:	A transitional diet between the Full Liquid Diet and the General Diet.
Examples of foods:	Foods that a patient can tolerate; fried foods, most raw fruits and vegetables, and very coarse breads and cereals may not be tolerated.
Adequacy:	This diet can be planned to provide all the nutrients necessary to be adequate.

Source: Chicago Dietetic Association, *Manual of Clinical Dietetics,* 2nd ed. Philadelphia, W.B. Saunders Company, 1981. Reprinted by permission.

TABLE 25-4 MECHANICAL SOFT DIET

Purpose:	To minimize the amount of chewing necessary for ingestion of food.
Use:	Used for people who have chewing difficulties due to poor or missing teeth, stroke, and oral surgery.
Examples of foods:	Allows same foods as the Regular Diet except that meat, poultry, and fish should be modified by chopping, grinding, or pureeing (straining) and served with enough broth or gravy to ease swallowing; fruits and vegetables should be cooked, mashed, or strained.
Adequacy:	This diet is adequate in all nutrients.

Source: Chicago Dietetic Association, *Manual of Clinical Dietetics,* 2nd ed. Philadelphia, W.B. Saunders Company, 1981. Reprinted by permission.

SAMPLE MENU FOR A FULL LIQUID DIET

Exchange	
	Breakfast
1 fruit	$\frac{1}{2}$ cup orange juice
1 bread	$\frac{1}{2}$ cup farina
	(cereal rich in protein and easily digested)
1 milk	1 cup milk
1 fat	1 tbsp light cream
	4 tsp sugar
	Mid-Morning Snack
	$\frac{1}{2}$ cup custard
	Lunch
	6 oz strained cream soup
	$\frac{1}{2}$ cup jello
1 fat	2 tbsp light cream
	8 oz eggnog
	1 cup tea
	2 tsp sugar
	Mid-Afternoon Snack
	$\frac{1}{2}$ cup vanilla pudding
	$\frac{1}{2}$ cup grape juice
	Dinner
	6 oz beef broth
	$\frac{1}{2}$ cup ice cream
1 milk	1 cup skim milk
2 fruit	$\frac{2}{3}$ cup apple juice
	1 cup coffee
1 fat	2 tbsp light cream
	2 tsp sugar
	Bedtime Snack
	10 oz malted milk shake
	$\frac{1}{2}$ cup jello

Analysis and Comments

- An analysis of this menu shows that it contains 2 milk, 0 vegetable, 3 fruit, 1 bread, 0 meat, and 3 fat.

- In addition to the individual milk exchanges, milk is present in the puddings, eggnog, cream soup, and malted milk. Milk is important to provide some protein, since there are no meat exchanges. Additional protein can be gained by incorporating nonfat dry milk into foods such as milk and puddings.

- If the diet is to be given to a lactose-intolerant person, lactose-free supplements are available.

- The one bread exchange is a cereal (farina) that is easily digested and contains primarily carbohydrates.

- Many of the foods on the menu are from the miscellaneous group (e.g., eggnog, malted milk, pudding, ice cream, and custard) and supply primarily carbohydrates. In addition to these foods, oral supplements that are low in residue, high in protein, and high in calories can be given.

- This menu is inadequate in niacin, folacin, and iron. If the above-mentioned supplements are given, the diet may be adequate in all nutrients.

Source: Menu adapted from Chicago Dietetic Association, *Manual of Clinical Dietetics,* 2nd ed. Philadelphia: W.B. Saunders Company, 1981. Reprinted by permission.

DIET THERAPY FOR BURN PATIENTS

Body surface area (BSA) An estimate of the total body surface area. This measurement is important in burn situations for determining the level of nutritional care.

Small burns Burns that cover less than 20% of the BSA.

A person who has received extensive burns is in a hypermetabolic state. The body systems are stressed to the point where their energy needs can be met only by metabolizing fat and protein stores. As a result of this situation, plus exposure of areas of the body to bacteria, the person will experience tissue catabolism and rapid loss of body mass. Nutritional support is critical for survival and healing for a person who has been burned over 20% or more of the body.

The aggressiveness and importance of nutritional support depend on how seriously the person is burned. A person whose burns cover less than 20% of the **body surface area (BSA)** has what many consider to be **small burns.** This person can usually recover adequately on a regular diet. However, a person who has burns covering more than 20% of the BSA usually needs very aggressive nutritional support. The specifics of the diet depend upon the three stages of burn care.

NUTRITIONAL SUPPORT FOR STAGE 1 OF BURN CARE

Loss of fluids is a major concern immediately after a serious burn. The loss of fluids and edema at the burn site result from loss of skin, loss of fluids from exposed blood vessels, and shifting of fluids from tissue spaces. As a result of the fluid loss, the person's blood volume decreases, which may result in shock and decreased urinary output. In addition to incurring a major problem from fluid loss during the first 48 hours after a burn, the person may also develop a potassium excess and a sodium deficit. The potassium excess results from its release from damaged cells. The sodium deficit results from a shift of sodium out of the body in the edematous fluid. **Metabolic acidosis** may occur as a result of a shift of bicarbonate ions out of the blood with sodium. The nutritional support and the reasons for stage 1 of burn care are as follows:

Metabolic acidosis An acidic state of the blood as a result of the accumulation of ketones.

Nutritional Support	Reasons for Stage 1
Replacement of fluids and electrolytes	Primarily important to prevent irreversible shock and renal shutdown. From 3 to 5 liters of fluid generally are needed to replace fluid losses per day.
	Saline lactated Ringer's solution (sodium chloride, potassium chloride, and calcium chloride) is used to replace lost electrolytes.
Replacement of bicarbonate ions	Helps to prevent metabolic acidosis.
Replacement of glucose and amino acids	Counteracts tissue catabolism.

Generally, nutritional support for stage 1 is supplied parenterally for 1–3 days or until the risk of shock is over and fluid and electrolyte levels are stabilized. Oral feeding is not normally used, since **paralytic ileus** normally occurs in stage 1.

Paralytic ileus Absence of peristalsis.

Antibiotics are usually prescribed to protect against infection, and a tetanus shot is usually given.

NUTRITIONAL SUPPORT FOR STAGE 2 OF BURN CARE

After stabilization of the fluid and electrolyte levels, there is a period of increased diuresis. This is an indication that the replacement therapy has been effective. In addition, tissue wasting is reversed and oral feeding can begin, since paralytic ileus usually ceases and normal peristalsis is present.

During stage 2, nutritional support is important for wound care and closure and for prevention and treatment of complications, including infection. In order to achieve these goals, the diet is high in kilocalories, protein, vitamins, minerals and electrolytes. The details of the diet are as follows:

High kilocalories

Adults

25 kcal/kg (preburn body weight) + (40 kcal × % BSA burned)

Example: 58-kg woman with 50% BSA

25 kcal × 58 kg + (40 kcal × 50)

1,450 kcal + 2,000 kcal = 3,450 kcal total daily requirement

or

60 kcal/kg preburn weight/day

60 kcal × 58 kg = 3,480 kcal/day

High protein

2 to 3 g protein per kilogram of preburn body weight per day. This compares with 0.8 g per kilogram of preburn body weight for an unburned person.

Example:

58 kg × 3 g/kg/day = 175 g protein per day.

This high level of protein is needed to establish a positive nitrogen balance to allow healing of the wounds and synthesis of antibodies to fight infection.

High vitamins

Two standard multivitamin tablets per day plus 1–2 g vitamin C.

The B complex vitamins are important for metabolism of the nutrients. Vitamin C is important for the synthesis of collagen, which is critical for the synthesis of new tissues.

Minerals

Generally, adequate amounts are provided by the high protein and kilocalorie intake. However, sodium and potassium levels especially need to be monitored because of diuresis. High intakes of zinc appear to promote more rapid wound healing, and a high protein intake should provide an adequate amount.

Fluids

Fluid intake should be based on output, which may be significant as a result of increased diuresis. However, it is important to avoid excessive water intake to the point of water intoxication.

In order to achieve these high levels of nutrients, oral feeding usually has to be supplemented with tube feedings and parenteral nutrition. Frequent small feedings are used to increase compliance with the diet, since the patient usually is in pain, depressed, anorexic, and subjected to many dressing changes. Constipation is a common problem and can be reduced by increasing the intake of fluid, fiber, fruit, and vegetables. Anemia is a common problem due to blood losses and reduced bone marrow activity. Transfusion has been found to be more effective than drug and diet therapy in treating anemia.

Infection is almost always a problem with burn treatment; therefore, antibiotics are usually added to the intravenous solutions.

Stage 2 continues until the burned area is covered with new tissue or until skin grafting begins.

NUTRITIONAL SUPPORT FOR STAGE 3 OF BURN CARE

Stage 3 is characterized by reconstruction, with grafting and plastic surgery occurring during this time. Optimal nutritional care is important during this time for these procedures to be successful. The diet generally does not have to contain as high a level of nutrients as it does during stage 2, since by this time the metabolism is usually back to normal.[3]

CASE STUDY: SEVERE BURN PATIENT

Mrs. G is a 57-year-old woman who was admitted to the hospital with severe full-thickness (third-degree) and partial-thickness (second-degree) burns over 60% of her body. A physical examination reveals that she is in acute distress.

Physical Findings	Normal Values
Height: 5 ft 4 in.	
Weight: 121 lb	114–127 lbs (medium frame)
Blood pressure: $\dfrac{106 \text{ mm Hg}}{80 \text{ mm Hg}}$	$\dfrac{95\text{–}140 \text{ mm Hg}}{60\text{–}90 \text{ mm Hg}}$
Pulse: 128 beats/min	60–80 beats/min
Laboratory Findings	
Serum sodium: 125 mEq/liter	135–145 mEq/liter
Serum potassium: 5.8 mEq/liter	3.5–5.5 mEq/liter

Serum albumin: 2.6 g/dl	3.5–5.0 g/dl
Hematocrit: 53%	38–47%
Serum bicarbonate: 14 mEq/liter	20–30 mEq/liter

Using the information above and in this chapter, answer the following questions.

1. The potassium excess results from _____ and the sodium deficit from _____.
   A. destruction of kidneys—destruction of cells
   B. decreased urination—edema
   C. release from damaged cells—loss in edematous fluid
   D. none of these

2. Nutritional support for stage 1 of burn care consists of
   1. high kilocalories
   3. high protein
   2. replacement of fluids and electrolytes
   4. replacement of bicarbonate ions
      A. 1, 2, 3 B. 1, 3 C. 2, 4 D. 4 E. all of these

3. The best feeding method for stage 1 of burn care is _____ because _____ normally is present.
   A. enteral—destruction of blood vessels (eliminating parenteral nutrition)
   B. parenteral—paralytic ileus (absence of peristalsis)
   C. oral—malnutrition
   D. parenteral—destruction of the upper gastrointestinal tract

4. During stage 2 of burn care for Mrs. G, based on physical findings, her protein intake should be _____ and her energy intake should be _____ kcal.
   A. 110–165 g—3,775
   B. 44–55 g—2,400
   C. 150–235 g—1,375
   D. 23–35 g—1,683

5. In order to achieve the levels of nutrients necessary for stage 2 of Mrs. G's recovery, oral feeding usually has to be supplemented with _____ and _____.
   A. increased fluid intake—a high level of vitamin C
   B. increased minerals—increased antibiotics
   C. tube feedings—parenteral nutrition
   D. none of these

6. Mrs. G. is experiencing constipation; the following compensatory changes are made in her diet:

    1. increased fiber   3. increased fruit
    2. high protein   4. high fat
       A. 1, 2, 3   B. 1, 3   C. 2, 4   D. 4   E. all of these

OUTLINE

PREOPERATIVE NUTRITION

This is important to meet the metabolic stress of surgery, improve wound healing, and increase resistance to infection.

Two major nutritional problems in the preoperative period are undernutrition and obesity.

Nutrients are important to an undernourished person.

Kilocalories
Kilocalories are important to resist the stress of surgery. They may have to be provided by total parenteral nutrition.

Protein
The person who is deficient in protein is more susceptible to shock, anesthesia toxicity to the liver, edema at the site of incision, and infection.

Vitamins and Minerals
A deficiency of vitamins hinders carbohydrate metabolism. A deficiency of potassium may cause malfunction of the heart; a deficiency of calcium and sodium may cause abnormal muscle and nerve activity.

Preoperative problems for the obese person:

- Decreased effects of some anesthetic agents
- Greater strain on the heart
- Increased chance of infection due to decreased resistance

PREOPERATIVE DIET

If adequate time exists, an undernourished patient can benefit from a high-kilocalorie, high-protein, high-carbohydrate diet; tube feeding or parenteral nutrition may be required for people who cannot eat orally.

Twenty-four hours before surgery, the diet should provide nutrients that cannot be stored—glucose, B complex vitamins, and vitamin C. A high fluid intake is also valuable.

Eight hours before surgery, all fluids and foods are withheld to reduce regurgitation and aspiration.

A restricted-residue diet is given for 2 or 3 days before surgery on the gastrointestinal tract; many facilities use synthetic low-residue and residue free diets during this period.

POSTOPERATIVE DIET

The immediate concern is to replace lost fluids and electrolytes; initially, they are replaced parenterally or by tubes, since the patient is often nauseated and vomiting.

Once peristaltic contractions return, the physician often orders the following diet progression: clear liquid → full liquid → soft diet → regular diet.

DIET THERAPY FOR BURN PATIENTS

Aggressive diet therapy is important for people burned over 20% or more of their body surface area (BSA); if the burn is smaller, the person usually can recover well with a regular diet.

Nutritional Support for Stage 1 of Burn Care
The immediate concern after a burn is loss of fluids, which may result in shock and renal failure. The person may develop a potassium excess and a sodium deficit; metabolic acidosis may also occur.

- Replacement of fluids and electrolytes prevents shock.
- Replacement of bicarbonate ions helps prevent metabolic acidosis.
- Replacement of glucose and amino acids counteracts tissue catabolism.

Generally, support is supplied parenterally for 1–3 days or until the risk of shock is over and fluid and electrolytes are stabilized. Food is usually not supplied orally due to paralytic ileus (absence of peristalsis).

Nutritional Support for Stage 2 of Burn Care
There is increased diuresis (urination), and tissue wasting begins to decrease.

Nutritional support is important for wound care, closure, and prevention and treatment of complications, especially infection.

- High kilocalories
  25 kcal/kg (preburn body weight) + (40 kcal × % BSA burned) or 60 kcal/kg (preburn weight)
- High protein
  2 to 3 g protein/kg (preburn body weight)/day
- High vitamin intake
  Two standard multivitamins per day plus 1 to 2 g vitamin C per day.
- Minerals
  Generally, adequate amounts will be provided by the high protein and kilocalorie intakes.
- Fluids
  Based on fluid output and should be monitored carefully to prevent dehydration and water intoxication.

Nutritional Support for Stage 3 of Burn Care
Optimal nutritional care is important for grafting and plastic surgery.

REVIEW QUESTIONS

TRUE (A) OR FALSE (B)

Questions 1–15

1. Two major nutritional problems in the preoperative period are undernutrition and obesity.
2. A major problem an undernourished person faces in surgery if he or she is deficient in proteins is shock.
3. Obesity interferes with surgery by hindering muscle and nerve activity.
4. A preoperative diet high in kilocalories, protein, and carbohydrate, is of benefit even if consumed for only a week.
5. Nutrients should be given to a presurgery patient up to the time of surgery for maximum benefit.
6. Following surgery a common diet progression is soft diet → clear liquid → regular → full liquid.
7. Aggressive nutritional support is important for all burn patients, no matter what percent of their body surface area (BSA) is burned.
8. Nutritional support immediately after a burn prevents shock and decreases urinary output.
9. Immediately, after a burn the person may develop a potassium excess and a sodium deficit.
10. Replacement of bicarbonate ions in nutritional support for stage 1 of burn care is important to counteract tissue catabolism.
11. Oral feeding is started almost immediately after a burn in order to instill the maximum amount of nutrients into the body.
12. During stage 2 of nutritional support for burn care, the most important factor to correct is increased diuresis.
13. The high-kilcalorie diet for stage 2 is often calculated at the rate of 60 kcal/kg preburn weight/day.
14. The kilocalorie intake given in question 13 can be provided only by oral intake.
15. Vitamin C should be given in amounts of 1–2 g/day for the synthesis of collagen.

DISCUSSION QUESTIONS

1. Describe how kilocalories, proteins, vitamins, and minerals are important in the preoperative nutrition of an undernourished person.
2. Describe a postoperative diet progression.
3. Discuss the major nutritional concern in stage 1 of burn care. Discuss why stage 1 is frequently characterized by a potassium excess and a sodium deficit.
4. Name three replacement solutions that are administered in stage 1 of burn care and state the function of each.
5. Explain the basic importance of nutritional support during stage 2 of burn care.
6. Using the kilocalorie burn formula, calculate the number of kilocalories required for a man who had a preburn body weight of 68 kg and had 43% of his BSA burned.
7. Describe the amounts of protein, vitamins, minerals, and fluids for stage 2 of burn care.

REFERENCES

1. L.H. Bodinski, *The Nurse's Guide to Diet Therapy*. New York: John Wiley & Sons, 1982, pp. 140–142.
2. M.E. Shils and H.T. Randell, "Diet and nutrition in the care of the surgical patient." In R.S. Goodhart and M.E. Shils, eds.: *Modern Nutrition in Health and Disease*, 6th ed. Philadelphia: Lea and Febiger, 1980.
3. L.S. Brunner and D.S. Suddarth, *Textbook of Medical Surgical Nursing*, 5th ed. Philadelphia: J.B. Lippincott Co., 1984, pp. 1203–1224.

26 NUTRITION AND MENTAL HEALTH

OBJECTIVES

Upon completion of this chapter, you should be able to:

1. Compare the characteristic signs and causes of marasmus and kwashiorkor.

2. Discuss the behavioral changes that result from marasmus and kwashiorkor in children.

3. Discuss the Feingold hypothesis about what causes hyperactivity in children, symptoms of hyperactivity, and the Feingold Kaiser-Permanente diet.

4. Describe the orthomolecular approach to the treatment of schizophrenia.

5. Describe pellagra and schizophrenia in terms of causes and treatment.

6. Give and describe three examples of secondary malnutrition that result from the toxic effects of alcohol.

7. Name the vitamins and minerals that are often deficient in alcoholics.

8. Compare and contrast the symptoms of Wernicke's syndrome and Korsakoff's syndrome.

9. Name the possible cause and treatment of Alzheimer's disease.

10. Describe the cause and treatment of tardive dyskinesia.

INTRODUCTION

Nutrition and its interrelationship with mental health is important and has received increasing attention during the last two decades. It is now recognized that nutrition is important to the therapeutic treatment and prevention of mental illness. In addition, nutrition can influence a person's mood and behavior.

Mental as well as physical health is a worldwide problem. In 1978 the World Health Organization estimated that 40 million people in the world suffer from severe mental illness, and over 80 million suffer from alcohol and drug addiction, mental retardation, and organic brain disorders. In addition, another 80 million suffer from neuroses.[1]

This chapter presents examples of mental illness and their relationship to nutrition.

MALNUTRITION AND BEHAVIOR

Marasmus and kwashiorkor, as types of malnutrition, were discussed in Chapters 5 and 15. These two types of malnutrition are not a problem for children in the United States and other developed countries. However, in South America, southern Africa, India, the Middle East, and the Far East, marasmus and kwashiorkor are public health problems.

MARASMUS

Attention deficit disorders (ADD) Disorders such as hyperkinesia that can be seen in children.

As a result of marasmus, the infant's brain does not develop properly. The immediate behavioral changes are apathy and withdrawal. Intermediate behavioral problems involve reductions in intellectual performance and retarded development of language skills. Long-term behavioral problems include **attention-deficit disorders (ADD),** poor school performance, and abnormal behavior in school.[2]

KWASHIORKOR

As with marasmus, a kwashiorkor infant will experience immediate behavioral problems of apathy and withdrawal. In addition, the child will have the same long-range problems of poor school performance and abnormal behavior in school.

HYPERKINESIS (HYPERACTIVITY) AND ITS RELATION TO FOOD ADDITIVES AND HIGH SUGAR INTAKE

Hyperactivity Abnormally increased activity that is often referred to as *hyperkinesia* in children.

Salicylate-like Analgesic or pain-relieving compounds.

In 1975 Dr. B.F. Feingold published a book entitled *Why Your Child Is Hyperactive.* Dr. Feingold proposed that much of the **hyperactivity** that accompanies learning disabilities could be attributed to **salicylate-like** natural compounds in foods and artificial food flavors and colors. Dr. Feingold claimed that 40–70% of hyperactive children who were treated with the Feingold Kaiser-Permanente (K-P) diet demonstrated a marked reduction in hyperactive behavior.[3] Dr. Feingold's claims were considered to be very important, since hyperactive children are personally, educationally, and socially disruptive. Some of the characteristics of a hyperkinetic child are hyperactivity, short attention span, poor power of concentration, impulsiveness, and the inability to delay gratification. Currently, the American Psychiatric Association categorizes these symptoms as attention deficit disorder (ADD) with or without concurrent hyperactivity. This condition is treated by pediatricians, family practitioners, and child psychiatrists with various forms of psychological treatments as well as with stimulant drugs, with only modest success.

Dr. Feingold's K-P diet is an exclusion one. It excludes 21 fruits and vegetables that Feingold says contain natural salicylates. In addition, all foods that contain artificial color and flavor are prohibited, with 54 foods included in his book as examples. Dr. Feingold's hypothesis is that hyperactive children have genetic variations, not abnormalities, that predispose them to the behaviors described. In order to verify Feingold's claims, many studies have been done. Most of them do not verify Dr. Feingold's claims. However, some researchers believe that the additive-free diet has no apparent harmful effects and that some hyperactive children may actually benefit from it.[4]

Another popular theory about the cause of hyperactivity focuses on high sugar intake. Studies do not conclusively prove the validity of this theory.[5] More research needs to be conducted on this relationship.

VITAMIN THERAPY AND MENTAL DISORDERS

Schizophrenia A mental illness characterized by withdrawal from reality and disturbances in thought and behavior.

SCHIZOPHRENIA AND THE ORTHOMOLECULAR APPROACH

Schizophrenia is a mental illness that is characterized by withdrawal from reality and by disturbances in thought and behavior. The **ortho-**

Orthomolecular approach
An approach that consists of giving large doses of vitamins, especially niacin (vitamin B₃, nicotinic acid) and vitamin C (ascorbic acid) to schizophrenic patients.

molecular approach, as a mode of treatment for schizophrenia, was pioneered by Dr. Linus Pauling in 1973.[6] The term *orthomolecular* essentially means "right molecules" and is the essence of the approach. Pauling and others theorized that large doses of certain vitamins would provide increased amounts of the right molecules to the brain, where chemical imbalances cause schizophrenia.

The American Psychiatric Association Task Force reviewed the research of Pauling and others and concluded that this approach by itself (without accompanying standard **antipsychotic** medication) does not provide any benefit to schizophrenic patients.[1] In addition to being ineffective, the megadoses of niacin, one of the vitamins given, may produce niacin toxicity, characterized by clouding of consciousness, fever, flushing, dryness of skin, increased pigmentation, nausea, diarrhea, and abnormal liver function.[7]

Antipsychotic Drugs that control the symptoms of mental disorders but not the causes.

PELLAGRA AND SCHIZOPHRENIA

As discussed in Chapter 6, pellagra can result from a niacin deficiency, with dementia (a mental disorder) being one of the possible results. Frequently, the mental disorder is schizophrenic in nature. Administering niacin can alleviate the other symptoms of pellagra (dermatitis and diarrhea), in addition to the schizophrenic behavior. However, the amounts of niacin administered frequently are less than 1 g/day. This is in comparison to the megadose levels of at least 3–6 g/day recommended by the orthomolecular supporters for correction of schizophrenia.

ALCOHOLISM AND NUTRITION

Primary malnutrition
Malnutrition that results from diet alone. Alcoholics often suffer from primary malnutrition as a result of an inadequate diet.

Secondary malnutrition
Malnutrition that results from impaired use of nutrients. It is often seen in alcoholics and results from the toxic effects of alcohol on the liver and the gastrointestinal tract.

Alcohol is both a food and a drug. Alcohol is recognized as a food, since it supplies 7 kcal/g. As a drug, it has mood-altering effects. While alcohol provides energy, it does not provide nutrients like protein, vitamins, and minerals. It is not surprising, then, that alcoholics frequently have nutritional deficiencies. One reason for the deficiencies is that alcoholics frequently eat very little. One reason for the low intake of food is that alcohol interferes with the hunger and appetite sensations. In addition, they often go on long drinking bouts in which they substitute alcohol for food. Malnutrition in alcoholics resulting from lack of food is classified as **primary malnutrition. Secondary malnutrition** in alcoholics results from the toxic effects of alcohol on the liver, as well as on other gastrointestinal tract organs and processes. Some examples are as follows:

Pancreatitis: Alcohol-induced inflammation of the pancreas resulting in decreased secretion of enzymes and insulin (see Chapter 20 for details of pancreatitis).

Anemias: Malabsorption of nutrients and decreased synthesis of transferrin (see Chapter 8 for details of transferrin and iron transport).

Fatty liver: Triglyceride accumulation in liver cells (see Chapter 20 for details of fatty liver).

Hypoglycemia: Decreased food intake and depletion of glycogen stores.

Cirrhosis: Development of scar tissue due to the direct effect of alcohol and fatty infiltration. (See Chapter 20 for details of cirrhosis).

Peripheral neuritis Degenerative changes in the peripheral nerves.

The brain is frequently affected by thiamin deficiencies, with **peripheral neuritis** (degenerative changes in peripheral nerves) and **Wernicke's syndrome** being the results.

Wernicke's syndrome A nervous condition that results form a thiamin deficiency.

EFFECTS OF ALCOHOL ON VITAMIN AND MINERAL NUTRITION

Alcoholics frequently have deficiencies of the vitamins thiamin, niacin, folacin, vitamin B_6, and vitamin B_{12}. The basic reason is that alcohol interferes with their absorption. In addition, the use of folacin is decreased, which can lead to anemia.

Absorption of fat-soluble vitamins is often impaired in alcoholics. Due to damage to the liver, alcoholics may have reduced storage of vitamin A, which can lead to night blindness and deterioration of the mucous membranes.

Low potassium levels in alcoholics are common due to potassium loss in urine. If they are severe enough, abnormalities in heart rhythms can occur. Edema in alcoholics results from retention of sodium and water.

ALCOHOL-NUTRITIONAL DISEASES

Wernicke-Korsakoff Disease

Diplopia Double vision.

Nystagmus Rapid movement of the eyeballs.

Ataxia Uncoordinated gait.

Wernicke-Korsakoff disease results from a thiamin deficiency. Wernicke's syndrome and Korsakoff's psychosis are thought to be different phases of the same disease. Wernicke's syndrome is characterized initially by **diplopia,** which results from damage to the third or sixth cranial nerve, **nystagmus,** and **ataxia.** In addition, the patient frequently already has peripheral neuritis, with pain and tingling in the feet and legs being examples. If treatment is not initiated when these symptoms appear, the alcoholic's mental state frequently deteriorates to drowsiness, sleepiness, and a daze.

The treatment of Wernicke's syndrome is thiamin replacement. As little as 2 mg of the vitamin injected intravenously will rapidly restore normal eye movements and vision. However, most clinicians use doses of 50–100 mg daily. In addition, some researchers have found that a magnesium deficiency accompanies Wernicke's syndrome and hinders thiamin treatment.[8] In practice, a multiple vitamin preparation including all the B vitamins is usually administered, since the alcoholic is usually deficient in many vitamins including thiamin.

The symptoms of Korsakoff's psychosis often appear in alcoholics who are recovering from Wernicke's syndrome. The chief defects are memory loss, an inability to learn new information, and **confabulation.** Treatment is the same as for Wernicke's syndrome. However, recovery of complete memory generally occurs in only a small percentage of cases, since permanent brain damage is often the reason for the symptoms of Korsakoff's psychosis.[9] (*See Case Study: Alcoholic Patient, at end of chapter, for reinforcement of and application of information related to alcoholism.*)

Confabulation Recitation of imaginary experiences to fill gaps in memory.

DEMENTIA

Dementia is a major health problem of the elderly and is the leading cause of the first admission to state mental hospitals.[8] **Senile dementia** occurs in about 4% of people over the age of 65. Mental disorders occurring in younger people are called **presenile dementias,** with **Alzheimer's disease** being the most common.

Senile dementia Dementia that occurs in people over the age of 65.

Presenile dementias Mental disorders occurring in people below the age of 65.

ALZHEIMER'S DISEASE

Alzheimer's disease is the most common senile disorder, but in some individuals it occurs when they are in their forties and fifties. The current theory about the cause of Alzheimer's disease focuses on a depletion of the neurotransmitter **acetylcholine** by certain nerve cells in the brain. Acetylcholine is composed partly of the compound **choline,** which can be synthesized in the body from the amino acids serine and methionine. Choline is also a component of the phospholipid lecithin.

Alzheimer's disease A condition that results form a depletion of acetylcholine and causes losses of neurons in the brain.

Acetylcholine A neurotransmitter that transmits nerve impulses between certain types of neurons.

This depletion is accompanied by degenerative changes and losses of neurons in the **basal region** of the frontal lobe of the brain. Symptoms include lessening of mental alertness, impairment of memory of recent events, untidiness, impaired judgment, agitation, and periods of confusion.

Choline A compound that is synthesized in the body from serine and methionine.

Therapeutic treatment of Alzheimer's disease by some researchers has involved oral administration of choline and lecithin (phosphatidylcholine). It should be emphasized that in clinical studies only phosphatidylcholine is an effective source of choline; lecithin, sold in health food

Basal region A region located at the base of the brain.

stores, provides only negligible amounts of choline. The administration of lecithin to control Alzheimer's disease has not shown significant improvement in dementia.

TARDIVE DYSKINESIA

Tardive dyskinesia A condition that occurs in patients with mental disorders as a side effect of long-term treatment with antipsychotic drugs.

The symptoms of tardive dyskinesia include uncontrollable movements of the mouth, face, and tongue, as well as rapid, jerky, and involuntary movements of the trunk and extremities.

Tardive dyskinesia is believed to be partly due to an imbalance of acetylcholine. As with Alzheimer's disease, treatment with choline and lecithin has been tried, but with more success.[1]

EATING DISORDERS

Two eating disorders that are related to mental and behavioral factors are anorexia nervosa and bulimia, which are discussed in Chapter 10.

CASE STUDY: ALCOHOLIC PATIENT

Mr. G is a 58-year-old alcoholic who has been hospitalized for alcohol withdrawal. Anthropometric and laboratory measurements indicate that he is suffering from primary and secondary malnutrition. Mr. G is receiving the following medications for his withdrawal:

Medications	Possible Adverse Nutritional Effects
Antianxiety drug: benzodiazepines (Librium)	Gastrointestinal distress
Tranquilizer: chlorpromazine (Thorazine)	Gastrointestinal distress
Hypnotic: flurazepam (Dalmane)	None
Anticonvulsant: diphenylhydantoin (Dilantin)	Decreased taste sensation, decreased absorption of vitamin B_{12}, folic acid, and calcium

1. The primary malnutrition Mr. G is suffering from is a result of
_____.

A. the toxic effects of alcohol on his gastrointestinal tract organs

B. cirrhosis

C. pancreatitis

D. lack of food

2. The secondary malnutrition Mr. G is suffering from may be a result of _____.

   1. pancreatitis   3. fatty liver
   2. anemia   4. cirrhosis
      A. 1, 2, 3 B. 1, 3   C. 2, 4   D. 4   E. all of these

3. Mr. G is being administered a multivitamin complex. Some of the vitamins that are commonly deficient in alcoholics are

   1. thiamin   3. folacin
   2. niacin   4. vitamin B_{12}
      A. 1, 2, 3 B. 1, 3   C. 2, 4   D. 4   E. all of these

4. Mr. G has been complaining of double vision, nystagmus (rapid movement of the eyeballs), ataxia, and pain and tingling in the feet and legs. These symptoms indicate that he may be suffering from _____ and the cause is _____.

   A. Wernicke's syndrome   thiamin deficiency
   B. Korsakoff's psychosis   vitamin C deficiency
   C. dementia   depletion of acetylcholine
   D. Alzheimer's disease   lack of choline

5. In order to reduce the nutritional side effects of the medications, librium and thorazine, they should be consumed _____.

   A. several hours before meals
   B. 30 minutes before or with meals
   C. with water only as opposed to with milk
   D. none of these

6. Mr. G is experiencing some edema, which is an indication that he has an imbalance of _____.

   A. B complex vitamins
   B. potassium
   C. sodium and water
   D. water-soluble vitamins

7. Alcohol is recognized as a food because it _____.

   A. supplies nutrients
   B. supplies 7 kcal/g
   C. is nutritious
   D. none of these

OUTLINE

INTRODUCTION

Nutrition is important to the therapeutic treatment and prevention of mental illness.
  Mental illness is a problem worldwide

- 40 million people suffer from severe mental illness
- Over 80 million people worldwide suffer from alcohol and drug addiction, mental retardation, and organic brain disorders.

MALNUTRITION AND BEHAVIOR

Marasmus
The brain does not develop properly, and immediate behavioral changes are apathy and withdrawal. Intermediate behavioral problems include reductions in intellectual performance and retarded development of language skills. Long-term behavioral problems are attention-deficit disorders, poor school performance, and abnormal behavior in school.

Kwashiorkor
Behavioral problems are essentially the same as those of marasmus due to inadequate development of the brain.

HYPERKINESIS (HYPERACTIVITY) AND ITS RELATION TO FOOD ADDITIVES AND HIGH SUGAR INTAKE

The Feingold hypothesis states that the cause of hyperkinesis or hyperactivity in children is salicylate-like natural compounds in foods and artificial foods.
  The characteristics of hyperactivity (attention deficit disorder are hyperactivity, short attention span, poor power of concentration, impulsiveness, and the inability to delay gratification.
  The Feingold K-P diet excludes 21 fruits and vegetables that contain salicylates (analgesic, or pain relieving, compounds) and artificial colors and flavors.
  Most studies do not verify Dr. Feingold's claims.
  High sugar intake as a cause of hyperactivity has not been verified.

VITAMIN THERAPY AND MENTAL DISORDERS

Schizophrenia and the Orthomolecular Approach
Schizophrenia, a mental illness characterized by withdrawal from reality and disturbances in thought and behavior, was proposed to be helped by an orthomolecular approach. It was theorized that large doses of certain vitamins would provide increased amounts of the "right molecules" to the brain, where chemical imbalances caused schizophrenia. The American Psychiatric Association Task Force concluded that this treatment without antipsychotic medications did not provide any benefit.

Pellagra and Schizophrenia
Pellagra can result from a niacin deficiency, producing schizophrenic condition. Administering niacin in quantities of less than 1 g/day can help alleviate schizophrenic behavior.

ALCOHOLISM AND NUTRITION

Alcohol is both a food and a drug. Alcoholics frequently experience primary malnutrition as a result of consuming very little food. Secondary malnutrition results from toxic effects of alcohol on the liver as well as on other gastrointestinal tract organs and processes (e.g., pancreatitis, anemias, fatty liver, hypoglycemia, and cirrhosis).

Effects of Alcohol on Vitamin and Mineral Nutrition
Alcohol can affect the absorption of vitamins, thiamin, niacin, folacin, vitamin B_6, and vitamin B_{12}.
  In addition, the use of folacin is decreased.
  Absorption of fat-soluble vitamins is often impaired in alcoholics, leading to reduced storage of vitamin A.
  Low potassium levels in alcoholics are common due to potassium losses in urine.

Alcohol-Nutritional Diseases
Wernicke-Korsakoff Disease
Wernicke's syndrome results from a thiamin deficiency; it is characterized by double vision (diplopia), nystagmus (rapid movement of the eyeballs), and ataxia (uncoordinated gait). Treatment: thiamin replacement with as little as 2 mg injected intravenously can restore normal eye movements. In practice, 50–100 mg daily or multiple vitamin preparations are administered.
  The symptoms of Korsakoff's psychosis often appear in alcoholics who are recovering from Wernicke's syndrome. They include memory loss, inability to learn new things, and confabulation (recitation of imaginary experiences to fill gaps in memory). The treatment is the same as for Wernicke's syndrome.

DEMENTIA

Dementia is a severe mental disorder involving impairment of mental ability.

Senile dementia occurs in about 4% of people over age of 65.

Presenile dementia occurs in younger people, with Alzheimer's disease being the most common form.

Alzheimer's Disease

The disease may occur in individuals when they are in their forties and fifties.

Cause: the current theory concerns a depletion of the neurotransmitter acetylcholine by certain nerve cells in the brain.

Symptoms: lessening of mental alertness, impairment of memory of recent events, untidiness, impaired judgment, agitation, and periods of confusion.

Treatment: oral administration of choline and lecithin (phosphatidylcholine) by some researchers; most studies have not shown significant improvement of dementia.

Tardive Dyskinesia

The condition occurs in some patients with mental disorders as a side effect of long-term treatment with antipsychotic drugs.

Symptoms: uncontrollable movements of the mouth, face, and tongue, as well as rapid, jerky, and involuntary movements of the trunk and extremities.

Cause and treatment: believed to be partly caused by an imbalance of acetylcholine; treatment with choline and lecithin has been successful.

REVIEW QUESTIONS

TRUE (A) OR FALSE (B)

Questions 1–7

1. Marasmus and kwashiorkor cause not only physical problems but also changes in mental behavior.
2. Hyperkinetic or hyperactive children show distinct improvement when placed on the Feingold exclusion diet, which excludes foods containing natural sources of salicylates (analgesic, or pain reducing, compounds).
3. The orthomolecular approach by itself has not been shown to provide any benefit to schizophrenic patients.
4. Dementia associated with pellagra, a disease caused by a niacin deficiency, has been shown to decrease this problem, as well as the other symptoms of pellagra (dermatitis and diarrhea).
5. While alcoholics often have abnormal mental behavior, they seldom have nutritional deficiencies.
6. Wernicke-Korsakoff disease results from deficiencies of water- and fat-soluble vitamins, and treatment involves administration of them in megadose quantities.
7. Alzheimer's disease is rare and is theorized to result from a deficiency of niacin.

DISCUSSION QUESTIONS

1. Discuss the Feingold hypothesis as to what causes hyperactivity in children, the symptoms, and the Feingold Kaiser-Permanente diet.
2. Describe the orthomolecular approach to the treatment of schizophrenia.
3. Give and describe three examples of secondary malnutrition that can result from the toxic effects of alcohol.
4. State the possible cause and treatment of Alzheimer's disease.

REFERENCES

1. J.C. Coleman, J.N. Butcher, and R.C. Carson, *Abnormal Psychology and Modern Life*, 7th ed. Glenview, Ill.: Scott, Foresman, and Co., 1984, p. 696.
2. J.R. Galler, F. Ramsey, G. Solimano, W.E. Lowell and E. Mason, "The influence of early malnutrition on subsequent behavioral development. I. Degree of impairment in intellectual performance." *Journal of Child Psychiatry*, 22, 8–15 (1983).
3. K.A. Kavale and S.R. Forness, "Hyperactivity and diet treatment: A meta-analysis of the Feingold hypothesis." *Journal of Learning Disabilities*, 16(6), 324–329 (1983).
4. M.A. Lipton and J.P. Mayo, "Diet and hyperkinesis—an update." *Journal of the American Dietetic Association*, 83(2), 132–134 (1983).
5. R.J. Prinz, W.A. Roberts and E. Hantman, "Dietary correlates of hyperactive behavior in children." *Journal of Consulting Clinical Psychology*, 48, 760 (1980).
6. L. Pauling and D. Hawkins, *Orthomolecular Psychiatry*. San Francisco: W.H. Freeman and Co., Publishers, 1973.
7. J.R. Galler, ed. *Nutrition and Behavior*. New York: Plenum Press, 1984, p. 217.
8. N.J. Estes and M.E. Heinemann, *Alcoholism: Development, Consequences, and Interventions*, 2nd ed. St. Louis: C.V. Mosby Co., 1982, p. 150.
9. E.K. Lindvig, *Nutrition and Mental Health*. Moscow: The University Press of Idaho, 1979, p. 112.

APPENDIXES

A. EXCHANGE LISTS FOR MEAL PLANNING

B. DIETARY FIBER IN SELECTED FOODS

C. CHOLESTEROL CONTENT OF FOODS

D. SUPPLEMENTAL FOOD CHOICES FOR CALORIE-CONTROLLED DIETS

E. ALCOHOLIC BEVERAGES IN CALORIE-CONTROLLED DIETS

F. DRUG–NUTRIENT INTERACTIONS

G. NUTRITIVE VALUES OF THE EDIBLE PART OF FOODS

H. RELATIVE RATIOS OF POLYUNSATURATED AND SATURATED FAT (P:S RATIO) IN REPRESENTATIVE FOODS

I. SODIUM AND POTASSIUM CONTENT OF FOODS

J. PHYSICAL GROWTH NCHS PERCENTILES

K. MID-UPPER-ARM CIRCUMFERENCE PERCENTILES (CM)

L. TRICEPS SKINFOLD PERCENTILES (MM)

M. RECOMMENDED ENERGY INTAKE

N. CONVERSION TABLES

O. RECOMMENDED FOOD INTAKE FOR GOOD NUTRITION FOR CHILDREN AND ADOLESCENTS

P. LEVELS OF NUTRITIONAL ASSESSMENT FOR INFANTS AND CHILDREN

Q. NUTRITION HISTORY: BIRTH TO 24 MONTHS

R. RANGE OF AVERAGE WATER REQUIREMENT OF CHILDREN AT DIFFERENT AGES UNDER ORDINARY CONDITIONS

APPENDIX A: EXCHANGE LISTS FOR MEAL PLANNING

LIST 1 MILK EXCHANGES (INCLUDES NONFAT, LOW-FAT, AND WHOLE MILK)[a]

This list shows the kinds and amounts of milk or milk products to use for one milk exchange. Those appearing in **bold type** are **nonfat.** Low-fat and whole milk contain saturated fat.

Nonfat fortified milk

Skim or nonfat milk	1 cup
Powdered (nonfat dry, before adding liquid)	$\frac{1}{3}$ cup
Canned, evaporated skim milk	$\frac{1}{2}$ cup
Buttermilk made from skim milk	1 cup
Yogurt made from skim milk (plain, unflavored)	1 cup

Low-fat fortified milk

1% fat fortified milk	1 cup
(add $\frac{1}{2}$ fat exchange or 25 kcal)	
2% fat fortified milk	1 cup
(add 1 fat exchange or 45 kcal)	
Yogurt made from 2% fortified milk (plain, unflavored)	1 cup
(add 1 fat exchange or 45 kcal)	

Whole Milk (add 2 fat exchanges or 90 kcal)

Whole milk	1 cup
Canned, evaporated whole milk	$\frac{1}{2}$ cup
Buttermilk made from whole milk	1 cup
Yogurt made from whole milk (plain, unflavored)	1 cup

[a]One exchange of milk contains 12 g of carbohydrate, 8 g of protein, a trace of fat, and 80 kcal.

LIST 2 VEGETABLE EXCHANGES[a]

This list shows the kinds of vegetables to use for one
vegetable exchange. One exchange is ½ cup.

Asparagus	Greens
Bean sprouts	Mustard
	Spinach
Beets	Turnip
Broccoli	Mushrooms
Brussels sprouts	Okra
Cabbage	Onions
Carrots	Rhubarb
Cauliflower	Rutabaga
Celery	Sauerkraut
Eggplant	String beans, green or yellow
Green pepper	Summer squash
Greens	Tomatoes
Beet	Tomato juice
Chards	Turnips
Collards	Vegetable juice cocktail
Dandelion	Zucchini
Kale	

The following raw vegetables may be used as desired:

Chicory	Lettuce
Chinese cabbage	Parsley
Cucumbers	Pickles, dill
Endive	Radishes
Escarole	Watercress

Starchy vegetables are found in the Bread Exchange List.

[a]One exchange of vegetables contains about 5 g of carbohydrate, 2 g of
protein, and 25 kcal.

LIST 3 FRUIT EXCHANGES[a]

This list shows the kinds and amounts of fruits to use for one fruit exchange.

Apple	1 small	Mango	$\frac{1}{2}$ small
Apple juice	$\frac{1}{3}$ cup	Melon	
Applesauce (unsweetened)	$\frac{1}{2}$ cup	Cantaloupe	$\frac{1}{4}$ small
Apricots, fresh	2 medium	Honeydew	$\frac{1}{8}$ medium
Apricots, dried	4 halves	Watermelon	1 cup
Banana	$\frac{1}{2}$ small	Nectarine	1 small
Berries		Orange	1 small
Blackberries	$\frac{1}{2}$ cup	Orange juice	$\frac{1}{2}$ cup
Blueberries	$\frac{1}{2}$ cup	Papaya	$\frac{3}{4}$ cup
Raspberries	$\frac{1}{2}$ cup	Peach	1 medium
Strawberries	$\frac{3}{4}$ cup	Pear	1 small
Cherries	10 large	Persimmon, native	1 medium
Cider	$\frac{1}{3}$ cup	Pineapple	$\frac{1}{2}$ cup
Dates	2	Pineapple juice	$\frac{1}{3}$ cup
Figs, fresh	1	Plums	2 medium
Figs, dried	1	Prunes	2 medium
Grapefruit	$\frac{1}{2}$	Prune juice	$\frac{1}{4}$ cup
Grapefruit juice	$\frac{1}{2}$ cup	Raisins	2 tbsp
Grapes	12	Tangerine	1 medium
Grape juice	$\frac{1}{4}$ cup		

Cranberries may be used as desired if no sugar is added.

[a]One exchange of fruit contains 10 g of carbohydrate and 40 kcal

LIST 4 BREAD EXCHANGES (INCLUDES BREAD, CEREAL, AND STARCHY VEGETABLES)[a]

This list shows the kinds and amounts of **breads, cereals, starchy vegetables,** and prepared foods to use for one bread exchange. Those that appear in **bold type** are **low-fat.**

Bread

White (including French and Italian)	1 slice
Whole wheat	1 slice
Rye or pumpernickel	1 slice
Raisin	1 slice
Bagel, small	$\frac{1}{2}$
English muffin, small	$\frac{1}{2}$
Plain roll, bread	1
Frankfurter roll	$\frac{1}{2}$
Hamburger bun	$\frac{1}{2}$
Dried bread crumbs	3 tbsp
Tortilla, 6 in.	1

Cereal

Bran flakes	$\frac{1}{2}$ cup
Other ready-to-eat unsweetened cereal	$\frac{3}{4}$ cup
Puffed cereal (unfrosted)	1 cup
Cereal (cooked)	$\frac{1}{2}$ cup
Grits (cooked)	$\frac{1}{2}$ cup
Rice or barley (cooked)	$\frac{1}{2}$ cup
Pasta (cooked), Spaghetti, noodles, Macaroni	$\frac{1}{2}$ cup
Popcorn (popped, no fat added, large kernel)	3 cups
Cornmeal (dry)	2 tbsp
Flour	$2\frac{1}{2}$ tbsp
Wheat germ	$\frac{1}{4}$ cup

Crackers

Arrowroot	3
Graham, $2\frac{1}{2}$-in. sq.	2
Matzoth, 4 × 6 in.	$\frac{1}{2}$
Oyster	20
Pretzels, $3\frac{1}{8}$ in. long × $\frac{1}{8}$ in. dia.	25
Rye wafers, 2 × $3\frac{1}{2}$ in.	3
Saltines	6
Soda, $2\frac{1}{2}$ in. sq.	4

Dried beans, peas, and lentils

Beans, peas, lentils (dried and cooked)	$\frac{1}{2}$ cup
Baked beans, no pork (canned)	$\frac{1}{4}$ cup

Starchy vegetables

Corn	$\frac{1}{3}$ cup
Corn on cob	1 small
Lima beans	$\frac{1}{2}$ cup
Parsnips	$\frac{2}{3}$ cup
Peas, green (canned or frozen)	$\frac{1}{2}$ cup
Potato, white	1 small
Potato (mashed)	$\frac{1}{2}$ cup
Pumpkin	$\frac{3}{4}$ cup
Winter squash, acorn or butternut	$\frac{1}{2}$ cup
Yam or sweet potato	$\frac{1}{4}$ cup

Prepared Foods

Biscuit 2 in. dia. (add 1 fat exchange or 45 kcal)	1
Corn bread, 2 × 2 × 1 in. (add 1 fat exchange or 45 kcal)	1
Corn muffin, 2 in. dia. (add 1 fat exchange or 45 kcal)	1
Crackers, round butter type (add 1 fat exchange or 45 kcal)	5
Muffin, plain small (add 1 fat exchange or 45 kcal)	1
Potatoes, french fried, length 2 to $3\frac{1}{2}$ in. (add 1 fat exchange or 45 kcal)	8
Potato or corn chips (add 2 fat exchanges or 45 kcal)	15
Pancake, 5 or $\frac{1}{2}$ in. (add 1 fat exchange or 45 kcal)	1
Waffle, 5 × $\frac{1}{2}$ in. (add 1 fat exchange or 45 kcal)	1

[a]One exchange of bread contains 15 g of carbohydrate, 2 g of protein and 70 kcal

LIST 5 MEAT EXCHANGES

LEAN MEAT[a]

This list shows the kinds and amounts of lean meat and other protein-rich foods to use for one low-fat meat exchange. Trim off all visible fat.

Beef:	Baby beef (very lean), chipped beef, chuck, flank steak, tenderloin, plate ribs, plate skirt steak, round (bottom, top), all cuts rump, spare ribs, tripe	1 oz
Lamb:	Leg, rib, sirloin, loin (roast and chops), shank, shoulder	1 oz
Pork:	Leg (whole rump, center shank), ham, smoked (center slices)	1 oz
Veal:	Leg, loin, rib, shank, shoulder, cutlets	1 oz
Poultry:	Meat *without skin* of chicken, turkey, cornish hen, guinea hen, pheasant	1 oz
Fish:	Any fresh or frozen	1 oz
	Canned salmon, tuna, mackerel, crab and lobster,	$\frac{1}{4}$ cup
	clams, oysters, scallops, shrimp,	5 or 1 oz
	sardines, drained	3
Cheeses containing less than 5% butterfat		1 oz
Cottage cheese, dry and 2% butterfat		$\frac{1}{4}$ cup
Dried beans and peas (add 1 bread exchange or 45 kcal)		$\frac{1}{2}$ cup

MEDIUM-FAT MEAT[b]

This list shows the kinds and amounts of medium-fat meat and other protein-rich foods to use for one medium-fat meat exchange. Trim off all visible fat.

Beef:	Ground (15% fat), corned beef (canned), rib eye, round (ground commercial)	1 oz
Pork:	Loin (all cuts tenderloin), shoulder arm (picnic), shoulder blade, Boston butt, Canadian bacon, boiled ham	1 oz
Liver, heart, kidney, and sweetbreads (these are high in cholesterol)		1 oz
Cottage cheese, creamed		$\frac{1}{4}$ cup
Cheese:	Mozzarella, Ricotta, farmer's cheese, Neufchatel,	1 oz
	Parmesan	3 tbsp
Egg (high in cholesterol)		1
Peanut butter (add 2 additional fat exchanges or 90 kcal)		2 tbsp

LIST 5 *(Continued)*

HIGH-FAT MEAT[c]

This list shows the kinds and amounts of high-fat meat and other protein-rich foods to use for one high-fat meat exchange. Trim off all visible fat.

Beef:	Brisket, corned beef (brisket), ground beef (more than 20% fat), hamburger (commercial), chuck (ground commercial), roasts (rib), steaks (club and rib)	1 oz
Lamb:	Breast	1 oz
Pork:	Spare ribs, loin (back ribs), pork (ground), country-style ham, deviled ham	1 oz
Veal:	Breast	1 oz
Poultry:	Capon, duck (domestic), goose	1 oz
Cheese:	Cheddar types	1 oz
Cold cuts		$4\frac{1}{2} \times \frac{1}{8}$ in. slice
Frankfurter		1 small

[a]One exchange of lean meat (1 oz) contains 7 g of protein, 3 g of fat, and 55 kcal.
[b]One exchange of medium-fat meat (1 oz) contains 7 g of protein, 5 g of fat, and 75 kcal.
[c]One exchange of high-fat meat (1 oz) contains 7 g of protein, 8 g of fat, and 100 kcal.

LIST 6 FAT EXCHANGES[a]

This list shows the kinds and amounts of fat-containing foods to use for one fat exchange. To plan a diet low in saturated fat, select only those exchanges that appear in **bold type.** They are **polyunsaturated.**

Margarine, soft, tub or stick[a]	1 tsp
Avocado (4 in. in diameter)[b]	$\frac{1}{8}$
Oil, corn, cottonseed, safflower, soy, sunflower	1 tsp
Oil, olive[b]	1 tsp
Oil, peanut[b]	1 tsp
Olives[b]	5 small
Almonds[b]	10 whole
Pecans[b]	2 large whole
Peanuts[b]	
Spanish	20 whole
Virginia	10 whole
Walnuts	6 small
Nuts, other[b]	6 small
Margarine, regular stick	1 tsp
Butter	1 tsp
Bacon fat	1 tsp
Bacon, crisp	1 strip
Cream, light	2 tbsp
Cream, sour	2 tbsp
Cream, heavy	1 tbsp
Cream cheese	1 tbsp
French dressing[c]	1 tbsp
Italian dressing[c]	1 tbsp
Lard	1 tsp
Mayonnaise[c]	1 tsp
Salad dressing, mayonnaise type***	2 tsp
Salt pork	$\frac{3}{4}$-in. cube

One exchange of fat contains 5 g of fat and 45 kcal.

[a]Made with corn, cottonseed, safflower, soy, or sunflower oil only.

[b]Fat content is primarily monounsaturated.

[c]If made with corn, cottonseed, safflower, soy, or sunflower oil, can be used on a fat-modified diet.

The exchange lists from the Exchange Lists for Meal Planning were prepared by committees of the American Diabetes Association, Inc., and The American Dietetic Association in cooperation with the National Institute of Arthritis, Metabolism and Digestive Diseases and the National Heart and Lung Institute, National Institutes of Health, Public Health Service, U.S. Department of Health, Education, and Welfare.

APPENDIX B: DIETARY FIBER IN SELECTED FOODS (g/100 g)

Food	Total Dietary Fiber
Breads	
Brown	5.11
White	2.72
Wholemeal	8.50
Cereals	
All-Bran	26.7
Cornflakes	11.0
Grapenuts	7.00
Rice Krispies	4.47
Puffed Wheat	15.41
Sugar Puffs	6.08
Shredded Wheat	12.26
Special K	5.45
Flour	
Bran	44.0
Brown	7.87
White	3.15
Fruits	
Apples	
Flesh	1.42
Peel only	3.71
Bananas	1.75
Cherries	1.24
Grapefruit (canned)[a]	0.44
Mandarin oranges (canned)[a]	0.29
Mangoes (canned)[a]	1.00
Peaches	2.28
Pears	
Flesh	2.44
Peel only	8.59
Plums	1.52
Rhubarb (raw)	1.78
Strawberries (raw)	2.12
Nuts	
Brazils	7.73
Peanuts	9.30
Preserves	
Jam, strawberry	1.12
Marmalade	0.71
Peanut butter	7.55
Pickle	1.53

APPENDIX B: *(Continued)*

Food	Total Dietary Fiber
Vegetables	
Beans, baked (canned)	7.27
Broccoli tops (boiled)	4.10
Brussels sprouts (boiled)	2.86
Cabbage (boiled)	2.83
Carrots (boiled)	3.70
Cauliflower (boiled)	1.80
Corn	
Cooked	4.74
Canned[b]	5.69
Lettuce (raw)	1.53
Onions (raw)	2.10
Parsnips (raw)	4.90
Peas	
Frozen (raw)	7.75
Garden (canned)[b]	6.28
Processed (canned)[b]	7.85
Peppers (cooked)	0.93
Potato (raw)	3.51
Tomato (fresh)	1.40
Turnips (raw)	2.20

Source: D.A.T. Southgate, B. Bailey, E. Collinsun, and A. F. Walker, "Dietary fiber in selected foods," *Journal of Human Nutrition 30,* (1976).

[a]Fruit and syrup.
[b]Drained.

APPENDIX C: CHOLESTEROL VALUE OF SELECTED FOODS[a,b]

Food	Cholesterol (mg)	Food	Cholesterol (mg)
Milk		Eggs	
Whole, 3.5% fat (1 cup)	34	Whole (large size)	252
Nonfat (skim) (1 cup)	5	White of egg	0
Low-fat (1 cup)	22	Yolk of egg	252
Cheese		Meat, poultry, fish, shellfish, related products	
Blue or Roquefort type (1 cu in.)	15	Bacon (2 slices)	16
Camembert (1 wedge)	35	Beef (lean only) (2.5 oz)	66
Cheddar (1 cu in.)	17	Hamburger, broiled, lean (3 oz)	77
Cottage cheese, creamed (1 pkg)	65	Rib roast, oven cooked, lean and fat (3 oz)	80
Cottage cheese, uncreamed (1 pkg)	24	Rib roast, oven cooked, lean only (1.8 oz)	46
Cream cheese (1 pkg, 3 oz)	94	Steak, broiled, lean and fat (6 oz)	160
Parmesan (1 tbsp)	5	Steak, broiled, lean only (6 oz)	153
Swiss cheese (1 cu in.)	15	Corned beef (3 oz)	85
Processed cheese (1 cu in.)	16	Chicken, flesh only, broiled (3 oz)	74
American pasteurized process cheese food (1 tbsp)	10	Chicken, breast, fried (with bone), (3 oz)	75
American process cheese spread (1 oz)	18	Chicken, breast, fried (flesh and skin only) (2.7 oz)	68
Cream		Chili con carne, canned, with beans (1 cup)	77
Half-and-half (1 tbsp)	6	Chili con carne, canned, without beans (1 cup)	153
Light, coffee or table (1 tbsp)	10	Lamb chop, broiled with bone (1 chop) (4.8 oz)	74
Sour (1 tbsp)	8	Roast leg of lamb, lean and fat (3 oz)	83
Whipped topping (1 cup), pressurized	51	Roast lam shoulder, lean and fat (3 oz)	83
Milk beverages		Beef liver, fried (2 oz)	250
Cocoa, homemade (1 cup)	35	Roast ham, lean and fat (3 oz)	76
Chocolate-flavored drink (skim milk) (1 cup)	20	Boiled ham, sliced (2 oz)	51
Milk desserts		Canned, spiced or unspiced ham (2 oz)	51
Custard, baked (1 cup)	278	Pork chop, thick with bone (1 chop) (3.5 oz)	59
Ice cream, regular (1 cup)	53		
Ice milk, hardened (1 cup)	26		
Ice milk, soft serve (1 cup)	36		
Yogurt (made from partially skimmed milk) (1 cup)	17		
Yogurt (made from whole milk) (1 cup)	30		
Yogurt (sweetened with fruit added) (1 cup)	15		

APPENDIX C: (Continued)

Food	Cholesterol (mg)	Food	Cholesterol (mg)
Pork chop, lean only (1 chop) (1.7 oz)	42	Yellow cake (1 piece)	36
Bologna (2 slices)	26	Brownies with nuts (1 brownie)	17
Braunschweiger (2 slices)	20	Doughnuts, cake type (1)	27
Frankfurter, heated (1 frank)	56	Macaroni and cheese, baked (1 cup)	42
Pork links, cooked (2 links)	26		
Salami, dry type (1 oz)	28	Muffins (1)	21
Vienna sausage, canned (1 sausage)	16	Egg noodles (1 cup)	50
		Pancakes (1 cake)	20
Veal cutlet (3 oz)	86	Apple pie (1 piece)	0
Veal roast (3 oz)	86	Custard pie (1 piece)	137
Bluefish, baked (3 oz)	60	Lemon meringue pie (1 piece)	112
Clams, raw (3 oz)	43		
Clams, canned (3 oz)	86	Mince pie (1 piece)	16
Crabmeat, canned (3 oz)	86	Pecan pie (1 piece)	57
Fishsticks, frozen (2 sticks)	46	Pumpkin pie (1 piece)	79
Haddock, fried (3 oz)	51	Spaghetti with meat balls and tomato sauce (1 cup)	75
Ocean perch, fried (3 oz)	51		
Oysters, raw (1 cup)	120	Spaghetti with meat balls and tomato sauce, canned (1 cup)	39
Salmon, pink, canned (3 oz)	30		
Sardines, Atlantic (3 oz)	119		
Shrimp, canned (3 oz)	128	Waffles (1)	45
Tuna, canned in oil (3 oz)	55	Fats and oils	
Grain products[c]		Butter (1 tbsp)	35
Angel-food cake (whole cake) (1 cake)	0	Butter (1 pat)	13
		Whipped butter (1 tbsp)	22
Devil's-food cake with chocolate icing (1 cake)	531	Whipped butter (1 pat)	10
		Lard (1 tbsp)	12
Cupcake (1)	17	Mayonnaise, regular (1 tbsp)	8
Gigerbread (1 cake)	6	Sugars and sweets	
White layer cake with chocolate icing (1 cake)	23	Chocolate candy, milk, plain (1 oz)	21
Boston cream pie (1 piece)	33	Miscellaneous items	
Fruitcake, dark (1 slice)	7	Chocolate pudding (1 cup)	30
Pound cake (1 slice)	30	Vanilla pudding (1 cup)	35
Sponge cake (1 piece)	162	Tapioca cream pudding (1 cup)	159
Yellow cake without icing (1 piece)	26		

Source: F.J. Stare and M. McWilliams, *Living Nutrition*, 4th ed. New York: John Wiley & Sons, Inc., © 1984. Reprinted by permission.

Note: Letters a and b designate items that have the same chemical composition for the edible portion but differ in the amount of refuse. The data in column B apply to 100 g of the edible portion of the item, although it may be purchased with the refuse indicated in column D and described or implied in column A.

APPENDIX D: SUPPLEMENTAL FOOD CHOICES FOR CALORIE-CONTROLLED DIETS

Items	Portion Size	Exchange
Angel food cake	$\frac{1}{20}$ slice	1 starch
Animal Crackers	7	1 starch
Arrow Root Biscuits	3	1 starch
Bread pudding (raisins)[a]	$\frac{1}{2}$ cup	1 starch, $\frac{1}{2}$ milk, 1 fruit
Brown-edged wafers	3	1 starch
Chili dog	1	$1\frac{1}{2}$ starch, $1\frac{1}{2}$ high-fat meat, 2 fat
Cool Whip	1 tbsp	free
Cream puff shell	1	1 starch
Corn dog	1	1 starch, 1 high-fat meat, 2 fat
Custard[a]	$\frac{1}{2}$ cup	$\frac{1}{2}$ starch, 1 milk, 2 fat
Doughnut, plain cake type, 2 in.	1	1 starch, 1 fat
Doughnut, plain yeast type, $3\frac{3}{4}$ in.	1	1 starch, 1 fat
Dressing	$\frac{1}{3}$ cup	1 starch, 1 fat
Frozen yogurt, vanilla[a]	$\frac{1}{2}$ cup	1 starch
Frozen yogurt, on a stick, uncoated[a]	1	1 starch
Fruit cake	1 slice (3 × 3 × $\frac{1}{2}$ in.)	1 starch, 1 fruit, 1 fat
Fruit-flavored gelatin, Jello	$\frac{1}{2}$ cup	1 starch
Gingersnaps	3	1 starch
Gravy	2 tbsp	1 fat
Ice cream, regular vanilla[a]	$\frac{1}{2}$ cup	1 starch, 2 fat
Ice cream cone only[a]	1	$\frac{1}{2}$ bread
Ice milk, vanilla[a]	$\frac{1}{2}$ cup	1 starch, 1 fat
Lady Fingers	2	1 starch
Lorna Doones[a]	3	1 starch, 1 fat
Malted powder, plain dry	2 tbsp	1 starch
Marshmallows[a]	2	1 starch
Mince pie[a]	$\frac{1}{8}$ 9-in. pie	1 starch, 3 fat, $3\frac{1}{2}$ fruit
Pecan pie[a]	$\frac{1}{8}$ 9-in. pie	1 starch, 4 fat, 1 meat, 4 fruit
Pudding, any flavor, regular[a]	$\frac{1}{4}$ cup	1 starch
Pumpkin pie[a]	$\frac{1}{8}$ 9-in. pie	1 starch, 2 fat, $\frac{1}{2}$ meat, 1 fruit
Sherbet[a]	$\frac{1}{2}$ cup	1 starch
Social Tea biscuit	4	1 starch
Soft ice cream (with cone)[a]	1 very small	1 starch
Soft serve ice milk (without cone)[a]	$\frac{1}{2}$ cup	1 starch, 1 fat

APPENDIX D: *(Continued)*

Items	Portion Size	Exchange
Sponge Cake	$\frac{1}{20}$ slice	1 starch
Strawberries	$\frac{3}{4}$ cup	1 fruit
Submarine sandwich: 8-in. roll made of ham, provolone cheese, salami, lettuce, tomato	1	3 starch, 1 vegetable, 3 high-fat meat, 1 fat
8-in. roll made of roast beef, cheese, lettuce, tomato	1	3 starch, 2 vegetable, 2 meat
Sweet potatoes	$\frac{1}{4}$ cup	1 starch
Sweet potato pie[a]	$\frac{1}{8}$ 9-in. pie	1 starch, 2 fat, $\frac{1}{4}$ meat, 1 fruit
Vanilla wafers	5	1 starch
White sauce	$\frac{1}{4}$ cup	$\frac{1}{2}$ starch, 1 fat

Source: Adapted from J.A. Pennington and H.N. Church, *Food Values of Portions Commonly Used,* 14th ed. New York: Harper & Row, 1983.

[a]High in simple sugars.

Note: Those foods in **bold type** are low in cholesterol.

APPENDIX E: ALCOHOLIC BEVERAGES
IN CALORIE-CONTROLLED DIETS

Item	Measure	Exchange	Kilocalories (kcal)
Ale, mild	8 oz	$\frac{1}{2}$ bread, $1\frac{1}{2}$ fat	100
Beer (4.5% by volume)	12 oz	1 bread, 2 fat	160
Brandy or cognac	1 oz	$1\frac{1}{2}$ fat	70
Cider, fermented	6 oz	$1\frac{1}{2}$ fat	70
Cordials: anisette, Curacao, Apricot brandy, Benedictine	$\frac{2}{3}$ oz	$\frac{1}{2}$ bread, 1 fat	80
Daiquiri	$3\frac{1}{2}$ oz	$\frac{1}{2}$ bread, 2 fat	125
Eggnog, Christmas type	3 oz	1 bread, 4 fat	250
Liquor: gin, rum, scotch, etc.	$1\frac{1}{2}$ oz	3 fat	135
Manhattan	$3\frac{1}{2}$ oz	$\frac{1}{2}$ bread, 3 fat	170
Martini	$3\frac{1}{2}$ oz	3 fat	135
Old-Fashioned	4 oz	$\frac{1}{2}$ bread, $3\frac{1}{2}$ fat	190
Port or Muscatelle	$3\frac{1}{2}$ oz	1 bread, 2 fat	160
Tom Collins			
Regular mixer	10 oz	$\frac{1}{2}$ bread, $3\frac{1}{2}$ fat	190
Artificially sweetened mixer	10 oz	$3\frac{1}{2}$ fat	160
Sherry, dry	3 oz	$\frac{1}{2}$ bread, 2 fat	125
Wine, dry table, 12% alcohol (champagne, sauterne, chablis)	3 oz	$1\frac{1}{2}$ fat	70

Source: Adapted from C.F. Adams and M. Richardson, *Nutritive Value of Foods*. Home and Garden Bulletin 72, Agricultural Research Service. Washington, D.C.: U.S. Department of Agriculture, 1970.

APPENDIX F: DRUG–NUTRIENT INTERACTIONS

TABLE 1 MINERAL DEPLETION CAUSED BY DRUGS

Drug or Drug Group	Minerals Depleted
Diuretics	
Thiazide (e.g., hydrochlorothiazide)	Potassium, magnesium, zinc
Loop (e.g., furosemide)	Potassium, magnesium, zinc, calcium
Glucocorticoids (e.g., prednisone)	Calcium, potassium
Chelating agents (e.g., penicillamine)	Zinc, copper
Cancer chemotherapeutic agents (heavy metal) (e.g., cisplatinum)	Magnesium, zinc
Ethanol	Potassium, magnesium, zinc
Laxatives (e.g., phenolphthalein)	Potassium, calcium
Antacids (e.g., aluminum hydroxide)	Phosphate

TABLE 2 DRUGS THAT ARE BETTER ABSORBED ON AN EMPTY STOMACH

Penicillin G (oral)	Isoniazid
Cephalexin	Tetracycline
Erythromycin (stearate)	Aspirin
Phenacetin	Theophylline

DRUGS THAT ARE BETTER ABSORBED WITH FOOD OR MILK

Erythomycin (ethylate)	Nitrofurantoin
Propanolol	Griseofulvin
Chlorothiazide	Prednisone
Indocin	Levodopa
K-Lor	K-Lyte

TABLE 3 RECOMMENDED VITAMIN/MINERAL SUPPLEMENTS DURING DRUG THERAPY

Drug Group	Recommended Supplement
Tetracyclines	Calcium
Phenytoin	Vitamin D, vitamin K
Sulfasalazine	Folic acid
Aspirin	Folic acid, ascorbic acid, iron
Indomethacin	Iron
Isoniazid	Vitamin B_6, niacin, vitamin D
Mineral oil	Vitamin A, vitamin D
Antacids	Folic acid
Penacillamine	Vitamin B_6
Cholestyramine	Vitamin A
Colestipol	Vitamin D, vitamin K, folic acid

TABLE 4 ADVERSE NUTRITIONAL OUTCOMES OF OVER-THE-COUNTER (OTC) USE AND ABUSE

Drug Group	Drug	Nutritional Impairment
Antacids	Sodium bicarbonate	Sodium overload
	Calcium carbonate	Milk alkali syndrome
		Folate malabsorption
	Aluminum hydroxide	Aluminum toxicity
		Phosphate depletion
	Magnesium hydroxide	Magnesium overload
		Phosphate depletion
		Osteomalacia
Laxatives	Phenolphthalein	Hypokalemia
	Bisacodyl	Malabsorption
	Senna	↓ Osteomalacia
		Protein-losing enteropathy
		↓ Hypoalbuminea
	Mineral oil	Vitamin A, D, K depletion
Nonnarcotic analgesics	Aspirin	Iron deficiency

Source: Adapted from "Food, nutrition and pharmacology," *Seminars in Nutrition*, 4(4), 5–13 (1985).

APPENDIX G: NUTRITIVE VALUES TO THE EDIBLE PART OF FOODS

				Nutrients in Indicated Quantity			
Item No. (A)	Foods, approximate measures, units, and weight (edible part unless footnote indicate otherwise) (B)		g	Water (C) %	Food Energy (D) kcal	Pro-tein (E) g	Fat (F) g

Key to Abbreviations:
% = Percent   g = Grams   IU = International Units
kcal = Kilocalories   mg = Milligrams   TR = Trace

Dairy Products (Cheese, Cream, Imitation Cream, Milk & Related Products)

Butter. See Fats, oils; related products, items 103–108.

Cheese

Natural

1	Blue	1 oz	28	42	100	6	8
2	Camembert (3 wedges per 4-oz container).	1 wedge	38	52	115	8	9
	Cheddar						
3	Cut pieces	1 oz	28	37	115	7	9
4		1 cu in	17.2	37	70	4	6
5	Shredded	1 cup	113	37	455	28	37
	Cottage (curd not pressed down)						
	Creamed (cottage cheese, 4% fat)						
6	Large curd	1 cup	225	79	235	28	10
7	Small curd	1 cup	210	79	220	26	9
8	Low fat (2%)	1 cup	226	79	205	31	4
9	Low fat (1%)	1 cup	226	82	165	28	2
10	Uncreamed (cottage cheese dry curd, less than ½% fat).	1 cup	145	80	125	25	1
11	Cream	1 oz	28	54	100	2	10
	Mozzarella, made with:						
12	Whole milk	1 oz	28	48	90	6	7
13	Part skim milk	1 oz	28	49	80	8	5
	Parmesan, grated						
14	Cup, not pressed down	1 cup	100	18	455	42	30
15	Tablespoon	1 tbsp	5	18	25	2	2
16	Ounce	1 oz	28	18	130	12	9
17	Provolone	1 oz	28	41	100	7	8
	Ricotta, made with:						
18	Whole milk	1 cup	246	72	430	28	32

Source: C. F. Adams, and M. Richardson, *Nutritive Value of Foods,* Home and Garden Bulletin 72, Agricultural Research Service, U.S. Department of Agriculture, Washington, D.C., revised 1982.

Note: Dashes (—) denote lack of reliable data for a constituent believed to be present in measurable amount.

							Nutrients in Indicated Quantity					
Fatty Acids												
	Unsaturated											
Satu-rated (Total) (G) g	Oleic (H) g	Lino-leic (I) g	Carbo-hydrate (J) g	Calcium (K) mg	Phos-phorus (L) mg	Iron (M) mg	Potas-sium (N) mg	Vitamin A Value (O) I.U.	Thiamin (P) mg	Ribo-flavin (Q) mg	Niacin (R) mg	Ascorbic Acid (S) mg
5.3	1.9	0.2	1	150	110	0.1	73	200	0.01	0.11	0.3	0
5.8	2.2	0.2	TR	147	132	0.1	71	350	0.01	0.19	0.2	0
6.1	2.1	0.2	TR	204	145	0.2	28	300	0.01	0.11	TR	0
3.7	1.3	0.1	TR	124	88	0.1	17	180	TR	0.06	TR	0
24.2	8.5	0.7	1	815	579	0.8	111	1,200	0.03	0.42	0.1	0
6.4	2.4	0.2	6	135	297	0.3	190	370	0.05	0.37	0.3	TR
6.0	2.2	0.2	6	126	277	0.3	177	340	0.04	0.34	0.3	TR
2.8	1.0	0.1	8	155	340	0.4	217	160	0.05	0.42	0.3	TR
1.5	0.5	0.1	6	138	302	0.3	193	80	0.05	0.37	0.3	TR
0.4	0.1	TR	3	46	151	0.3	47	40	0.04	0.21	0.2	0
6.2	2.4	0.2	1	23	30	0.3	34	400	TR	0.06	TR	0
4.4	1.7	0.2	1	163	117	0.1	21	260	TR	0.08	TR	0
3.1	1.2	0.1	1	207	149	0.1	27	180	0.01	0.10	TR	0
19.1	7.7	0.3	4	1,376	807	1.0	107	700	0.05	0.39	0.3	0
1.0	0.4	TR	TR	69	40	TR	5	40	TR	0.02	TR	0
5.4	2.2	0.1	1	390	229	0.3	30	200	0.01	0.11	0.1	0
4.8	1.7	0.1	1	214	141	0.1	39	230	0.01	0.09	TR	0
20.4	7.1	0.7	7	509	389	0.9	257	1,210	0.03	0.48	0.3	0

(Continued)

APPENDIX G: *(Continued)*

				Nutrients in Indicated Quantity			
Item No. (A)	Foods, approximate measures, units, and weight (edible part unless footnote indicate otherwise) (B)		g	Water (C) %	Food Energy (D) kcal	Pro-tein (E) g	Fat (F) g

Dairy Products (Cheese, Cream, Imitation Cream, Milk & Related Products)							
	Cheese—Continued						
	Natural—Continued						
	Ricotta, made with:—Continued						
19	Part skim milk	1 cup	246	74	340	28	19
20	Romano	1 oz	28	31	110	9	8
21	Swiss	1 oz	28	37	105	8	8
	Pasteurized process cheese						
22	American	1 oz	28	39	105	6	9
23	Swiss	1 oz	28	42	95	7	7
24	Pasteurized process cheese food, American.	1 oz	28	43	95	6	7
25	Pasteurized process cheese spread, American	1 oz	28	48	80	5	6
	Cream, sweet						
26	Half-and-half (cream and milk)	1 cup	242	81	315	7	28
27		1 tbsp	15	81	20	TR	2
28	Light, coffee, or table	1 cup	240	74	470	6	46
29		1 tbsp	15	74	30	TR	3
30	Light	1 cup	239	64	700	5	74
31		1 tbsp	15	64	45	TR	5
32	Heavy	1 cup	238	58	820	5	88
33		1 tbsp	15	58	80	TR	6
34	Whipped topping, (pressurized)	1 cup	60	61	155	2	13
35		1 tbsp	3	61	10	TR	1
36	Cream, sour	1 cup	230	71	495	7	48
37		1 tbsp	12	71	25	TR	3
	Cream products, imitation (made with vegetable fat)						
	Sweet						
	Creamers						
38	Liquid (frozen)	1 cup	245	77	335	2	24
39		1 tbsp	15	77	20	TR	1
40	Powdered	1 cup	94	2	515	5	33
41		1 tsp	2	2	10	TR	1
	Whipped topping						
42	Frozen	1 cup	75	50	240	1	19
43		1 tbsp	4	50	15	TR	1

[1]Vitamin A value is largely from beta-carotene used for coloring. Riboflavin value for items 40–41 apply to product with added riboflavin.

| | Fatty Acids | | | | | | | | | | | | |
| | | Unsaturated | | | | | | | | | | | |
Satu-rated (Total) (G) g	Oleic (H) g	Lino-leic (I) g	Carbo-hydrate (J) g	Calcium (K) mg	Phos-phorus (L) mg	Iron (M) mg	Potas-sium (N) mg	Vitamin A Value (O) I.U.	Thiamin (P) mg	Ribo-flavin (Q) mg	Niacin (R) mg	Ascorbic Acid (S) mg
12.1	4.7	0.5	13	669	449	1.1	308	1,060	0.05	0.46	0.2	0
—	—	—	1	302	215	—	—	160	—	0.11	TR	0
5.0	1.7	0.2	1	272	171	TR	31	240	0.01	0.10	TR	0
5.6	2.1	0.2	TR	174	211	0.1	46	340	0.01	0.10	TR	0
4.5	1.7	0.1	1	219	216	0.2	61	230	TR	0.08	TR	0
4.4	1.7	0.1	2	163	130	0.2	79	260	0.01	0.13	TR	0
3.8	1.5	0.1	2	159	202	0.1	69	220	0.01	0.12	TR	0
17.3	7.0	0.6	10	254	230	0.2	314	260	0.08	0.36	0.2	2
1.1	0.4	TR	1	16	14	TR	19	20	0.01	0.02	TR	TR
28.8	11.7	1.0	9	231	192	0.1	292	1,730	0.08	0.36	0.1	2
1.8	0.7	0.1	1	14	12	TR	18	110	TR	0.02	TR	TR
46.2	18.3	1.5	7	166	146	0.1	231	2,690	0.06	0.30	0.1	1
2.9	1.1	0.1	TR	10	9	TR	15	170	TR	0.02	TR	TR
54.8	22.2	2.0	TR	154	149	TR	179	3,500	0.05	0.26	0.1	1
3.5	1.4	0.1	TR	10	9	TR	11	220	TR	0.02	TR	TR
8.3	3.4	0.3	7	61	54	TR	88	550	0.02	0.04	TR	0
0.4	0.2	TR	TR	3	3	TR	4	30	TR	TR	TR	0
30.0	12.1	1.1	10	268	195	0.1	331	1,820	0.08	0.34	0.2	2
1.6	0.6	0.1	1	14	10	TR	17	90	TR	0.02	TR	TR
22.8	0.3	TR	28	23	157	0.1	467	[1]220	0	0	0	0
1.4	TR	0	2	1	10	TR	29	[1]10	0	0	0	0
30.6	0.9	TR	52	21	397	0.1	763	[1]190	0	0.16	0	0
0.7	TR	0	1	TR	8	TR	16	[1]TR	0	[1]TR	0	0
16.3	1.0	0.2	17	5	6	0.1	14	[1]650	0	0	0	0
0.9	0.1	TR	1	TR	TR	TR	1	[1]30	0	0	0	0

(Continued)

APPENDIX G: (Continued)

Nutrients in Indicated Quantity

Item No. (A)	Foods, approximate measures, units, and weight (edible part unless footnote indicate otherwise) (B)		g	Water (C) %	Food Energy (D) kcal	Pro- tein (E) g	Fat (F) g
Dairy Products (Cheese, Cream, Imitation Cream, Milk & Related Products)							
	Cream products, imitation (made with vegetable fat—Continued						
	Sweet—Continued						
	Whipped topping—Continued						
44	Powdered, made with whole milk	1 cup	80	67	150	3	10
45		1 tbsp	4	67	10	TR	TR
46	Pressurized	1 cup	70	60	185	1	16
47		1 tbsp	4	60	10	TR	1
48	Sour dressing (imitation sour cream) made with nonfat dry milk	1 cup	235	75	415	8	39
49		1 tbsp	12	75	20	TR	2
	Ice cream. See Milk desserts, frozen (items 75–80)						
	Ice milk. See Milk desserts, frozen (items 81–83)						
	Milk						
	Fluid						
50	Whole (3.3% fat)	1 cup	244	88	150	8	8
	Lowfat (2%)						
51	No milk solids added	1 cup	244	89	120	8	5
	Milk solids added						
52	Label claims less than 10 g of protein per cup	1 cup	245	89	125	9	5
53	Label claim 10 or more grams of protein per cup (protein fortified).	1 cup	246	88	135	10	5
	Lowfat (1%)						
54	No milk solids added	1 cup	244	90	100	8	3
	Milk solids added						
55	Label claim less than 10 g of protein per cup	1 cup	245	90	105	9	2
56	Label claim 10 or more grams of protein per cup (protein fortified)	1 cup	246	89	120	10	3
57	Nonfat (skim)						
	No milk solids added	1 cup	245	91	85	8	TR
	Milk solids added						
58	Label claim less than 10 g of protein per cup	1 cup	245	90	90	9	1
59	Label claim 10 or more grams of protein per cup (protein fortified)	1 cup	246	89	100	10	1

[2]Applies to product without added vitamin A. With added vitamin A, value is 500 International Units (IU).

| | Fatty Acids | | | | | | | | | | | |
| | | Unsaturated | | | | | | | | | | |
Satu-rated (Total) (G) g	Oleic (H) g	Lino-leic (I) g	Carbo-hydrate (J) g	Calcium (K) mg	Phos-phorus (L) mg	Iron (M) mg	Potas-sium (N) mg	Vitamin A Value (O) I.U.	Thiamin (P) mg	Ribo-flavin (Q) mg	Niacin (R) mg	Ascorbic Acid (S) mg
8.5	0.6	0.1	13	72	69	TR	121	[1]290	0.02	0.09	TR	1
0.4	TR	TR	1	4	3	TR	6	[1]10	TR	TR	TR	TR
13.2	1.4	0.2	11	4	13	TR	13	[1]330	0	0	0	0
0.8	0.1	TR	1	TR	1	TR	1	[1]20	0	0	0	0
31.2	4.4	1.1	11	286	205	0.1	380	[1]20	0.09	0.38	0.2	2
1.6	0.2	0.1	1	14	10	TR	19	[1]TR	0.01	0.02	TR	TR
5.1	2.1	0.2	11	291	228	0.1	370	[2]310	0.09	0.40	0.2	2
2.9	1.2	0.1	12	297	232	0.1	377	500	0.10	0.40	0.2	2
2.9	1.2	0.1	12	313	245	0.1	397	500	0.10	0.42	0.2	2
3.0	1.2	0.1	14	352	276	0.1	447	500	0.11	0.48	0.2	2
1.6	0.7	0.1	12	300	235	0.1	381	500	0.10	0.41	0.2	2
1.5	0.6	0.1	12	313	245	0.1	397	500	0.10	0.42	0.2	2
1.8	0.7	0.1	14	349	273	0.1	444	500	0.11	0.47	0.2	2
0.3	0.1	TR	12	302	247	0.1	406	500	0.09	0.37	0.2	2
0.4	0.1	TR	12	316	255	0.1	418	500	0.10	0.43	0.2	2
0.4	0.1	TR	14	352	275	0.1	446	500	0.11	0.48	0.2	3

(Continued)

APPENDIX G: *(Continued)*

Nutrients in Indicated Quantity

Item No. (A)	Foods, approximate measures, units, and weight (edible part unless footnotes indicate otherwise) (B)		g	Water (C) %	Food Energy (D) kcal	Pro-tein (E) g	Fat (F) g
Dairy Products (Cheese, Cream, Imitation Cream, Milk & Related Products)—Con.							
	Milk—Continued						
	Fluid—Continued						
60	Buttermilk	1 cup	245	90	100	8	2
	Canned						
	Evaporated, unsweetened						
61	Whole milk	1 cup	252	74	340	17	19
62	Skim milk	1 cup	255	79	200	19	1
63	Sweetened, condensed	1 cup	306	27	980	24	27
	Dried						
64	Buttermilk	1 cup	120	3	465	41	7
	Nonfat instant						
65	Envelope, net wt., 3.2 oz[5]	1 envelope	91	4	325	32	1
66	Cup[7]	1 cup	68	4	245	24	TR
	Milk beverages						
	Chocolate milk (commercial)						
67	Regular	1 cup	250	82	210	8	8
68	Lowfat (2%)	1 cup	250	84	180	8	5
69	Lowfat (1%)	1 cup	250	85	160	8	3
70	Eggnog (commercial)	1 cup	254	74	340	10	19
	Malted milk, home prepared with 1 cup of whole milk and 2 to 3 heaping tsp of malted milk powder (about ¾ oz)						
71	Chocolate +¾ oz of powder	1 cup of milk	265	81	235	9	9
72	Natural +¾ oz of powder	1 cup of milk	265	81	235	11	10
	Shakes, thick[8]						
73	Chocolate, container, net wt., 10.6 oz	1 container	300	72	355	9	8
74	Vanilla, container, net wt., 11 oz	1 container	313	74	350	12	9

[3]Applies to product without vitamin A added.
[4]Applies to product with added vitamin A. Without added vitamin A, value is 20 IU.
[5]Yields 1 qt of fluid milk when reconstituted according to package directions.
[6]Applies to product with added vitamin A.
[7]Weight applies to product with label claim of 1⅓ cups equal to 3.2 oz.
[8]Applies to products made from thick shake mixes and that do not contain added ice cream. Products made from milk shake mixes are higher in fat and usually contain added ice cream.

| | Fatty Acids | | | | | | | | | | | |
| | Unsaturated | | | | | | | | | | | |
Saturated (Total) (G) g	Oleic (H) g	Linoleic (I) g	Carbohydrate (J) g	Calcium (K) mg	Phosphorus (L) mg	Iron (M) mg	Potassium (N) mg	Vitamin A Value (O) I.U.	Thiamin (P) mg	Riboflavin (Q) mg	Niacin (R) mg	Ascorbic Acid (S) mg
1.3	0.5	TR	12	285	219	0.1	371	[3]80	0.08	0.38	0.1	2
11.6	5.3	0.4	25	657	510	0.5	764	[3]610	0.12	0.80	0.5	5
0.3	0.1	TR	29	738	497	0.7	845	[4]1,000	0.11	0.79	0.4	3
16.8	6.7	0.7	166	868	775	0.6	1,136	[3]1,000	0.28	1.27	0.6	8
4.3	1.7	0.2	59	1,421	1,119	0.4	1,910	[3]260	0.47	1.90	1.1	7
0.4	0.1	TR	47	1,120	896	0.3	1,552	[6]2,160	0.38	1.59	0.8	5
0.3	0.1	TR	35	837	670	0.2	1,160	[6]1,610	0.28	1.19	0.6	4
5.3	2.2	0.2	26	280	251	0.6	417	[3]300	0.09	0.41	0.3	2
3.1	1.3	0.1	26	284	254	0.6	422	500	0.10	0.42	0.3	2
1.5	0.7	0.1	26	287	257	0.6	426	500	0.10	0.40	0.2	2
11.3	5.0	0.6	34	330	278	0.5	420	890	0.09	0.48	0.3	4
5.5	—	—	29	304	265	0.5	500	330	0.14	0.43	0.7	2
6.0	—	—	27	347	307	0.3	529	380	0.20	0.54	1.3	2
5.0	2.0	0.2	63	396	378	0.9	672	260	0.14	0.67	0.4	0
5.9	2.4	0.2	56	457	361	0.3	572	360	0.09	0.61	0.5	0

Nutrients in Indicated Quantity

(Continued)

APPENDIX G: *(Continued)*

					Nutrients in Indicated Quantity		

Item No. (A)	Foods, approximate measures, units, and weight (edible part unless footnote indicate otherwise) (B)		g	Water (C) %	Food Energy (D) kcal	Pro-tein (E) g	Fat (F) g
Dairy Products (Cheese, Cream, Imitation Cream, Milk & Related Products)—Con.							
	Milk desserts, frozen						
	Ice cream						
	Regular (about 11% fat)						
75	Hardened	½ gal	1,064	61	2,155	38	115
76		1 cup	133	61	270	5	14
77		3-fl oz	50	61	100	2	5
78	Soft serve (frozen custard)	1 cup	173	60	375	7	23
79	Rich (about 16% fat), hardened.	½ gal	1,188	59	2,805	33	190
80		1 cup	148	59	350	4	24
	Ice milk						
81	Hardened (about 4.3% fat)	½ gal	1,048	69	1,470	41	45
82		1 cup	131	69	185	5	6
83	Soft serve (about 2.6% fat)	1 cup	175	70	225	8	5
84	Sherbet (about 2% fat)	½ gal	1,542	66	2,160	17	31
85		1 cup	193	66	270	2	4
	Milk desserts, other						
86	Custard, baked	1 cup	265	77	305	14	15
	Puddings						
	From home recipe						
	Starch base						
87	Chocolate	1 cup	260	66	385	8	12
88	Vanilla (blancmange)	1 cup	255	76	285	9	10
89	Tapioca cream	1 cup	165	72	220	8	8
	From mix (chocolate) and milk						
90	Regular (cooked)	1 cup	260	70	320	9	8
91	Instant	1 cup	260	69	325	8	7
	Yogurt						
	With added milk solids						
	Made with lowfat milk						
92	Fruit-flavored[9]	1 8 oz. container	227	75	230	10	3
93	Plain	1 container	227	85	145	12	4
94	Made with nonfat milk	1 8 oz. container	227	85	125	13	TR
	Without added milk solds						
95	Made with whole milk	1 8 oz. container	227	88	140	8	7

[9]Content of fat, vitamin A, and carbohydrate varies. Consult the label when precise values are needed for special diets.
[10]Applies to product made with milk containing no added vitamin A.

								Nutrients in Indicated Quantity					
Fatty Acids													
	Unsaturated												
Satu-rated (Total) (G) g	Oleic (H) g	Lino-leic (I) g	Carbo-hydrate (J) g	Calcium (K) mg	Phos-phorus (L) mg	Iron (M) mg	Potas-sium (N) mg	Vitamin A Value (O) I.U.	Thiamin (P) mg	Ribo-flavin (Q) mg	Niacin (R) mg	Ascorbic Acid (S) mg
---	---	---	---	---	---	---	---	---	---	---	---	---
71.3	28.8	2.6	254	1,406	1,075	1.0	2,052	4,340	0.42	2.63	1.1	6
8.9	3.6	0.3	32	176	134	0.1	257	540	0.05	0.33	0.1	1
3.4	1.4	0.1	12	66	51	TR	96	200	0.02	0.12	0.1	TR
13.5	5.9	0.6	38	236	199	0.4	338	790	0.08	0.45	0.2	1
118.3	47.8	4.3	256	1,213	927	0.8	1,771	7,200	0.36	2.27	0.9	5
14.7	6.0	0.5	32	151	115	0.1	221	900	0.04	0.28	0.1	1
28.1	11.3	1.0	232	1,409	1,035	1.5	2,117	1,710	0.61	2.78	0.9	6
3.5	1.4	0.1	29	176	129	0.1	265	210	0.08	0.35	0.1	1
2.9	1.2	0.1	38	274	202	0.3	412	180	0.12	0.54	0.2	1
19.0	7.7	0.7	469	827	594	2.5	1,585	1,480	0.26	0.71	1.0	31
2.4	1.0	0.1	59	103	74	0.3	198	190	0.03	0.09	0.1	4
6.8	5.4	0.7	29	297	310	1.1	387	930	0.11	0.50	0.3	1
7.6	3.3	0.3	67	250	255	1.3	445	390	0.05	0.36	0.3	1
6.2	2.5	0.2	41	298	232	TR	352	410	0.08	0.41	0.3	2
4.1	2.5	0.5	28	173	180	0.7	223	480	0.07	0.30	0.2	2
4.3	2.6	0.2	59	265	247	0.8	354	340	0.05	0.39	0.3	2
3.6	2.2	0.3	63	374	237	1.3	335	340	0.08	0.39	0.3	2
1.8	0.6	0.1	42	343	269	0.2	439	[10]120	0.08	0.40	0.2	1
2.3	0.8	0.1	16	415	326	0.2	531	[10]150	0.10	0.49	0.3	2
0.3	0.1	TR	17	452	355	0.2	579	[10]20	0.11	0.53	0.3	2
4.8	1.7	0.1	11	274	215	0.1	351	280	0.07	0.32	0.2	1

(Continued)

APPENDIX G: *(Continued)*

Nutrients in Indicated Quantity

Item No. (A)	Foods, approximate measures, units, and weight (edible part unless footnote indicate otherwise) (B)		g	Water (C) %	Food Energy (D) kcal	Pro- tein (E) g	Fat (F) g
Eggs							
	Eggs, large (24 oz per dozen)						
	Raw						
96	Whole, without shell	1 egg	50	75	80	6	6
97	White	1 white	33	88	15	3	TR
98	Yolk	1 yolk	17	49	65	3	6
	Cooked						
99	Fried in butter	1 egg	46	72	85	5	6
100	Hard-cooked, shell removed	1 egg	50	75	80	6	6
101	Poached	1 egg	50	74	80	6	6
102	Scrambled (milk added) in butter. Also omelet	1 egg	64	76	95	6	7
Fats, Oils, Related Products							
	Butter						
	Regular (1 brick or 4 sticks per lb)						
103	Stick ($\frac{1}{2}$ cup)	1 stick	113	16	815	1	92
104	Tablespoon (about $\frac{1}{8}$ stick)	1 tbsp	14	16	100	TR	12
105	Pat (1 in square, $\frac{1}{3}$ in high; 90 per lb)	1 pat	5	16	35	TR	4
	Whipped (6 sticks or two 8-oz containers per lb).						
106	Stick ($\frac{1}{2}$ cup)	1 stick	76	16	540	1	61
107	Tablespoon (about $\frac{1}{8}$ stick)	1 tbsp	9	16	65	TR	8
108	Pat ($1\frac{1}{4}$ in square, $\frac{1}{3}$ in high; 120 per lb)	1 pat	4	16	25	TR	3
109	Fats, cooking (vegetable shortenings)	1 cup	200	0	1,770	0	200
110		1 tbsp	13	0	110	0	13
111	Lard	1 cup	205	0	1,850	0	205
112		1 tbsp	13	0	115	0	13
	Margarine						
	Regular (1 brick or 4 sticks per lb)						
113	Stick ($\frac{1}{2}$ cup)	1 stick	113	16	815	1	92
114	Tablespoon (about $\frac{1}{8}$ stick)	1 tbsp	14	16	100	TR	12
115	Pat (1 in square, $\frac{1}{3}$ in. high; 90 per lb)	1 pat	5	16	35	TR	4
116	Soft, two 8-oz containers per lb	1 container	227	16	1,635	1	184
117		1 tbsp	14	16	100	TR	12
	Whipped (6 sticks per lb)						
118	Stick ($\frac{1}{2}$ cup)	1 stick	76	16	545	TR	61

[11]Based on year-round average.

[12]Based on average vitamin A content of fortified margarine. Federal specifications for fortified margarine require a minimum of 15,000 International Units (IU) of vitamin A per pound.

					Nutrients in Indicated Quantity							
Fatty Acids												
	Unsaturated											
Satu-rated (Total) (G) g	Oleic (H) g	Lino-leic (I) g	Carbo-hydrate (J) g	Calcium (K) mg	Phos-phorus (L) mg	Iron (M) mg	Potas-sium (N) mg	Vitamin A Value (O) I.U.	Thiamin (P) mg	Ribo-flavin (Q) mg	Niacin (R) mg	Ascorbic Acid (S) mg
1.7	2.0	0.6	1	28	90	1.0	65	260	0.04	0.15	TR	0
0	0	0	TR	4	4	TR	45	0	TR	0.09	TR	0
1.7	2.1	0.6	TR	26	86	0.9	15	310	0.04	0.07	TR	0
2.4	2.2	0.6	1	26	80	0.9	58	290	0.03	0.13	TR	0
1.7	2.0	0.6	1	28	90	1.0	65	260	0.04	0.14	TR	0
1.7	2.0	0.6	1	28	90	1.0	65	260	0.04	0.13	TR	0
2.8	2.3	0.6	1	47	97	0.9	85	310	0.04	0.16	TR	0
57.3	23.1	2.1	TR	27	26	0.2	29	[11]3,470	0.01	0.04	TR	0
7.2	2.9	0.3	TR	3	3	TR	4	[11]430	TR	TR	TR	0
2.5	1.0	0.1	TR	1	1	TR	1	[11]150	TR	TR	TR	0
38.2	15.4	1.4	TR	18	17	0.1	20	[11]2,310	TR	0.03	TR	0
4.7	1.9	0.2	TR	2	2	TR	2	[11]290	TR	TR	TR	0
1.9	0.8	0.1	TR	1	1	TR	1	[11]120	0	TR	TR	0
48.8	88.2	48.4	0	0	0	0	0	—	0	0	0	0
3.2	5.7	3.1	0	0	0	0	0	—	0	0	0	0
81.0	83.8	20.5	0	0	0	0	0	0	0	0	0	0
5.1	5.3	1.3	0	0	0	0	0	0	0	0	0	0
16.7	42.9	24.9	TR	27	26	0.2	29	[12]3,750	0.01	0.04	TR	0
2.1	5.3	3.1	TR	3	3	TR	4	[12]470	TR	TR	TR	0
0.7	1.9	1.1	TR	1	1	TR	1	[12]170	TR	TR	TR	0
32.5	71.5	65.4	TR	53	52	0.4	59	[12]7,500	0.01	0.08	0.1	0
2.0	4.5	4.1	TR	3	3	TR	4	[12]470	TR	TR	TR	0
11.2	28.7	16.7	TR	18	17	0.1	20	[12]2,500	TR	0.03	TR	0

(Continued)

APPENDIX G: (Continued)

Item No. (A)	Foods, approximate measures, units, and weight (edible part unless footnote indicate otherwise) (B)		Water (C) %	Food Energy (D) kcal	Pro- tein (E) g	Fat (F) g
		g				
Fats, Oils, Related Products—Con.						
	Margarine—Continued						
	Whipped (6 sticks per lb)—Continued						
119	Tablespoon (about ⅛ stick)	1 tbsp	9	16	70	TR	8
	Oils, salad or cooking						
120	Corn	1 cup	218	0	1,925	0	218
121		1 tbsp	14	0	120	0	14
122	Olive	1 cup	216	0	1,910	0	216
123		1 tbsp	14	0	120	0	14
124	Peanut	1 cup	216	0	1,910	0	216
125		1 tbsp	14	0	120	0	14
126	Safflower	1 cup	218	0	1,925	0	218
127		1 tbsp	14	0	120	0	14
128	Soybean oil, hydrogenated (partially hardened)	1 cup	218	0	1,925	0	218
129		1 tbsp	14	0	120	0	14
130	Soybean-cottonseed oil blend, hydrogenated	1 cup	218	0	1,925	0	218
131		1 tbsp	14	0	120	0	14
	Salad dressings						
	Commercial						
	Blue cheese						
132	Regular	1 tbsp	15	32	75	1	8
133	Low calorie (5 cal/tsp)	1 tbsp	16	84	10	TR	1
	French						
134	Regular	1 tbsp	16	39	65	TR	6
135	Low calorie (5 cal/tsp)	1 tbsp	16	77	15	TR	1
	Italian						
136	Regular	1 tbsp	15	28	85	TR	9
137	Low calorie (2 cal/tsp)	1 tbsp	15	90	10	TR	1
138	Mayonnaise	1 tbsp	14	15	100	TR	11
	Mayonnaise type						
139	Regular	1 tbsp	15	41	65	TR	6
140	Low calorie (8 cal/tsp)	1 tbsp	16	81	20	TR	2
141	Tartar sauce, regular	1 tbsp	14	34	75	TR	8
	Thousand Island						
142	Regular	1 tbsp	16	32	80	TR	8
143	Low calorie (10 cal/tsp)	1 tbsp	15	68	25	TR	2

Nutrients in Indicated Quantity

							Nutrients in Indicated Quantity					
Fatty Acids												
	Unsaturated											
Satu-rated (Total) (G) g	Oleic (H) g	Lino-leic (I) g	Carbo-hydrate (J) g	Calcium (K) mg	Phos-phorus (L) mg	Iron (M) mg	Potas-sium (N) mg	Vitamin A Value (O) I.U.	Thiamin (P) mg	Ribo-flavin (Q) mg	Niacin (R) mg	Ascorbic Acid (S) mg
1.4	3.6	2.1	TR	2	2	TR	2	[12]310	TR	TR	TR	0
27.7	53.6	125.1	0	0	0	0	0	—	0	0	0	0
1.7	3.3	7.8	0	0	0	0	0	—	0	0	0	0
30.7	154.4	17.7	0	0	0	0	0	—	0	0	0	0
1.9	9.7	1.1	0	0	0	0	0	—	0	0	0	0
37.4	98.5	67.0	0	0	0	0	0	—	0	0	0	0
2.3	6.2	4.2	0	0	0	0	0	—	0	0	0	0
20.5	25.9	159.8	0	0	0	0	0	—	0	0	0	0
1.3	1.6	10.0	0	0	0	0	0	—	0	0	0	0
31.8	93.1	75.6	0	0	0	0	0	—	0	0	0	0
2.0	5.8	4.7	0	0	0	0	0	—	0	0	0	0
38.2	63.0	99.6	0	0	0	0	0	—	0	0	0	0
2.4	3.9	6.2	0	0	0	0	0	—	0	0	0	0
1.6	1.7	3.8	1	12	11	TR	6	30	TR	0.02	TR	TR
0.5	0.3	TR	1	10	8	TR	5	30	TR	0.01	TR	TR
1.1	1.3	3.2	3	2	2	0.1	13	—	—	—	—	—
0.1	0.1	0.4	2	2	2	0.1	13	—	—	—	—	—
1.6	1.9	4.7	1	2	1	TR	2	TR	TR	TR	TR	—
0.1	0.1	0.4	TR	TR	1	TR	2	TR	TR	TR	TR	—
2.0	2.4	5.6	TR	3	4	0.1	5	40	TR	0.01	TR	—
1.1	1.4	3.2	2	2	4	TR	1	30.	TR	TR	TR	—
0.4	0.4	1.0	2	3	4	TR	1	40	TR	TR	TR	—
1.5	1.8	4.1	1	3	4	0.1	11	30	TR	TR	TR	TR
1.4	1.7	4.0	2	2	3	0.1	18	50	TR	TR	TR	TR
0.4	0.4	1.0	2	2	3	0.1	17	50	TR	TR	TR	TR

(Continued)

APPENDIX G: (Continued)

Item No. (A)	Foods, approximate measures, units, and weight (edible part unless footnote indicate otherwise) (B)		g	Water (C) %	Food Energy (D) kcal	Pro- tein (E) g	Fat (F) g
Fats, Oils, Related Products—Con.							
	Salad dressings—Continued						
	From home recipe						
144	Cooked type[13]	1 tbsp	16	68	25	1	2
Fish, Shellfish, Meat, Poultry; Related Products							
	Fish and Shellfish						
145	Bluefish, baked with butter or margarine	3 oz	85	68	135	22	4
	Clams						
146	Raw, meat only	3 oz	85	82	65	11	1
147	Canned, solids and liquid	3 oz	85	86	45	7	1
148	Crabmeat (white or king), canned, not pressed down	1 cup	135	77	135	24	3
149	Fish sticks, breaded, cooked, frozen (stick, 4 by 1 by ½ in)	1 fish stick	28	66	50	5	3
150	Haddock, breaded, fried[14]	3 oz	85	66	140	17	5
151	Ocean perch, breaded, fried[14]	1 fillet	85	59	195	16	11
152	Oysters, raw, meat only (13–19 medium Selects)	1 cup	240	85	160	20	4
153	Salmon, pink, canned, solids and liquid	3 oz	85	71	120	17	5
154	Sardines, Atlantic, canned in oil, drained solids	3 oz	85	62	175	20	9
155	Scallops, frozen, breaded, fried, reheated	6 scallops	90	60	175	16	8
156	Shad, baked with butter or margarine, bacon	3 oz	85	64	170	20	10
	Shrimp						
157	Canned meat	3 oz	85	70	100	21	1
158	French fried[16]	3 oz	85	57	190	17	9
159	Tuna, canned in oil, drained solids	3 oz	85	61	170	24	7
160	Tuna salad[17]	1 cup	205	70	350	30	22
	Meat and meat products						
161	Bacon, (20 slices per lb, raw), broiled or fried, crisp	2 slices	15	8	85	4	8
	Beef,[18] cooked						
	Cuts braised, simmered or pot roasted						
162	Lean and fat (piece, 2½ by 2½ by ¾ in)	3 oz	85	53	245	23	16

[13]Fatty acid values apply to product made with regular-type margarine.
[14]Dipped in egg, milk or water, and breadcrumbs; fried in vegetable shortening.
[15]If bones are discarded, value for calcium will be greatly reduced.
[16]Dipped in egg, breadcrumbs, and flour or batter.
[17]Prepared with tuna, celery, salad dressing (mayonnaise type), pickle, onion, and egg.
[18]Outer layer of fat on the cut was removed to within approximately ½ in. of the lean. Deposits of fat within the cut were not removed.

					Nutrients in Indicated Quantity							

Fatty Acids												
	Unsaturated											
Satu-rated (Total) (G) g	Oleic (H) g	Lino-leic (I) g	Carbo-hydrate (J) g	Calcium (K) mg	Phos-phorus (L) mg	Iron (M) mg	Potas-sium (N) mg	Vitamin A Value (O) I.U.	Thiamin (P) mg	Ribo-flavin (Q) mg	Niacin (R) mg	Ascorbic Acid (S) mg
0.5	0.6	0.3	2	14	15	0.1	19	80	0.01	0.03	TR	TR
—	—	—	0	25	244	0.6	—	40	0.09	0.08	1.6	—
—	—	—	2	59	138	5.2	154	90	0.08	0.15	1.1	8
0.2	TR	TR	2	47	116	3.5	119	—	0.01	0.09	0.9	—
0.6	0.4	0.1	1	61	246	1.1	149	—	0.11	0.11	2.6	—
—	—	—	2	3	47	0.1	—	0	0.01	0.02	0.5	—
1.4	2.2	1.2	5	34	210	1.0	296	—	0.03	0.06	2.7	2
2.7	4.4	2.3	6	28	192	1.1	242	—	0.10	0.10	1.6	—
1.3	0.2	0.1	8	226	343	13.2	290	740	0.34	0.43	6.0	—
0.9	0.8	0.1	0	[15]167	243	0.7	307	60	0.03	0.16	6.8	—
3.0	2.5	0.5	0	372	424	2.5	502	190	0.02	0.17	4.6	—
—	—	—	9	—	—	—	—	—	—	—	—	—
—	—	—	0	20	266	0.5	320	30	0.11	0.22	7.3	—
0.1	0.1	TR	1	98	224	2.6	104	50	0.01	0.03	1.5	—
2.3	3.7	2.0	9	61	162	1.7	195	—	0.03	0.07	2.3	—
1.7	1.7	0.7	0	7	199	1.6	—	70	0.04	0.10	10.1	—
4.3	6.3	6.7	7	41	291	2.7	—	590	0.08	0.23	10.3	2
2.5	3.7	0.7	TR	2	34	0.5	35	0	0.08	0.05	0.8	—
6.8	6.5	0.4	0	10	114	2.9	184	30	0.04	0.18	3.6	—

(Continued)

APPENDIX G: *(Continued)*

Item No. (A)	Foods, approximate measures, units, and weight (edible part unless footnotes indicate otherwise) (B)		g	Water (C) %	Food Energy (D) kcal	Protein (E) g	Fat (F) g
Fish, Shellfish, Meat, Poultry; Related Products—Con.							
	Meat and meat products—Continued						
	Beef,[18] cooked—Continued						
	Cuts braised, simmered or pot roasted—Continued						
163	Lean only from item 162	2.5 oz	72	62	140	22	5
	Ground beef, broiled:						
164	Lean with 10% fat	3-oz patty	85	60	185	23	10
165	Lean with 21% fat	2.9-oz patty	82	54	235	20	17
	Roast, oven cooked, no liquid added						
	Relatively fat, such as rib						
166	Lean and fat (2 pieces, 4⅛ by 2¼ by ¼ in)	3 oz	85	40	375	17	33
167	Lean only from item 166	1.8 oz	51	57	125	14	7
	Relatively lean, such as heel of round						
168	Lean and fat (2 pieces, 4⅛ by 2¼ by ¼ in)	3 oz	85	62	165	25	7
169	Lean only from item 168	2.8 oz	78	65	125	24	3
	Steak						
	Relatively fat-sirloin, broiled						
170	Lean and fat (piece, 2½ by 2½ by ¾ in.)	3 oz	85	44	330	20	27
171	Lean only from item 170	2.0 oz	56	59	115	18	4
	Relatively lean-round, braised						
172	Lean and fat (piece, 4⅛ by 2¼ by ½ in.)	3 oz	85	55	220	24	13
173	Lean only from item 172	2.4 oz	68	61	130	21	4
	Beef, canned						
174	Corned beef	3 oz	85	59	185	22	10
175	Corned beef hash	1 cup	220	67	400	19	25
176	Beef, dried, chipped	2½-oz jar	71	48	145	24	4
177	Beef and vegetable stew	1 cup	245	82	220	16	11
178	Beef potpie ((home recipe), baked[19] (piece, ⅓ of 9-in. diam. pie).	1 piece	210	55	515	21	30
179	Chili con carne with beans, canned	1 cup	255	72	340	19	16
180	Chop suey with beef and pork (home recipe)	1 cup	250	75	300	26	17
181	Heart, beef, lean, braised	3 oz	85	61	160	27	5
	Lamb, cooked						
	Chop, rib (cut 3 per lb with bone), broiled						
182	Lean and fat	3.1 oz	89	43	360	18	32

[18]Outer layer of fat on the cut was removed to within approximately ½ in of the lean. Deposits of fat within the cut were not removed.
[19]Crust made with vegetable shortening and enriched flour.

| | Fatty Acids | | | | | | | | | | | |
| | | Unsaturated | | | | | | | | | | |
Satu-rated (Total) (G) g	Oleic (H) g	Lino-leic (I) g	Carbo-hydrate (J) g	Calcium (K) mg	Phos-phorus (L) mg	Iron (M) mg	Potas-sium (N) mg	Vitamin A Value (O) I.U.	Thiamin (P) mg	Ribo-flavin (Q) mg	Niacin (R) mg	Ascorbic Acid (S) mg
2.1	1.8	0.2	0	10	108	2.7	176	10	0.04	0.17	3.3	—
4.0	3.9	0.3	0	10	196	3.0	261	20	0.08	0.20	5.1	—
7.0	6.7	0.4	0	9	159	2.6	221	30	0.07	0.17	4.4	—
14.0	13.6	0.8	0	8	158	2.2	189	70	0.05	0.13	3.1	—
3.0	2.5	0.3	0	6	131	1.8	161	10	0.04	0.11	2.6	—
2.8	2.7	0.2	0	11	208	3.2	279	10	0.06	0.19	4.5	—
1.2	1.0	0.1	0	10	199	3.0	268	TR	0.06	0.18	4.3	—
11.3	11.1	0.6	0	9	162	2.5	220	50	0.05	0.15	4.0	—
1.8	1.6	0.2	0	7	146	2.2	202	10	0.05	0.14	3.6	—
5.5	5.2	0.4	0	10	213	3.0	272	20	0.07	0.19	4.8	—
1.7	1.5	0.2	0	9	182	2.5	238	10	0.05	0.16	4.1	—
4.9	4.5	0.2	0	17	90	3.7	—	—	0.01	0.20	2.9	—
11.9	10.9	0.5	24	29	147	4.4	440	—	0.02	0.20	4.6	—
2.1	2.0	0.1	0	14	287	3.6	142	—	0.05	0.23	2.7	0
4.9	4.5	0.2	15	29	184	2.9	613	2,400	0.15	0.17	4.7	17
7.9	12.8	6.7	39	29	149	3.8	334	1,720	0.30	0.30	5.5	6
7.5	6.8	0.3	31	82	321	4.3	594	150	0.08	0.18	3.3	—
8.5	6.2	0.7	13	60	248	4.8	425	600	0.28	0.38	5.0	33
1.5	1.1	0.6	1	5	154	5.0	197	20	0.21	1.04	6.5	1
14.8	12.1	1.2	0	8	139	1.0	200	—	0.11	0.19	4.1	—

(Continued)

APPENDIX G: *(Continued)*

Item No. (A)	Foods, approximate measures, units, and weight (edible part unless footnote indicate otherwise) (B)		Water (C) %	Food Energy (D) kcal	Pro- tein (E) g	Fat (F) g
		g				
Fish, Shellfish, Meat, Poultry; Related Products—Con.						
	Meat and meat products—Continued					
	Lamb, cooked—Continued					
	Chop, rib (cut 3 per lb with bone), broiled— Continued					
183	Lean only from item 182	2 oz	57	60	120	16	6
	Leg, roasted					
184	Lean and fat (2 pieces, 4⅛ by 2¼ by ¼ in.)	3 oz	85	54	235	22	16
185	Lean only from item 184	2.5 oz	71	62	130	20	5
	Shoulder, roasted					
186	Lean and fat (3 pieces, 2½ by 2½ by ¼ in.)	3 oz	85	50	285	18	23
187	Lean only from item 186	2.3 oz	64	61	130	17	6
188	Liver, beef, fried[20] (slice, 6½ by 2⅜ by ⅜ in.)	3 oz	85	56	195	22	9
	Pork, cured, cooked					
189	Ham, light cure, lean and fat, roasted (2 pieces, 4⅛ by 2¼ by ¼ in.)[22]	3 oz	85	54	245	18	19
	Luncheon meat					
190	Boiled ham, slice (8 per 8-oz pkg.)	1 oz	28	59	65	5	5
	Canned, spiced or unspiced					
191	Slice, approx. 3 by 2 by ½ in.	1 slice	60	55	175	9	15
	Pork, fresh,[18] cooked					
	Chop, loin (cut 3 per lb with bone), broiled					
192	Lean and fat	2.7 oz	78	42	305	19	25
193	Lean only from item 192	2 oz	56	53	150	17	9
	Roast, oven cooked, no liquid added					
194	Lean and fat (piece, 2½ by 2½ by ¾ in.)	3 oz	85	46	310	21	24
195	Lean only from item 194	2.4 oz	68	55	175	20	10
	Shoulder cut, simmered					
196	Lean and fat (3 pieces, 2½ by 2½ by ¼ in.)	3 oz	85	46	320	20	26
197	Lean only from item 196	2.2 oz	63	60	135	18	6
	Sausages (see also Luncheon meat (items 190–191))					
198	Bologna, slice (8 per 8-oz pkg.)	1 slice	28	56	85	3	8
199	Braunschweiger, slice (6 per 6-oz pkg.)	1 slice	28	53	90	4	8
200	Brown and serve (10–11 per 8-oz pkg.), browned	1 link	17	40	70	3	6

[20]Regular-type margarine used.
[21]Value varies widely.
[22]About one-fourth of the outer layer of fat on the cut was removed. Deposits of fat within the cut were not removed.

	Fatty Acids											
		Unsaturated										
Saturated (Total) (G) g	Oleic (H) g	Linoleic (I) g	Carbohydrate (J) g	Calcium (K) mg	Phosphorus (L) mg	Iron (M) mg	Potassium (N) mg	Vitamin A Value (O) I.U.	Thiamin (P) mg	Riboflavin (Q) mg	Niacin (R) mg	Ascorbic Acid (S) mg
2.5	2.1	0.2	0	6	121	1.1	174	—	0.09	0.15	3.4	—
7.3	6.0	0.6	0	9	177	1.4	241	—	0.13	0.23	4.7	—
2.1	1.8	0.2	0	9	169	1.4	227	—	0.12	0.21	4.4	—
10.8	8.8	0.9	0	9	146	1.0	206	—	0.11	0.20	4.0	—
3.6	2.3	0.2	0	8	140	1.0	193	—	0.10	0.18	3.7	—
2.5	3.5	0.9	5	9	405	7.5	323	[21]45,390	0.22	3.56	14.0	23
6.8	7.9	1.7	0	8	146	2.2	199	0	0.40	0.15	3.1	—
1.7	2.0	0.4	0	3	47	0.8	—	0	0.12	0.04	0.7	—
5.4	6.7	1.0	1	5	65	1.3	133	0	0.19	0.13	1.8	—
8.9	10.4	2.2	0	9	209	2.7	216	0	0.75	0.22	4.5	—
3.1	3.6	0.8	0	7	181	2.2	192	0	0.63	0.18	3.8	—
8.7	10.2	2.2	0	9	218	2.7	233	0	0.78	0.22	4.8	—
3.5	4.1	0.8	0	9	211	2.6	224	0	0.73	0.21	4.4	—
9.3	10.9	2.3	0	9	118	2.6	158	0	0.46	0.21	4.1	—
2.2	2.6	0.6	0	8	111	2.3	146	0	0.42	0.19	3.7	—
3.0	3.4	0.5		2	36	0.5	65	—	0.05	0.06	0.7	—
2.6	3.4	0.8	1	3	69	1.7	—	1,850	0.05	0.41	2.3	—
2.3	2.8	0.7	—	—	—	—	—	—	—	—	—	—

(Continued)

APPENDIX G: *(Continued)*

Item No. (A)	Foods, approximate measures, units, and weight (edible part unless footnotes indicate otherwise) (B)		Water (C) %	Food Energy (D) kcal	Pro- tein (E) g	Fat (F) g
		g				
Fish, Shellfish, Meat, Poultry; Related Products—Con.						
	Meat and meat products—Continued						
	Sausages (see also Luncheon meat (items 190–191))—Continued						
201	Deviled ham, canned	1 tbsp	13	51	45	2	4
202	Frankfurter (8 per 1-lb pkg.), cooked (reheated)	1 frankfurter	56	57	170	7	15
203	Meat, potted (beef, chicken, turkey), canned	1 tbsp	13	61	30	2	2
204	Pork link (16 per 1-lb pkg.), cooked	1 link	13	35	60	2	6
	Salami						
205	Dry type, slice (12 per 4-oz pkg.)	1 slice	10	30	45	2	4
206	Cooked type, slice (8 per 8-oz pkg.)	1 slice	28	51	90	5	7
207	Vienna sausage (7 per 4-oz can)	1 sausage	16	63	40	2	3
	Veal, medium fat, cooked, bone removed						
208	Cutlet (4⅛ by 2¼ by ½ in.), braised or broiled	3 oz	85	60	185	23	9
209	Rib (2 pieces, 4⅛ by 2¼ by ¼ in.), roasted	3 oz	85	55	230	23	14
	Poultry and poultry products						
	Chicken, cooked						
210	Breast, fried,[23] bones removed, ½ breast (3.3 oz with bones).	2.8 oz	79	58	160	26	5
211	Drumstick, fried,[23] bones removed (2 oz with bones)	1.3 oz	38	55	90	12	4
212	Half broiler, broiled, bones removed (10.4 oz with bones)	6.2 oz	176	71	240	42	7
213	Chicken, canned, boneless	3 oz	85	65	170	18	10
214	Chicken a la king, cooked (home recipe)	1 cup	245	68	470	27	34
215	Chicken and noodles, cooked (home recipe)	1 cup	240	71	365	22	18
	Chicken chow mein						
216	Canned	1 cup	250	89	95	7	TR
217	From home recipe	1 cup	250	78	255	31	10
218	Chicken potpie (home recipe), baked,[19] piece (⅓ or 9-in. diam. pie)	1 piece	232	57	545	23	31
	Turkey, roasted, flesh without skin						
219	Dark meat, piece, 2½ by 1⅝ by ¼ in.	4 pieces	85	61	175	26	7
220	Light meat, piece, 4 by 2 by ¼ in.	2 pieces	85	62	150	28	3
	Light and dark meat						
221	Chopped or diced	1 cup	140	61	265	44	9
222	Pieces (1 slice white meat, 4 by 2 by ¼ in with 2 slices dark meat, 2½ by 1⅝ by ¼ in)	3 pieces	85	61	160	27	5

[23]Vegetable shortening used.

						Nutrients in Indicated Quantity						
Fatty Acids												
Saturated (Total) (G) g	Unsaturated		Carbo-hydrate (J) g	Calcium (K) mg	Phos-phorus (L) mg	Iron (M) mg	Potas-sium (N) mg	Vitamin A Value (O) I.U.	Thiamin (P) mg	Ribo-flavin (Q) mg	Niacin (R) mg	Ascorbic Acid (S) mg
	Oleic (H) g	Lino-leic (I) g										
1.5	1.8	0.4	0	1	12	0.3	—	0	0.02	0.01	0.2	—
5.6	6.5	1.2	1	3	57	0.8	—	—	0.08	0.11	1.4	—
—	—	—	0	—	—	—	—	—		0.03	0.2	—
2.1	2.4	0.5		1	21	0.3	35	0	0.10	0.04	0.5	—
1.6	1.6	0.1		1	28	0.4	—	—	0.04	0.03	0.5	—
3.1	3.0	0.2		3	57	0.7	—	—	0.07	0.07	1.2	—
1.2	1.4	0.2		1	24	0.3	—	—	0.01	0.02	0.4	—
4.0	3.4	0.4	0	9	196	2.7	258	—	0.06	0.21	4.6	—
6.1	5.1	0.6	0	10	211	2.9	259	—	0.11	0.26	6.6	—
1.4	1.8	1.1	1	9	218	1.3	—	70	0.04	0.17	11.6	—
1.1	1.3	0.9		6	89	0.9	—	50	0.03	0.15	2.7	—
2.2	2.5	1.3	0	16	355	3.0	483	160	0.09	0.34	15.5	—
3.2	3.8	2.0	0	18	210	1.3	117	200	0.03	0.11	3.7	3
2.7	14.3	3.3	12	127	358	2.5	404	1,130	0.10	0.42	5.4	12
5.9	7.1	3.5	26	26	247	2.2	149	430	0.05	0.17	4.3	
—	—	—	18	45	35	1.3	418	150	0.05	0.10	1.0	13
2.4	3.4	3.1	10	58	293	2.5	473	280	0.08	0.23	4.3	10
11.3	10.9	5.6	42	70	232	3.0	343	3,090	0.34	0.31	5.5	5
2.1	1.5	1.5	0	—	—	2.0	338	—	0.03	0.20	3.6	—
0.9	0.6	0.7	0	—	—	1.0	349	—	0.04	0.12	9.4	—
2.5	1.7	1.8	0	11	351	2.5	514	—	0.07	0.25	10.8	—
1.5	1.0	1.1	0	7	213	1.5	312	—	0.04	0.15	6.5	—

(Continued)

APPENDIX G: *(Continued)*

Item No. (A)	Foods, approximate measures, units, and weight (edible part unless footnote indicate otherwise) (B)		g	Water (C) %	Food Energy (D) kcal	Pro-tein (E) g	Fat (F) g
Fruits and Fruit Products							
	Apples, raw, unpeeled, without cores:						
223	2¾-in diam. (about 3 per lb with cores)	1 apple	138	84	80	TR	1
224	3¼ in diam. (about 2 per lb with cores)	1 apple	212	84	125	TR	1
225	Applejuice, bottled or canned[24]	1 cup	248	88	120	TR	TR
	Applesauce, canned						
226	Sweetened	1 cup	255	76	230	1	TR
227	Unsweetened	1 cup	244	89	100	TR	TR
	Apricots						
228	Raw, without pits (about 12 per lb with pits)	3 apricots	107	85	55	1	TR
229	Canned in heavy sirup (halves and sirup)	1 cup	258	77	220	2	TR
	Dried						
230	Uncooked (28 large or 37 medium halves per cup)	1 cup	130	25	340	7	1
231	Cooked, unsweetened, fruit and liquid	1 cup	250	76	215	4	1
232	Apricot nectar, canned	1 cup	251	85	145	1	TR
	Avocados, raw, whole, without skins and seeds						
233	California, mid- and late-winter (with skin and seed, 3⅛-in diam.; wt., 10 oz)	1 avocado	216	74	370	5	37
234	Florida, late summer and fall (with skin and seed, 3⅝-in. diam.; wt., 1 lb).	1 avocado	304	78	390	4	33
235	Banana without peel (about 2.6 per lb with peel)	1 banana	119	76	100	1	TR
236	Banana flakes	1 tbsp	6	3	20	TR	TR
237	Blackberries, raw	1 cup	144	85	85	2	1
238	Blueberries, raw	1 cup	145	83	90	1	1
	Cantaloup. See Muskmelons (item 271)						
	Cherries						
239	Sour (tart), red, pitted, canned, water pack.	1 cup	244	88	105	2	TR
240	Sweet, raw, without pits and stems.	10 cherries	68	80	45	1	TR
241	Cranberry juice cocktail, bottled, sweetened.	1 cup	253	83	165	TR	TR
242	Cranberry sauce, sweetened, canned, strained.	1 cup	277	62	405	TR	1
	Dates						
243	Whole, without pits	10 dates	80	23	220	2	TR
244	Chopped	1 cup	178	23	490	4	1

[24]Also applies to pasteurized apple cider.
[25]Applies to product without added ascorbic acid. For value of product with added ascorbic acid, refer to label.
[26]Based on product with label claim of 45% of U.S. RDA in 6 fl oz.
[27]Based on product with label claim of 100% of U.S. RDA in 6 fl oz.

Nutrients in Indicated Quantity												
Fatty Acids												
	Unsaturated											
Satu-rated (Total) (G) g	Oleic (H) g	Lino-leic (I) g	Carbo-hydrate (J) g	Calcium (K) mg	Phos-phorus (L) mg	Iron (M) mg	Potas-sium (N) mg	Vitamin A Value (O) I.U.	Thiamin (P) mg	Ribo-flavin (Q) mg	Niacin (R) mg	Ascorbic Acid (S) mg
—	—	—	20	10	14	0.4	152	120	0.04	0.03	0.1	6
—	—	—	31	15	21	0.6	233	190	0.06	0.04	0.2	8
—	—	—	30	15	22	1.5	250	—	0.02	0.05	0.2	[25]2
—	—	—	61	10	13	1.3	166	100	0.05	0.03	0.1	[25]3
—	—	—	26	10	12	1.2	190	100	0.05	0.02	0.1	[25]2
—	—	—	14	18	25	0.5	301	2,890	0.03	0.04	0.6	11
—	—	—	57	28	39	0.8	604	4,490	0.05	0.05	1.0	10
—	—	—	86	87	140	7.2	1,273	14,170	0.01	0.21	4.3	16
—	—	—	54	55	88	4.5	795	7,500	0.01	0.13	2.5	8
—	—	—	37	23	30	0.5	379	2,380	0.03	0.03	0.5	[26]36
5.5	22.0	3.7	13	22	91	1.3	1,303	630	0.24	0.43	3.5	30
6.7	15.7	5.3	27	30	128	1.8	1,836	880	0.33	0.61	4.9	43
—	—	—	26	10	31	0.8	440	230	0.06	0.07	0.8	12
—	—	—	5	2	6	0.2	92	50	0.01	0.01	0.2	
—	—	—	19	46	27	1.3	245	290	0.04	0.06	0.6	30
—	—	—	22	22	19	1.5	117	150	0.04	0.09	0.7	20
—	—	—	26	37	32	0.7	317	1,660	0.07	0.05	0.5	12
—	—	—	12	15	13	0.3	129	70	0.03	0.04	0.3	7
—	—	—	42	13	8	0.8	25	TR	0.03	0.03	0.1	[27]81
—	—	—	104	17	11	0.6	83	60	0.03	0.03	0.1	6
—	—	—	58	47	50	2.4	518	40	0.07	0.08	1.8	0
—	—	—	130	105	112	5.3	1,153	90	0.16	0.18	3.9	0

APPENDIX G: *(Continued)*

Item No. (A)	Foods, approximate measures, units, and weight (edible part unless footnote indicate otherwise) (B)		g	Water (C) %	Food Energy (D) kcal	Pro- tein (E) g	Fat (F) g
Fruits and Fruit Products—Con.							
245	Fruit cocktail, canned, in heavy sirup	1 cup	255	80	195	1	TR
	Grapefruit						
	Raw, medium, 3¾-in diam. (about 1 lb 1 oz)						
246	Pink or red	½ grapefruit[28]	241	89	50	1	TR
247	White	½ grapefruit[28]	241	89	45	1	TR
248	Canned, sections with sirup	1 cup	254	81	180	2	TR
	Grapefruit juice						
249	Raw, pink, red, or white	1 cup	246	90	95	1	TR
	Canned, white						
250	Unsweetened	1 cup	247	89	100	1	TR
251	Sweetened	1 cup	250	86	135	1	TR
	Frozen, concentrate, unsweetened						
252	Undiluted, 6-fl oz can	1 can	207	62	300	4	1
253	Diluted with 3 parts water by volume	1 cup	247	89	100	1	TR
254	Dehydrated crystals, prepared with water (1 lb yields about 1 gal).	1 cup	247	90	100	1	TR
	Grapes, European type (adherent skin), raw						
255	Thompson Seedless	10 grapes	50	81	35	TR	TR
256	Tokay and Emperor, seeded types	10 grapes[30]	60	81	40	TR	TR
	Grape juice						
257	Canned or bottled	1 cup	253	83	165	1	TR
	Frozen concentrate, sweetened						
258	Undiluted, 6-fl oz can	1 can	216	53	395	1	TR
259	Diluted with 3 parts water by volume	1 cup	250	86	135	1	TR
260	Grape drink, canned	1 cup	250	86	135	TR	TR
261	Lemon, raw, size 165, without peel and seeds (about 4 per lb with peels and seeds)	1 lemon	74	90	20	1	TR
	Lemon juice						
262	Raw	1 cup	244	91	60	1	TR

[28]Weight includes peel and membranes between sections. Without these parts, the weight of the edible portion is 123 g for item 246 and 118 g for item 247.

[29]For white-fleshed varieties, value is about 20 International Units (I.U.) per cup; for red-fleshed varieties, 1,080 I.U.

[30]Weight includes seeds. Without seeds, weight of the edible portion is 57 g.

[31]Applies to product without added ascorbic acid. With added ascorbic acid, based on claim that 6 fl oz of reconstituted juice contain 45% or 50% of the U.S. RDA, value in milligrams is 108 or 120 for a 6-fl oz can (item 258), 36 or 40 for 1 cup of diluted juice (item 259).

[32]For products with added thiamin and riboflavin but without added ascorbic acid, values in milligrams would be 0.60 for thiamin, 0.80 for riboflavin, and trace for ascorbic acid. For products with only ascorbic acid added, value varies with the brand. Consult the label.

								Nutrients in Indicated Quantity					
Fatty Acids													
	Unsaturated												
Satu-rated (Total) (G) g	Oleic (H) g	Lino-leic (I) g	Carbo-hydrate (J) g	Calcium (K) mg	Phos-phorus (L) mg	Iron (M) mg	Potas-sium (N) mg	Vitamin A Value (O) I.U.	Thiamin (P) mg	Ribo-flavin (Q) mg	Niacin (R) mg	Ascorbic Acid (S) mg
—	—	—	50	23	31	1.0	411	360	0.05	0.03	1.0	5
—	—	—	13	20	20	0.5	166	540	0.05	0.02	0.2	44
—	—	—	12	19	19	0.5	159	10	0.05	0.02	0.2	44
—	—	—	45	33	36	0.8	343	30	0.08	0.05	0.5	76
—	—	—	23	22	37	0.5	399	([29])	0.10	0.05	0.5	93
—	—	—	24	20	35	1.0	400	20	0.07	0.05	0.5	84
—	—	—	32	20	35	1.0	405	30	0.08	0.05	0.5	78
—	—	—	72	70	124	0.8	1,250	60	0.29	0.12	1.4	286
—	—	—	24	25	42	0.2	420	20	0.10	0.04	0.5	96
—	—	—	24	22	40	0.2	412	20	0.10	0.05	0.5	91
—	—	—	9	6	10	0.2	87	50	0.03	0.02	0.2	2
—	—	—	10	7	11	0.2	99	60	0.03	0.02	0.2	2
—	—	—	42	28	30	0.8	293	—	0.10	0.05	0.5	[25]TR
—	—	—	100	22	32	0.9	255	40	0.13	0.22	1.5	[31]32
—	—	—	33	8	10	0.3	85	10	0.05	0.08	0.5	[31]10
—	—	—	35	8	10	0.3	88	—	[32]0.03	[32]0.03	0.3	([32])
—	—	—	6	19	12	0.4	102	10	0.03	0.01	0.1	39
—	—	—	20	17	24	0.5	344	50	0.07	0.02	0.2	112

(Continued)

APPENDIX G: *(Continued)*

Item No. (A)	Foods, approximate measures, units, and weight *(edible part unless footnotes indicate otherwise)* (B)		g	Water (C) %	Food Energy (D) kcal	Pro-tein (E) g	Fat (F) g
Fruits and Fruit Products—Con.							
	Lemon juice—Continued						
263	Canned, or bottled, unsweetened	1 cup	244	92	55	1	TR
264	Frozen, single strength, unsweetened, 6-fl oz can	1 can	183	92	40	1	TR
	Lemonade concentrate, frozen						
265	Undiluted, 6-fl oz can	1 can	219	49	425	TR	TR
266	Diluted with 4⅓ parts water by volume	1 cup	248	89	105	TR	TR
	Limeade concentrate, frozen						
267	Undiluted, 6-fl oz can	1 can	218	50	410	TR	TR
268	Diluted with 4⅓ parts water by volume	1 cup	247	89	100	TR	TR
	Limejuice						
269	Raw	1 cup	246	90	65	1	TR
270	Canned, unsweetened	1 cup	246	90	65	1	TR
	Muskmelons, raw, with rind, without seed cavity						
271	Cantaloup, orange-fleshed (with rind and seed cavity, 5-in. diam., 2⅓ lb)	½ melon with rind[33]	477	91	80	2	TR
272	Honeydew (with rind and seed cavity, 6½-in. diam., 5¼ lb)	1/10 melon with rind[33]	226	91	50	1	TR
	Oranges, all commercial varieties, raw						
273	Whole, 2⅝-in diam., without peel and seeds (about 2½ per lb with peel and seeds)	1 orange	131	86	65	1	TR
274	Sections without membrane	1 cup	180	86	90	2	TR
	Orange juice						
275	Raw, all varieties	1 cup	248	88	110	2	TR
276	Canned, unsweetened	1 cup	249	87	120	2	TR
	Frozen concentrate						
277	Undiluted, 6-fl oz can	1 can	213	55	360	5	TR
278	Diluted with 3 parts water by volume	1 cup	249	87	120	2	TR
279	Dehydrated crystals, prepared with water (1 lb yields about 1 gal)	1 cup	248	88	115	1	TR
	Orange and grapefruit juice						
	Frozen concentrate						
280	Undiluted, 6-fl oz can	1 can	210	59	330	4	1
281	Diluted with 3 parts water by volume	1 cup	248	88	110	1	TR
282	Papayas, raw, ½-in cubes	1 cup	140	89	55	1	TR

[33]Weight includes rind. Without rind, the weight of the edible portion is 272 g for item 271 and 149 g for item 272.

| | Fatty Acids | | | | | | | | | | | |
| | | Unsaturated | | | | | | | | | | |
Satu-rated (Total) (G) g	Oleic (H) g	Lino-leic (I) g	Carbo-hydrate (J) g	Calcium (K) mg	Phos-phorus (L) mg	Iron (M) mg	Potas-sium (N) mg	Vitamin A Value (O) I.U.	Thiamin (P) mg	Ribo-flavin (Q) mg	Niacin (R) mg	Ascorbic Acid (S) mg
							Nutrients in Indicated Quantity					
—	—	—	19	17	24	0.5	344	50	0.07	0.02	0.2	102
—	—	—	13	13	16	0.5	258	40	0.05	0.02	0.2	81
—	—	—	112	9	13	0.4	153	40	0.05	0.06	0.7	66
—	—	—	28	2	3	0.1	40	10	0.01	0.02	0.2	17
—	—	—	108	11	13	0.2	129	TR	0.02	0.02	0.2	26
—	—	—	27	3	3	TR	32	TR	TR	TR	TR	6
—	—	—	22	22	27	0.5	256	20	0.05	0.02	0.2	79
—	—	—	22	22	27	0.5	256	20	0.05	0.02	0.2	52
—	—	—	20	38	44	1.1	682	9,240	0.11	0.08	1.6	90
—	—	—	11	21	24	0.6	374	60	0.06	0.04	0.9	34
—	—	—	16	54	26	0.5	263	260	0.13	0.05	0.5	66
—	—	—	22	74	36	0.7	360	360	0.18	0.07	0.7	90
—	—	—	26	27	42	0.5	496	500	0.22	0.07	1.0	124
—	—	—	28	25	45	1.0	496	500	0.17	0.05	0.7	100
—	—	—	87	75	126	0.9	1,500	1,620	0.68	0.11	2.8	360
—	—	—	29	25	42	0.2	503	540	0.23	0.03	0.9	120
—	—	—	27	25	40	0.5	518	500	0.20	0.07	1.0	109
—	—	—	78	61	99	0.8	1,308	800	0.48	0.06	2.3	302
—	—	—	26	20	32	0.2	439	270	0.15	0.02	0.7	102
—	—	—	14	28	22	0.4	328	2,450	0.06	0.06	0.4	78

(Continued)

APPENDIX G: *(Continued)*

Item No. (A)	Foods, approximate measures, units, and weight (edible part unless footnote indicate otherwise) (B)		g	Water (C) %	Food Energy (D) kcal	Pro- tein (E) g	Fat (F) g
	Fruits and Fruit Products—Con.						
	Peaches						
	Raw						
283	Whole, 2½-in diam., peeled, pitted (about 4 per lb with peels and pits)	1 peach	100	89	40	1	TR
284	Sliced	1 cup	170	89	65	1	TR
	Canned, yellow-fleshed, solids and liquid (halves or slices)						
285	Sirup pack	1 cup	256	79	200	1	TR
286	Water pack	1 cup	244	91	75	1	TR
	Dried						
287	Uncooked	1 cup	160	25	420	5	1
288	Cooked, unsweetened, halves and juice	1 cup	250	77	205	3	1
	Frozen, sliced, sweetened						
289	10-oz container	1 container	284	77	250	1	TR
290	Cup	1 cup	250	77	220	1	TR
	Pears						
	Raw, with skin, cored						
291	Bartlett, 2½-in diam. (about 2½ per lb with cores and stems)	1 pear	164	83	100	1	1
292	Bosc, 2½-in diam. (about 3 per lb with cores and stems)	1 pear	141	83	85	1	1
293	D'Anjou, 3-in diam. (about 2 per lb with cores and stems)	1 pear	200	83	120	1	1
294	Canned, solids and liquid, sirup pack, heavy (halves or slices)	1 cup	255	80	195	1	1
	Pineapple						
295	Raw, diced	1 cup	155	85	80	1	TR
	Canned, heavy sirup pack, solids and liquid						
296	Crushed, chunks, tidbits	1 cup	255	80	190	1	TR
	Slices and liquid						
297	Large	1 slice; 2¼ tbsp of liquid	105	80	80	TR	TR
298	Medium	1 slice; 1¼ tbsp of liquid	58	80	45	TR	TR
299	Pineapple juice, unsweetened, canned	1 cup	250	86	140	1	TR

[34]Represents yellow-fleshed varieties. For white-fleshed varieties, value is 50 International Units (I.U.) for 1 peach, 90 I.U. for 1 cup of slices.
[35]Value represents products with added ascorbic acid. For products without added ascorbic acid, value in milligrams is 116 for a 10-oz container, 103 for 1 cup.

	Nutrients in Indicated Quantity												
Fatty Acids													
	Unsaturated												
Satu-rated (Total) (G) g	Oleic (H) g	Lino-leic (I) g	Carbo-hydrate (J) g	Calcium (K) mg	Phos-phorus (L) mg	Iron (M) mg	Potas-sium (N) mg	Vitamin A Value (O) I.U.	Thiamin (P) mg	Ribo-flavin (Q) mg	Niacin (R) mg	Ascorbic Acid (S) mg
—	—	—	10	9	19	0.5	202	[34]1,330	0.02	0.05	1.0	7
—	—	—	16	15	32	0.9	343	[34]2,260	0.03	0.09	1.7	12
—	—	—	51	10	31	0.8	333	1,100	0.03	0.05	1.5	8
—	—	—	20	10	32	0.7	334	1,100	0.02	0.07	1.5	7
—	—	—	109	77	187	9.6	1,520	6,240	0.02	0.30	8.5	29
—	—	—	54	38	93	4.8	743	3,050	0.01	0.15	3.8	5
—	—	—	64	11	37	1.4	352	1,850	0.03	0.11	2.0	[35]116
—	—	—	57	10	33	1.3	310	1,630	0.03	0.10	1.8	[35]103
—	—	—	25	13	18	0.5	213	30	0.03	0.07	0.2	7
—	—	—	22	11	16	0.4	83	30	0.03	0.06	0.1	6
—	—	—	31	16	22	0.6	260	40	0.04	0.08	0.2	8
—	—	—	50	13	18	0.5	214	10	0.03	0.05	0.3	3
—	—	—	21	26	12	0.8	226	110	0.14	0.05	0.3	26
—	—	—	49	28	13	0.8	245	130	0.20	0.05	0.5	18
—	—	—	20	12	5	0.3	101	50	0.08	0.02	0.2	7
—	—	—	11	6	3	0.2	56	30	0.05	0.01	0.1	4
—	—	—	34	38	23	0.8	373	130	0.13	0.05	0.5	[27]80

(Continued)

APPENDIX G: *(Continued)*

					Nutrients in Indicated Quantity	

Item No. (A)	Foods, approximate measures, units, and weight (edible part unless footnotes indicate otherwise) (B)			Water (C) %	Food Energy (D) kcal	Protein (E) g	Fat (F) g
			g				
Fruits and Fruit Products—Con.							
	Plums						
	Raw, without pits						
300	Japanese and hybrid (2⅛-in diam., about 6½ per lb with pits)	1 plum	66	87	30	TR	TR
301	Prune-type (1½-in diam., about 15 per lb with pits)	1 plum	28	79	20	TR	TR
	Canned, heavy sirup pack (Italian prunes), with pits and liquid						
302	Cup	1 cup[36]	272	77	215	1	TR
303	Portion	3 plums; 2¾ tbsp of liquid[36]	140	77	110	1	TR
	Prunes, dried, "softenized," with pits						
304	Uncooked	4 extra large or 5 large prunes[36]	49	28	110	1	TR
305	Cooked, unsweetened, all sizes, fruit and liquid	1 cup[36]	250	66	255	2	1
306	Prune juice, canned or bottled	1 cup	256	80	195	1	TR
	Raisins, seedless						
307	Cup, not pressed down	1 cup	145	18	420	4	TR
308	Packet, ½ oz (1½ tbsp)	1 packet	14	18	40	TR	TR
	Raspberries, red						
309	Raw, capped, whole	1 cup	123	84	70	1	1
310	Frozen, sweetened, 10-oz container	1 container	284	74	280	2	1
	Rhubarb, cooked, added sugar						
311	From raw	1 cup	270	63	380	1	TR
312	From frozen, sweetened	1 cup	270	63	385	1	1
	Strawberries						
313	Raw, whole berries, capped	1 cup	149	90	55	1	1
	Frozen, sweetened						
314	Sliced, 10-oz container	1 container	284	71	310	1	1
315	Whole, 1-lb container (about 1¾ cups)	1 container	454	76	415	2	1
316	Tangerine, raw, 2⅜-in diam., size 176, without peel (about 4 per lb with peels and seeds)	1 tangerine	86	87	40	1	TR
317	Tangerine juice, canned, sweetened	1 cup	249	87	125	1	TR
318	Watermelon, raw, 4 by 8 in wedge with rind and seeds (1/16 of 32⅔-lb melon, 10 by 16 in.)	1 wedge[37]	926	93	110	2	1

[36]Weight includes pits. After removal of the pits, the weight of the edible portion is 258 g for item 302, 133 g for item 303, 43 g for item 304, and 213 g for item 305.

[37]Weight includes rind and seeds. Without rind and seeds, weight of the edible portion is 426 g.

	Fatty Acids												
		Unsaturated		Nutrients in Indicated Quantity									
Satu-rated (Total) (G) g	Oleic (H) g	Lino-leic (I) g	Carbo-hydrate (J) g	Calcium (K) mg	Phos-phorus (L) mg	Iron (M) mg	Potas-sium (N) mg	Vitamin A Value (O) I.U.	Thiamin (P) mg	Ribo-flavin (Q) mg	Niacin (R) mg	Ascorbic Acid (S) mg
---	---	---	---	---	---	---	---	---	---	---	---	---
—	—	—	8	8	12	0.3	112	160	0.02	0.02	0.3	4
—	—	—	6	3	5	0.1	48	80	0.01	0.01	0.1	1
—	—	—	56	23	26	2.3	367	3,130	0.05	0.05	1.0	5
—	—	—	29	12	13	1.2	189	1,610	0.03	0.03	0.5	3
—	—	—	29	22	34	1.7	298	690	0.04	0.07	0.7	1
—	—	—	67	51	79	3.8	695	1,590	0.07	0.15	1.5	2
—	—	—	49	36	51	1.8	602	—	0.03	0.03	1.0	5
—	—	—	112	90	146	5.1	1,106	30	0.16	0.12	0.7	1
—	—	—	11	9	14	0.5	107	TR	0.02	0.01	0.1	TR
—	—	—	17	27	27	1.1	207	160	0.04	0.11	1.1	31
—	—	—	70	37	48	1.7	284	200	0.06	0.17	1.7	60
—	—	—	97	211	41	1.6	548	220	0.05	0.14	0.8	16
—	—	—	98	211	32	1.9	475	190	0.05	0.11	0.5	16
—	—	—	13	31	31	1.5	244	90	0.04	0.10	0.9	88
—	—	—	79	40	48	2.0	318	90	0.06	0.17	1.4	151
—	—	—	107	59	73	2.7	472	140	0.09	0.27	2.3	249
—	—	—	10	34	15	0.3	108	360	0.05	0.02	0.1	27
—	—	—	30	44	35	0.5	440	1,040	0.15	0.05	0.2	54
—	—	—	27	30	43	2.1	426	2,510	0.13	0.13	0.9	30

(Continued)

APPENDIX G: *(Continued)*

Item No. (A)	Foods, approximate measures, units, and weight (edible part unless footnote indicate otherwise) (B)		g	Water (C) %	Food Energy (D) kcal	Pro-tein (E) g	Fat (F) g
Grain Products							
	Bagel, 3-in diam.						
319	Egg	1 bagel	55	32	165	6	2
320	Water	1 bagel	55	29	165	6	1
321	Barley, pearled, light, uncooked	1 cup	200	11	700	16	2
	Biscuits, baking powder, 2-in diam. (enriched flour, vegetable shortening)						
322	From home recipe	1 biscuit	28	27	105	2	5
323	From mix	1 biscuit	28	29	90	2	3
	Breadcrumbs (enriched)[38]						
324	Dry, grated	1 cup	100	7	390	13	5
	Soft. See White bread (items 349–350).						
	Breads						
325	Boston brown bread, canned, slice, $3\frac{1}{4}$ by $\frac{1}{2}$ in.[38]	1 slice	45	45	95	2	1
	Cracked-wheat bread ($\frac{3}{4}$ enriched wheat flour, $\frac{1}{4}$ cracked wheat):[38]						
326	Loaf, 1 lb	1 loaf	454	35	1,195	39	10
327	Slice (18 per loaf)	1 slice	25	35	65	2	1
	French or vienna bread, enriched:[38]						
328	Loaf, 1 lb	1 loaf	454	31	1,315	41	14
	Slice						
329	French (5 by $2\frac{1}{2}$ by 1 in)	1 slice	35	31	100	3	1
330	Vienna ($4\frac{3}{4}$ by 4 by $\frac{1}{2}$ in).	1 slice	25	31	75	2	1
	Italian bread, enriched:						
331	Loaf, 1 lb	1 loaf	454	32	1,250	41	4
332	Slice, $4\frac{1}{2}$ by $3\frac{1}{4}$ by $\frac{3}{4}$ in.	1 slice	30	32	85	3	TR
	Raisin bread, enriched:[38]						
333	Loaf, 1 lb	1 loaf	454	35	1,190	30	13
334	Slice (18 per loaf)	1 slice	25	35	65	2	1
	Rye bread						
	American, light ($\frac{2}{3}$ enriched wheat flour, $\frac{1}{3}$ rye flour)						
335	Loaf, 1 lb	1 loaf	454	36	1,100	41	5
336	Slice ($4\frac{3}{4}$ by $3\frac{3}{4}$ by $\frac{7}{16}$ in)	1 slice	25	36	60	2	TR

[38]Made with vegetable shortening.
[39]Applies to product made with white cornmeal. With yellow cornmeal, value is 30 International Units (I.U.).

| | Fatty Acids | | | | | | | | | | | |
| | | Unsaturated | | | | | | | | | | |
Satu-rated (Total) (G) g	Oleic (H) g	Lino-leic (I) g	Carbo-hydrate (J) g	Calcium (K) mg	Phos-phorus (L) mg	Iron (M) mg	Potas-sium (N) mg	Vitamin A Value (O) I.U.	Thiamin (P) mg	Ribo-flavin (Q) mg	Niacin (R) mg	Ascorbic Acid (S) mg
0.5	0.9	0.8	28	9	43	1.2	41	30	0.14	0.10	1.2	0
0.2	0.4	0.6	30	8	41	1.2	42	0	0.15	0.11	1.4	0
0.3	0.2	0.8	158	32	378	4.0	320	0	0.24	0.10	6.2	0
1.2	2.0	1.2	13	34	49	0.4	33	TR	0.08	0.08	0.7	TR
0.6	1.1	0.7	15	19	65	0.6	32	TR	0.09	0.08	0.8	TR
1.0	1.6	1.4	73	122	141	3.6	152	TR	0.35	0.35	4.8	TR
0.1	0.2	0.2	21	41	72	0.9	131	390	0.06	0.04	0.7	0
2.2	3.0	3.9	236	399	581	9.5	608	TR	1.52	1.13	14.4	TR
0.1	0.2	0.2	13	22	32	0.5	34	TR	0.08	0.06	0.8	TR
3.2	4.7	4.6	251	195	386	10.0	408	TR	1.80	1.10	15.0	TR
0.2	0.4	0.4	19	15	30	0.8	32	TR	0.14	0.08	1.2	TR
0.2	0.3	0.3	14	11	21	0.6	23	TR	0.10	0.06	0.8	TR
0.6	0.3	1.5	256	77	349	10.0	336	0	1.80	1.10	15.0	0
TR	TR	0.1	17	5	23	0.7	22	0	0.12	0.07	1.0	0
3.0	4.7	3.9	243	322	395	10.0	1,057	TR	1.70	1.07	10.7	TR
0.2	0.3	0.2	13	18	22	0.6	58	TR	0.09	0.06	0.6	TR
0.7	0.5	2.2	236	340	667	9.1	658	0	1.35	0.98	12.9	0
TR	TR	0.1	13	19	37	0.5	36	0	0.07	0.05	0.7	0

(Continued)

APPENDIX G: *(Continued)*

| | | | | | Nutrients in Indicated Quantity | | |
| | | | | | | | |

Item No. (A)	Foods, approximate measures, units, and weight (edible part unless footnote indicate otherwise) (B)			Water (C) %	Food Energy (D) kcal	Pro- tein (E) g	Fat (F) g
			g				
Grain Products—Con.							
	Rye bread—Continued						
	Pumpernickel ($\frac{2}{3}$ rye flour, $\frac{1}{3}$ enriched wheat flour)						
337	Loaf, 1 lb	1 loaf	454	34	1,115	41	5
338	Slice (5 by 4 by $\frac{3}{8}$ in)	1 slice	32	34	80	3	TR
	White bread, enriched[38]						
	Soft-crumb type						
339	Loaf, 1 lb	1 loaf	454	36	1,225	39	15
340	Slice (18 per loaf)	1 slice	25	36	70	2	1
341	Slice, toasted	1 slice	22	25	70	2	1
342	Slice (22 per loaf)	1 slice	20	36	55	2	1
343	Slice, toasted	1 slice	17	25	55	2	1
344	Loaf, $1\frac{1}{2}$ lb	1 loaf	680	36	1,835	59	22
345	Slice (24 per loaf)	1 slice	28	36	75	2	1
346	Slice, toasted	1 slice	24	25	75	2	1
347	Slice (28 per loaf)	1 slice	24	36	65	2	1
348	Slice, toasted	1 slice	21	25	65	2	1
349	Cubes	1 cup	30	36	80	3	1
350	Crumbs	1 cup	45	36	120	4	1
	Firm-crumb type						
351	Loaf, 1 lb	1 loaf	454	35	1,245	41	17
352	Slice (20 per loaf)	1 slice	23	35	65	2	1
353	Slice, toasted	1 slice	20	24	65	2	1
354	Loaf, 2 lb	1 loaf	907	35	2,495	82	34
355	Slice (34 per loaf)	1 slice	27	35	75	2	1
356	Slice, toasted	1 slice	23	24	75	2	1
	Whole-wheat bread						
	Soft-crumb type[38]						
357	Loaf, 1 lb	1 loaf	454	36	1,095	41	12
358	Slice (16 per loaf)	1 slice	28	36	65	3	1
359	Slice, toasted	1 slice	24	24	65	3	1
	Firm-crumb type[38]						
360	Loaf, 1 lb	1 loaf	454	36	1,100	48	14
361	Slice (18 per loaf)	1 slice	25	36	60	3	1
362	Slice, toasted	1 slice	21	24	60	3	1

								Nutrients in Indicated Quantity				
Fatty Acids												
	Unsaturated											
Satu-rated (Total) (G) g	Oleic (H) g	Lino-leic (I) g	Carbo-hydrate (J) g	Calcium (K) mg	Phos-phorus (L) mg	Iron (M) mg	Potas-sium (N) mg	Vitamin A Value (O) I.U.	Thiamin (P) mg	Ribo-flavin (Q) mg	Niacin (R) mg	Ascorbic Acid (S) mg
0.7	0.5	2.4	241	381	1,039	11.8	2,059	0	1.30	0.93	8.5	0
0.1	TR	0.2	17	27	73	0.8	145	0	0.09	0.07	0.6	0
3.4	5.3	4.6	229	381	440	11.3	476	TR	1.80	1.10	15.0	TR
0.2	0.3	0.3	13	21	24	0.6	26	TR	0.10	0.06	0.8	TR
0.2	0.3	0.3	13	21	24	0.6	26	TR	0.08	0.06	0.8	TR
0.2	0.2	0.2	10	17	19	0.5	21	TR	0.08	0.05	0.7	TR
0.2	0.2	0.2	10	17	19	0.5	21	TR	0.06	0.05	0.7	TR
5.2	7.9	6.9	343	571	660	17.0	714	TR	2.70	1.65	22.5	TR
0.2	0.3	0.3	14	24	27	0.7	29	TR	0.11	0.07	0.9	TR
0.2	0.3	0.3	14	24	27	0.7	29	TR	0.09	0.07	0.9	TR
0.2	0.3	0.2	12	20	23	0.6	25	TR	0.10	0.06	0.8	TR
0.2	0.3	0.2	12	20	23	0.6	25	TR	0.08	0.06	0.8	TR
0.2	0.3	0.3	15	25	29	0.8	32	TR	0.12	0.07	1.0	TR
0.3	0.5	0.5	23	38	44	1.1	47	TR	0.18	0.11	1.5	TR
3.9	5.9	5.2	228	435	463	11.3	549	TR	1.80	1.10	15.0	TR
0.2	0.3	0.3	12	22	23	0.6	28	TR	0.09	0.06	0.8	TR
0.2	0.3	0.3	12	22	23	0.6	28	TR	0.07	0.06	0.8	TR
7.7	11.8	10.4	455	871	925	22.7	1,097	TR	3.60	2.20	30.0	TR
0.2	0.3	0.3	14	26	28	0.7	33	TR	0.11	0.06	0.9	TR
0.2	0.3	0.3	14	26	28	0.7	33	TR	0.09	0.06	0.9	TR
2.2	2.9	4.2	224	381	1,152	13.6	1,161	TR	1.37	0.45	12.7	TR
0.1	0.2	0.2	14	24	71	0.8	72	TR	0.09	0.03	0.8	TR
0.1	0.2	0.2	14	24	71	0.8	72	TR	0.07	0.03	0.8	TR
2.5	3.3	4.9	216	449	1,034	13.6	1,238	TR	1.17	0.54	12.7	TR
0.1	0.2	0.3	12	25	57	0.8	68	TR	0.06	0.03	0.7	TR
0.1	0.2	0.3	12	25	57	0.8	68	TR	0.05	0.03	0.7	TR

(Continued)

APPENDIX G: (Continued)

					Nutrients in Indicated Quantity		

Item No. (A)	Foods, approximate measures, units, and weight (edible part unless footnotes indicate otherwise) (B)		g	Water (C) %	Food Energy (D) kcal	Pro- tein (E) g	Fat (F) g
Grain Products—Con.							
	Breakfast cereals						
	Hot type, cooked						
	Corn (hominy) grits, degermed						
363	Enriched	1 cup	245	87	125	3	TR
364	Unenriched	1 cup	245	87	125	3	TR
365	Farina, quick-cooking, enriched	1 cup	245	89	105	3	TR
366	Oatmeal or rolled oats	1 cup	240	87	130	5	2
367	Wheat, rolled	1 cup	240	80	180	5	1
368	Wheat, whole-meal	1 cup	245	88	110	4	1
	Ready-to-eat:						
369	Bran flakes (40% bran), added sugar, salt, iron, vitamins	1 cup	35	3	105	4	1
370	Bran flakes with raisins, added sugar, salt, iron, vitamins	1 cup	50	7	145	4	1
	Corn flakes						
371	Plain, added sugar, salt, iron, vitamins.	1 cup	25	4	95	2	TR
372	Sugar-coated, added salt, iron, vitamins	1 cup	40	2	155	2	TR
373	Corn, oat flour, puffed, added sugar, salt, iron, vitamins	1 cup	20	4	80	2	1
374	Corn, shredded, added sugar, salt, iron, thiamin, niacin	1 cup	25	3	95	2	TR
375	Oats, puffed, added sugar, salt, minerals, vitamins	1 cup	25	3	100	3	1
	Rice, puffed						
376	Plain, added iron, thiamin, niacin	1 cup	15	4	60	1	TR
377	Presweetened, added salt, iron, vitamins	1 cup	28	3	115	1	0
378	Wheat flakes, added sugar, salt, iron, vitamins	1 cup	30	4	105	3	TR
	Wheat, puffed						
379	Plain, added iron, thiamin, niacin	1 cup	15	3	55	2	TR
380	Presweetened, added salt, iron, vitamins	1 cup	38	3	140	3	TR

[40]Applies to white varieties. For yellow varieties, value is 150 International Units (I.U.).
[41]Applies to products that do not contain di-sodium phosphate. If di-sodium phosphate is an ingredient, value is 162 mg.
[42]Value may range from less than 1 mg to about 8 mg depending on the brand. Consult the label.
[43]Applies to product with added nutrient. Without added nutrient, value is trace.
[44]Value varies with the brand. Consult the label.
[45]Applies to product with added nutrient. Without added nutrient, value is trace.

| Fatty Acids | | | | | | | | | | | | |
Saturated (Total) (G) g	Unsaturated Oleic (H) g	Unsaturated Linoleic (I) g	Carbohydrate (J) g	Calcium (K) mg	Phosphorus (L) mg	Iron (M) mg	Potassium (N) mg	Vitamin A Value (O) I.U.	Thiamin (P) mg	Riboflavin (Q) mg	Niacin (R) mg	Ascorbic Acid (S) mg
TR	TR	0.1	27	2	25	0.7	27	[40]TR	0.10	0.07	1.0	0
TR	TR	0.1	27	2	25	0.2	27	[40]TR	0.05	0.02	0.5	0
TR	TR	0.1	22	147	[41]113	([42])	25	0	0.12	0.07	1.0	0
0.4	0.8	0.9	23	22	137	1.4	146	0	0.19	0.05	0.2	0
—	—	—	41	19	182	1.7	202	0	0.17	0.07	2.2	0
—	—	—	23	17	127	1.2	118	0	0.15	0.05	1.5	0
—	—	—	28	19	125	5.6	137	1,540	0.46	0.52	6.2	0
—	—	—	40	28	146	7.9	154	[43]2,200	([44])	([44])	([44])	0
—	—	—	21	([44])	9	([44])	30	([44])	([44])	([44])	([44])	[45]13
—	—	—	37	1	10	([44])	27	1,760	0.53	0.60	7.1	[45]21
—	—	—	16	4	18	5.7	—	880	0.26	0.30	3.5	11
—	—	—	22	1	10	0.6	—	0	0.33	0.05	4.4	13
—	—	—	19	44	102	4.0	—	1,100	0.33	0.38	4.4	13
—	—	—	13	3	14	0.3	15	0	0.07	0.01	0.7	0
—	—	—	26	3	14	([44])	43	[45]1,240	([44])	([44])	([44])	[45]15
—	—	—	24	12	83	4.8	81	1,320	0.40	0.45	5.3	16
—	—	—	12	4	48	0.6	51	0	0.08	0.03	1.2	0
—	—	—	33	7	52	([44])	63	1,680	0.50	0.57	6.7	[45]20

Nutrients in Indicated Quantity

(Continued)

APPENDIX G: *(Continued)*

Nutrients in Indicated Quantity

Item No. (A)	Foods, approximate measures, units, and weight (edible part unless footnote indicate otherwise) (B)		g	Water (C) %	Food Energy (D) kcal	Pro- tein (E) g	Fat (F) g
Grain Products—Con.							
	Breakfast cereals—Continued						
	Ready-to-eat—Continued						
381	Wheat, shredded, plain	1 oblong biscuit or $\frac{1}{2}$ cup spoon-size biscuits	25	7	90	2	1
382	Wheat germ, without salt and sugar, toasted	1 tbsp	6	4	25	2	1
383	Buckwheat flour, light, sifted	1 cup	98	12	340	6	1
384	Bulgur, canned, seasoned	1 cup	135	56	245	8	4
	Cake icings. See Sugars and Sweets (items 532–536)						
	Cakes made from cake mixes with enriched flour[46]						
	Angelfood						
385	Whole cake ($9\frac{3}{4}$-in diam. tube cake)	1 cake	635	34	1,645	36	1
386	Piece, $\frac{1}{12}$ of cake	1 piece	53	34	135	3	TR
	Coffee cake						
387	Whole cake ($7\frac{3}{4}$ by $5\frac{5}{8}$ by $1\frac{1}{4}$ in)	1 cake	430	30	1,385	27	41
388	Piece, $\frac{1}{6}$ of cake	1 piece	72	30	230	5	7
	Cupcakes, made with egg, milk, $2\frac{1}{2}$-in diam.						
389	Without icing	1 cupcake	25	26	90	1	3
390	With chocolate icing	1 cupcake	36	22	130	2	5
	Devil's food with chocolate icing						
391	Whole, 2 layer cake (8- or 9-in diam.)	1 cake	1,107	24	3,755	49	136
392	Piece, $\frac{1}{16}$ of cake	1 piece	69	24	235	3	8
393	Cupcake, $2\frac{1}{2}$-in diam.	1 cupcake	35	24	120	2	4
	Gingerbread						
394	Whole cake (8-in square)	1 cake	570	37	1,575	18	39
395	Piece, $\frac{1}{9}$ of cake	1 piece	63	37	175	2	4
	White, 2 layer with chocolate icing						
396	Whole cake (8- or 9-in. diam.)	1 cake	1,140	21	4,000	44	122
397	Piece $\frac{1}{16}$ of cake	1 piece	71	21	250	3	8
	Yellow, 2 layer with chocolate icing						
398	Whole cake (8- or 9-in. diam.)	1 cake	1,108	26	3,735	45	125
399	Piece, $\frac{1}{16}$ of cake	1 piece	69	26	235	3	8

[46]Excepting angelfood cake, cakes were made from mixes containing vegetable shortening; icings, with butter.

		Nutrients in Indicated Quantity										

Fatty Acids												
	Unsaturated											
Satu-rated (Total) (G) g	Oleic (H) g	Lino-leic (I) g	Carbo-hydrate (J) g	Calcium (K) mg	Phos-phorus (L) mg	Iron (M) mg	Potas-sium (N) mg	Vitamin A Value (O) I.U.	Thiamin (P) mg	Ribo-flavin (Q) mg	Niacin (R) mg	Ascorbic Acid (S) mg
—	—	—	20	11	97	0.9	87	0	0.06	0.03	1.1	0
—	—	—	3	3	70	0.5	57	10	0.11	0.05	0.3	1
0.2	0.4	0.4	78	11	86	1.0	314	0	0.08	0.04	0.4	0
—	—	—	44	27	263	1.9	151	0	0.08	0.05	4.1	0
—	—	—	377	603	756	2.5	381	0	0.37	0.95	3.6	0
—	—	—	32	50	63	0.2	32	0	0.03	0.08	0.3	0
11.7	16.3	8.8	225	262	748	6.9	469	690	0.82	0.91	7.7	1
2.0	2.7	1.5	38	44	125	1.2	78	120	0.14	0.15	1.3	TR
0.8	1.2	0.7	14	40	59	0.3	21	40	0.05	0.05	0.4	TR
2.0	1.6	0.6	21	47	71	0.4	42	60	0.05	0.06	0.4	TR
50.0	44.9	17.0	645	653	1,162	16.6	1,439	1,660	1.06	1.65	10.1	1
3.1	2.8	1.1	40	41	72	1.0	90	100	0.07	0.10	0.6	TR
1.6	1.4	0.5	20	21	37	0.5	46	50	0.03	0.05	0.3	TR
9.7	16.6	10.0	291	513	570	8.6	1,562	TR	0.84	1.00	7.4	TR
1.1	1.8	1.1	32	57	63	0.9	173	TR	0.09	0.11	0.8	TR
48.2	46.4	20.0	716	1,129	2,041	11.4	1,322	680	1.50	1.77	12.5	2
3.0	2.9	1.2	45	70	127	0.7	82	40	0.09	0.11	0.8	TR
47.8	47.8	20.3	638	1,008	2,017	12.2	1,208	1,550	1.24	1.67	10.6	2
3.0	3.0	1.3	40	63	126	0.8	75	100	0.08	0.10	0.7	TR

(Continued)

APPENDIX G: *(Continued)*

Item No. (A)	Foods, approximate measures, units, and weight (edible part unless footnote indicate otherwise) (B)		g	Water (C) %	Food Energy (D) kcal	Pro-tein (E) g	Fat (F) g
	Grain Products—Con.						
	Cakes made from home recipes using enriched flour[47]						
	Boston cream pie with custard filling						
400	Whole cake (8-in. diam.)	1 cake	825	35	2,490	41	78
401	Piece, $\frac{1}{12}$ of cake	1 piece	69	35	210	3	6
	Fruitcake, dark						
402	Loaf, 1-lb ($7\frac{1}{2}$ by 2 by $1\frac{1}{2}$ in.)	1 loaf	454	18	1,720	22	69
403	Slice, $\frac{1}{30}$ of loaf	1 slice	15	18	55	1	2
	Plain, sheet cake						
	Without icing						
404	Whole cake (9-in. square)	1 cake	777	25	2,830	35	108
405	Piece, $\frac{1}{9}$ of cake	1 piece	86	25	315	4	12
	With uncooked white icing						
406	Whole cake (9-in. square)	1 cake	1,096	21	4,020	37	129
407	Piece, $\frac{1}{9}$ of cake	1 piece	121	21	445	4	14
	Pound[49]						
408	Loaf, $8\frac{1}{2}$ by $3\frac{1}{2}$ by $3\frac{1}{4}$ in.	1 loaf	565	16	2,725	31	170
409	Slice, $\frac{1}{17}$ of loaf	1 slice	33	16	160	2	10
	Spongecake:						
410	Whole cake ($9\frac{3}{4}$-in diam. tube cake)	1 cake	790	32	2,345	60	45
411	Piece, $\frac{1}{12}$ of cake	1 piece	66	32	195	5	4
	Cookies made with enriched flour[50,51]						
	Brownies with nuts						
	Home-prepared, $1\frac{3}{4}$ by $1\frac{3}{4}$ by $\frac{7}{8}$ in.						
412	From home recipe	1 brownie	20	10	95	1	6
413	From commercial recipe	1 brownie	20	11	85	1	4
414	Frozen, with chocolate icing,[52] $1\frac{1}{2}$ by $1\frac{3}{4}$ by $\frac{7}{8}$ in.	1 brownie	25	13	105	1	5

[47]Excepting spongecake, vegetable shortening used for cake portion; butter, for icing. If butter or margarine used for cake portion, vitamin A values would be higher.

[48]Applies to product made with a sodium aluminum-sulfate type baking powder. With a low-sodium type baking powder containing potassium, value would be about twice the amount shown.

[49]Equal weights of flour, sugar, eggs, and vegetable shortening.

[50]Products are commercial unless otherwise specified.

[51]Made with enriched flour and vegetable shortening except for macaroons which do not contain flour or shortening.

[52]Icing made with butter.

	Nutrients in Indicated Quantity											
Fatty Acids												
	Unsaturated											
Saturated (Total) (G) g	Oleic (H) g	Linoleic (I) g	Carbohydrate (J) g	Calcium (K) mg	Phosphorus (L) mg	Iron (M) mg	Potassium (N) mg	Vitamin A Value (O) I.U.	Thiamin (P) mg	Riboflavin (Q) mg	Niacin (R) mg	Ascorbic Acid (S) mg
23.0	30.1	15.2	412	553	833	8.2	[48]734	1,730	1.04	1.27	9.6	2
1.9	2.5	1.3	34	46	70	0.7	[48]61	140	0.09	0.11	0.8	TR
14.4	33.5	14.8	271	327	513	11.8	2,250	540	0.72	0.73	4.9	2
0.5	1.1	0.5	9	11	17	0.4	74	20	0.02	0.02	0.2	TR
29.5	44.4	23.9	434	497	793	8.5	[48]614	1,320	1.21	1.40	10.2	2
3.3	4.9	2.6	48	55	88	0.9	[48]68	150	0.13	0.15	1.1	TR
42.2	49.5	24.4	694	548	822	8.2	[48]669	2,190	1.22	1.47	10.2	2
4.7	5.5	2.7	77	61	91	0.8	[48]74	240	0.14	0.16	1.1	TR
42.9	73.1	39.6	273	107	418	7.9	345	1,410	0.90	0.99	7.3	0
2.5	4.3	2.3	16	6	24	0.5	20	80	0.05	0.06	0.4	0
13.1	15.8	5.7	427	237	885	13.4	687	3,560	1.10	1.64	7.4	TR
1.1	1.3	0.5	36	20	74	1.1	57	300	0.09	0.14	0.6	TR
1.5	3.0	1.2	10	8	30	0.4	38	40	0.04	0.03	0.2	TR
0.9	1.4	1.3	13	9	27	0.4	34	20	0.03	0.02	0.2	TR
2.0	2.2	0.7	15	10	31	0.4	44	50	0.03	0.03	0.2	TR

(Continued)

APPENDIX G: (Continued)

Item No. (A)	Foods, approximate measures, units, and weight (edible part unless footnotes indicate otherwise) (B)		g	Water (C) %	Food Energy (D) kcal	Pro- tein (E) g	Fat (F) g
Grain Products—Con.							
	Cookies made with enriched flour[50,51]—Continued						
	Chocolate chip						
415	Commercial, 2¼-in. diam., ⅜ in. thick	4 cookies	42	3	200	2	9
416	From home recipe, 2⅓-in. diam.	4 cookies	40	3	205	2	12
417	Fig bars, square (1⅝ by 1⅝ by ⅜ in.) or rectangular (1½ by 1¾ by ½ in.)	4 cookies	56	14	200	2	3
418	Gingersnaps, 2-in diam., ¼ in thick	4 cookies	28	3	90	2	2
419	Macaroons, 2¾-in diam., ¼ in thick	2 cookies	38	4	180	2	9
420	Oatmeal with raisins, 2⅝-in diam., ¼ in thick	4 cookies	52	3	235	3	8
421	Plain, prepared from commercial chilled dough, 2½-in diam., ¼ in thick	4 cookies	48	5	240	2	12
422	Sandwich type (chocolate or vanilla), 1¾-in diam., ⅜ in thick	4 cookies	40	2	200	2	9
423	Vanilla wafers, 1¾-in diam., ¼ in. thick.	10 cookies	40	3	185	2	6
	Cornmeal						
424	Whole-ground, unbolted, dry form	1 cup	122	12	435	11	5
425	Bolted (nearly whole-grain), dry form	1 cup	122	12	440	11	4
	Degermed, enriched						
426	Dry form	1 cup	138	12	500	11	2
427	Cooked	1 cup	240	88	120	3	TR
	Degermed, unenriched						
428	Dry form	1 cup	138	12	500	11	2
429	Cooked	1 cup	240	88	120	3	TR
	Crackers[38]						
430	Graham, plain, 2½-in square	2 crackers	14	6	55	1	1
431	Rye wafers, whole-grain, 1⅞ by 3½ in.	2 wafers	13	6	45	2	TR
432	Saltines, made with enriched flour	4 crackers	11	4	50	1	1
	Danish pastry (enriched flour), plain without fruit or nuts:[54]						
433	Packaged ring, 12 oz	1 ring	340	22	1,435	25	80
434	Round piece, about 4¼-in diam. by 1 in.	1 pastry	65	22	275	5	15
435	Ounce	1 oz	28	22	120	2	7
	Doughnuts, made with enriched flour:[38]						
436	Cake type, plain, 2½-in diam., 1 in high	1 doughnut	25	24	100	1	5
437	Yeast-leavened, glazed, 3¾-in diam., 1¼ in high	1 doughnut	50	26	205	3	11

[53]Applies to yellow varieties; white varieties contain only a trace.
[54]Contains vegetable shortening and butter.

								Nutrients in Indicated Quantity				
Fatty Acids												
	Unsaturated											
Satu-rated (Total) (G) g	*Oleic (H) g*	*Lino-leic (I) g*	*Carbo-hydrate (J) g*	*Calcium (K) mg*	*Phos-phorus (L) mg*	*Iron (M) mg*	*Potas-sium (N) mg*	*Vitamin A Value (O) I.U.*	*Thiamin (P) mg*	*Ribo-flavin (Q) mg*	*Niacin (R) mg*	*Ascorbic Acid (S) mg*
2.8	2.9	2.2	29	16	48	1.0	56	50	0.10	0.17	0.9	TR
3.5	4.5	2.9	24	14	40	0.8	47	40	0.06	0.06	0.5	TR
0.8	1.2	0.7	42	44	34	1.0	111	60	0.04	0.14	0.9	TR
0.7	1.0	0.6	22	20	13	0.7	129	20	0.08	0.06	0.7	0
—	—	—	25	10	32	0.3	176	0	0.02	0.06	0.2	0
2.0	3.3	2.0	38	11	53	1.4	192	30	0.15	0.10	1.0	TR
3.0	5.2	2.9	31	17	35	0.6	23	30	0.10	0.08	0.9	0
2.2	3.9	2.2	28	10	96	0.7	15	0	0.06	0.10	0.7	0
—	—	—	30	16	25	0.6	29	50	0.10	0.09	0.8	0
0.5	1.0	2.5	90	24	312	2.9	246	[53]620	0.46	0.13	2.4	0
0.5	0.9	2.1	91	21	272	2.2	303	[53]590	0.37	0.10	2.3	0
0.2	0.4	0.9	108	8	137	4.0	166	[53]610	0.61	0.36	4.8	0
TR	0.1	0.2	26	2	34	1.0	38	[53]140	0.14	0.10	1.2	0
0.2	0.4	0.9	108	8	137	1.5	166	[53]610	0.19	0.07	1.4	0
TR	0.1	0.2	26	2	34	0.5	38	[53]140	0.05	0.02	0.2	0
0.3	0.5	0.3	10	6	21	0.5	55	0	0.02	0.08	0.5	0
—	—	—	10	7	50	0.5	78	0	0.04	0.03	0.2	0
0.3	0.5	0.4	8	2	10	0.5	13	0	0.05	0.05	0.4	0
24.3	31.7	16.5	155	170	371	6.1	381	1,050	0.97	1.01	8.6	TR
4.7	6.1	3.2	30	33	71	1.2	73	200	0.18	0.19	1.7	TR
2.0	2.7	1.4	13	14	31	0.5	32	90	0.08	0.08	0.7	TR
1.2	2.0	1.1	13	10	48	0.4	23	20	0.05	0.05	0.4	TR
3.3	5.8	3.3	22	16	33	0.6	34	25	0.10	0.10	0.8	0

(Continued)

APPENDIX G: (Continued)

				Nutrients in Indicated Quantity		
Item No. (A)	Foods, approximate measures, units, and weight (edible part unless footnote indicate otherwise) (B)	g	Water (C) %	Food Energy (D) kcal	Pro- tein (E) g	Fat (F) g

Grain Products—Con.

	Macaroni, enriched, cooked (cut lengths, elbows, shells)					
438	Firm stage (hot)	1 cup	130	64	190	7	1
	Tender stage					
439	Cold macaroni	1 cup	105	73	115	4	TR
440	Hot macaroni	1 cup	140	73	155	5	1
	Macaroni (enriched) and cheese:					
441	Canned[55]	1 cup	240	80	230	9	10
442	From home recipe (served hot)[56]	1 cup	200	58	430	17	22
	Muffins made with enriched flour:[38]					
	From home recipe					
443	Blueberry, 2⅜-in diam., 1½ in high	1 muffin	40	39	110	3	4
444	Bran	1 muffin	40	35	105	3	4
445	Corn (enriched degermed cornmeal and flour), 2⅜-in. diam., 1½ in high	1 muffin	40	33	125	3	4
446	Plain, 3-in diam., 1½ in high	1 muffin	40	38	120	3	4
	From mix, egg, milk					
447	Corn, 2⅜-in diam., 1½ in high[58]	1 muffin	40	30	130	3	4
448	Noodles (egg noodles), enriched, cooked	1 cup	160	71	200	7	2
449	Noodles, chow mein, canned	1 cup	45	1	220	6	11
	Pancakes, (4-in diam.)[38]					
450	Buckwheat, made from mix (with buckwheat and enriched flours), egg and milk added	1 cake	27	58	55	2	2
	Plain					
451	Made from home recipe using enriched flour	1 cake	27	50	60	2	2
452	Made from mix with enriched flour, egg and milk added	1 cake	27	51	60	2	2
	Pies, piecrust made with enriched flour, vegetable shortening (9-in diam.)					
	Apple					
453	Whole	1 pie	945	48	2,420	21	105
454	Sector, ⅓ of pie	1 sector	135	48	345	3	15

[55]Made with corn oil.
[56]Made with regular margarine.
[57]Applies to product made with yellow cornmeal.
[58]Made with enriched degermed cornmeal and enriched flour.

Nutrients in Indicated Quantity

Saturated (Total) (G) g	Oleic (H) g	Linoleic (I) g	Carbohydrate (J) g	Calcium (K) mg	Phosphorus (L) mg	Iron (M) mg	Potassium (N) mg	Vitamin A Value (O) I.U.	Thiamin (P) mg	Riboflavin (Q) mg	Niacin (R) mg	Ascorbic Acid (S) mg
—	—	—	39	14	85	1.4	103	0	0.23	0.13	1.8	0
—	—	—	24	8	53	0.9	64	0	0.15	0.08	1.2	0
—	—	—	32	11	70	1.3	85	0	0.20	0.11	1.5	0
4.2	3.1	1.4	26	199	182	1.0	139	260	0.12	0.24	1.0	TR
8.9	8.8	2.9	40	362	322	1.8	240	860	0.20	0.40	1.8	TR
1.1	1.4	0.7	17	34	53	0.6	46	90	0.09	0.10	0.7	TR
1.2	1.4	0.8	17	57	162	1.5	172	90	0.07	0.10	1.7	TR
1.2	1.6	0.9	19	42	68	0.7	54	[57]120	0.10	0.10	0.7	TR
1.0	1.7	1.0	17	42	60	0.6	50	40	0.09	0.12	0.9	TR
1.2	1.7	0.9	20	96	152	0.6	44	[57]100	0.08	0.09	0.7	TR
—	—	—	37	16	94	1.4	70	110	0.22	0.13	1.9	0
—	—	—	26	—	—	—	—	—	—	—	—	—
0.8	0.9	0.4	6	59	91	0.4	66	60	0.04	0.05	0.2	TR
0.5	0.8	0.5	9	27	38	0.4	33	30	0.06	0.07	0.5	TR
0.7	0.7	0.3	9	58	70	0.3	42	70	0.04	0.06	0.2	TR
27.0	44.5	25.2	360	76	208	6.6	756	280	1.06	0.79	9.3	9
3.9	6.4	3.6	51	11	30	0.9	108	40	0.15	0.11	1.3	2

(Continued)

APPENDIX G: *(Continued)*

Item No. (A)	Foods, approximate measures, units, and weight (edible part unless footnote indicate otherwise) (B)		g	Water (C) %	Food Energy (D) kcal	Protein (E) g	Fat (F) g
Grain Products—Con.							
	Pies, piecrust made with enriched flour, vegetable shortening (9-in diam.)—Continued						
	Banana cream						
455	Whole	1 pie	910	54	2,010	41	85
456	Sector, ⅟ of pie	1 sector	130	54	285	6	12
	Blueberry						
457	Whole	1 pie	945	51	2,285	23	102
458	Sector, ⅟ of pie	1 sector	135	51	325	3	15
	Cherry						
459	Whole	1 pie	945	47	2,465	25	107
460	Sector, ⅟ of pie	1 sector	135	47	350	4	15
	Custard						
461	Whole	1 pie	910	58	1,985	56	101
462	Sector, ⅟ of pie	1 sector	130	58	285	8	14
	Lemon meringue						
463	Whole	1 pie	840	47	2,140	31	86
464	Sector, ⅟ of pie	1 sector	120	47	305	4	12
	Mince						
465	Whole	1 pie	945	43	2,560	24	109
466	Sector, ⅟ of pie	1 sector	135	43	365	3	16
	Peach						
467	Whole	1 pie	945	48	2,410	24	101
468	Sector, ⅟ of pie	1 sector	135	48	345	3	14
	Pecan						
469	Whole	1 pie	825	20	3,450	42	189
470	Sector, ⅟ of pie	1 sector	118	20	495	6	27
	Pumpkin						
471	Whole	1 pie	910	59	1,920	36	102
472	Sector, ⅟ of pie	1 sector	130	59	275	5	15
473	Piecrust (home recipe) made with enriched flour and vegetable shortening, baked	1 pie shell, 9 in diam.	180	15	900	11	60
474	Piecrust mix with enriched flour and vegetable shortening, 10-oz pkg. prepared and baked	Piecrust for 2 crust pie 9-in diam.	320	19	1,485	20	93
475	Pizza (cheese) baked, 4¾-in sector; ⅛ of 12-in diam. pie.[19]	1 sector	60	45	145	6	4
	Popcorn, popped						
476	Plain, large kernel	1 cup	6	4	25	1	TR

Nutrients in Indicated Quantity												
Fatty Acids												
	Unsaturated											
Satu-rated (Total) (G) g	Oleic (H) g	Lino-leic (I) g	Carbo-hydrate (J) g	Calcium (K) mg	Phos-phorus (L) mg	Iron (M) mg	Potas-sium (N) mg	Vitamin A Value (O) I.U.	Thiamin (P) mg	Ribo-flavin (Q) mg	Niacin (R) mg	Ascorbic Acid (S) mg
26.7	33.2	16.2	279	601	746	7.3	1,847	2,280	0.77	1.51	7.0	9
3.8	4.7	2.3	40	86	107	1.0	264	330	0.11	0.22	1.0	1
24.8	43.7	25.1	330	104	217	9.5	614	280	1.03	0.80	10.0	28
3.5	6.2	3.6	47	15	31	1.4	88	40	0.15	0.11	1.4	4
28.2	45.0	25.3	363	132	236	6.6	992	4,160	1.09	0.84	9.8	TR
4.0	6.4	3.6	52	19	34	0.9	142	590	0.16	0.12	1.4	TR
33.9	38.5	17.5	213	874	1,028	8.2	1,247	2,090	0.79	1.92	5.6	0
4.8	5.5	2.5	30	125	147	1.2	178	300	0.11	0.27	0.8	0
26.1	33.8	16.4	317	118	412	6.7	420	1,430	0.61	0.84	5.2	25
3.7	4.8	2.3	45	17	59	1.0	60	200	0.09	0.12	0.7	4
28.0	45.9	25.2	389	265	359	13.3	1,682	20	0.96	0.86	9.8	9
4.0	6.6	3.6	56	38	51	1.9	240	TR	0.14	0.12	1.4	1
24.8	43.7	25.1	361	95	274	8.5	1,408	6,900	1.04	0.97	14.0	28
3.5	6.2	3.6	52	14	39	1.2	201	990	0.15	0.14	2.0	4
27.8	101.0	44.2	423	388	850	25.6	1,015	1,320	1.80	0.95	6.9	TR
4.0	14.4	6.3	61	55	122	3.7	145	190	0.26	0.14	1.0	TR
37.4	37.5	16.6	223	464	628	7.3	1,456	22,480	0.78	1.27	7.0	TR
5.4	5.4	2.4	32	66	90	1.0	208	3,210	0.11	0.18	1.0	TR
14.8	26.1	14.9	79	25	90	3.1	89	0	0.47	0.40	5.0	0
22.7	39.7	23.4	141	131	272	6.1	179	0	1.07	0.79	9.9	0
1.7	1.5	0.6	22	86	89	1.1	67	230	0.16	0.18	1.6	4
TR	0.1	0.2	5	1	17	0.2	—	—	—	0.01	0.1	0

(Continued)

APPENDIX G: (*Continued*)

				Nutrients in Indicated Quantity		
Item No. (A)	Foods, approximate measures, units, and weight (edible part unless footnotes indicate otherwise) (B)		Water (C) %	Food Energy (D) kcal	Pro-tein (E) g	Fat (F) g
		g				
	Grain Products—Con.					
	Popcorn, popped—Continued					
477	With oil (coconut) and salt added, large kernel	1 cup	9	3	40	1	2
478	Sugar coated	1 cup	35	4	135	2	1
	Pretzels, made with enriched flour					
479	Dutch, twisted, 2¾ by 2⅝ in.	1 pretzel	16	5	60	2	1
480	Thin, twisted, 3¼ by 2¼ by ¼ in.	10 pretzels	60	5	235	6	3
481	Stick, 2¼ in long	10 pretzels	3	5	10	TR	TR
	Rice, white, enriched					
482	Instant, ready-to-serve, hot	1 cup	165	73	180	4	TR
	Long grain					
483	Raw	1 cup	185	12	670	12	1
484	Cooked, served hot	1 cup	205	73	225	4	TR
	Parboiled					
485	Raw	1 cup	185	10	685	14	1
486	Cooked, served hot	1 cup	175	73	185	4	TR
	Rolls, enriched:[38]					
	Commercial					
487	Brown-and-serve (12 per 12-oz pkg.), browned	1 roll	26	27	85	2	2
488	Cloverleaf or pan, 2½-in diam., 2 in. high	1 roll	28	31	85	2	2
489	Frankfurter and hamburger (8 per 11½-oz pkg.)	1 roll	40	31	120	3	2
490	Hard, 3¾-in diam., 2 in high	1 roll	50	25	155	5	2
491	Hoagie or submarine, 11½ by 3 by 2½ in.	1 roll	135	31	390	12	4
	From home recipe					
492	Cloverleaf, 2½-in diam., 2 in high	1 roll	35	26	120	3	3
	Spaghetti, enriched, cooked:					
493	Firm stage, "al dente," served hot	1 cup	130	64	190	7	1
494	Tender stage, served hot	1 cup	140	73	155	5	1
	Spaghetti (enriched) in tomato sauce with cheese					
495	From home recipe	1 cup	250	77	260	9	9
496	Canned	1 cup	250	80	190	6	2
	Spaghetti (enriched) with meat balls and tomato sauce					
497	From home recipe	1 cup	248	70	330	19	12

[59]Product may or may not be enriched with riboflavin. Consult the label.

						Nutrients in Indicated Quantity						
Fatty Acids													
	Unsaturated												
Satu-rated (Total) (G) g	Oleic (H) g	Lino-leic (I) g	Carbo-hydrate (J) g	Calcium (K) mg	Phos-phorus (L) mg	Iron (M) mg	Potas-sium (N) mg	Vitamin A Value (O) I.U.	Thiamin (P) mg	Ribo-flavin (Q) mg	Niacin (R) mg	Ascorbic Acid (S) mg
1.5	0.2	0.2	5	1	19	0.2	—	—	—	0.01	0.2	0
0.5	0.2	0.4	30	2	47	0.5	—	—	—	0.02	0.4	0
—	—	—	12	4	21	0.2	21	0	0.05	0.04	0.7	0
—	—	—	46	13	79	0.9	78	0	0.20	0.15	2.5	0
—	—	—	2	1	4	TR	4	0	0.01	0.01	0.1	0
TR	TR	TR	40	5	31	1.3	—	0	0.21	(59)	1.7	0
0.2	0.2	0.2	149	44	174	5.4	170	0	0.81	0.06	6.5	0
0.1	0.1	0.1	50	21	57	1.8	57	0	0.23	0.02	2.1	0
0.2	0.1	0.2	150	111	370	5.4	278	0	0.81	0.07	6.5	0
0.1	0.1	0.1	41	33	100	1.4	75	0	0.19	0.02	2.1	0
0.4	0.7	0.5	14	20	23	0.5	25	TR	0.10	0.06	0.9	TR
0.4	0.6	0.4	15	21	24	0.5	27	TR	0.11	0.07	0.9	TR
0.5	0.8	0.6	21	30	34	0.8	38	TR	0.16	0.10	1.3	TR
0.4	0.6	0.5	30	24	46	1.2	49	TR	0.20	0.12	1.7	TR
0.9	1.4	1.4	75	58	115	3.0	122	TR	0.54	0.32	4.5	TR
0.8	1.1	0.7	20	16	36	0.7	41	30	0.12	0.12	1.2	
—	—	—	39	14	85	1.4	103	0	0.23	0.13	1.8	0
—	—	—	32	11	70	1.3	85	0	0.20	0.11	1.5	0
2.0	5.4	0.7	37	80	135	2.3	408	1,080	0.25	0.18	2.3	13
0.5	0.3	0.4	39	40	88	2.8	303	930	0.35	0.28	4.5	10
3.3	6.3	0.9	39	124	236	3.7	665	1,590	0.25	0.30	4.0	22

(Continued)

APPENDIX G: *(Continued)*

| | | | | | *Nutrients in Indicated Quantity* | | | |

Item No. (A)	Foods, approximate measures, units, and weight (edible part unless footnote indicate otherwise) (B)		g	Water (C) %	Food Energy (D) kcal	Pro- tein (E) g	Fat (F) g
	Grain Products—Con.						
	Spaghetti (enriched) with meatballs and tomato sauce—Continued						
498	Canned	1 cup	250	78	260	12	10
499	Toaster pastries	1 pastry	50	12	200	3	6
	Waffles, made with enriched flour, 7-in diam.[38]						
500	From home recipe	1 waffle	75	41	210	7	7
501	From mix, egg and milk added	1 waffle	75	42	205	7	8
	Wheat flours						
	All-purpose or family flour, enriched						
502	Sifted, spooned	1 cup	115	12	420	12	1
503	Unsifted, spooned	1 cup	125	12	455	13	1
504	Cake or pastry flour, enriched, sifted, spooned	1 cup	96	12	350	7	1
505	Self-rising, enriched, unsifted, spooned	1 cup	125	12	440	12	1
506	Whole-wheat, from hard wheats, stirred	1 cup	120	12	400	16	2
	Legumes (Dry), Nuts, Seeds; Related Products						
	Almonds, shelled						
507	Chopped (about 130 almonds)	1 cup	130	5	775	24	70
508	Slivered, not pressed down (about 115 almonds).	1 cup	115	5	690	21	62
	Beans, dry						
	Common varieties as Great Northern, navy, and others						
	Cooked, drained						
509	Great Northern	1 cup	180	69	210	14	1
510	Pea (navy)	1 cup	190	69	225	15	1
	Canned, solids and liquid						
	White with:						
511	Frankfurters (sliced)	1 cup	255	71	365	19	18
512	Pork and tomato sauce	1 cup	255	71	310	16	7
513	Pork and sweet sauce	1 cup	255	66	385	16	12
514	Red kidney	1 cup	255	76	230	15	1
515	Lima, cooked, drained	1 cup	190	64	260	16	1
516	Blackeye peas, dry, cooked (with residual cooking liquid)	1 cup	250	80	190	13	1
517	Brazil nuts, shelled (6–8 large kernels)	1 oz	28	5	185	4	19
518	Cashew nuts, roasted in oil	1 cup	140	5	785	24	64

[60]Value varies with the brand. Consult the label.

	Nutrients in Indicated Quantity											
Fatty Acids												
	Unsaturated											
Satu-rated (Total) (G) g	Oleic (H) g	Lino-leic (I) g	Carbo-hydrate (J) g	Calcium (K) mg	Phos-phorus (L) mg	Iron (M) mg	Potas-sium (N) mg	Vitamin A Value (O) I.U.	Thiamin (P) mg	Ribo-flavin (Q) mg	Niacin (R) mg	Ascorbic Acid (S) mg
2.2	3.3	3.9	29	53	113	3.3	245	1,000	0.15	0.18	2.3	5
—	—	—	36	[60]54	[60]67	1.9	[60]74	500	0.16	0.17	2.1	([60])
2.3	2.8	1.4	28	85	130	1.3	109	250	0.17	0.23	1.4	TR
2.8	2.9	1.2	27	179	257	1.0	146	170	0.14	0.22	0.9	TR
0.2	0.1	0.5	88	18	100	3.3	109	0	0.74	0.46	6.1	0
0.2	0.1	0.5	95	20	109	3.6	119	0	0.80	0.50	6.6	0
0.1	0.1	0.3	76	16	70	2.8	91	0	0.61	0.38	5.1	0
0.2	0.1	0.5	93	331	583	3.6	—	0	0.80	0.50	6.6	0
0.4	0.2	1.0	85	49	446	4.0	444	0	0.66	0.14	5.2	0
5.6	47.7	12.8	25	304	655	6.1	1,005	0	0.31	1.20	4.6	TR
5.0	42.2	11.3	22	269	580	5.4	889	0	0.28	1.06	4.0	TR
—	—	—	38	90	266	4.9	749	0	0.25	0.13	1.3	0
—	—	—	40	95	281	5.1	790	0	0.27	0.13	1.3	0
—	—	—	32	94	303	4.8	668	330	0.18	0.15	3.3	TR
2.4	2.8	0.6	48	138	235	4.6	536	330	0.20	0.08	1.5	5
4.3	5.0	1.1	54	161	291	5.9	—	—	0.15	0.10	1.3	—
—	—	—	42	74	278	4.6	673	10	0.13	0.10	1.5	—
—	—	—	49	55	293	5.9	1,163	—	0.25	0.11	1.3	—
—	—	—	35	43	238	3.3	573	30	0.40	0.10	1.0	—
4.8	6.2	7.1	3	53	196	1.0	203	TR	0.27	0.03	0.5	—
12.9	36.8	10.2	41	53	522	5.3	650	140	0.60	0.35	2.5	—

(Continued)

APPENDIX G: *(Continued)*

Item No. (A)	Foods, approximate measures, units, and weight (edible part unless footnotes indicate otherwise) (B)		Water (C) %	Food Energy (D) kcal	Pro- tein (E) g	Fat (F) g
		g				
Legumes (Dry), Nuts, Seeds; Related Products						
	Coconut meat, fresh					
519	Piece, about 2 by 2 by ½ in.	1 piece	45	51	155	2	16
520	Shredded or grated, not pressed down	1 cup	80	51	275	3	28
521	Filberts (hazelnuts), chopped (about 80 kernels)	1 cup	115	6	730	14	72
522	Lentils, whole, cooked	1 cup	200	72	210	16	TR
523	Peanuts, roasted in oil, salted (whole, halves, chopped)	1 cup	144	2	840	37	72
524	Peanut butter	1 tbsp	16	2	95	4	8
525	Peas, split, dry, cooked	1 cup	200	70	230	16	1
526	Pecans, chopped or pieces (about 120 large halves)	1 cup	118	3	810	11	84
527	Pumpkin and squash kernels, dry, hulled	1 cup	140	4	775	41	65
528	Sunflower seeds, dry, hulled	1 cup	145	5	810	35	69
	Walnuts					
	Black:					
529	Chopped or broken kernels	1 cup	125	3	785	26	74
530	Ground (finely)	1 cup	80	3	500	16	47
531	Persian or English, chopped (about 60 halves)	1 cup	120	4	780	18	77
Sugars and Sweets						
	Cake icings					
	Boiled, white					
532	Plain	1 cup	94	18	295	1	0
533	With coconut	1 cup	166	15	605	3	13
	Uncooked					
534	Chocolate made with milk and butter	1 cup	275	14	1,035	9	38
535	Creamy fudge from mix and water	1 cup	245	15	830	7	16
536	White	1 cup	319	11	1,200	2	21
	Candy					
537	Caramels, plain or chocolate	1 oz	28	8	115	1	3
	Chocolate					
538	Milk, plain	1 oz	28	1	145	2	9
539	Semisweet, small pieces (60 per oz)	1 cup or 6-oz pkg	170	1	860	7	61
540	Chocolate-coated peanuts	1 oz	28	1	160	5	12
541	Fondant, uncoated (mints, candy corn, other)	1 oz	28	8	105	TR	1
542	Fudge, chocolate, plain	1 oz	28	8	115	1	3
543	Gum drops	1 oz	28	12	100	TR	TR

| | Fatty Acids | | | | | | | | | | | |
| | Unsaturated | | | | | | | | | | | |
Satu-rated (Total) (G) g	Oleic (H) g	Lino-leic (I) g	Carbo-hydrate (J) g	Calcium (K) mg	Phos-phorus (L) mg	Iron (M) mg	Potas-sium (N) mg	Vitamin A Value (O) I.U.	Thiamin (P) mg	Ribo-flavin (Q) mg	Niacin (R) mg	Ascorbic Acid (S) mg
						Nutrients in Indicated Quantity						
14.0	0.9	0.3	4	6	43	0.8	115	0	0.02	0.01	0.2	1
24.8	1.6	0.5	8	10	76	1.4	205	0	0.04	0.02	0.4	2
5.1	55.2	7.3	19	240	388	3.9	810	—	0.53	—	1.0	TR
—	—	—	39	50	238	4.2	498	40	0.14	0.12	1.2	0
13.7	33.0	20.7	27	107	577	3.0	971	—	0.46	0.19	24.8	0
1.5	3.7	2.3	3	9	61	0.3	100	—	0.02	0.02	2.4	0
—	—	—	42	22	178	3.4	592	80	0.30	0.18	1.8	—
7.2	50.5	20.0	17	86	341	2.8	712	150	1.01	0.15	1.1	2
11.8	23.5	27.5	21	71	1,602	15.7	1,386	100	0.34	0.27	3.4	—
8.2	13.7	43.2	29	174	1,214	10.3	1,334	70	2.84	0.33	7.8	—
6.3	13.3	45.7	19	TR	713	7.5	575	380	0.28	0.14	0.9	—
4.0	8.5	29.2	12	TR	456	4.8	368	240	0.18	0.09	0.6	—
8.4	11.8	42.2	19	119	456	3.7	540	40	0.40	0.16	1.1	2
0	0	0	75	2	2	TR	17	0	TR	0.03	TR	0
11.0	0.9	TR	124	10	50	0.8	277	0	0.02	0.07	0.3	0
23.4	11.7	1.0	185	165	305	3.3	536	580	0.06	0.28	0.6	1
5.1	6.7	3.1	183	96	218	2.7	238	TR	0.05	0.20	0.7	TR
12.7	5.1	0.5	260	48	38	TR	57	860	TR	0.06	TR	TR
1.6	1.1	0.1	22	42	35	0.4	54	TR	0.01	0.05	0.1	TR
5.5	3.0	0.3	16	65	65	0.3	109	80	0.02	0.10	0.1	TR
36.2	19.8	1.7	97	51	255	4.4	553	30	0.02	0.14	0.9	0
4.0	4.7	2.1	11	33	84	0.4	143	TR	0.10	0.05	2.1	TR
0.1	0.3	0.1	25	4	2	0.3	1	0	TR	TR	TR	0
1.3	1.4	0.6	21	22	24	0.3	42	TR	0.01	0.03	0.1	TR
—	—	—	25	2	TR	0.1	1	0	0	TR	TR	0

(Continued)

APPENDIX G: *(Continued)*

Item No. (A)	Foods, approximate measures, units, and weight (edible part unless footnote indicate otherwise) (B)		g	Water (C) %	Food Energy (D) kcal	Pro-tein (E) g	Fat (F) g
Sugars and Sweets							
	Candy—Continued						
544	Hard	1 oz	28	1	110	0	TR
545	Marshmallows	1 oz	28	17	90	1	TR
	Chocolate-flavored beverage powders (about 4 heaping tsp per oz)						
546	With nonfat dry milk	1 oz	28	2	100	5	1
547	Without milk	1 oz	28	1	100	1	1
548	Honey, strained or extracted	1 tbsp	21	17	65	TR	0
549	Jams and preserves	1 tbsp	20	29	55	TR	TR
550		1 packet	14	29	40	TR	TR
551	Jellies	1 tbsp	18	29	50	TR	TR
552		1 packet	14	29	40	TR	TR
	Sirups						
	Chocolate-flavored sirup or topping						
553	Thin type	1 fl oz or 2 tbsp	38	32	90	1	1
554	Fudge type	1 fl oz or 2 tbsp	38	25	125	2	5
	Molasses, cane						
555	Light (first extraction)	1 tbsp	20	24	50	—	—
556	Blackstrap (third extraction)	1 tbsp	20	24	45	—	—
557	Sorghum	1 tbsp	21	23	55	—	—
558	Table blends, chiefly corn, light and dark	1 tbsp	21	24	60	0	0
	Sugars						
559	Brown, pressed down	1 cup	220	2	820	0	0
	White						
560	Granulated	1 cup	200	1	770	0	0
561		1 tbsp	12	1	45	0	0
562		1 packet	6	1	23	0	0
563	Powdered, sifted, spooned into cup.	1 cup	100	1	385	0	0
Vegetable and Vegetable Products							
	Asparagus, green:						
	Cooked, drained						
	Cuts and tips, 1½- to 2-in lengths						
564	From raw	1 cup	145	94	30	3	TR
565	From frozen	1 cup	180	93	40	6	TR
	Spears, ½-in diam. at base:						
566	From raw	4 spears	60	94	10	1	TR

| | Fatty Acids | | | | | | | | | | | |
| | | | | | | | | | | | | |

							Nutrients in Indicated Quantity					
	Fatty Acids											
		Unsaturated										
Satu-rated (Total) (G) g	Oleic (H) g	Lino-leic (I) g	Carbo-hydrate (J) g	Calcium (K) mg	Phos-phorus (L) mg	Iron (M) mg	Potas-sium (N) mg	Vitamin A Value (O) I.U.	Thiamin (P) mg	Ribo-flavin (Q) mg	Niacin (R) mg	Ascorbic Acid (S) mg
—	—	—	28	6	2	0.5	1	0	0	0	0	0
—	—	—	23	5	2	0.5	2	0	0	TR	TR	0
0.5	0.3	TR	20	167	155	0.5	227	10	0.04	0.21	0.2	1
0.4	0.2	TR	25	9	48	0.6	142	—	0.01	0.03	0.1	0
0	0	0	17	1	1	0.1	11	0	TR	0.01	0.1	TR
—	—	—	14	4	2	0.2	18	TR	TR	0.01	TR	TR
—	—	—	10	3	1	0.1	12	TR	TR	TR	TR	TR
—	—	—	13	4	1	0.3	14	TR	TR	0.01	TR	1
—	—	—	10	3	1	0.2	11	TR	TR	TR	TR	1
0.5	0.3	TR	24	6	35	0.6	106	TR	0.01	0.03	0.2	0
3.1	1.6	0.1	20	48	60	0.5	107	60	0.02	0.08	0.2	TR
—	—	—	13	33	9	0.9	183	—	0.01	0.01	TR	—
—	—	—	11	137	17	3.2	585	—	0.02	0.04	0.4	—
—	—	—	14	35	5	2.6	—	—	—	0.02	TR	—
0	0	0	15	9	3	0.8	1	0	0	0	0	0
0	0	0	212	187	42	7.5	757	0	0.02	0.07	0.4	0
0	0	0	199	0	0	0.2	6	0	0	0	0	0
0	0	0	12	0	0	TR	TR	0	0	0	0	0
0	0	0	6	0	0	TR	TR	0	0	0	0	0
0	0	0	100	0	0	0.1	3	0	0	0	0	0
—	—	—	5	30	73	0.9	265	1,310	0.23	0.26	2.0	38
—	—	—	6	40	115	2.2	396	1,530	0.25	0.23	1.8	41
—	—	—	2	13	30	0.4	110	540	0.10	0.11	0.8	16

(Continued)

APPENDIX G: *(Continued)*

Item No. (A)	Foods, approximate measures, units, and weight (edible part unless footnotes indicate otherwise) (B)		g	Water (C) %	Food Energy (D) kcal	Pro- tein (E) g	Fat (F) g
Vegetable and Vegetable Products—Con.							
	Blackeye peas, immature seeds, cooked and drained						
585	From raw	1 cup	165	72	180	13	1
586	From frozen	1 cup	170	66	220	15	1
	Broccoli, cooked, drained						
	From raw						
587	Stalk, medium size	1 stalk	180	91	45	6	1
588	Stalks cut into $\frac{1}{2}$-in. pieces	1 cup	155	91	40	5	TR
	From frozen:						
589	Stalk, $4\frac{1}{2}$ to 5 in. long	1 stalk	30	91	10	1	TR
590	Chopped	1 cup	185	92	50	5	1
	Brussels sprouts, cooked, drained:						
591	From raw, 7–8 sprouts ($1\frac{1}{4}$- to $1\frac{1}{2}$-in. diam.)	1 cup	155	88	55	7	1
592	From frozen	1 cup	155	89	50	5	TR
	Cabbage						
	Common varieties						
	Raw						
593	Coarsely shredded or sliced	1 cup	70	92	15	1	TR
594	Finely shredded or chopped	1 cup	90	92	20	1	TR
595	Cooked, drained	1 cup	145	94	30	2	TR
596	Red, raw, coarsely shredded or sliced	1 cup	70	90	20	1	TR
597	Savoy, raw, coarsely shredded or sliced	1 cup	70	92	15	2	TR
598	Cabbage, celery (also called *pe-tsai* or *wongbok*), raw, 1-in pieces	1 cup	75	95	10	1	TR
599	Cabbage, white mustard (also called *bokchoy* or *pakchoy*), cooked, drained	1 cup	170	95	25	2	TR
	Carrots						
	Raw, without crowns and tips, scraped						
600	Whole, $7\frac{1}{2}$ by $1\frac{1}{8}$ in, or strips, $2\frac{1}{2}$ to 3 in long	1 carrot or 18 strips	72	88	30	1	TR
601	Grated	1 cup	110	88	45	1	TR
602	Cooked (crosswise cuts), drained	1 cup	155	91	50	1	TR
	Canned						
603	Sliced, drained solids	1 cup	155	91	45	1	TR
604	Strained or junior (baby food)	1 oz ($1\frac{3}{4}$ to 2 tbsp)	28	92	10	TR	TR
	Cauliflower						
605	Raw, chopped	1 cup	115	91	31	3	TR

Nutrients in Indicated Quantity												
Fatty Acids												
	Unsaturated											
Satu-rated (Total) (G) g	Oleic (H) g	Lino-leic (I) g	Carbo-hydrate (J) g	Calcium (K) mg	Phos-phorus (L) mg	Iron (M) mg	Potas-sium (N) mg	Vitamin A Value (O) I.U.	Thiamin (P) mg	Ribo-flavin (Q) mg	Niacin (R) mg	Ascorbic Acid (S) mg
—	—	—	30	40	241	3.5	625	580	0.50	0.18	2.3	28
—	—	—	40	43	286	4.8	573	290	0.68	0.19	2.4	15
—	—	—	8	158	112	1.4	481	4,500	0.16	0.36	1.4	162
—	—	—	7	136	96	1.2	414	3,880	0.14	0.31	1.2	140
—	—	—	1	12	17	0.2	66	570	0.02	0.03	0.2	22
—	—	—	9	100	104	1.3	392	4,810	0.11	0.22	0.9	105
—	—	—	10	50	112	1.7	423	810	0.12	0.22	1.2	135
—	—	—	10	33	95	1.2	457	880	0.12	0.16	0.9	126
—	—	—	4	34	20	0.3	163	90	0.04	0.04	0.2	33
—	—	—	5	44	26	0.4	210	120	0.05	0.05	0.3	42
—	—	—	6	64	29	0.4	236	190	0.06	0.06	0.4	48
—	—	—	5	29	25	0.6	188	30	0.06	0.04	0.3	43
—	—	—	3	47	38	0.6	188	140	0.04	0.06	0.2	39
—	—	—	2	32	30	0.5	190	110	0.04	0.03	0.5	19
—	—	—	4	252	56	1.0	364	5,270	0.07	0.14	1.2	26
—	—	—	7	27	26	0.5	246	7,930	0.04	0.04	0.4	6
—	—	—	11	41	40	0.8	375	12,100	0.07	0.06	0.7	9
—	—	—	11	51	48	0.9	344	16,280	0.08	0.08	0.8	9
—	—	—	10	47	34	1.1	186	23,250	0.03	0.05	0.6	3
—	—	—	2	7	6	0.1	51	3,690	0.01	0.01	0.1	1
—	—	—	6	29	64	1.3	339	70	0.13	0.12	0.8	90

(Continued)

APPENDIX G: *(Continued)*

				Nutrients in Indicated Quantity			

Item No. (A)	Foods, approximate measures, units, and weight (edible part unless footnote indicate otherwise) (B)		g	Water (C) %	Food Energy (D) kcal	Pro-tein (E) g	Fat (F) g
Vegetable and Vegetable Products—Con.							
	Cauliflower—Continued						
	Cooked, drained						
606	From raw (flower buds)	1 cup	125	93	30	3	TR
607	From frozen (flowerets)	1 cup	180	94	30	3	TR
	Celery, Pascal type, raw						
608	Stalk, large outer, 8 by 1½ in, at root end	1 stalk	40	94	5	TR	TR
609	Pieces, diced	1 cup	120	94	20	1	TR
	Collards, cooked, drained						
610	From raw (leaves without stems)	1 cup	190	90	65	7	1
611	From frozen (chopped)	1 cup	170	90	50	5	1
	Corn, sweet						
	Cooked, drained						
612	From raw, ear 5 by 1¾ in	1 ear[61]	140	74	70	2	1
	From frozen						
613	Ear, 5 in long	1 ear[61]	229	73	120	4	1
614	Kernels	1 cup	165	77	130	5	1
	Canned:						
615	Cream style	1 cup	256	76	210	5	2
	Whole kernel						
616	Vacuum pack	1 cup	210	76	175	5	1
617	Wet pack, drained solids	1 cup	165	76	140	4	1
	Cowpeas. See Blackeye peas (Items 585–586)						
	Cucumber slices, ⅛ in thick (large, 2⅛-in diam.; small, 1¾-in diam.)						
618	With peel	6 large or 8 small slices		95	5	TR	TR
619	Without peel	6½ large or 9 small pieces	28	96	5	TR	TR
620	Dandelion greens, cooked, drained	1 cup	105	90	35	2	1
621	Endive, curly (including escarole), raw, small pieces	1 cup	50	93	10	1	TR
	Kale, cooked, drained						
622	From raw (leaves without stems and midribs)	1 cup	110	88	45	5	1
623	From frozen (leaf style)	1 cup	130	91	40	4	1

[61]Weight includes cob. Without cob, weight is 77 g for item 612, 126 g for item 613.
[62]Based on yellow varieties. For white varieties, value is trace.

| | Fatty Acids | | | | | | | | | | | |
| | Unsaturated | | | | | | | | | | | |
Satu-rated (Total) (G) g	Oleic (H) g	Lino-leic (I) g	Carbo-hydrate (J) g	Calcium (K) mg	Phos-phorus (L) mg	Iron (M) mg	Potas-sium (N) mg	Vitamin A Value (O) I.U.	Thiamin (P) mg	Ribo-flavin (Q) mg	Niacin (R) mg	Ascorbic Acid (S) mg
—	—	—	5	26	53	0.9	258	80	0.11	0.10	0.8	69
—	—	—	6	31	68	0.9	373	50	0.07	0.09	0.7	74
—	—	—	2	16	11	0.1	136	110	0.01	0.01	0.1	4
—	—	—	5	47	34	0.4	409	320	0.04	0.04	0.4	11
—	—	—	10	357	99	1.5	498	14,820	0.21	0.38	2.3	144
—	—	—	10	299	87	1.7	401	11,560	0.10	0.24	1.0	56
—	—	—	16	2	69	0.5	151	[62]310	0.09	0.08	1.1	7
—	—	—	27	4	121	1.0	291	[62]440	0.18	0.10	2.1	9
—	—	—	31	5	120	1.3	304	[62]580	0.15	0.10	2.5	8
—	—	—	51	8	143	1.5	248	[62]840	0.08	0.13	2.6	13
—	—	—	43	6	153	1.1	204	[62]740	0.06	0.13	2.3	11
—	—	—	33	8	81	0.8	160	[62]580	0.05	0.08	1.5	7
—	—	—	1	7	8	0.3	45	70	0.01	0.01	0.1	3
—	—	—	1	5	5	0.1	45	TR	0.01	0.01	0.1	3
—	—	—	7	147	44	1.9	244	12,290	0.14	0.17	—	19
—	—	—	2	41	27	0.9	147	1,650	0.04	0.07	0.3	5
—	—	—	7	206	64	1.8	243	9,130	0.11	0.20	1.8	102
—	—	—	7	157	62	1.3	251	10,660	0.08	0.20	0.9	49

(Continued)

APPENDIX G: *(Continued)*

Item No. (A)	Foods, approximate measures, units, and weight (edible part unless footnote indicate otherwise) (B)		Water (C) %	Food Energy (D) kcal	Pro- tein (E) g	Fat (F) g
		g				
Vegetable and Vegetable Products—Con.						
	Lettuce, raw						
	Butterhead, as Boston types						
624	Head, 5-in diam.	1 head[63]	220	95	25	2	TR
625	Leaves	1 outer or 2 inner or 3 heart leaves	15	95	TR	TR	TR
	Crisphead, as Iceberg						
626	Head, 6-in diam.	1 head[64]	567	96	70	5	1
627	Wedge, ¼ of head	1 wedge	135	96	20	1	TR
628	Pieces, chopped or shredded	1 cup	55	96	5	TR	TR
629	Looseleaf (bunching varieties including romaine or cos), chopped or shredded pieces	1 cup	55	94	10	1	TR
630	Mushrooms, raw, sliced or chopped	1 cup	70	90	20	2	TR
631	Mustard greens, without stems and midribs, cooked, drained	1 cup	140	93	30	3	1
632	Okra pods, 3 by ⅜ in, cooked	10 pods	106	91	30	2	TR
	Onions						
	Mature						
	Raw						
633	Chopped	1 cup	170	89	65	3	TR
634	Sliced	1 cup	115	89	45	2	TR
635	Cooked (whole or sliced), drained	1 cup	210	92	60	3	TR
636	Young green, bulb (⅜ in diam.) and white portion of top	6 onions	30	88	15	TR	TR
637	Parsley, raw, chopped	1 tbsp	4	85	TR	TR	TR
638	Parsnips, cooked (diced or 2-in. lengths)	1 cup	155	82	100	2	1
	Peas, green						
	Canned						
639	Whole, drained solids	1 cup	170	77	150	8	1
640	Strained (baby food)	1 oz (1¾ to 2 tbsp)	28	86	15	1	TR
641	Frozen, cooked, drained	1 cup	160	82	110	8	TR
642	Peppers, hot, red, without seeds, dried (ground chili powder, added seasonings)	1 tsp	2	9	5	TR	TR

[63]Weight includes refuse of outer leaves and core. Without these parts, weight is 163 g.

[64]Weight includes core. Without core, weight is 539 g.

[65]Value based on white-fleshed varieties. For yellow-fleshed varieties, value is International Units (I.U.) is 70 for item 633, 50 for item 634, and 80 for item 635.

| | Fatty Acids | | | | | | | | | | | |
| | Unsaturated | | | | | | | | | | | |
Satu-rated (Total) (G) g	Oleic (H) g	Lino-leic (I) g	Carbo-hydrate (J) g	Calcium (K) mg	Phos-phorus (L) mg	Iron (M) mg	Potas-sium (N) mg	Vitamin A Value (O) I.U.	Thiamin (P) mg	Ribo-flavin (Q) mg	Niacin (R) mg	Ascorbic Acid (S) mg
—	—	—	4	57	42	3.3	430	1,580	0.10	0.10	0.5	13
—	—	—	TR	5	4	0.3	40	150	0.01	0.01	TR	1
—	—	—	16	108	118	2.7	943	1,780	0.32	0.32	1.6	32
—	—	—	4	27	30	0.7	236	450	0.08	0.08	0.4	8
—	—	—	2	11	12	0.3	96	180	0.03	0.03	0.2	3
—	—	—	2	37	14	0.8	145	1,050	0.03	0.04	0.2	10
—	—	—	3	4	81	0.6	290	TR	0.07	0.32	2.9	2
—	—	—	6	193	45	2.5	308	8,120	0.11	0.20	0.8	67
—	—	—	6	98	43	0.5	184	520	0.14	0.19	1.0	21
—	—	—	15	46	61	0.9	267	[65]TR	0.05	0.07	0.3	17
—	—	—	10	31	41	0.6	181	[65]TR	0.03	0.05	0.2	12
—	—	—	14	50	61	0.8	231	[65]TR	0.06	0.06	0.4	15
—	—	—	3	12	12	0.2	69	TR	0.02	0.01	0.1	8
—	—	—	TR	7	2	0.2	25	300	TR	0.01	TR	6
—	—	—	23	70	96	0.9	587	50	0.11	0.12	0.2	16
—	—	—	29	44	129	3.2	163	1,170	0.15	0.10	1.4	14
—	—	—	3	3	18	0.3	28	140	0.02	0.03	0.3	3
—	—	—	19	30	138	3.0	216	960	0.43	0.14	2.7	21
—	—	—	1	5	4	0.3	20	1,300	TR	0.02	0.2	TR

Nutrients in Indicated Quantity

(Continued)

APPENDIX G: *(Continued)*

Item No. (A)	Foods, approximate measures, units, and weight (edible part unless footnotes indicate otherwise) (B)		g	Water (C) %	Food Energy (D) kcal	Pro- tein (E) g	Fat (F) g
	Vegetable and Vegetable Products—Con.						
	Peppers, sweet (about 5 per lb, whole), stem and seeds removed						
643	Raw	1 pod	74	93	15	1	TR
644	Cooked, boiled, drained	1 pod	73	95	15	1	TR
	Potatoes, cooked						
645	Baked, peeled after baking (about 2 per lb, raw)	1 potato	156	75	145	4	TR
	Boiled (about 3 per lb, raw):						
646	Peeled after boiling	1 potato	137	80	105	3	TR
647	Peeled before boiling	1 potato	135	83	90	3	TR
	French-fried, strip, 2 to 3½ in long						
648	Prepared from raw	10 strips	50	45	135	2	7
649	Frozen, oven heated	10 strips	50	53	110	2	4
650	Hashed brown, prepared from frozen	1 cup	155	56	345	3	18
	Mashed, prepared from—						
	Raw						
651	Milk added	1 cup	210	83	135	4	2
652	Milk and butter added	1 cup	210	80	195	4	9
653	Dehydrated flakes (without milk), water, milk, butter, and salt added.	1 cup	210	79	195	4	7
654	Potato chips, 1¾ by 2½ in oval cross section	10 chips	20	2	115	1	8
655	Potato salad, made with cooked salad dressing	1 cup	250	76	250	7	7
656	Pumpkin, canned	1 cup	245	90	80	2	1
657	Radishes, raw (prepackaged) stem ends, rootless cut off	4 radishes	18	95	5	TR	TR
658	Sauerkraut, canned, solids and liquid	1 cup	235	93	40	2	TR
	Southern peas. See Blackeye peas (items 585–586)						
	Spinach						
659	Raw, chopped	1 cup	55	91	15	2	TR
	Cooked, drained						
660	From raw	1 cup	180	92	40	5	1
	From frozen						
661	Chopped	1 cup	205	92	45	6	1
662	Leaf	1 cup	190	92	45	6	1
663	Canned, drained solids	1 cup	205	91	50	6	1

						Nutrients in Indicated Quantity						

Fatty Acids												
Saturated (Total)	Unsaturated		Carbo-hydrate	Calcium	Phosphorus	Iron	Potassium	Vitamin A Value	Thiamin	Riboflavin	Niacin	Ascorbic Acid
(G)	Oleic (H)	Linoleic (I)	(J)	(K)	(L)	(M)	(N)	(O)	(P)	(Q)	(R)	(S)
g	g	g	g	mg	mg	mg	mg	I.U.	mg	mg	mg	mg
—	—	—	4	7	16	0.5	157	310	0.06	0.06	0.4	94
—	—	—	3	7	12	0.4	109	310	0.05	0.05	0.4	70
—	—	—	33	14	101	1.1	782	TR	0.15	0.07	2.7	31
—	—	—	23	10	72	0.8	556	TR	0.12	0.05	2.0	22
—	—	—	20	8	57	0.7	385	TR	0.12	0.05	1.6	22
1.7	1.2	3.3	18	8	56	0.7	427	TR	0.07	0.04	1.6	11
1.1	0.8	2.1	17	5	43	0.9	326	TR	0.07	0.01	1.3	11
4.6	3.2	9.0	45	28	78	1.9	439	TR	0.11	0.03	1.6	12
0.7	0.4	TR	27	50	103	0.8	548	40	0.17	0.11	2.1	21
5.6	2.3	0.2	26	50	101	0.8	525	360	0.17	0.11	2.1	19
3.6	2.1	0.2	30	65	99	0.6	601	270	0.08	0.08	1.9	11
2.1	1.4	4.0	10	8	28	0.4	226	TR	0.04	0.01	1.0	3
2.0	2.7	1.3	41	80	160	1.5	798	350	0.20	0.18	2.8	28
—	—	—	19	61	64	1.0	588	15,680	0.07	0.12	1.5	12
—	—	—	1	5	6	0.2	58	TR	0.01	0.01	0.1	5
—	—	—	9	85	42	1.2	329	120	0.07	0.09	0.5	33
—	—	—	2	51	28	1.7	259	4,460	0.06	0.11	0.3	28
—	—	—	6	167	68	4.0	583	14,580	0.13	0.25	0.9	50
—	—	—	8	232	90	4.3	683	16,200	0.14	0.31	0.8	39
—	—	—	7	200	84	4.8	688	15,390	0.15	0.27	1.0	53
—	—	—	7	242	53	5.3	513	16,400	0.04	0.25	0.6	29

(Continued)

APPENDIX G: *(Continued)*

Item No. (A)	Foods, approximate measures, units, and weight (edible part unless footnote indicate otherwise) (B)		g	Water (C) %	Food Energy (D) kcal	Pro-tein (E) g	Fat (F) g
Vegetable and Vegetable Products—Con.							
	Squash, cooked						
664	Summer (all varieties), diced, drained	1 cup	210	96	30	2	TR
665	Winter (all varieties), baked, mashed	1 cup	205	81	130	4	1
	Sweet potatoes						
	Cooked (raw, 5 by 2 in.; about 2½ per lb)						
666	Baked in skin, peeled	1 potato	114	64	160	2	1
667	Boiled in skin, peeled	1 potato	151	71	170	3	1
668	Candied, 2½ by 2-in piece	1 piece	105	60	175	1	3
	Canned						
669	Solid pack (mashed)	1 cup	255	72	275	5	1
670	Vacuum pack, piece 2¾ by 1 in.	1 piece	40	72	45	1	TR
	Tomatoes						
671	Raw, 2⅗-in diam. (3 per 12 oz pkg.)	1 tomato[66]	135	94	25	1	TR
672	Canned, solids and liquid	1 cup	241	94	50	2	TR
673	Tomato catsup	1 cup	273	69	290	5	1
674		1 tbsp	15	69	15	TR	TR
	Tomato juice, canned						
675	Cup	1 cup	243	94	45	2	TR
676	Glass (6 fl oz)	1 glass	182	94	35	2	TR
677	Turnips, cooked, diced	1 cup	155	94	35	1	TR
	Turnip greens, cooked, drained						
678	From raw (leaves and stems)	1 cup	145	94	30	3	TR
679	From frozen (chopped)	1 cup	165	93	40	4	TR
680	Vegetables, mixed, frozen, cooked	1 cup	182	83	115	6	1
Miscellaneous Items							
	Baking powders for home use						
	Sodium aluminum sulfate						
681	With monocalcium phosphate monohydrate	1 tsp	3.0	2	5	TR	TR

[66]Weight includes cores and stem ends. Without these parts, weight is 123 g.

[67]Based on year-round average. For tomatoes marketed from November through May, value is about 12 mg; from June through October, 32 mg.

[68]Applies to product without calcium salts added. Value for products with calcium salts added may be as much as 63 mg for whole tomatoes, 241 mg for cut forms.

								Nutrients in Indicated Quantity					
Fatty Acids													
	Unsaturated												
Satu-rated (Total) (G) g	Oleic (H) g	Lino-leic (I) g	Carbo-hydrate (J) g	Calcium (K) mg	Phos-phorus (L) mg	Iron (M) mg	Potas-sium (N) mg	Vitamin A Value (O) I.U.	Thiamin (P) mg	Ribo-flavin (Q) mg	Niacin (R) mg	Ascorbic Acid (S) mg
—	—	—	7	53	53	0.8	296	820	0.11	0.17	1.7	21
—	—	—	32	57	98	1.6	945	8,610	0.10	0.27	1.4	27
—	—	—	37	46	66	1.0	342	9,230	0.10	0.08	0.8	25
—	—	—	40	48	71	1.1	367	11,940	0.14	0.09	0.9	26
2.0	0.8	0.1	36	39	45	0.9	200	6,620	0.06	0.04	0.4	11
—	—	—	63	64	105	2.0	510	19,890	0.13	0.10	1.5	36
—	—	—	10	10	16	0.3	80	3,120	0.02	0.02	0.2	6
—	—	—	6	16	33	0.6	300	1,110	0.07	0.05	0.9	[67]28
—	—	—	10	[68]14	46	1.2	523	2,170	0.12	0.07	1.7	41
—	—	—	69	60	137	2.2	991	3,820	0.25	0.19	4.4	41
—	—	—	4	3	8	0.1	54	210	0.01	0.01	0.2	2
—	—	—	10	17	44	2.2	552	1,940	0.12	0.07	1.9	39
—	—	—	8	13	33	1.6	413	1,460	0.09	0.05	1.5	29
—	—	—	8	54	37	0.6	291	TR	0.06	0.08	0.5	34
—	—	—	5	252	49	1.5	—	8,270	0.15	0.33	0.7	68
—	—	—	6	195	64	2.6	246	11,390	0.08	0.15	0.7	31
—	—	—	24	46	115	2.4	348	9,010	0.22	0.13	2.0	15
0	0	0	1	58	87	—	5	0	0	0	0	0

(Continued)

APPENDIX G: *(Continued)*

Item No. (A)	Foods, approximate measures, units, and weight (edible part unless footnote indicate otherwise) (B)		*g*	*Water (C) %*	*Food Energy (D) kcal*	*Pro-tein (E) g*	*Fat (F) g*
Miscellaneous Items—Con.							
	Baking powders for home use—Continued						
	Sodium aluminum sulfate—Continued						
682	With monocalcium phosphate monohydrate, calcium sulfate	1 tsp	2.9	1	5	TR	TR
683	Straight phosphate	1 tsp	3.8	2	5	TR	TR
684	Low sodium	1 tsp	4.3	2	5	TR	TR
685	Barbecue sauce	1 cup	250	81	230	4	17
	Beverages, alcoholic						
686	Beer	12 fl oz	360	92	150	1	0
	Gin, rum, vodka, whisky:						
687	80-proof	1½-fl oz jigger	42	67	95	—	—
688	86-proof	1½-fl oz jigger	42	64	105	—	—
689	90-proof	1½-fl oz jigger	42	62	110	—	—
	Wines						
690	Dessert	3½-fl oz glass	103	77	140	TR	0
691	Table	3½-fl oz glass	102	86	85	TR	0
	Beverages, carbonated, sweetened, nonalcoholic						
692	Carbonated water	12 fl oz	366	92	115	0	0
693	Cola type	12 fl oz	369	90	145	0	0
694	Fruit-flavored sodas and Tom Collins mixer	12 fl oz	372	88	170	0	0
695	Ginger ale	12 fl oz	366	92	115	0	0
696	Root beer	12 fl oz	370	90	150	0	0
	Chili powder. See Peppers, hot, red (item 642)						
	Chocolate						
697	Bitter or baking	1 oz	28	2	145	3	15
	Semisweet, see Candy, chocolate (item 539).						
698	Gelatin, dry	1, 7-g envelope	7	13	25	6	TR
699	Gelatin dessert prepared with gelatin dessert powder and water	1 cup	240	84	140	4	0
700	Mustard, prepared, yellow	1 tsp or individual serving pouch or cup.	5	80	5	TR	TR
	Olives, pickled, canned:						
701	Green	4 medium or 3 extra large or 2 giant.[69]	16	78	15	TR	2
702	Ripe, Mission	3 small or 2 large[69]	10	73	15	TR	2

[69]Weight includes pits. Without pits, weight is 13 g for item 701, 9 g for item 702.

												Nutrients in Indicated Quantity

Fatty Acids											
	Unsaturated										
Satu-rated (Total) (G) g	Oleic (H) g	Lino-leic (I) g	Carbo-hydrate (J) g	Calcium (K) mg	Phos-phorus (L) mg	Iron (M) mg	Potas-sium (N) mg	Vitamin A Value (O) I.U.	Thiamin (P) mg	Ribo-flavin (Q) mg	Niacin (R) mg	Ascorbic Acid (S) mg
---	---	---	---	---	---	---	---	---	---	---	---	---
0	0	0	1	183	45	—	—	0	0	0	0	0
0	0	0	1	239	359	—	6	0	0	0	0	0
0	0	0	2	207	314	—	471	0	0	0	0	0
2.2	4.3	10.0	20	53	50	2.0	435	900	0.03	0.03	0.8	13
0	0	0	14	18	108	TR	90	—	0.01	0.11	2.2	—
0	0	0	TR	—	—	—	1	—	—	—	—	—
0	0	0	TR	—	—	—	1	—	—	—	—	—
0	0	0	TR	—	—	—	1	—	—	—	—	—
0	0	0	8	8	—	—	77	—	0.01	0.02	0.2	—
0	0	0	4	9	10	0.4	94	—	TR	0.01	0.1	—
0	0	0	29	—	—	—	—	0	0	0	0	0
0	0	0	37	—	—	—	—	0	0	0	0	0
0	0	0	45	—	—	—	—	0	0	0	0	0
0	0	0	29	—	—	—	0	0	0	0	0	0
0	0	0	39	—	—	—	0	0	0	0	0	0
8.9	4.9	0.4	8	22	109	1.9	235	20	0.01	0.07	0.4	0
0	0	0	0	—	—	—	—	—	—	—	—	—
0	0	0	34	—	—	—	—	—	—	—	—	—
—	—	—	TR	4	4	0.1	7	—	—	—	—	—
0.2	1.2	0.1	TR	8	2	0.2	7	40	—	—	—	—
0.2	1.2	0.1	TR	9	1	0.1	2	10	TR	TR	—	—

(Continued)

APPENDIX G: *(Continued)*

Item No. (A)	Foods, approximate measures, units, and weight (edible part unless footnotes indicate otherwise) (B)			Water (C) %	Food Energy (D) kcal	Pro- tein (E) g	Fat (F) g

Nutrients in Indicated Quantity

Item No. (A)	Foods (B)		g	Water (C) %	Food Energy (D) kcal	Pro-tein (E) g	Fat (F) g
	Miscellaneous Items—Con.						
	Pickles, cucumber						
703	Dill, medium, whole, 3¾ in long, 1¼-in diam.	1 pickle	65	93	5	TR	TR
704	Fresh-pack, slices 1½-in diam., ¼ in thick	2 slices	15	79	10	TR	TR
705	Sweet, gherkin, small, whole, about 2½ in long, ¾-in diam.	1 pickle	15	61	20	TR	TR
706	Relish, finely chopped, sweet	1 tbsp	15	63	20	TR	TR
	Popcorn. See items 476–478						
707	Popsicle, 3-fl oz size	1 popsicle	95	80	70	0	0
	Soups						
	Canned, condensed						
	Prepared with equal volume of milk						
708	Cream of chicken	1 cup	245	85	180	7	10
709	Cream of mushroom	1 cup	245	83	215	7	14
710	Tomato	1 cup	250	84	175	7	7
	Prepared with equal volume of water						
711	Bean with pork	1 cup	250	84	170	8	6
712	Beef broth, bouillon, consomme	1 cup	240	96	30	5	0
713	Beef noodle	1 cup	240	93	65	4	3
714	Clam chowder, Manhattan type (with tomatoes, without milk)	1 cup	245	92	80	2	3
715	Cream of chicken	1 cup	240	92	95	3	6
716	Cream of mushroom	1 cup	240	90	135	2	10
717	Minestrone	1 cup	245	90	105	5	3
718	Split pea	1 cup	245	85	145	9	3
719	Tomato	1 cup	245	91	90	2	3
720	Vegetable beef	1 cup	245	92	80	5	2
721	Vegetarian	1 cup	245	92	80	2	2
	Dehydrated						
722	Bouillon cube, ½ in.	1 cube	4	4	5	1	TR
	Mixes:						
	Unprepared						
723	Onion	1½-oz pkg.	43	3	150	6	5
	Prepared with water						
724	Chicken noodle	1 cup	240	95	55	2	1
725	Onion	1 cup	240	96	35	1	1
726	Tomato vegetable with noodles	1 cup	240	93	65	1	1

Nutrients in Indicated Quantity												
Fatty Acids												
	Unsaturated											
Satu-rated (Total) (G) g	Oleic (H) g	Lino-leic (I) g	Carbo-hydrate (J) g	Calcium (K) mg	Phos-phorus (L) mg	Iron (M) mg	Potas-sium (N) mg	Vitamin A Value (O) I.U.	Thiamin (P) mg	Ribo-flavin (Q) mg	Niacin (R) mg	Ascorbic Acid (S) mg
—	—	—	1	17	14	0.7	130	70	TR	0.01	TR	4
—	—	—	3	5	4	0.3	—	20	TR	TR	TR	1
—	—	—	5	2	2	0.2	—	10	TR	TR	TR	1
—	—	—	5	3	2	0.1	—	—	—	—	—	—
0	0	0	18	0	—	TR	—	0	0	0	0	0
4.2	3.6	1.3	15	172	152	0.5	260	610	0.05	0.27	0.7	2
5.4	2.9	4.6	16	191	169	0.5	279	250	0.05	0.34	0.7	1
3.4	1.7	1.0	23	168	155	0.8	418	1,200	0.10	0.25	1.3	15
1.2	1.8	2.4	22	63	128	2.3	395	650	0.13	0.08	1.0	3
0	0	0	3	TR	31	0.5	130	TR	TR	0.02	1.2	—
0.6	0.7	0.8	7	7	48	1.0	77	50	0.05	0.07	1.0	TR
0.5	0.4	1.3	12	34	47	1.0	184	880	0.02	0.02	1.0	—
1.6	2.3	1.1	8	24	34	0.5	79	410	0.02	0.05	0.5	TR
2.6	1.7	4.5	10	41	50	0.5	98	70	0.02	0.12	0.7	TR
0.7	0.9	1.3	14	37	59	1.0	314	2,350	0.07	0.05	1.0	—
1.1	1.2	0.4	21	29	149	1.5	270	440	0.25	0.15	1.5	1
0.5	0.5	1.0	16	15	34	0.7	230	1,000	0.05	0.05	1.2	12
—	—	—	10	12	49	0.7	162	2,700	0.05	0.05	1.0	—
—	—	—	13	20	39	1.0	172	2,940	0.05	0.05	1.0	—
—	—	—	TR	—	—	—	4	—	—	—	—	—
1.1	2.3	1.0	23	42	49	0.6	238	30	0.05	0.03	0.3	6
—	—	—	8	7	19	0.2	19	50	0.07	0.05	0.5	TR
—	—	—	6	10	12	0.2	58	TR	TR	TR	TR	2
—	—	—	12	7	19	0.2	29	480	0.05	0.02	0.5	5

(Continued)

APPENDIX G: *(Continued)*

Nutrients in Indicated Quantity

Item No. (A)	Foods, approximate measures, units, and weight (edible part unless footnote indicate otherwise) (B)		g	Water (C) %	Food Energy (D) kcal	Pro-tein (E) g	Fat (F) g
Miscellaneous Items—Con.							
727	Vinegar, cider	1 tbsp	15	94	TR	TR	0
728	White sauce, medium, with enriched flour	1 cup	250	73	405	10	31
	Yeast						
729	Baker's, dry, active	1 pkg	7	5	20	3	TR
730	Brewer's, dry	1 tbsp	8	5	25	3	TR

[70]Value may vary from 6 to 60 mg.

| | Fatty Acids | | | | | | | | | | | |
| | Unsaturated | | | | | | | | | | | |
Satu-rated (Total) (G) g	Oleic (H) g	Lino-leic (I) g	Carbo-hydrate (J) g	Calcium (K) mg	Phos-phorus (L) mg	Iron (M) mg	Potas-sium (N) mg	Vitamin A Value (O) I.U.	Thiamin (P) mg	Ribo-flavin (Q) mg	Niacin (R) mg	Ascorbic Acid (S) mg
0	0	0	1	1	1	0.1	15	—	—	—	—	—
19.3	7.8	0.8	22	288	233	0.5	348	1,150	0.12	0.43	0.7	2
—	—	—	3	3	90	1.1	140	TR	0.16	0.38	2.6	TR
—	—	—	3	[70]17	140	1.4	152	TR	1.25	0.34	3.0	TR

Nutrients in Indicated Quantity

APPENDIX H: RELATIVE RATIOS
OF POLYUNSATURATED FAT AND SATURATED
FAT (P/S RATIO) IN REPRESENTATIVE FOODS

P/S Ratio	Foods
High >2.5:1	Almonds Corn oil Cottonseed oil Mayonnaise (made with oils in this group) Safflower oil Sesame oil Soft margarines Soybean oil Sunflower oil Walnuts
Medium high 2:1	Chicken Fish Peanut oil Semisolid margarines
Medium 1:1	Beef heart and liver Hydrogenated or hardened vegetable oils (shortenings, special products) Pecans Peanuts, peanut butter Solid margarines
Low 0.1–0.5:1	Chicken liver Lamb Lard Olive oil Palm oil Pork Veal
Very low <0.1:1	Beef Butter, cream Coconut oil Egg yolk Whole milk and milk products

APPENDIX I: SODIUM AND POTASSIUM CONTENT OF FOODS

Food	Approximate Amount	Weight (gm)	Sodium (mEq)	Potassium (mEq)
Meat Group				
Meat (cooked)				
Beef	1 oz	30	0.8	2.8
Ham	1 oz	30	14.3	2.6
Lamb	1 oz	30	0.9	2.2
Pork	1 oz	30	0.9	3.0
Veal	1 oz	30	1.0	3.8
Liver	1 oz	30	2.4	3.2
Sausage, pork	2 links	40	16.5	2.8
Beef, dried	2 slices	20	37.0	1.0
Cold cuts	1 slice	45	25.0	2.7
Frankfurters	1	50	24.0	3.0
Fowl				
Chicken	1 oz	30	1.0	3.0
Goose	1 oz	30	1.6	4.6
Duck	1 oz	30	1.0	2.2
Turkey	1 oz	30	1.2	2.8
Egg	1	50	2.7	1.8
Fish	1 oz	30	1.0	2.6
Salmon				
Fresh	$\frac{1}{4}$ cup	30	0.6	2.3
Canned	$\frac{1}{4}$ cup	30	4.6	2.6
Tuna				
Fresh	$\frac{1}{4}$ cup	30	0.5	2.2
Canned	$\frac{1}{4}$ cup	30	10.4	2.3
Sardines	3 medium	35	12.5	4.5
Shellfish				
Clams	5 small	50	2.6	2.3
Lobster	1 small tail	40	3.7	1.8
Oysters	5 small	70	2.1	1.5
Scallops	1 large	50	5.7	6.0
Shrimp	5 small	30	1.8	1.7
Cheese				
Cheese, American or Cheddar type	1 slice	30	9.1	0.6
Cheese foods	1 slice	30	15.0	0.8
Cheese spreads	2 tbsp	30	15.0	0.8
Cottage cheese	$\frac{1}{4}$ cup	50	5.0	1.1
Peanut butter	2 tbsp	30	7.8	5.0
Peanuts, unsalted	25	25	—	4.5

(Continued)

APPENDIX I: *(Continued)*

Food	Approximate Amount	Weight (gm)	Sodium (mEq)	Potassium (mEq)
Fat Group				
Avocado	$\frac{1}{8}$	30	—	4.6
Bacon	1 slice	5	2.2	0.6
Butter or margarine	1 tsp	5	2.2	—
Cooking fat	1 tsp	5	—	—
Cream				
Half and half	2 tbsp	30	0.6	1.0
Sour	2 tbsp	30	0.4	—
Whipped	2 tbsp	15	0.3	1.0
Cream cheese	1 tbsp	15	1.7	—
Mayonnaise	1 tsp	5	1.3	—
Nuts				
Almonds, slivered	5 (2 tsp)	6	—	0.8
Pecans	4 halves	5	—	0.8
Walnuts	5 halves	10	—	1.0
Oil, salad	1 tsp	5	—	—
Olives, green	3 medium	30	31.3	0.4
Bread Group				
Bread	1 slice	25	5.5	0.7
Biscuit	1 (2-in. diameter)	35	9.6	0.7
Muffin	1 (2-in. diameter)	35	7.3	1.2
Cornbread	1 ($1\frac{1}{2}$-in. cube)	35	11.3	1.7
Roll	1 (2-in. diameter)	25	5.5	0.6
Bun	1	30	6.6	0.7
Pancake	1 (4-in. diameter)	45	8.8	1.1
Waffle	$\frac{1}{2}$ square	35	8.5	1.0
Cereals				
Cooked	$\frac{2}{3}$ cup	140	8.7	2.0
Dry, flake	$\frac{2}{3}$ cup	20	8.7	0.6
Dry, puffed	$1\frac{1}{2}$ cups	20	—	1.5
Shredded wheat	1 biscuit	20	—	2.2
Crackers				
Graham	3	20	5.8	2.0
Melba toast	4	20	5.5	0.7
Oyster	20	20	9.6	0.6
Ritz	6	20	9.5	0.5
Rye-Krisp	3	30	11.5	3.0
Saltines	6	20	9.6	0.6
Soda	3	20	9.6	0.6
Dessert				
Commercial gelatin	$\frac{1}{2}$ cup	100	2.2	—
Ice cream	$\frac{1}{2}$ cup	75	2.0	3.0

APPENDIX I: (Continued)

Food	Approximate Amount	Weight (gm)	Sodium (mEq)	Potassium (mEq)
Sherbet	$\frac{1}{3}$ cup	50	—	—
Angel food cake	$1\frac{1}{2} \times 1\frac{1}{2}$ i.	25	3.0	0.6
Sponge cake	$1\frac{1}{2} \times 1\frac{1}{2}$ in.	25	1.8	0.6
Vanilla wafers	5	15	1.7	—
Floor products				
Cornstarch	2 tbsp	15	—	—
Macaroni	$\frac{1}{4}$ cup	50	—	0.8
Noodles	$\frac{1}{4}$ cup	50	—	0.6
Rice	$\frac{1}{4}$ cup	50	—	0.9
Spaghetti	$\frac{1}{4}$ cup	50	—	0.8
Tapioca	2 tbsp	15	—	—
Vegetable Group[a]				
Artichokes	1 large bud	100	1.3	7.7
Asparagus				
Cooked	$\frac{1}{2}$ cup	100	—	4.7
Canned[b]	$\frac{1}{2}$ cup	100	10.0	3.6
Frozen	$\frac{1}{2}$ cup	100	—	5.5
Beans, dried (cooked)	$\frac{1}{2}$ cup	90	—	10.0
Beans, lima	$\frac{1}{2}$ cup	90	—	9.5
Bean sprouts	$\frac{1}{2}$ cup	100	—	4.0
Beans, green or wax				
Fresh or frozen	$\frac{1}{2}$ cup	100	—	4.0
Canned[b]	$\frac{1}{2}$ cup	100	10.0	2.5
Beet greens	$\frac{1}{2}$ cup	100	3.0	8.5
Beets	$\frac{1}{2}$ cup	100	1.8	5.0
Broccoli	$\frac{1}{2}$ cup	100	—	7.0
Brussels sprouts	$\frac{2}{3}$ cup	100	—	7.6
Cabbage, cooked	$\frac{1}{2}$ cup	100	0.6	4.2
Raw	1 cup	100	0.9	6.0
Carrots, cooked	$\frac{1}{2}$ cup	100	1.4	5.7
Raw	1 large	100	2.0	8.8
Cauliflower, cooked	1 cup	100	0.4	5.2
Celery, raw	1 cup	100	5.4	9.0
Chard, Swiss	$\frac{3}{5}$ cup	100	3.7	8.0
Collards	$\frac{1}{2}$ cup	100	0.8	6.0
Corn				
Canned[b]	$\frac{1}{3}$ cup	80	8.0	2.0
Fresh	$\frac{1}{2}$ ear	100	—	2.0
Frozen	$\frac{1}{3}$ cup	80	—	3.7
Cress, garden (cooked)	$\frac{1}{2}$ cup	100	0.5	7.2
Cucumber	1 medium	100	0.3	4.0

(Continued)

APPENDIX I: *(Continued)*

Food	Approximate Amount	Weight (gm)	Sodium (mEq)	Potassium (mEq)
Vegetable Group[a] (Continued)				
Dandelion greens	½ cup	100	2.0	6.0
Eggplant	½ cup	100	—	3.8
Hominy (dry)	¼ cup	36	4.1	—
Kale, cooked	¾ cup	100	2.0	5.6
Frozen	½ cup	100	1.0	5.0
Kohlrabi	⅔ cup	100	—	6.6
Leeks, raw	3–4	100	—	9.0
Lettuce	varies	100	0.4	4.5
Mushrooms, raw	4 large	100	0.7	10.6
Mustard greens	½ cup	100	0.8	4.4
Okra	½ cup	100	—	4.4
Onions, cooked	½ cup	100	—	2.8
Parsnips	⅔ cup	100	0.3	9.7
Peas				
Canned[b]	½ cup	100	10.0	1.2
Dried	½ cup	90	1.5	6.8
Fresh	½ cup	100	—	2.5
Frozen	½ cup	100	2.5	1.7
Pepper, green or red				
Cooked	½ cup	100	—	5.5
Raw	1	100	0.5	4.0
Popcorn	1 cup	15	—	—
Potato				
Potato chips	1 oz	30	13.0	3.7
White, baked	½ cup	100	—	13.0
White, boiled	½ cup	100	—	7.3
Sweet, baked	¼ cup	50	0.4	4.0
Pumpkin	½ cup	100	—	6.3
Radishes	10	100	0.8	8.0
Rutabagas	½ cup	100	—	4.4
Sauerkraut	⅔ cup	100	32.0	3.5
Spinach	½ cup	100	2.2	8.5
Squash	½ cup	100	—	3.5
Squash, winter				
Baked	½ cup	100	—	12.0
Boiled	½ cup	100	—	6.5
Tomatoes	½ cup	100	—	6.5
Tomato juice	½ cup	100	0.7	3.8
Turnip greens	½ cup	100	0.7	3.8
Turnips	½ cup	100	1.5	4.8

APPENDIX I: *(Continued)*

Food	Approximate Amount	Weight (gm)	Sodium (mEq)	Potassium (mEq)
Milk Group				
Whole milk	1 cup	240	5.2	8.8
Evaporated whole milk	½ cup	120	6.0	9.2
Powdered whole milk	¼ cup	30	5.2	10.0
Buttermilk	1 cup	240	13.6	8.5
Skim milk	1 cup	240	5.2	8.8
Powdered skim milk	¼ cup	30	6.9	13.5
Fruit Group				
Figs				
Canned	½ cup	120	—	4.6
Dried	1 small	15	—	2.5
Fresh	1 large	60	—	5.0
Fruit cocktail	½ cup	120	—	5.0
Grapes				
Canned	⅓ cup	80	—	2.2
Fresh	15	80	—	3.2
Juice				
Bottled	¼ cup	60	—	2.8
Frozen	⅓ cup	80	—	2.4
Grapefruit				
Fresh	½ medium	120	—	3.6
Juice	½ cup	120	—	4.1
Sections	¾ cup	150	—	5.1
Mandarin orange	¾ cup	200	—	6.5
Mango	½ small	70	—	3.4
Melon				
Cantaloupe	½ small	200	—	13.0
Honeydew	¼ medium	200	—	13.0
Watermelon	½ slice	200	—	5.0
Nectarine	1 medium	80	—	6.0
Orange				
Fresh	1 medium	100	—	5.1
Juice	½ cup	120	—	5.7
Sections	½ cup	100	—	5.1
Papaya	½ cup	120	—	7.0
Peach				
Canned	½ cup	120	—	4.0
Dried	2 halves	20	—	5.0
Fresh	1 medium	120	—	6.2
Nectar	½ cup	120	—	2.4

(Continued)

APPENDIX I: (Continued)

Food	Approximate Amount	Weight (gm)	Sodium (mEq)	Potassium (mEq)
Fruit Group (Continued)				
Pear				
Canned	½ cup	120	—	2.5
Dried	2 halves	20	—	3.0
Fresh	1 small	80	—	2.6
Nectar	⅓ cup	80	—	0.9
Pineapple				
Canned	½ cup	120	—	3.0
Fresh	½ cup	80	—	3.0
Juice	⅓ cup	80	—	3.0
Plums				
Canned	½ cup	120	—	4.5
Fresh	2 medium	80	—	4.1
Prunes	2 medium	15	—	2.6
Juice	¼ cup	60	—	3.6
Raisins	1 tbsp	15	—	2.9
Rhubarb	½ cup	100	—	6.5
Tangerines				
Fresh	2 small	100	—	3.2
Juice	½ cup	120	—	5.5
Sections	½ cup	100	—	3.2

Source: Reproduced with permission from *Mayo Clinic Diet Manual,* 4th ed. Philadelphia: W.B. Saunders Company, 1971.

[a]Value for products without added salt.

[b]Estimated average based on addition of salt, approximately 0.6% of the finished product.

Note: To convert mEq to mg multiply mEq by 23 (sodium) or 39 (potassium) mEq $\times$ 23 = mg of sodium mEq $\times$ 39 = mg of potassium.

APPENDIX J: PHYSICAL GROWTH NCHS PERCENTILES

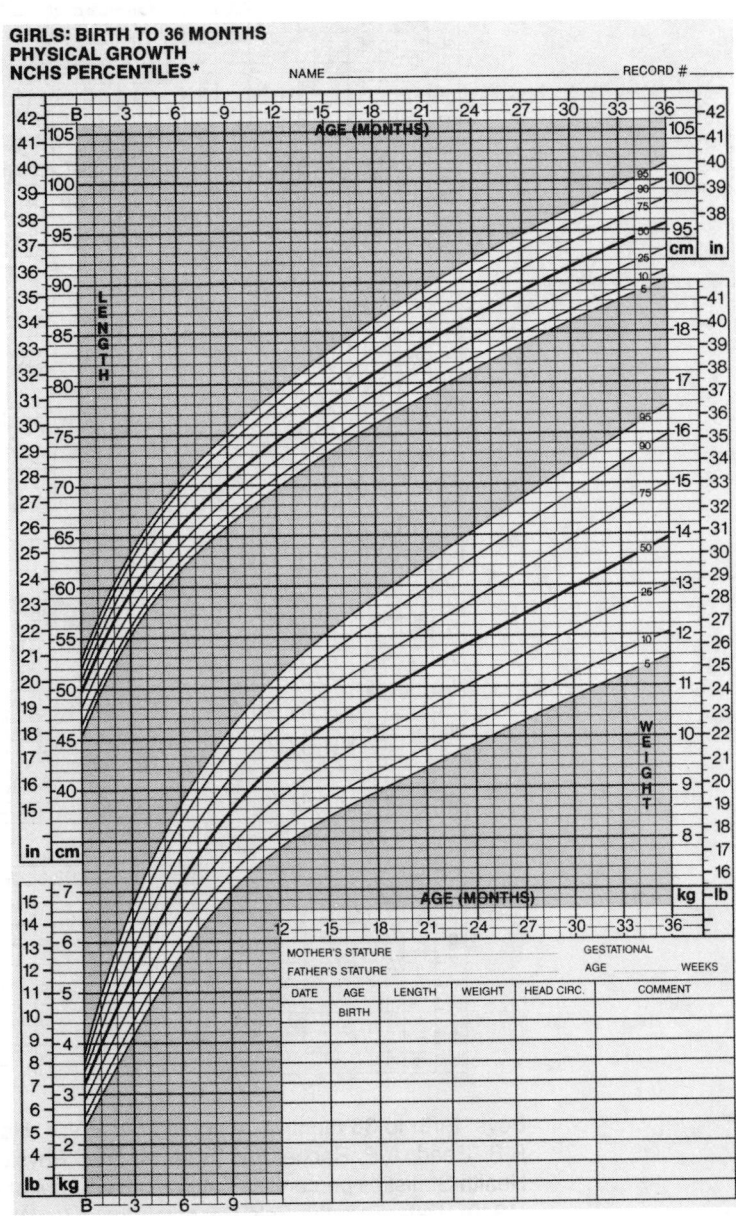

Girls: Birth to 36 months. Adapted from P.V.V. Hamill, T.A. Drizd, C.L. Johnson, R.B. Reed, A.F. Roche, and W.M. Moore: "Physical growth: National Center for Health Statistics percentiles." *American Journal of Clinical Nutrition, 32,* 607–629 (1979). Data from the Fels Research Institute, Wright State University School of Medicine, Yellow Springs, Ohio. © 1982 Ross Laboratories

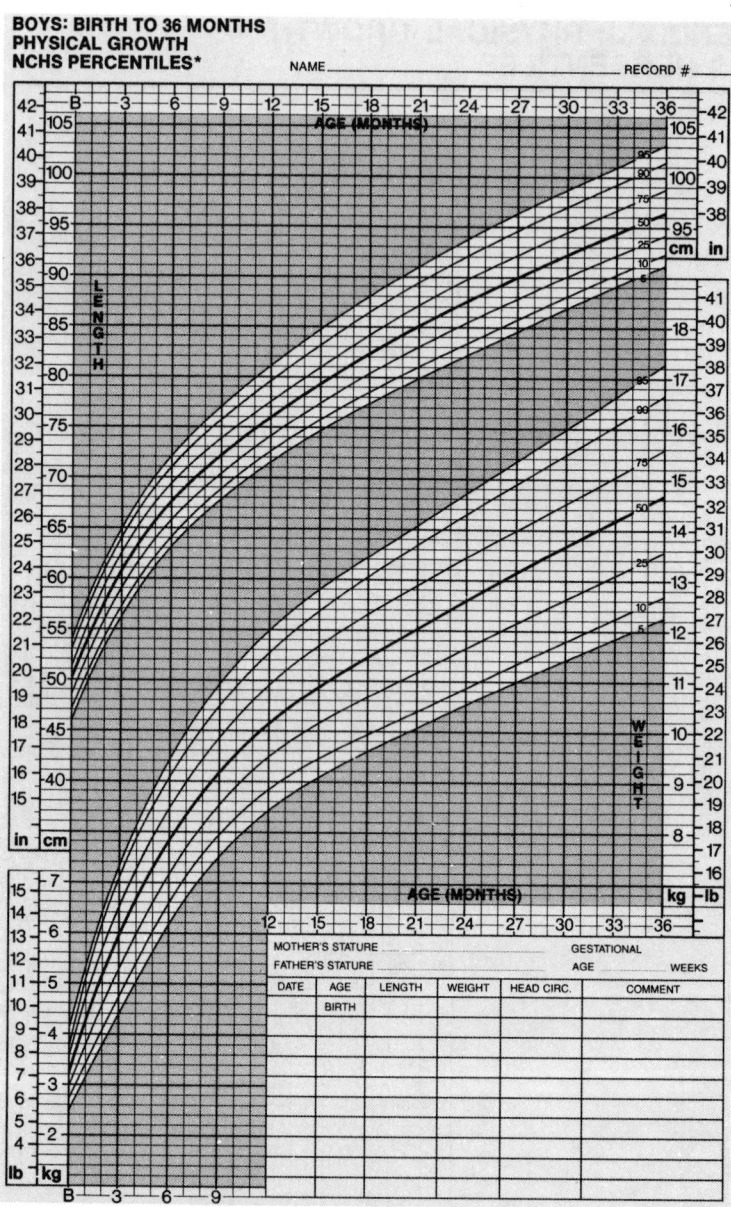

Boys: Birth to 36 months. Adapted from P.V.V. Hamill, T.A. Drizd, C.L. Johnson, R.B. Reed, A.F. Roche, and W.M. Moore: "Physical growth: National Center for Health Statistics percentiles." *American Journal of Clinical Nutrition, 32,* 607–629 (1979). Data from the Fels Research Institute, Wright State University School of Medicine, Yellow Springs, Ohio. © 1982 Ross Laboratories

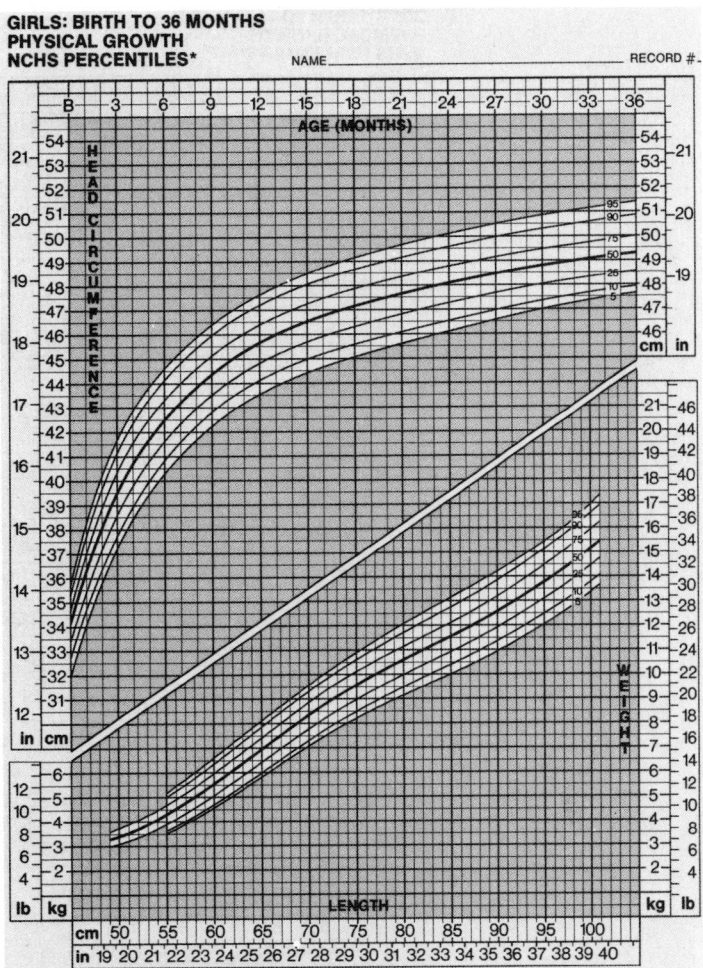

Girls: Birth to 36 months. Adapted from P.V.V. Hamill, T.A. Drizd, C.L. Johnson, R.B. Reed, A.F. Roche, and W.M. Moore: "Physical growth: National Center for Health Statistics percentiles." *American Journal of Clinical Nutrition, 32,* 607–629 (1979). Data from the Fels Research Institute, Wright State University School of Medicine, Yellow Springs, Ohio. © 1982 Ross Laboratories

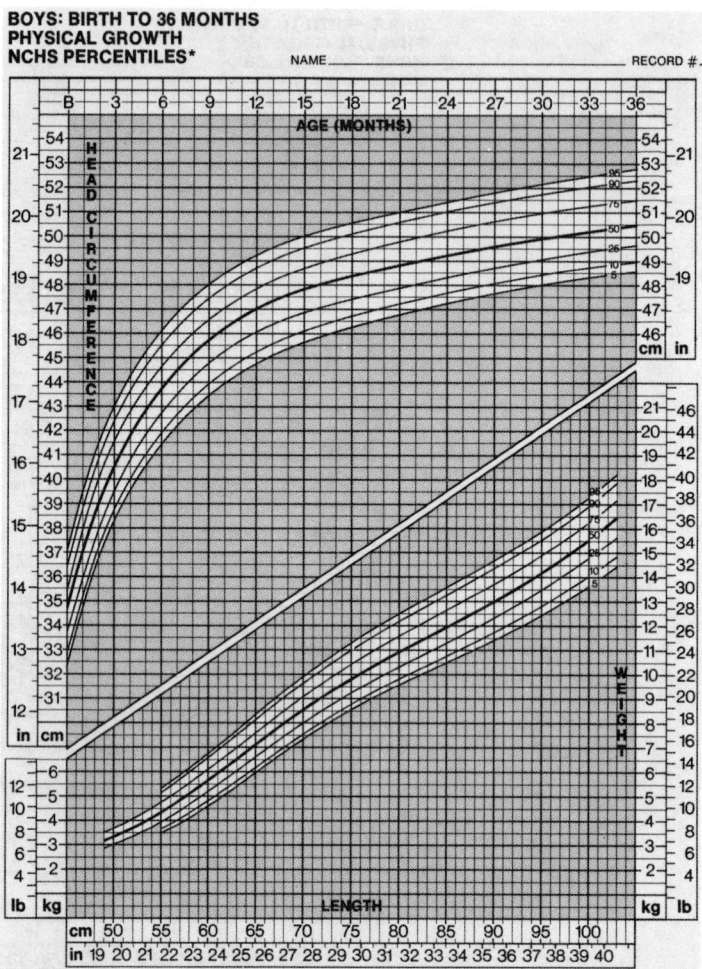

Boys: Birth to 36 months. Adapted from P.V.V. Hamill, T.A. Drizd, C.L. Johnson, R.B. Reed, A.F. Roche, and W.M. Moore: "Physical growth: National Center for Health Statistics percentiles." *American Journal of Clinical Nutrition, 32,* 607–629 (1979). Data from the Fels Research Institute, Wright State University School of Medicine, Yellow Springs, Ohio. © 1982 Ross Laboratories

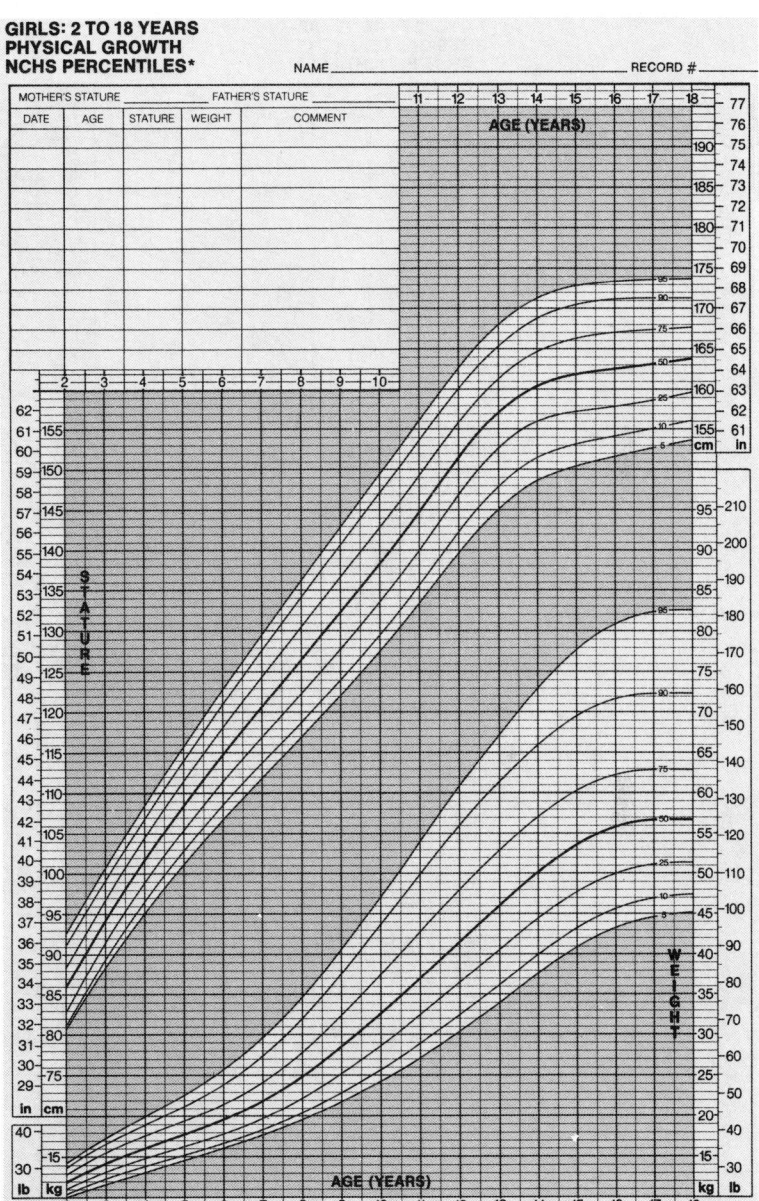

Girls: 2 to 18 years. Adapted from P.V.V. Hamill, T.A. Drizd, C.L. Johnson, R.B. Reed, A.F. Roche, and W.M. Moore: "Physical growth: National Center for Health Statistics percentiles." *American Journal of Clinical Nutrition, 32,* 607–629 (1979). Data from the National Center for Health Statistics (NCHS) Hyattsville, Md. © 1982 Ross Laboratories

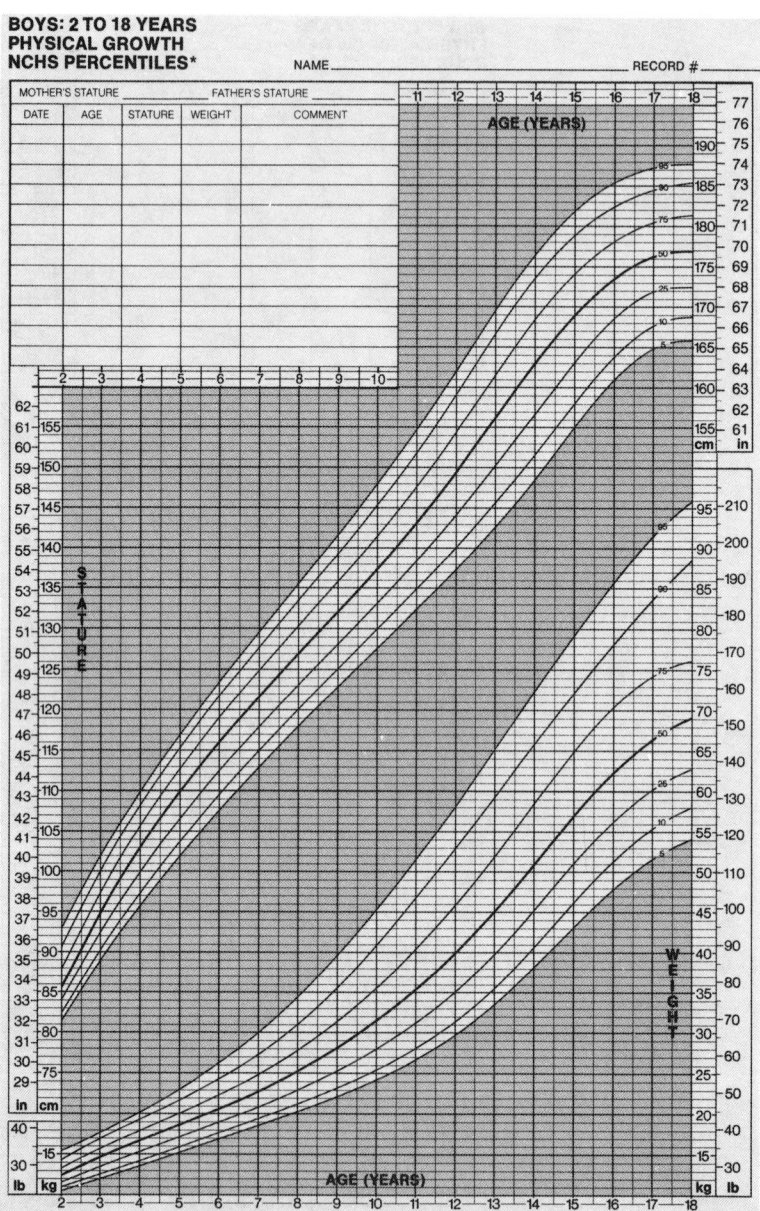

Boys: 2 to 18 years. Adapted from P.V.V. Hamill, T.A. Drizd, C.L. Johnson, R.B. Reed, A.F. Roche, and W.M. Moore: "Physical growth: National Center for Health Statistics percentiles." *American Journal of Clinical Nutrition, 32,* 607–629 (1979). Data from the National Center for Health Statistics (NCHS) Hyattsville, Md. © 1982 Ross Laboratories

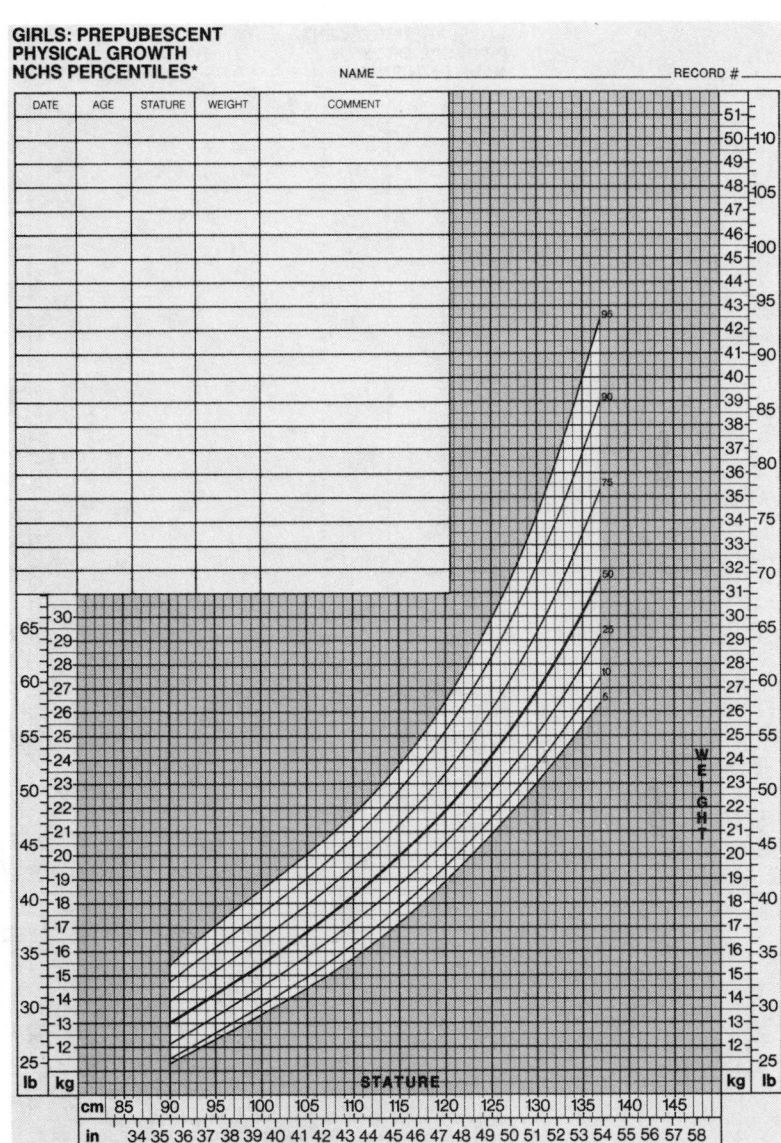

Girls: Prepubescent. Adapted from P.V.V. Hamill, T.A. Drizd, C.L. Johnson, R.B. Reed, A.F. Roche, and A.M. Moore: "Physical growth: National Center for Health Statistics percentiles." *American Journal of Clinical Nutrition, 32,* 607–629 (1979). Data from the National Center for Health Statistics (NCHS) Hyattsville, Md. © 1982 Ross Laboratories

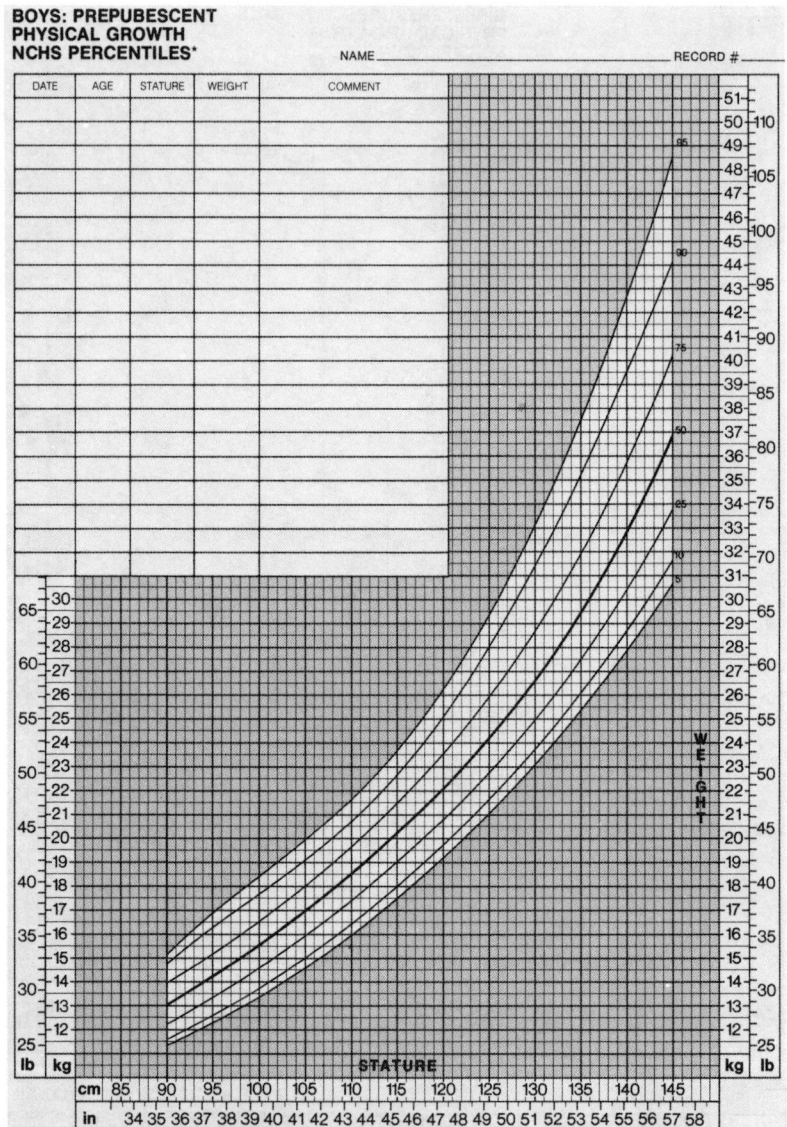

Boys: Prepubescent. Adapted from P.V.V. Hamill, T.A. Drizd, C.L. Johnson, R.B. Reed, A.F. Roche, and W.M. Moore: "Physical growth: National Center for Health Statistics percentiles." *American Journal of Clinical Nutrition, 32,* 607–629 (1979). Data from the National Center for Health Statistics (NCHS) Hyattsville, Md. © 1982 Ross Laboratories

APPENDIX K: MID-UPPER-ARM CIRCUMFERENCE PERCENTILES (cm)[a]

	Female Percentiles					Male Percentiles				
Age (yr)	5th	25th	50th	75th	95th	5th	25th	50th	75th	95th
1	13.8	14.8	15.6	16.4	17.7	14.2	15.0	15.9	17.0	18.3
2	14.2	15.2	16.0	16.7	18.4	14.1	15.3	16.2	17.0	18.5
3	14.3	15.8	16.7	17.5	18.9	15.0	16.0	16.7	17.5	19.0
4	14.9	16.0	16.9	17.7	19.1	14.9	16.2	17.1	18.0	19.2
5	15.3	16.5	17.5	18.5	21.1	15.3	16.7	17.5	18.5	20.4
6	15.6	17.0	17.6	18.7	21.1	15.5	16.7	17.9	18.8	22.8
7	16.4	17.4	18.3	19.9	23.1	16.2	17.7	18.7	20.1	23.0
8	16.8	18.3	19.5	21.4	26.1	16.2	17.7	19.0	20.2	24.5
9	17.8	19.4	21.1	22.4	26.0	17.5	18.7	20.0	21.7	25.7
10	17.4	19.3	21.0	22.8	26.5	18.1	19.6	21.0	23.1	27.4
11	18.5	20.8	22.4	24.8	30.3	18.6	20.2	22.3	24.4	28.0
12	19.4	21.6	23.7	25.6	29.4	19.3	21.4	23.2	25.4	30.3
13	20.2	22.3	24.3	27.1	33.8	19.4	22.8	24.7	26.3	30.1
14	21.4	23.7	25.2	27.2	32.2	22.0	23.7	25.3	28.3	32.3
15	20.8	23.9	25.4	27.9	32.2	22.2	24.4	26.4	28.4	32.0
16	21.8	24.1	25.8	28.3	33.4	24.4	26.2	27.8	30.3	34.3
17	22.0	24.1	26.4	29.5	35.0	24.6	26.7	28.5	30.8	34.7
18	22.2	24.1	25.8	28.1	32.5	24.5	27.6	29.7	32.1	37.9
19–25	21.1	24.7	26.5	29.0	34.5	26.2	28.8	30.8	33.1	37.2
25–35	23.3	25.6	27.7	30.4	36.8	27.1	30.0	31.9	34.2	37.5
35–45	24.1	26.7	29.0	31.7	37.8	27.8	30.5	32.6	34.5	37.4
45–55	24.2	27.4	29.9	32.8	38.4	26.7	30.1	32.2	34.2	37.6
55–65	24.3	28.0	30.3	33.5	38.5	25.8	29.6	31.7	33.6	36.9
65–75	24.0	27.4	29.9	32.6	37.3	24.8	28.5	30.7	32.5	35.5

Source: Adapted from A.R. Frisancho: "New norms of upper limb fat and muscle areas for assessment of nutritional status," *American Journal of Clinical Nutrition, 34,* 2540 (1981). Copyright *American Journal of Clinical Nutrition,* American Society for Clinical Nutrition.

[a]Data derived from the Health and Nutrition Examination Survey data of 1971–1974, using same population samples as those of the National Center for Health Statistics (NCHS) growth percentiles for children.

APPENDIX L: TRICEPS SKINFOLD
PERCENTILES (mm)[a]

Age (yr)	Female Percentiles					Male Percentiles				
	5th	25th	50th	75th	95th	5th	25th	50th	75th	95th
1	6	8	10	12	16	6	8	10	12	16
2	6	9	10	12	16	6	8	10	12	15
3	7	9	11	12	15	6	8	10	11	15
4	7	8	10	12	16	6	8	9	11	14
5	6	8	10	12	18	6	8	9	11	15
6	6	8	10	12	16	5	7	8	10	16
7	6	9	11	13	18	5	7	9	12	17
8	6	9	12	15	24	5	7	8	10	16
9	8	10	13	16	22	6	7	10	13	18
10	7	10	12	17	27	6	8	10	14	21
11	7	10	13	18	28	6	8	11	16	24
12	8	11	14	18	27	6	8	11	14	28
13	8	12	15	21	30	5	7	10	14	26
14	9	13	16	21	28	4	7	9	14	24
15	8	12	17	21	32	4	6	8	11	24
16	10	15	18	22	31	4	6	8	12	22
17	10	13	19	24	37	5	6	8	12	19
18	10	15	18	22	30	4	6	9	13	24
19–25	10	14	18	24	34	4	7	10	15	22
25–35	10	16	21	27	37	5	8	12	16	24
35–45	12	18	23	29	38	5	8	12	16	23
45–55	12	20	25	30	40	6	8	12	15	25
55–65	12	20	25	31	38	5	8	11	14	22
65–75	12	18	24	29	36	4	8	11	15	22

Source: Adapted from A.R. Frisancho: New norms of upper limb fat and muscle areas for assessment of nutritional status. *American Journal of Clinical Nutrition, 34,* 2540 (1981). Copyright *American Journal of Clinical Nutrition,* American Society for Clinical Nutrition.

[a]Data derived from the Health and Nutrition Examination Survey data of 1971–1974, using same population samples as those of the National Center for Health Statistics (NCHS) growth percentiles for children.

APPENDIX M: RECOMMENDED ENERGY INTAKE

Age (years)	Weight (kg)	Weight (lb)	Height (cm)	Height (in.)	Energy needs[a] (cal)	Energy needs[a] (MJ)[b]
Infants						
0.0–0.5	6	13	60	24	kg × 115 (95–145)	kg × 0.48
0.5–1.0	9	20	71	28	kg × 105 (80–135)	kg × 0.44
Children						
1–3	13	29	90	35	1,300 (900–1,800)	5.5
4–6	20	44	112	44	1,700 (1,300–2,300)	7.1
7–10	28	62	132	52	2,400 (1,650–3,300)	10.1
Males						
11–14	45	99	157	62	2,700 (2,000–3,700)	11.3
15–18	66	145	176	69	2,800 (2,100–3,900)	11.8
19–22	70	154	177	70	2,900 (2,500–3,300)	12.2
23–50	70	154	178	70	2,700 (2,300–3,100)	11.3
51–75	70	154	178	70	2,400 (2,000–2,800)	10.1
76+	70	154	178	70	2,050 (1,650–2,450)	8.6
Females						
11–14	46	101	157	62	2,200 (1,500–3,000)	9.2
15–18	55	120	163	64	2,100 (1,200–3,000)	8.8
19–22	55	120	163	64	2,100 (1,700–2,500)	8.8
23–50	55	120	163	64	2,000 (1,600–2,400)	8.4
51–75	55	120	163	64	1,800 (1,400–2,200)	7.6
76+	55	120	163	64	1,600 (1,200–2,000)	6.7
Pregnant					+300	
Lactating					+500	

[a]The energy allowances for the young adults are for men and women doing light work. The allowances for the two older age groups represent mean energy needs over these age spans, allowing for a 2% decrease in basal (resting) metabolic rate per decade and a reduction in activity of 200 cal per day for men and women between 51 and 75 years, 500 cal for men over 75 years, and 400 cal for women over 75. The customary range of daily energy output, shown in parentheses, is based on a variation in energy needs of ±400 cal at any one age, emphasizing the wide range of energy intakes appropriate for any group of people. Energy allowances for children through age 18 are based on median energy intakes of children these ages followed in longitudinal growth studies. The values in parentheses are tenth and ninetieth percentiles of energy intake, to indicate the range of energy consumption among children of these ages.
[b]MJ stands for megajoules (1 MJ = 1,000 kJ).

APPENDIX N: CONVERSION TABLES

	To Change	To	Multiply By
W			
E			
I	Ounces	Grams	30[a]
G	Pounds	Kilograms	0.45
H	Grams	Ounces	0.035
T	Kilograms	Pounds	2.2
	Teaspoons	Milliliters	5
	Tablespoons	Milliliters	15
	Fluid ounces	Milliliters	30
V	Cups	Liters	0.24
O	Pints	Liters	0.47
L	Quarts	Liters	0.95
U	Gallons	Liters	3.8
M	Milliliters	Fluid ounces	0.03
E	Liters	Pints	2.1
	Liters	Quarts	1.06
	Liters	Gallons	0.26
L	Inches	Centimeters	2.5
E	Feet	Centimeters	30
N	Yards	Meters	0.9
G	Millimeters	Inches	0.04
T	Centimeters	Inches	0.4
H	Meters	Feet	3.3
	Meters	Yards	1.1

Source: Exchange Lists for Meal Planning. Copyright American Diabetes Association, Inc., The American Dietetic Association, 1976.

[a]The precise figure is 28.25. However, some dietitians find it more convenient to use 30.

APPENDIX O: RECOMMENDED FOOD INTAKE FOR GOOD NUTRITION[a] FOR CHILDREN AND ADOLESCENTS

Food Group	Servings/Day	1 Year	2–3 Years	4–5 Years	6–9 Years	10–12 Years	13–15 Years
			Average Size of Servings				
Milk and cheese (1.5 oz cheese = 1 C milk) (C = 1 cup − 8 oz or 240 g)	4	$\frac{1}{2}$ C	$\frac{1}{2}$–$\frac{3}{4}$ C	$\frac{3}{4}$ C	$\frac{3}{4}$–1 C	1 C	1 C
Meat group (protein foods)	3 or more						
Egg		1	1	1	1	1	1 or more
Lean meat, fish, poultry (liver once a week)		2 tbsp	2 tbsp	4 tbsp	2–3 oz (4–6 tbsp)	3–4 oz	4 oz or more
Peanut butter			1 tbsp	2 tbsp	2–3 tbsp	3 tbsp	3 tbsp
Fruits and vegetables Vitamin C source (citrus fruits, berries, tomato, cabbage, cantaloupe)	At least 4, including 1 or more (twice as much tomato as citrus)	$\frac{1}{3}$ C citrus	$\frac{1}{2}$ C	$\frac{1}{2}$ C	1 medium orange	1 medium orange	1 medium orange
Vitamin A source (green or yellow fruits and vegetables)	1 or more	2 tbsp	3 tbsp	4 tbsp ($\frac{1}{4}$ C)	$\frac{1}{4}$ C	$\frac{1}{3}$ C	$\frac{1}{2}$ C
Other vegetables (potato and legumes, etc.) or	2	2 tbsp	3 tbsp	4 tbsp ($\frac{1}{4}$ C)	$\frac{1}{3}$ C	$\frac{1}{2}$ C	$\frac{3}{4}$ C
Other fruits (apple, banana, etc.)		$\frac{1}{4}$ C	$\frac{1}{3}$ C	$\frac{1}{2}$ C	1 medium	1 medium	1 medium
Cereals (whole grain or enriched)	At least 4						
Bread		$\frac{1}{2}$ slice	1 slice	1$\frac{1}{2}$ slices	1–2 slices	2 slices	2 slices
Ready-to-eat cereals		$\frac{1}{2}$ oz	$\frac{3}{4}$ oz	1 oz	1 oz	1 oz	1 oz
Cooked cereal (including macaroni, spaghetti, rice, etc.)		$\frac{1}{4}$ C	$\frac{1}{3}$ C	$\frac{1}{2}$ C	$\frac{1}{2}$ C	$\frac{3}{4}$ C	1 C or more
Fats and carbohydrates	To meet caloric needs						
Butter, margarine, mayonnaise, oils 1 tbsp = 100 calories (kcal)		1 tbsp	1 tbsp	1 tbsp	2 tbsp	2 tbsp	2–4 tbsp

(Continued)

APPENDIX O: *(Continued)*

			Average Size of Servings				
Food Group	*Servings/Day*	*1 Year*	*2–3 Years*	*4–5 Years*	*6–9 Years*	*10–12 Years*	*13–15 Years*
Desserts and sweets: 100-calorie portions as follows: $\frac{1}{3}$ C pudding or ice cream 2–3 in. cookies, 1 oz cake, $1\frac{1}{3}$ oz pie, 2 tbsp jelly, jam, honey, sugar		1 portion	$1\frac{1}{2}$ portions	$1\frac{1}{2}$ portions	3 portions	3 portions	3–6 portions

Source: Reprinted with permission from V.C. Vaughan and R.J. McKay, editors, *Nelson Textbook of Pediatrics,* 10th ed., p. 159. © 1975 by the W. B. Saunders Company, Philadelphia.

[a]Based on food groups and the average size of servings at different age levels.

APPENDIX P: LEVELS OF NUTRITIONAL ASSESSMENT FOR INFANTS AND CHILDREN

Level of Approach[a]	History		Clinical Evaluation	Laboratory Evaluation
	Dietary	Medical and Socioeconomic		
		Birth to 24 Months		
Minimal	1. Source of iron 2. Vitamin supplement 3. Milk intake (type and amount)	1. Birth weight 2. Length of gestation 3. Serious or chronic illness 4. Use of medicines	1. Body weight and length 2. Gross defects	1. Hematocrit 2. Hemoglobin

Mid-level	1. Semiquantitative
	  a. Iron-cereal, meat, egg yolks, supplement
	  b. Energy nutrients
	  c. Micronutrients: calcium, niacin, riboflavin, vitamin C
	  d. Protein
	2. Food intolerances
	3. Baby foods: processed commercially, home cooked
		1. Family history: diabetes, tuberculosis
		2. Maternal: height, prenatal care
		3. Infant: immunizations, tuberculin test
			1. Head circumference
			2. Skin color, pallor, turgor
			3. Subcutaneous tissue paucity, excess
				1. RBC morphology
				2. Serum iron
				3. Total iron-binding capacity
				4. Sickle cell testing

In-depth level	1. Quantitative 24-hour recall 2. Dietary history	1. Prenatal details 2. Complications of delivery 3. Regular health supervision	1. Cranial bossing 2. Epiphyseal enlargement 3. Costochondral beading 4. Ecchymoses	Same as above, plus vitamin and appropriate enzyme assays, also protein and amino acids, hydroxyproline, etc., should be available
		For Ages 2 to 5 Years		
	Determine amount of intake	Probe about pica, medications	Add height at all levels, add arm circumference at all levels, add triceps skinfolds at in-depth level	Add serum lead at mid-level, add serum micronutrients (vitamin A, C, folate, etc.) at in-depth level

(Continued)

APPENDIX Q: (*Continued*)

INITIAL EVALUATION SUMMARY AND RECOMMENDATIONS

Adequacy of diet in terms of nutrients: _____

_____

_____

Anticipatory guidance (counseling needed for future developmental-nutritional needs)

_____

_____

_____

Follow-up: _____

_____

_____

_____

_____

Date: _____

Source: Reprinted with permission from Yolanda Gutierrez, M.S., Assistant Clinical Professor, Department of Family Health Care Nursing, University of California, San Francisco.

APPENDIX R: RANGE OF AVERAGE WATER REQUIREMENT OF CHILDREN AT DIFFERENT AGES UNDER ORDINARY CONDITIONS

Age	Average Body Weight (kg)	Total Water in 24 hours (ml)	Water per kg Body Weight in 24 hours (ml)
3 days	3.0	250–300	80–100
10 days	3.2	400–500	125–150
3 months	5.4	750–850	140–160
6 months	7.3	950–1,100	130–155
9 months	8.6	1,100–1,250	125–145
1 year	9.5	1,150–1,300	120–135
2 years	11.8	1,350–1,500	115–125
4 years	16.2	1,600–1,800	100–110
6 years	20.0	1,800–2,000	90–100
10 years	28.7	2,000–2,500	70–85
14 years	45.0	2,200–2,700	50–60
18 years	54.0	2,200–2,700	40–50

Source: Reprinted with permission from V.C. Vaughan, R.J. McKay, and R.E. Behrman, editors, *Nelson Textbook of Pediatrics,* 11th ed., Philadelphia: W.B. Saunders, 1979, p. 175.

GLOSSARY

Abscess Localized collection of pus in cavities formed by the disintegration of tissues.

Acetylcholine A neurotransmitter that transmits nerve impulses between certain types of neurons.

Acid ash diet A diet that includes foods that will form an acid urine.

Acidic An acid-forming substance. Some foods cause an acidic pH in the urine.

Acidosis A condition in which the pH of blood is below 7.35; can result in the denaturation of proteins.

Acid-base balance A balance of the amount of acid and base ions so that blood pH is within the normal range, 7.35–7.45.

Acid-resistant Something that is resistant to acid but susceptible to bases. An example is the enteric coating on some drugs.

Active transport Movement of molecules from a low concentration to a high concentration. Energy is required and involves carrier molecules.

Acute fulminating A condition that occurs suddenly with great intensity.

Acute glomerulonephritis A form of kidney disease that involves inflammation of the glomeruli.

Acute renal disease Sudden onset of kidney disease.

Acute renal failure Sudden onset of renal failure.

Acute respiratory failure (ARF) Inadequacy of the respiratory function in maintaining the body's need for an oxygen supply and for carbon dioxide removal while at rest.

Addison's disease A disease caused by insufficient secretion of adrenal hormones.

Adipose tissue Fat tissue.

Adolescence The period of life from 12 to about 20 years of age.

Adrenal gland A gland located on top of the kidneys that secretes several different hormones.

Adrenocorticotrophic hormone (ACTH) A hormone that is secreted by the anterior pituitary gland.

Adult respiratory distress syndrome (ARDS) A variety of acute lung lesions that cause deficient oxygenation of the blood.

Adult-onset obesity Obesity beginning in adulthood.

Aerobic respiration A process in cell respiration in which ATP molecules are synthesized and oxygen is required.

Air embolism Air bubbles in the blood as a result of air leaks through a catheter.

Albumin A blood protein that regulates the osmotic pressure of the blood.

Albuminuria Albumin in the urine.

Aldosterone A hormone secreted from the adrenal gland that regulates the levels of sodium and potassium.

Alimentary canal A muscular tube that extends from the mouth to the anus.

Alkalosis A condition in which the pH of blood is above 7.45; can result in the denaturation of proteins.

Alveolar surfactant A protein compound that is important in inflating the lungs.

Alzheimer's disease A condition that results from a depletion of acetylcholine and causes losses of neurons in the brain.

Amino acid The fundamental building block of proteins.

Amino acid content The number of essential amino acids present in a particular food.

Amino acid pool A region in which large numbers of amino acids are maintained, such as in the liver.

From the liver, the amino acids are distributed to the tissues.

Anabolic steroid Male hormone that is naturally secreted in large quantities during sexual maturity.

Anabolism A metabolic process whereby large molecules are synthesized from small ones.

Anaerobic (glycolysis) respiration A process in cell respiration in which ATP molecules are synthesized and oxygen is not required.

Anemia A condition in which the total quantity of red blood cells and hemoglobin is less than normal.

Angina pectoris Acute pain in the chest resulting from ischemia of the heart muscle.

Anhydrous Lacking water molecules; an example is anhydrous dextrose, which is found in food.

Anion Mineral that is negatively charged.

Anorexia A loss of appetite.

Anorexia nervosa A self-starvation disease that is characterized by severe disruption of the person's eating behavior.

Anthropometric measurement Measurement of the size, weight, and proportions of the human body.

Antiarrhythmic Agent that prevents variations of the normal heart rhythm.

Antibiotic Chemical substance produced by bacteria, yeasts, and molds that is damaging to other cells such as disease-producing bacteria.

Antibody Protein formed by the body to combat antigens.

Anticholinergic drug Drug that blocks the passage of impulses through the parasympathetic nerves.

Anticonvulsant Agent that suppresses convulsions; the drug Dilantin is an example of an anticonvulsant.

Antifungal An agent that destroys or checks the growth of fungi.

Antigen Foreign substance (usually a protein) that invades the body; can cause infections and allergic reactions.

Antihistamine Drug that counteracts inflammation or allergies.

Antihypertensive agent Agent that reduces high blood pressure.

Antineoplastic agent Cancer-fighting drug.

Antioxidant A compound that prevents oxidation.

Antipsychotic drugs Drugs that control the symptoms of mental disorders but not the causes.

Anti-inflammatory agent An agent that counteracts inflammation.

Anuria Less than 50 ml of urine per day excreted from the body.

Appetite A learned psychological response to food that is initiated for reasons other than the need for food.

Arachidonic A fatty acid that is derived from linoleic acid.

Ascending colon The portion of the large intestine that ascends upward on the right side of the body from the cecum to the liver.

Ascites The accumulation of fluids in the abdominal cavity.

Aseptic Free from infection or infectious material.

Aspiration pneumonia Regurgitation of the stomach contents and inhalation into the lungs.

Asthma A respiratory condition, characterized by recurrent attacks of wheezing, that may be due to bronchitis.

ATP Adenosine triphosphate. A high-energy compound that supplies energy for body processes.

Ataxia Uncoordinated gait.

Atelectasis A collapsed state of the lungs, which may involve all or part of the lungs.

Atheroma An abnormal mass of fatty or lipid material with a fibrous covering often found in the inner lining of arteries.

Atherosclerosis Accumulation of fatty plaques within medium-sized and large arteries.

Atrial arrhythmia Abnormal rhythm in the contractions of the atria in the heart.

Atrophy A decrease in the size of a normally developed organ.

Attention deficit disorder (ADD) Disorder such as hyperkinesia that can be seen in children.

Autodigestion Self-digestion.

Autoimmunity A condition in which the body forms antibodies against its own tissues.

Autosomal dominant trait A dominant gene that is present on one of the 22 pairs of genes known as *autosomes*.

Azotemia Presence of excess nitrogen in the blood.

Bacterial pneumonia A type of pneumonia in which the alveoli become filled with exudate that interferes with the exchange of gases.

Barrel chest An appearance of the chest often seen in people who suffer from chronic asthma attacks.

Basal energy expenditure (BEE) The amount of energy expended by a person at rest.

Basal metabolic rate The rate at which the body uses energy for maintenance of homeostasis at rest.

Basal region A region located at the base of the brain.

Basic A base-forming substance. Some foods cause a basic pH in the urine.

Behavior modification An approach to the correction of undesirable eating habits. This procedure involves the manipulation of environmental and behavioral variables.

Beta cell Cell in the pancreas that secretes insulin. These cells are often damaged in IDDM, causing an insulin deficiency.

Bile A fluid secreted by the liver that emulsifies fat molecules in the small intestine.

Bile salt Clear yellow or orange fluid secreted by the liver.

Biliary atresia Congenital destruction or closure of one or more bile ducts in the liver.

Bilirubin A pigment produced by the breakdown of heme and secreted into bile.

Binder compound Substance that inhibits absorption of calcium.

Binge eating Consumption of large amounts of food in a short period of time.

Biological value (BV) Measures the absorbed nitrogen that is retained for growth or maintenance and not excreted through the feces, urine, or skin.

Blackhead A plug of sebum within a hair follicle.

Bland diet A diet that restricts the use of many spicy foods.

Blood acidosis A condition in which blood pH is below 7.35. This condition can result from an excess amount of ketones.

Blood capillary Microscopic blood vessels through which nutrients and wastes are exchanged.

Blood lipid profile A measurement of the amounts of different classes of lipoproteins.

Blood urea nitrogen (BUN) Nitrogenous waste product formed in the liver when amino acids are deaminized.

Body composition The percentage of total body weight that is composed of fat, muscle, and water.

Body frame size The size of a person's body frame, with small, medium, and large being the three possibilities.

Body size Height and weight.

Body surface area (BSA) An estimate of the total body surface area. This measurement is important in burn situations for determining the level of nutritional care.

Bolus A round mass of food.

Bolus feeding Intermittent feeding of a formula as meals.

Bonding The formation of an emotional link between the mother and infant.

Bowman's capsule A proximal portion of a renal tubule that encloses the glomerulus of a nephron.

Bronchial pneumonia Inflammation of the bronchi in the lungs.

Bronchiogenic cancer A malignant tumor of the lung that originates in the epithelial lining of the bronchi.

Bronchitis Inflammation of the bronchi, the passageways to the lungs.

Buffer Compound in the blood that resists changes in pH with the addition of acids and bases.

Bulimarexia Purging of food.

Bulimia An enormous appetite that is satisfied by eating binges.

Cachexia A problem characterized by extreme weight loss, weakness, and severe wasting of tissues.

Calcidiol The inactive form of vitamin D that is stored in the liver.

Calcification The hardening of soft tissues due to an accumulation of calcium.

Calcitriol The active form of vitamin D.

Calcium antagonist Antiarrhythmic drug that is effective in managing some types of arrhythmias.

Calipers An instrument with two bent or curved legs. It is frequently used for measuring skinfold thickness.

Calorie (cal) The amount of heat required to raise the temperature of 1 g of water 1°C.

Carbohydrate Organic compound composed of carbon, hydrogen, and oxygen, with a 2:1 ratio of hydrogen to oxygen atoms.

Carcinogenic A cancer-causing substance.

Cardiotonic glycoside Drug that increases the strength of heart contractions.

Cardiovascular disease Disease of the blood vessels and the heart.

Carotene A precursor of vitamin A.

Caseous necrosis Necrosis of the tubules in which the dead tissue assumes a cheesy appearance.

Catabolic steroid Steroid hormone that promotes catabolism.

Catabolism A breakdown phase that involves oxidation (the loss of hydrogen atoms and energy) of glucose.

Catabolized Broken down.

Cathartic Laxative drugs.

Catheter A slender, flexible tube of rubber or plastic that is inserted into a channel such as a vein.

Cation Mineral that is positively charged.

Cecum The first portion of the large intestine to which the small intestine attaches and from which the appendix extends.

Celiac crisis An attack of watery diarrhea and vomiting.

Celiac disease A disease characterized by the degeneration and atrophy of the intestinal villi, induced by the ingestion of foods containing gluten.

Cellulose Fiber.

Celsius (C) A unit of temperature measurement on the Celsius scale.

Central vein A vein located in the center or midline of the body; an example is the superior vena cava.

Central vein total parenteral nutrition Infusion of nutrients through a catheter into the subclavian vein and their guidance into the superior vena cava.

Cephalin A phospholipid found in the body.

Cerebrovascular accident A rupture or blockage of a blood vessel in the brain.

Cheilosis Cracks at the corner of the mouth due to a deficiency of vitamin B_2.

Chemically defined (elemental) diet Formula that is composed of purified or synthetic nutrients.

Chlorophyll The green pigment found in most plant cells that is important for photosynthesis.

Cholecalciferol Chemical name for vitamin D.

Cholecystectomy Surgical removal of the gallbladder.

Cholecystitis An inflammation of the gallbladder that results from bacterial infection or gallstones.

Cholecystokinin A hormone that stimulates the gallbladder to contract and release bile.

Cholelithiasis The formation of stones in the gallbladder.

Cholesterol A lipid that is produced by the body and used in the synthesis of steroid hormones and excreted in bile.

Choline A compound that is synthesized in the body from serine and methionine amino acids.

Chromosome Rod-like structure that appears in the nucleus of the cell during mitosis. The chromosomes contain genes.

Chronic continuous A condition that persists for a long time and shows either little change or an extremely slow progression over a long period.

Chronic intermittent (recurrent) colitis A type of ulcerative colitis that is characterized by mild diarrhea and intermittent, slight bleeding.

Chronic obstructive pulmonary disease (COPD) A chronic, persistent obstruction of the air flow into the bronchi of the lung. Asthma, bronchitis, and emphysema are the main causes of this condition.

Chronic persistent hepatitis. An inflammation of the liver that may last for 4–8 months.

Chronic renal disease Gradual onset of kidney disease.

Chronic renal failure Gradual onset of renal failure.

Chylomicron Lipoprotein synthesized in the intestines that transports triglycerides through the lymph and blood to the liver.

Chyme Semifluid mass of food that is formed in the stomach and released into the duodenum.

Cirrhosis Inflammation and scarring of interstitial

(between parts) tissue; commonly occurs in liver tissue.

Citric acid cycle (Krebs Cycle) A series of aerobic respiration reactions that result in the release of hydrogen atoms and CO_2 molecules and the synthesis of one ATP molecule.

Clear liquid diet A diet limited to liquids such as broths, Jello, and strained fruit juices.

Clinical care process A series of activities (assessment, planning, implementation, and evaluation) used by health professionals to identify and meet patients' needs.

Coenzyme A small nonprotein molecule that combines with an inactive protein to make it an active enzyme.

Colic A spasm in an organ accompanied by pain.

Collagen A protein that is important in the structure of skin, teeth, bones, and muscle.

Collateral channel Vein that is used as detour routes from the liver connecting to veins from the lower esophagus.

Collecting duct A duct that carries urine from the distal convoluted tubule of the nephron to the pelvic region.

Colonic diverticulosis A condition characterized by small, sac-like herniations of the colon mucosa called diverticula.

Complementary protein supplementation A strategy that involves eating two or more foods that are complementary to each other in amino acids.

Complete protein Protein that contains all of the essential amino acids in amounts needed by the body.

Cone Receptor cell in the retina of the eye that is sensitive to bright light and colors.

Confabulation Recitation of imaginary experiences to fill gaps in memory.

Congenital lactase deficiency A rare inherited intolerance of lactase throughout life.

Congenital metabolic disorder An inherited metabolic disorder that a child is born with, such as phenylketonuria (PKU).

Congestive heart failure A failure of the heart to pump the blood adequately to the tissues. It results in an accumulation of blood and fluids in the tissues and therefore causes congestion.

Convulsion Involuntary spasm or contraction of groups of muscles.

Cor pulmonale Hypertrophy of the right side of the heart.

Cornea The outer covering of the eye.

Coronary artery Artery that supplies blood to the myocardium (heart tissue).

Cortisone A hormone secreted from the cortex region of the adrenal glands. It increases the blood glucose level.

Creatinine A nitrogenous waste that is formed from protein, muscle, and purine metabolism.

Creatinine clearance The rate at which the nitrogen compound creatinine is filtered out of the blood by the kidneys.

Creatinine height index A laboratory test that measures the amount of creatinine excreted in the urine. Creatinine results from muscle metabolism; therefore, it is indicative of the skeletal muscle mass.

Cretinism A condition caused by an iodine deficiency in an infant.

Crohn's disease An inflammatory disease that is located primarily in the ileum region of the small intestine and may extend into the large intestine.

Crude fiber The residue left after laboratory treatment of food with acid and alkali.

Culture The concept, skills, and broad-based characteristics of a given population.

Cushing's disease A condition caused by an excessive secretion of hormones from the cortex region of the adrenal glands.

Cyanotic Bluish color of the skin due to reduced level of oxygen.

Cystic duct A duct that drains bile from the gallbladder to the common bile duct.

Cystic fibrosis A hereditary disease characterized by secretion and accumulation of excessively thick mucus that blocks the secretion of pancreatic enzymes.

Cytochrome A molecule in the electron transport system.

DDT (dichloro diphenyl trichloroethane) An insecticide that is toxic to insects and humans. It has been found in human breast milk.

Deamination The removal of an amine group (NH_2) from each amino acid.

Decompensation The inability of the heart to maintain adequate circulation. It is characterized by edema, cyanosis, and dyspnea.

Decubiti Bed sores or skin ulcers that result from interference with blood circulation to the skin.

Dehydration An excess loss of fluids from tissues.

Deltoid muscle Triangular-shaped muscle at the cap of the shoulder. It is frequently used as a site of injections.

Dementia A severe mental disorder involving impairment of mental ability.

Demographic The study of human populations in terms of size, growth, density, and other vital statistics.

Denaturation A change in the chemical structure of a molecule; often occurs with protein molecules when certain conditions exist.

Densitometry A method of determining the body composition and body fatness of a person. The method involves measuring the body's specific gravity by immersing the individual in water.

Dental caries Decay or cavities of the teeth.

Deoxyribonucleic acid (DNA) A nucleic acid found in the cell nucleus. It contains genetic information for the synthesis of specific proteins.

Dermatitis Inflammation of the skin, evidenced by itching and redness.

Descending colon The portion of the large intestine that extends downward along the left side of the abdomen.

Developmental lactase deficiency A condition that results from a gradual decrease in lactase during childhood and adolescence.

Dextrin Product of starch digestion in the mouth.

Diabetes insipidus A type of diabetes that is caused by inadequate secretion of the antidiuretic hormone (ADH).

Diabetes mellitus Disease of the pancreas that causes inadequate secretion of insulin, thereby resulting in an inability to regulate blood glucose level normally.

Diabetic ketoacidosis (DKA) A buildup of ketones in the blood that results from uncontrolled IDDM.

Diabetic nephropathy Kidney disease caused by damage to blood vessels that results from diabetes.

Diabetic retinopathy Damage to the retinal blood capillaries as a result of diabetes.

Dialysate A fluid that bathes semipermeable dialysis membranes.

Dialysis The separation of small molecules from large ones by passage through a semipermeable membrane.

Diastolic The pressure created by the relaxation of the heart ventricles.

Diet therapy The use of modified diets to help a person overcome or cope with an illness or interrelated illnesses.

Dietary fiber Fiber resistant to the human digestive enzymes.

Diffusion Movement of molecules from high concentration to low concentration.

Digestibility Pertains to the ease of digestion.

Dipeptides Molecules composed of two amino acid.

Diplopia Double vision.

Disaccharide Double sugar.

Distal convoluted tubule The portion of the renal tubule that is farthest from Bowman's tubule. Some water reabsorption and secretion occur here.

Diuresis Increased urine flow.

Diuretics Agents that promote urine excretion and are used to alleviate edema.

Diverticulitis Inflammatory condition of diverticula caused by bacterial growth and action arising from food residues and fecal matter.

Diverticulosis Presence of diverticula (outpouching of the colon wall).

Dorsal plexus A network of veins located near the dorsal surface of the foot.

Dorsum The back or posterior surface of a body or part.

Drug Chemical substance that is intended to have a therapeutic effect on a patient.

Dumping syndrome A number of physical problems (nausea, vomiting, sweating, and palpitations) that develop from a gastrectomy. The problems develop when the stomach contents enter the duodenum too rapidly and large amounts of fluid shift out of the blood into the duodenum.

Duodenal ulcer A deterioration of the mucosal lining of the duodenum.

Duodenum First region of the small intestine.

Dysphagia Difficulty in swallowing.

Dyspnea Labored breathing.

Eclampsia High blood pressure accompanied by convulsions and coma.

Eczema Redness and small blisters on the skin.

Edema Accumulation of water in tissues.

Edematous Refers to a condition of edema.

Elderly People who are 65 years of age or older.

Electrolyte depletion A reduction in the amount of electrolytes below the normal level.

Electron transport system Composed of cytochrome molecules by which the pairs of hydrogen electrons released from glycolysis and citric acid cycles are carried.

Elemental formula Liquid formula that contains simple sugars and amino acids.

Emphysema A disease characterized by the gradual destruction of alveoli, enlargement of distal air spaces, and trapping of air.

Emulsifying agent Substance that increases the surface area of fats for ease of absorption.

Endotracheal tube An airway catheter inserted into the trachea that removes secretions and maintains an adequate air passageway.

End-stage renal disease (ESRD) The stage of chronic renal failure in which 90% of the kidney tissue is damaged.

Energy The capacity to do work.

Energy balance The amount of energy remaining in the body when energy output is subtracted from energy input.

Energy intake Energy supplied by the three energy nutrients: carbohydrates, fats, and proteins.

Enteral nutrition The movement of nutrients through the intestine into the blood.

Enteric Pertains to the small intestine. An enteric coat prevents the release and absorption of the drug until it reaches the small intestine.

Epigastric distress (pain) Pain and discomfort in the epigastrium region, which is the upper central region of the abdomen.

Epinephrine A hormone secreted by the adrenal gland in times of stress.

Epithelial Cells that form the outer layer of the skin.

Erythrocyte Red blood cell.

Erythropoiesis The synthesis of red blood cells.

Erythropoietin A hormone, secreted by the kidneys, that stimulates erythropoiesis.

Esophageal reflux Backward and upward flow of food through the esophagus.

Esophageal varices Dilation of esophageal veins.

Esophagotomy Introduction of a tube through the skin into the esophagus.

Essential amino acids Amino acids that must be present in the diet since they cannot be synthesized by the body.

Essential fatty acid A fatty acid (e.g., linoleic acid) that cannot be manufactured by the body in adequate quantities and, therefore, must be obtained from the diet.

Essential hypertension A type of hypertension for which there is no known cause.

Essential nutrient Compound that the body cannot synthesize.

Estrogen The female sex hormone secreted by the ovaries. It stimulates the development of the female secondary sex characteristics.

Etiology Cause.

Exacerbation Increased severity and complications.

Exogenous Outside of the body.

Extracellular Fluid outside cells, such as plasma and interstitial fluid.

Extrinsic factor A compound that refers to vitamin B_{12} and is formed outside the body.

Exudate Fluid with a high content of protein and cellular debris.

Fasting blood glucose/sugar (FBG or FBS) A blood glucose test performed on a person's blood after an overnight fast.

Fasting hypoglycemia A type of hypoglycemia that occurs either long after a meal, in the middle of the night, or before breakfast.

Fat cell hypothesis The theory that the body has the potential to accumulate an excess number of fat cells during three periods of life: the last 3 months of fetal development, the first 3 years of life, and adolescence.

Fat soluble Able to be dissolved in fats.

Fatty acid Chain of carbon and hydrogen atoms that functions as a building block of fat molecules.

Ferric Chemical form of iron, Fe^{3+}; a less absorbable form than ferrous iron.

Ferritin A form of iron that is stored in the liver, spleen, and bone marrow.

Ferrous Chemical form of iron, Fe^{2+}; more absorbable form than ferric iron.

Ferrous sulfate An oral iron supplement that is often given to correct iron deficiency anemia.

Fetal alcohol syndrome (FAS) Characterized by growth retardation, physical deformities, behavioral defects, and mental retardation in a baby born to an alcoholic mother.

Fever Elevation of body temperature above normal.

Fibrinogen A blood protein that contributes to blood clotting.

Filtrate A fluid present in Bowman's capsule. It is formed by filtration of blood in the glomeruli.

Fistula Abnormal tube-like passage within the body tissue, usually between two internal organs.

Flavin adenine dinucleotide (FAD) An electron transfer compound that transfers electrons and hydrogen atoms from the Krebs cycle through the cytochrome system to oxygen.

Flavin A chemical that is fluorescent.

Food diary A record of what a person eats, the mood he or she is in while eating, and the circumstances in which eating occurs.

Food fallacy False, deceptive idea about food and its effects in the body.

Food frequency record A method that is used to determine how many times per day, week, month, or year a person consumes certain foods from the Basic Four Food Groups.

Fortified The addition of nutrients to a food to make it richer than the unprocessed food.

Fructose Fruit sugar.

Functional hypoglycemia A type of hypoglycemia that occurs 3–4 hours after eating or in response to a meal.

Galactosemia A genetic disease in which galactose is not properly metabolized due to the lack of an enzyme.

Gallstone Stone-like mass that forms in the gallbladder.

Gangrene Death of body tissue due to a loss of the vascular supply, followed by bacterial invasion and putrefaction.

Gastrectomy Surgical removal of the stomach.

Gastric ulcer A deterioration of the gastric mucosa generally located along the lesser curvature of the stomach.

Gastritis Inflammation of the stomach lining.

Gastrostomy Feeding directly into the stomach through a specially created opening.

Generic Chemical name of a drug.

Gene The portion of DNA molecules that contains information necessary to synthesize an enzyme.

Genetic Congenital or inherited.

Giordano-Giovannetti (G-G) diet A diet used to treat chronic renal failure.

Globule Small mass of material. Fat globules are small masses of fat that result from the interaction of large fat masses with bile.

Glomerular filtration rate (GFR) The amount of filtrate formed.

Glomerulus A capillary tuft within the Bowman's capsule of a nephron.

Glossitis Smooth, purplish appearance of the tongue due to a deficiency of vitamin B_2.

Glucagon A hormone secreted by the pancreas.

Glucose tolerance factor A compound that helps to bind insulin to cell membranes.

Glucostatic theory The theory that when the blood glucose level is high, a person will feel full, and when it is low, the person will feel hungry.

Gluten A water-soluble protein found in wheat, rye, barley, and oats.

Gluten intolerance (gluten-induced enteropathy) A disorder in which gluten (protein) causes the destruction of intestinal villi, thereby preventing the absorption of fats and other nutrients.

Glyceride A fat, such as monoglyceride, diglyceride, and triglyceride.

Glycogen Branched-chain polysaccharide composed of glucose molecules.

Glycogenesis Synthesis of glycogen.

Glycogenolysis The catabolism of glycogen.

Glycolysated hemoglobin (HbA$_{1c}$) A test that measures the amount of hemoglobin to which glucose is attached.

Goal A statement of the desired outcome in a patient.

Goiter Abnormal enlargement of the thyroid gland due to an inbalance in the amount of the mineral iodine.

Goitrogen Substance that blocks the absorption or use of iodine.

Gout A metabolic disease characterized by an inability to metabolize purines and an elevated uric acid level in the blood.

Granuloma A tumor-like mass of granulation tissue.

Gravity-Drip method A method by which liquid formulas flow slowly by gravity through a nasogastric tube.

Gum A water-soluble, nonstructural polysaccharide.

Hematocrit A percentage of RBCs in a sample of whole blood.

Hematuria Blood in the urine.

Hemicellulose A polysaccharide that is similar to cellulose.

Hemochromatosis An inherited disease in which a person absorbs and deposits excessive amounts of iron in the liver.

Hemodialysis Circulation of arterial blood from the body into a machine called a dialyzer. Through diffusion and osmosis, nitrogenous wastes, excess fluid, and electrolytes are exchanged from the blood into the dialysate. The cleansed blood is then returned to the body.

Hemoglobin A protein molecule composed of four amino acid chains with one iron atom in each.

Hemolytic anemia A condition that results in the destruction of red blood cells (RBCs) at a faster than normal rate.

Hemolyzed Broken down.

Hemorrhage An escape of blood from a ruptured or damaged vessel.

Hemosiderin An insoluble form of iron that is stored in the liver.

Hemothorax Presence of blood in the chest.

Heparin An anticoagulant or substance that prevents blood clotting.

Hepatic cirrhosis The degeneration of liver cells with the formation of fibrous scar tissue.

Hepatic coma A coma that results from the buildup of ammonia, which increases as a result of the liver's inability to convert ammonia to urea.

Hepatic encephalopathy A condition caused by increased levels of ammonia in the blood, which leads to a malfunction of brain tissue.

Hepatic vein Vein that drains the blood from the liver into the inferior vena cava.

Hepatitis A viral infection that results in inflammation of the liver tissue.

Hiatal hernia A condition in which the stomach protrudes through an opening in the diaphragm through which the esophagus passes.

High-fiber diet A diet that contains large amounts of fiber (greater than 40 g) such as fresh fruits, vegetables, and bran cereals.

High-potassium diet A diet that contains foods that are rich in potassium such as bacon, bran, instant coffee, and oatmeal.

Hives Itching and burning swellings of the skin.

Human lymphocyte antigens (HLA) A lymphocyte (a type of white blood cell) that has an antigen attached to its surface.

Hunger An inborn instinct that causes a physiological response to the body's need for food.

Hydrochloric acid Acid secreted by cells in the stomach that changes pepsinogen to pepsin.

Hydrogen transport molecule Molecule in cell respiration that transports hydrogen atoms from glucose to cytochrome molecules.

Hydrogenation A process by which an unsaturated fat is changed to a solid saturated fat by forcing hydrogens into the substance.

Hydrolysate Solution with amino acids.

Hydrometry A method of determining the body composition and body fatness of a person. It involves injection of deuterium oxide (heavy water) into the body.

Hydrothorax Fluid in the chest.

Hyperactivity Abnormally increased activity that is often referred to as hyperkinesia in children.

Hyperaldosteronism An increased level of the hormone aldosterone.

Hyperalimentation Injection of hyperosmolar fluids directly into the superior vena cava vein.

Hyperammonemia Excess ammonia in the blood.

Hypercalcemia A condition in which the blood calcium level is elevated.

Hypercholesterolemia High level of cholesterol in the blood.

Hyperglycemia A condition characterized by an excess amount of glucose in the blood.

Hyperkalemia Elevated blood potassium levels.

Hyperlipidemia Elevated level of lipids in the blood.

Hyperlipoproteinemia Elevated blood lipoprotein level.

Hypermetabolic A high metabolic rate following problems like major trauma or burns.

Hyperosmolar hyperglycemic nonketotic coma (HHNK) A complication of type II or non-insulin-dependent diabetes mellitus. Hyperglycemia causes a loss of fluids and electrolytes that can result in coma and death.

Hyperparathyroidism An excessive secretion of the parathyroid hormone from the gland.

Hyperphosphatemia An excess of phosphate in the blood.

Hyperplasia A dramatic increase in the number of fat cells.

Hypertension Sustained high arterial blood pressure, either diastolic, systolic, or both.

Hyperthyroidism Excessive activity of the thyroid gland, which results in increased secretion of thyroxine.

Hypertonic A food or solution that has an osmolality of at least 340 mOsm or higher.

Hypertrophy An increase in the size of fat cells.

Hypervitaminosis A An excess amount of vitamin A that results in a toxicity condition.

Hypoalbuminemia A low level of albumin in the blood.

Hypochromic Pale in color.

Hypochromic microcytic anemia Anemic condition characterized by RBCs that are smaller in size and pale in color.

Hypoglycemia Abnormally low level of blood glucose.

Hypoglycemic agent A drug that decreases blood glucose levels.

Hypokalemia Decreased blood potassium levels.

Hyponatremia Deficiency of sodium in the blood.

Hypophosphatemia A deficiency of phosphates in the blood.

Hypothalamus An area at the base of the brain that contains centers of hunger and satiety and secretes the antidiuretic hormone.

Hypothyroidism Decreased activity of the thyroid gland which results in an underproduction of thyroxine.

Hypotonic A food or solution that has an osmolality of 240 mOsm or lower.

Hypovolemic shock Shock caused by low blood volume.

Hypoxia A decreased amount of oxygen available to the tissues.

Iatrogenic malnutrition Physician-induced malnutrition.

Ideal body weight The values that originated from the height and weight tables issued by the Metropolitan Life Insurance Company in 1942.

Ileocecal valve A valve that is located between the ileum and the cecum.

Ileostomy An opening into the ileum for drainage of fecal matter.

Ileum The terminal portion of the small intestine that is connected to the large intestine.

Inborn error of metabolism An inherited metabolic disorder.

Incomplete protein Protein lacking one or more of the essential amino acids.

Infancy The period from time of birth through the first year.

Inferior vena cava The vein that drains the blood from the lower part of the body to the right atrium of the heart.

Inorganic nutrient Substance that does not contain carbon atoms.

Insensible water loss Fluid lost through the skin, vomiting, diarrhea, and fever.

Insulin A hormone secreted by the pancreas that

aids in both the diffusion of glucose into the liver and muscle cells and the synthesis of glycogen.

Insulin resistance The deactivation of insulin.

Insulin shock (insulin reaction) A condition caused by a blood glucose level below 50 mg/dl.

Insulinoma A small noncancerous pancreatic tumor that causes secretion of an excessive amount of insulin.

Insulin-dependent diabetes mellitus (IDDM) A type of diabetes in which the person does not secrete enough insulin to control the blood glucose level.

Intermittent positive-pressure breathing The use of a ventilator for treatment of patients with inadequate breathing.

Interstitial Between parts. Interstitial fluid, which is located between cells, is an example.

Intestinal flora Bacteria in the large intestine.

Intestinal villi Small mucous projections lining the small intestine.

Intracellular Fluid within cells.

Intralipid A fat emulsion solution that is administered intravenously to supply essential fatty acids and kilocalories.

Intramuscular injections Injections of substances into muscles.

Intramuscularly Within a muscle.

Intrauterine devices (IUDS) Objects inserted into the uterus for contraceptive purposes.

Intrinsic Functional substances in blood or urine.

Intrinsic factor A protein that is secreted by the gastric mucosa and combines with vitamin B_{12}, thereby making its absorption possible.

Involution The contraction of the enlarged uterus after birth.

Iodine number Number of grams of iodine absorbed by 100 g of fat.

Ionize Chemical process by which substances break apart into ions.

Ion Atom or molecule that has either a positive or a negative charge.

Iron deficiency anemia A reduced number of RBCs that are smaller than normal.

Ischemia The lack of blood flow and oxygen to a body part that is often due to an obstruction of an artery, as in atherosclerosis.

Islet cell antibodies Antibodies formed in response to islet of Langerhan cell fragments.

Islets of Langerhans Irregular microscopic structures scattered throughout the pancreas. They are composed of alpha cells that secrete glucagon and beta cells that secrete insulin.

Isotonic A food or solution that has the approximate osmolality of body fluids: 300 mOsm.

Jaundice Yellow discoloration of the whites of the eyes and the skin due to build-up of bile in blood.

Jejunostomy Feeding directly into the jejunum region of the small intestine through a specially created opening.

Jejunum The region of the small intestine that extends from the duodenum to the ileum.

Juvenile-onset obesity Obesity beginning during the last 3 months of fetal life, the first 3 years of life, and adolescence.

Keratin A protein substance in hair and nails.

Keratinized To become hard or horny.

Ketoacidosis High blood level of ketones (acids).

Ketone Product of incomplete metabolism of fats (acetone is an example of a ketone).

Kidney stones The stones formed in the kidneys as a result of certain dietary and chemical changes.

Kilocalorie (kcal) A unit of energy measurement that is calculated and expressed in relation to nutrition. A *calorie* is often called a *small calorie*, since 1,000 small calories equal 1 kilocalorie.

Kwashiorkor A type of protein-calorie malnutrition that results from a decreased protein intake.

Lactation Production of milk by the mammary glands.

Lacteal Lymph vessel.

Lactose Milk sugar.

Lacto-ovo vegetarian A vegan diet that includes milk, eggs, and other dairy products.

Laennec's cirrhosis Cirrhosis caused by chronic alcoholism.

Large-vessel disease The development of atherosclerosis in various arteries.

Lecithin A phospholipid found in the body.

Left subclavian vein Vein that receives the majority of lymph and chylomicrons.

Legume Seed of plants such as kidney beans, soybeans, garden peas, and lima beans.

Lethargic Sluggishness, slowness, and sleepiness that often result from drugs.

Liberal diet A diet that allows a variety of foods.

Lignin A noncarbohydrate substance that functions as a structured bonding agent in plants.

Linoleic A PUFA that is obtained from food and serves as a precursor of arachidonic and linolenic acids.

Linolenic A fatty acid that is derived from linoleic acid.

Lipid A biological substance that has an oily or greasy touch and is insoluble in water. Lipids are soluble in organic solvents such as ether and alcohol.

Lipoatrophy Loss of fat at an injection site, resulting in indentation.

Lipoprotein Lipid with a protein coat around it.

Lipostatic theory The theory that the tissues, especially the fat tissues, signal the brain when the level of fat is increased above or decreased below a certain level.

Lipotropic factor Compound that contributes to the formation of lipoproteins that transports fats out of the liver.

Liquefaction Conversion into a liquid form.

Long chain fatty acid Fatty acid that is 18 to 20 carbon atoms in length.

Low birth weight (LBW) baby A baby that weighs less than 5.5 lb (2500 g.)

Low-residue diet A diet low in residue and fiber; it is also called a low-fiber diet.

Low-sodium diet A diet that allows no salt in cooking or at the table; all cured and canned meats are also eliminated.

Lumen Inner open space in a tube such as blood vessel or the intestine.

Luminal effect Change that occurs in the lumen of the small intestine.

Lymph Fluid in lymphatic vessels that originates in tissue spaces.

Lymphocytopenia A low level of lymphocytes that help provide immunity.

Macrocytic anemia A type of anemia in which red blood cells are larger than normal.

Major mineral Mineral that is present in the body in quantities greater than 5 g and is required at levels of 100 mg/day.

Maltose Malt sugar.

Mammary gland Specialized gland in the breast that secretes milk during pregnancy.

Marasmus A type of protein-calorie malnutrition that results from a deficiency of proteins and calories.

Massive (morbid) obesity Body weight that is more than 100% above the ideal weight.

Maturity-onset diabetes of youth (MODY) NIDDM that occurs in people under 40.

Mechanical soft diet Same as a soft diet.

Medium chain fatty acid Fatty acid that contains 14 to 16 carbon atoms.

Megaloblastic anemia Anemia characterized by large, immature, nucleated red blood cells called megaloblasts.

Menopause A permanent cessation of menstruation when ovaries, fallopian tubes, uterus, vagina, and breasts atrophy.

Metabolic acidosis An acidic state of the blood as a result of the accumulation of ketones.

Metabolic factor (internal) An internal factor that can lead to obesity.

Metabolism All chemical reactions that absorbed molecules undergo inside cells.

Metastasis The transfer of a cancerous tumor.

Microcytic An RBC that is smaller in size than normal.

Midarm muscle circumference (MAMC) A measurement of the circumference of the arm. Usually done approximately midway between the shoulder and elbow. Using the formula, it is a good indicator of lean body or muscle mass.

Milk anemia Anemia that results from feeding older infants only milk that is low in iron.

Milliosmole (mOsm) Equals 1/1,000th of an osmole.

Mineral Small, inorganic element that yields no energy.

Miscarriage (spontaneous abortion) Interrupted pregnancy before the seventh month.

Modified (therapeutic) A normal diet that has modifications of nutritional components.

Monoglyceride Glyceride that contains one fatty acid chain.

Monohydrous Containing one water molecule; an example is monohydrous dextrose, which contains one water molecule connected to a dextrose molecule.

Monosaccharide Simple sugar.

Monounsaturated fatty acid A fatty acid that contains one double bond.

Morning sickness Nausea and vomiting experienced by pregnant women.

Motility Spontaneous movement. The contractions of the gastrointestinal tract are an example.

Mucosal effect Change that occurs in the mucosal lining of the gastrointestinal tract or inactivation of enzyme systems.

Mucous membrane Membrane that lines the cavities that open to the outside of the body.

Myelin sheath A sheath, composed of fatty material, that surrounds and insulates some nerve fibers.

Myocardial infarction A condition in which a portion of the heart tissue becomes necrotic. Commonly referred to as a heart attack.

Myoglobin (heme iron) A protein molecule composed of four amino acid chains, with one iron atom in each that is found in muscle tissue.

Nasogastric Referring to a tube of soft rubber or plastic that is inserted through a nostril into the stomach. It is used to instill liquid foods or withdraw gastric contents.

Naturally occurring sugar Sugar found naturally in foods, such as glucose and fructose, as opposed to artificial sugar, such as sorbital and xylitol.

Necrosis Death of tissue.

Negative energy balance A situation in which energy expenditure is greater than energy input.

Negative nitrogen balance A state that occurs when more nitrogen is excreted than ingested.

Neoplasm Tumor.

Nephron The structural and functional unit of the kidney.

Nephrosis Kidney disease that is characterized by a large loss of proteins in the urine and edema.

Nephrotic syndrome A stage of kidney disease that is characterized by large losses of protein in the urine, severe edema, low serum protein levels, elevated levels of cholesterol and other serum lipids, and anemia.

Night blindness The inability to see well in dim light.

Nitrogen equilibrium Conditions in which the amount of nitrogen consumed is equal to the amount excreted.

Nitrogen-fixing bacteria Bacteria that can take in nitrogen from the air and soil and convert it into proteins.

Noncaloric Non-energy-yielding.

Nonessential amino acid Amino acid that can be synthesized by the adult body from carbohydrates, lipids, and other amino acids.

Nonessential fatty acid A fatty acid that is synthesized by the body if a person consumes adequate quantities of food containing carbon, hydrogen, and oxygen atoms.

Nontropical sprue An alternative term for adult celiac disease (malabsorption disorder).

Non-insulin-dependent diabetes mellitus (NIDDM) A type of diabetes mellitus that is not caused by an insulin deficiency but rather by the ineffectiveness of insulin in moving glucose into the cells.

Norepinephrine A neurotransmitter secreted by the sympathetic nerves and as a hormone secreted from the adrenal gland.

Normal diet A diet that consists of any and all foods and provides the RDAs and adequacy by means of the Four Food Group Plan.

Nutrition The combination of processes by which the body receives and utilizes the materials necessary to maintain homeostasis.

Nystagmus Rapid movement of the eyeballs.

Obesity Body weight that is 15–25% above ideal weight.

Objective A statement of a short-term specific step to be used to help achieve a goal.

Oliguria Diminished urine output.

Omenta A serous membrane attached to the visceral organs.

Opsin A protein pigment that combines with retinene in the rods to form rhodopsin.

Oral glucose tolerance test (OGTT) A blood glucose test in which a person fasts overnight and is then given a measured amount of glucose in an oral glucose drink.

Organic compound Substance that contains carbon atoms.

Orthomolecular approach An approach that consists of giving large doses of vitamins, especially niacin (vitamin B_3, nicotinic acid) and vitamin C (ascorbic acid) to schizophrenic patients.

Osmolality The number of osmoles per kilogram of solvent.

Osmole The standard unit of measure of osmotic pressure.

Osmosis The movement of water from a low-solute concentration to a high-solute concentration through a membrane permeable to water only.

Osmotic overload A condition that results in the movement of large amounts of water into the intestines from the blood.

Osmotic pressure Pressure on the cell membrane due to the inability of solutes to pass through it.

Osteomalacia The softening of the bones due to the loss of calcium or demineralization.

Osteoporosis A progressive demineralization of bones that results in the reduction of bone tissue.

Overfat Disproportionately high percentage of fat tissue.

Overt Open and observable.

Overweight Body weight that is more than 10% above ideal weight.

Oxalic acid An acid found in some foods such as cocoa, rhubarb, and spinach. It inhibits the absorption of calcium, iron, and magnesium.

Oxidized A chemical reaction in which an atom or molecule either loses hydrogen atoms and electrons or accepts oxygen.

Oxytocin A pituitary hormone that stimulates uterine contractions.

Palmar erythema Bright red palms.

Pancreatic amylase An enzyme secreted by the pancreas that breaks down dextrins into maltose.

Pancreatic enzyme deficiency A deficiency in the amount of enzymes secreted by the pancreas. This deficiency is especially a problem with pancreatic lipase, which breaks down triglycerides.

Pancreatitis Inflammation of the pancreas.

Paralytic ileus Absence of peristalsis.

Parenteral feeding Feeding that bypasses the intestine and is infused directly into the veins.

Parenteral Nutrition The movement of nutrients that bypass the intestine and are infused directly into the veins.

Partial gastrectomy An operation in which a portion of the stomach is removed. The remaining section is joined to the duodenum.

Pectin A water-soluble, nonstructural polysaccharide.

Pellagra A condition that is caused by a niacin deficiency.

Pelvic girdle A ring of bones in the pelvic region composed of two hip bones joined to the sacrum.

Pepsin A gastric enzyme that breaks down proteins into short chain polypeptides, proteoses, and peptides.

Peptic ulcer A deterioration or lesion in the mucosal lining of the stomach or duodenum.

Peptidase enzyme An enzyme that catalyzes the degradation of a harmful peptide.

Peptide bond Chemical bond that connects amino acids.

Peptone Intermediate-sized protein segment.

Perforation An opening through the gastric or duodenal wall.

Peripheral edema Excess accumulation of interstitial fluids within the extremities.

Peripheral neuritis Degenerative changes in the peripheral nerves.

Peripheral resistance Resistance to the passage of blood through small blood vessels, especially the arterioles.

Peripheral vein A vein near the skin surface in the arm and forearm.

Peristalsis Wavelike, muscular contractions that propel food and wastes through the gastrointestinal tract.

Peristaltic contraction Rhythmic wave of smooth muscle contraction.

Peritoneal dialysis Infusion of dialysate fluid through a tube into the abdominal cavity. Nitrogenous wastes, excess fluids, and electrolytes are exchanged from the blood through the peritoneum into the dialysate fluid. The fluid is then drained out.

Peritoneum membrane A membrane that covers most of the abdominal pelvic organs and through which exchange of nutrients and wastes occurs in peritoneal dialysis.

Permeability A state of being permeable, or allowing the passage of materials.

Pernicious anemia Anemia that results from a deficiency of vitamin B_{12} because of a lack of the intrinsic factor.

Phagocytic cell Cell that carries on phagocytosis, such as some white blood cells.

Pharmacologic dose Dose of a nutrient that exceeds the normal requirements to the point where drug-like effects are observed.

Pharmacologic effect A drug-like effect.

Phenothiazine tranquilizer Tranquilizers used in the treatment of severe mental illnesses.

Phenylalanine An essential amino acid.

Phenylalanine hydroxylase An enzyme that synthesizes tyrosine from phenylalanine.

Phenylketonuria (PKU) A disorder in an infant caused by the absence of the enzyme phenylalanine hydroxylase, which oxidizes phenylalanine to tyrosine.

Phlebitis Inflammation of a vein.

Phospholipid A lipid subclass. Each phospholipid is composed of two fatty acid molecules connected to a glycerol molecule.

Photophobia Sensitivity of the eyes to light and strain.

Physical activity The amount of energy expended by the body to contract the skeletal muscles in voluntary activities.

Physiological solution Solution in which the osmotic pressure exerted by the solutions is equal to that of body fluids.

Phytic acid A binder compound that forms an insoluble calcium complex.

Pimple Small, elevated area of pus containing lesions of the skin. It is often called a blackhead.

Placenta A structure present within the uterus of a pregnant woman that is connected to the developing fetus and exchanges wastes and nutrients.

Placental lactogen A hormone secreted by the placenta that enhances lactation and inhibits insulin activity in the mother.

Plaque Mound of lipid material, smooth muscle cells, and calcium.

Plateau Period during weight reduction in which the person is not losing weight.

Pleurisy Inflammation of the pleura membrane that lines and covers the lungs in the thoracic cavity.

Pneumonia An acute infection of the lung tissue.

Pneumothorax Air or gas in the chest.

Polychlorinated biphenyl (PCB) Chemical used in the manufacture of plastics. It is not biodegradable and has been found in breast milk.

Polycythemia A condition characterized by an excessive number of red blood cells.

Polydipsia Increased thirst.

Polyphagia Increased hunger.

Polysaccharide Complex sugar.

Polyunsaturated fatty acid A fatty acid that contains two or more double bonds.

Polyuria Increased urination.

Porosity The state of being porous.

Portal hypertension Abnormally increased pressure in the portal circulation.

Portal vein Vein that brings blood rich in nutrients into the liver. Blood from the intestines, stomach, and spleen drain into the portal vein.

Positive energy balance A situation in which energy input is greater than energy expenditure.

Positive nitrogen balance A state that occurs when more nitrogen is ingested than excreted.

Potassium-40 A radioactive isotope that is naturally present in the body, but in low quantities in fat tissue.

Preeclampsia Sudden high blood pressure or an increase of 20–30 mmHg in systolic pressure and 10–15 mmHg in diastolic pressure.

Pregnancy-induced hypertension (PIH) Formerly called toxemia of pregnancy and characterized by proteinuria, hypertension, and edema.

Premature (preterm) baby Birth of a baby prior to the 38th week of pregnancy.

Preschooler Child from 3 to 6 years of age.

Presenile dementia Mental disorder occurring in people under the age of 65.

Primary aldosteronism An excessive secretion of the hormone aldosterone from the adrenal gland. It is characterized by hypertension, hypokalemia, muscular weakness, and polydipsia.

Primary level Health care that is aimed at averting the occurrence of disease and protecting the health of the general public.

Primary malnutrition Malnutrition that results from diet alone. Alcoholics often suffer from primary malnutrition as a result of an inadequate diet.

Problem-oriented medical record (POMR) A communication tool that focuses on a patient's health problems and the structuring of cooperative health care plans to cope with the identified problems.

Progesterone A female hormone that is important in the menstrual cycle and in pregnancy.

Protein The most fundamental constituent of living matter. Proteins are essential for the growth and repair of animal tissue.

Protein efficiency ratio (PER) Measures the growth of rats in relation to the amounts of protein eaten.

Proteinuria The loss of protein in the urine.

Protein-calorie malnutrition (PCM) Malnutrition that is caused by deficits of calories, proteins, or both.

Protein-sparing solution A solution that supplies the needed kilocalories so that proteins can be spared as a source of kilocalories.

Proteoses Intermediate-sized protein segment.

Prothrombin A blood protein that contributes to blood clotting.

Proximal tubule The portion of the renal tubule attached to Bowman's capsule. Most reabsorption of nutrients occurs here.

Pruritis vulvae Itching of the external genitalia of the female.

Psychotherapeutic Drug used in the treatment of manic-depressive illness.

Psychotherapy Any of a number of related techniques for treating mental illness by psychological methods. It is often used in the second stage of treating anorexia nervosa.

PUFA Polyunsaturated fatty acids.

Pulmonary therapy Treatment of lung diseases.

Pyloric obstruction A condition in which the pyloric sphincter becomes scarred and stenosed (the opening is narrowed).

Pyloric sphincter valve A circular muscle that controls the movement of food from the pyloric region of the stomach into the duodenum.

Pyrosis Heartburn.

Pyruvic acid An end product of anaerobic respiration.

Quinone Chemical compound that includes vitamin K.

Quinidine intoxication A poisoned state due to a buildup of the drug quinidine.

Reactant A substance that interacts with other substances to produce products.

Reagent A substance that is used to produce a chemical reaction.

Rebound scurvy A condition that occurs when a pregnant woman takes megadoses of vitamin C, causing the fetus to adapt to the massive doses. After birth, without continued ingestion of vitamin C, the infant shows signs of scurvy.

Recombinant DNA DNA in bacteria that has genes spliced into the normal molecule. Frequently, human genes that produce insulin are spliced, thereby forming recombinant DNA insulin; it is also called artificial human insulin.

Recommended Dietary Allowances (RDAs) Recommended allowances of certain nutrients that are established by the Food and Nutrition Board of the National Academy of Sciences–National Research Council (NAS–NRC).

Reflectance photometer A special device that measures the intensity of light reflected through urine and thereby the amount of glucose that is present.

Reflux Regurgitation.

Regulatory factor (external) An external factor that can lead to obesity.

Regurgitation Backup of stomach contents through the esophagus.

Renal failure A condition in which kidney damage is severe enough that the kidneys no longer excrete the nitrogenous wastes or maintain the electrolytes in the blood.

Renal osteodystrophy A complication of end-stage

renal disease that is characterized by the loss of calcium from the bones and bone mass.

Renin A hormone that causes the formation of the compound angiotensin.

Repletion Restoration of body composition.

Respiratory failure A condition that develops when the blood pH becomes too acidic, the pCO_2 increases, and the PO_2 decreases.

Respiratory insufficiency A condition that results when the exchange of oxygen and carbon dioxide is insufficient for the body's needs during normal activities.

Retina The innermost layer of the eye that contains the visual receptors, rods, and cones.

Retinene A pigment that is derived from vitamin A and results from the breakdown of rhodopsin.

Retinol A form of vitamin A that is found in food.

Rheumatoid disease A disease that results in inflammation and degeneration of the connective tissues around joints.

Rhodopsin The compound secreted by the rods in the retina.

Rickets A condition caused by a deficiency of vitamin D that leads to decreased absorption of calcium by the bones.

Rod Receptor cell in the retina of the eye that is sensitive to dim light.

R-group The rest of the amino acid that is attached to the amine and acid portions of the molecule.

Saccharide Sugar unit.

Salicylate-like Analgesic or pain-relieving compounds.

Salivary amylase An enzyme secreted in the mouth that splits starch into smaller fragments.

Satiety A sensation of fullness that follows a meal.

Saturated fatty acid A fatty acid whose carbon atoms are linked by single bonds, and are bonded to as many hydrogen atoms as possible.

Schizophrenia A mental illness characterized by withdrawal from reality and disturbances in thought and behavior.

School-age child Child from 6 to 12 years of age.

Sclerosis Hardening of a vein.

Scurvy A disease that is characterized by weakness, skin degeneration, ulcerated gums, loss of teeth, and hemorrhages in the skin.

Sebaceous gland Gland in the skin that secretes the oily substance sebum.

Sebum An oily secretion of the sebaceous glands. It lubricates and waterproofs the skin and hair.

Secondary lactase deficiency A condition that may develop as a secondary problem in a person who has a disease of the small intestine such as celiac disease, Crohn's disease, or protein-calorie malnutrition.

Secondary level Health care that is utilized for early diagnosis of disease and prevention of further complications.

Secondary malnutrition Malnutrition that results from impaired use of nutrients. It is often seen in alcoholics and results from the toxic effects of alcohol on the liver and the gastrointestinal tract.

Senile dementia Dementia that occurs in people over the age of 65.

Sepsis Presence of pathogenic bacteria in the blood.

Septic abortion An abortion in which a uterine infection is spread to the general circulation.

Serosa The outer layer of the intestine.

Serous A fluid that lubricates body walls and organs that are coated with the fluid.

Serum albumin A protein in the blood that is important for the regulation of osmotic pressure.

Serum transferrin test A test that measures the amount of globulin protein that transports iron; a sensitive indicator of PCM.

Set point theory The theory that the body is programmed to maintain a certain amount of fat.

Severe obesity Body weight that is 30–100% above the ideal weight.

Serum glutamic oxaloacetic transaminase (SGOT) An enzyme found especially in the heart and liver. An elevated level in the blood is indicative of liver damage.

Serum glutamic pyruvic transaminase (SGPT) An enzyme found in several tissues including the liver. An elevated level in the blood is indicative of liver disease.

Short bowel Surgical shortening of the length of the small intestine. Normally done as a therapeutic procedure to aid person in losing weight.

Short chain fatty acid Fatty acid that contains 8 to 12 carbon atoms.

Sickle cell disease A disease characterized by abnormal hemoglobin that results in sickle-shaped red blood cells.

Sigmoid colon The S-shaped portion of the large intestine between the descending colon and the rectum.

Sippy diet A diet that consists of hourly feedings of whole milk and cream.

Small burns Burns that cover less than 20% of the body surface area.

Small-vessel disease (microangiopathies) A thickening of small vessels such as arterioles, venules, and capillaries.

SOAP: Subjective, objective, assessment, and planning. This is a format in which progress notes are written.

Sodium-potassium pump Protein carriers in cell membranes that transport sodium and potassium ions back to their original positions.

Soft diet A diet modified in consistency that includes high-protein liquid foods and solid foods low in fiber.

Solute A substance that dissolves in a solvent.

Solvent A fluid that causes a solute to dissolve and form a solution.

Specific dynamic effect The expenditure of energy when food is consumed.

Specific heat The amount of heat required to raise the temperature of 1 g of liquid 1°C (Celsius).

Spermatogenesis The production of sperm cells in the testes.

Spider angioma Spider-shaped blood vessels.

Spleen A large glandular organ composed of lymphatic tissue.

Sputum Mucous secretion from the lungs, bronchi, and trachea.

Steatorrhea Abnormally large amounts of fats in the feces.

Steroid hormone Hormone secreted by the adrenal cortex and other endocrine glands that has a typical steroid shape.

Sterol A subclass of lipids. Molecule is composed of four fused rings (cholesterol is an example of a sterol).

Stillborn infant A baby dead at birth.

Stimuli Changes in an environmental condition that cause a response.

Stroke A rupture or blockage of a blood vessel in the brain, resulting in loss of consciousness, paralysis, or other symptoms; it is also called a cerebrovascular accident.

Subclavian vein A vein in the shoulder region that is often used for insertion of a TPN catheter.

Subcutaneous Under the skin.

Subjective Conditions or changes perceived by the patient rather than by a health examiner.

Sucrose Table sugar.

Superior vena cava A vein that carries blood from the upper part of the body into the heart. A TPN catheter is guided into this vein from the subclavian vein.

Superior vena cava thrombosis A blood clot in the superior vena cava.

Synapse The junction between two neurons where an impulse is transmitted.

Synergistic The combined effect is greater than the sum of the parts.

Synovial A fluid that lubricates bones articulating in joints.

Systemic flushing Redness throughout the body as a whole.

Systolic Pressure created by the contraction of the heart ventricles as blood is pumped into the arteries.

Tachycardia Rapid and irregular heartbeat.

Tardive dyskinesia A condition that occurs in patients with mental disorders as a side effect of long-term treatment with antipsychotic drugs.

Target organ Organ that is stimulated by hormones.

Tertiary level Health care that is designed to educate a patient for the maximum use of his or her remaining capacities.

Testicular degeneration Degeneration of the testes.

Testosterone The male sex hormone secreted by the testes. It stimulates the development of male secondary sex characteristics.

Tetany Continuous, forceful muscle contraction.

Tetracycline An antibiotic that is effective against

microorganisms such as gram-positive and gram-negative bacteria.

Therapeutic nutrition Nutritional care that is used to help a person cope with an illness.

Thoracic cavity Chest cavity.

Threshold level The amount of nutrients that will be reabsorbed into the blood of the nephrons. When this level is reached, no more reabsorption of the nutrients will occur.

Thrombosis Blood clot formation.

Thyroid gland An endocrine gland located below the larynx and in front of the trachea. Secretes thyroxine and triiodothyronine hormones.

Thyroxine (T_4) A thyroid hormone that regulates the body's metabolism. Each thyroxin molecule contains four iodine atoms; therefore, it is designated as T_4.

Toddler Child from 1 to 3 years of age.

Tooth mottling Brown discoloration of the teeth.

Total colectomy Removal of the colon.

Total iron-binding capacity A measurement of the percentage of saturation of transferrin. It evaluates the amount of extra iron that can be carried.

Total parenteral nutrition (TPN) Infusion of solutions composed of dextrose for energy, amino acids for tissue synthesis, fats for energy, and essential fatty acids plus vitamins and minerals.

Toxicity The quality of being poisonous; a condition that can result from consumption of excess amounts of some vitamins.

Trace mineral Mineral that is present in the body in quantities of less than 5 g.

Transferrin (nonheme iron) A combination of iron and a globulin protein; important as the transport form of iron.

Transverse colon The portion of the large intestine that extends across the abdomen from the right to the left.

Triceps A muscle located on the back of the upper arm.

Triceps skinfold thickness Measurement of skin thickness over the triceps brachii muscle; a good indicator of overall fatness.

Tricyclic antidepressant Drug used in the treatment of depression. The drug is thought to work

by increasing the amount of norepineprhine and serotonin.

Triglyceride A lipid compound composed of three fatty acids attached to a glycerol molecule.

Triiodothyronine (T_3) A thyroid hormone that regulates the body's metabolism. Each triiodothyronine molecule contains three iodine atoms; therefore, it is designated as T_3.

Trimester A period of 3 months.

Tripeptide Molecule composed of three amino acid molecules.

Tryptophan An amino acid.

Tubercle A small, rounded nodule produced by the bacterium *Mycobacterium tuberculosis*.

Tuberculosis A bacterial infectious disease caused by the bacterium *Mycobacterium tuberculosis*.

24-hour recall A recounting of the kinds and amounts of food consumed during the 24 hours preceding the interview.

Tyrosine A nonessential amino acid.

U100 insulin 100 units per milliter of insulin.

Ulcerative colitis A disease of the large intestine that is characterized by inflammation of the intestinal mucosa and ulcers.

Underweight Body weight that is more than 10% below the ideal weight.

Unproductive No expulsion of sputum.

Unsaturated fatty acid A fatty acid whose carbon atoms are linked by double or triple bonds, and therefore are not bonded to as many hydrogen atoms as possible.

Urea A nitrogen waste product that results from the metabolism or deamination of amino acids and is excreted in the urine.

Uremic syndrome A complex of symptoms that result from an extremely high level of nitrogenous wastes in the blood.

U.S. RDAs Nutrient recommendations established by the U.S. Food and Drug Administration (FDA) that are used as a standard for nutritional labeling.

Usual body weight (UBW) The normal or usual weight of a person.

Usual intake pattern A recounting of the foods that a person first eats or drinks during the day.

Vagus nerve The tenth cranial nerve. It stimulates gastric glands in the stomach to secrete hydrochloric acid and pepsin enzyme.

Vasodilation Increased diameter or size of blood vessels.

Vegan Pure vegetarian diet that uses no animal or dairy products.

Ventilation The ability to move air into and out of the lungs.

Ventricular arrhythmia Abnormal rhythm in the contraction of the ventricles in the heart.

Viscosity The tendency for a fluid to resist flowing.

Vitamin Organic substance that is essential for normal metabolism, growth, and development of the body. It does not generate energy.

Water soluble Refers to substances that dissolve in water. Fats become water soluble when a protein coat is secreted around them.

Wernicke-Korsakoff disease A mental disorder caused by a thiamin deficiency.

Wernicke's syndrome A condition that results from a thiamin deficiency.

Xerophthalmia A condition in which the cornea becomes thickened and opaque.

ANSWERS TO REVIEW QUESTIONS

CHAPTER 1

1. B	7. A	13. A
2. A	8. A	14. B
3. B	9. D	15. D
4. B	10. B	16. D
5. B	11. E	17. B
6. A	12. C	

CHAPTER 2

1. B	13. B	25. D
2. A	14. A	26. E
3. B	15. A	27. A
4. B	16. B	28. C
5. A	17. B	29. B
6. A	18. A	30. C
7. A	19. A	31. A
8. B	20. D	32. D
9. B	21. E	33. B
10. B	22. B	34. A
11. B	23. C	35. B
12. A	24. A	

CHAPTER 3

1. B	14. B	27. C
2. B	15. A	28. E
3. A	16. B	29. D
4. A	17. B	30. D
5. A	18. A	31. C
6. B	19. A	32. C
7. B	20. A	33. B
8. B	21. A	34. A
9. A	22. B	35. B
10. B	23. B	36. C
11. A	24. B	37. C
12. A	25. A	
13. B	26. B	

CHAPTER 4

1. A	5. A	9. A
2. A	6. B	10. A
3. B	7. B	11. A
4. B	8. B	12. B

CHAPTER 5

13. A	20. C	27. A
14. A	21. B	28. C
15. B	22. E	29. B
16. B	23. B	30. A
17. A	24. E	31. B
18. A	25. E	
19. D	26. D	

1. B	16. B	31. E
2. A	17. B	32. D
3. B	18. A	33. A
4. A	19. A	34. A
5. B	20. A	35. B
6. B	21. B	36. B
7. B	22. C	37. A
8. B	23. E	38. B
9. A	24. B	39. B
10. A	25. B	40. A
11. A	26. D	41. B
12. B	27. A	42. C
13. A	28. B	43. A
14. B	29. E	44. D
15. A	30. A	45. A

CHAPTER 6

1. B	17. A	33. E
2. B	18. B	34. B
3. A	19. B	35. E
4. A	20. A	36. A
5. A	21. A	37. B
6. B	22. A	38. A
7. A	23. B	39. D
8. B	24. A	40. C
9. B	25. B	41. A
10. B	26. B	42. D
11. A	27. C	43. B
12. A	28. E	44. E
13. B	29. C	45. C
14. B	30. A	46. A
15. B	31. E	
16. A	32. E	

CHAPTER 7

1. A	13. A	25. B
2. A	14. B	26. B
3. B	15. B	27. D
4. B	16. B	28. C
5. A	17. A	29. B
6. B	18. A	30. A
7. B	19. B	31. C
8. B	20. A	32. C
9. A	21. A	33. B
10. A	22. C	34. B
11. A	23. D	
12. B	24. B	

CHAPTER 8

1. A	11. A	21. A
2. B	12. B	22. C
3. B	13. B	23. E
4. B	14. B	24. B
5. A	15. B	25. D
6. A	16. E	26. C
7. B	17. B	27. E
8. A	18. B	28. B
9. A	19. D	29. A
10. B	20. C	

CHAPTER 9

1. B	9. B	17. E
2. B	10. A	18. E
3. A	11. B	19. B
4. A	12. A	20. A
5. B	13. E	21. C
6. A	14. C	22. B
7. A	15. E	23. C
8. A	16. B	24. A

CHAPTER 10

1. A	6. B	11. A
2. B	7. B	12. A
3. A	8. A	13. B
4. A	9. A	14. B
5. B	10. B	15. B

16. A	24. A	32. D
17. A	25. A	33. E
18. B	26. E	34. D
19. A	27. D	35. E
20. B	28. B	36. C
21. B	29. C	37. A
22. B	30. C	38. B
23. A	31. D	

CHAPTER 11

1. B	10. B	19. D
2. A	11. A	20. A
3. A	12. A	21. A
4. B	13. B	22. D
5. B	14. A	23. C
6. B	15. B	24. B
7. A	16. B	25. E
8. A	17. A	
9. A	18. C	

CHAPTER 12

1. A	10. B	19. B
2. A	11. B	20. A
3. B	12. B	21. B
4. B	13. B	22. E
5. B	14. A	23. E
6. B	15. A	24. B
7. B	16. B	25. C
8. A	17. A	
9. A	18. B	

CHAPTER 13

1. A	10. B	19. B
2. A	11. A	20. C
3. B	12. A	21. D
4. B	13. A	22. D
5. B	14. A	23. B
6. A	15. B	24. E
7. B	16. B	25. D
8. A	17. C	26. A
9. A	18. A	

CHAPTER 14

1. B	9. B	17. D
2. B	10. A	18. A
3. A	11. A	19. C
4. A	12. B	20. E
5. B	13. B	21. C
6. A	14. B	22. D
7. A	15. D	
8. A	16. E	

CHAPTER 15

1. A	12. B	23. D
2. B	13. B	24. E
3. B	14. A	25. E
4. A	15. A	26. E
5. A	16. B	27. E
6. B	17. A	28. C
7. B	18. B	29. D
8. B	19. C	30. A
9. A	20. A	31. B
10. A	21. B	
11. A	22. A	

CHAPTER 16

1. B	10. B	19. E
2. B	11. A	20. D
3. A	12. A	21. B
4. A	13. B	22. C
5. A	14. A	23. A
6. B	15. A	24. E
7. A	16. E	25. E
8. B	17. D	
9. B	18. D	

CHAPTER 17

1. A	10. A	19. A
2. B	11. A	20. B
3. A	12. B	21. D
4. B	13. B	22. D
5. B	14. B	23. B
6. A	15. A	24. A
7. B	16. C	25. E
8. B	17. E	
9. B	18. E	

CHAPTER 18

1. B	19. B	37. A
2. B	20. B	38. A
3. B	21. A	39. D
4. A	22. A	40. D
5. A	23. B	41. C
6. B	24. A	42. B
7. A	25. B	43. A
8. A	26. B	44. B
9. B	27. A	45. B
10. A	28. A	46. A
11. B	29. A	47. B
12. A	30. B	48. C
13. A	31. B	49. A
14. A	32. B	50. B
15. B	33. A	51. A
16. B	34. A	52. B
17. A	35. B	53. B
18. A	36. A	54. A

CHAPTER 19

1. A	15. B	29. E
2. A	16. B	30. D
3. B	17. B	31. B
4. B	18. A	32. C
5. B	19. B	33. A
6. A	20. A	34. C
7. B	21. A	35. B
8. A	22. B	36. D
9. A	23. B	37. A
10. B	24. A	38. C
11. B	25. A	39. C
12. A	26. A	40. E
13. A	27. A	
14. A	28. E	

CHAPTER 20

1. A	14. A	27. B
2. B	15. A	28. C
3. A	16. A	29. A
4. B	17. B	30. B
5. A	18. B	31. E
6. B	19. A	32. A
7. B	20. A	33. B
8. A	21. B	34. E
9. A	22. B	35. C
10. B	23. A	36. B
11. A	24. B	37. B
12. B	25. A	38. E
13. B	26. A	

CHAPTER 21

1. B	15. B	29. E
2. A	16. A	30. A
3. A	17. A	31. C
4. B	18. B	32. B
5. A	19. A	33. B
6. A	20. A	34. A
7. B	21. B	35. C
8. B	22. B	36. B
9. A	23. B	37. B
10. A	24. A	38. B
11. A	25. B	39. C
12. B	26. A	40. A
13. B	27. E	41. D
14. B	28. C	

CHAPTER 22

1. B	10. B	19. C
2. B	11. A	20. E
3. A	12. A	21. A
4. A	13. B	22. D
5. B	14. A	23. B
6. B	15. B	24. B
7. A	16. A	25. C
8. B	17. B	26. D
9. B	18. C	

CHAPTER 23

1. B	10. A	19. A
2. A	11. B	20. D
3. A	12. A	21. E
4. B	13. B	22. D
5. B	14. A	23. A
6. B	15. A	24. B
7. A	16. B	25. C
8. A	17. B	26. C
9. A	18. B	

CHAPTER 24

1. B	6. A	11. B
2. B	7. A	12. A
3. A	8. B	13. A
4. B	9. B	
5. A	10. A	

CHAPTER 25

1. A	6. B	11. B
2. A	7. B	12. B
3. B	8. A	13. A
4. A	9. A	14. B
5. B	10. B	15. A

CHAPTER 26

1. A	4. A	7. B
2. B	5. B	
3. A	6. B	

INDEX

Abscess, 467
Absorption, defined, 56
Acetylcholine, 155, 612
Acid ash diet, 573
Acid-base balance, defined, 169
Acidic substances, 363
Acidosis, defined, 100
Acid-resistance, *see* Enteric coating
Acid-resistant coating on drugs, 362
Acne, 289
  food fallacies about, 14
Active transport, digestion, 56
Acute glomerulonephritis, 562–563
  dietary and drug treatment, 563
Acute renal disease, 562
Acute renal failure, 566
  diet and drug therapy, 567
Acute respiratory failure (ARF), 545
Addison's disease, 180
Adenosine triphosphate, *see* ATP
    (Adenosine triphosphate)
Adipose tissue, 84
Adolescence:
  iron deficiency anemia, 199
  mineral needs, 289
  nutrition, 287–290
    problems, 290
  protein needs, 289
  recommended food intake,
    729–730
Adrenal gland, 156
Adrenocorticotrophic hormones
    (ACTH), obesity and,
    249–250
Adult diabetes, *see* Non-insulin-
    dependent diabetes
    mellitus (NDDM)
Adult-onset obesity, 244
Adult respiratory distress
    syndrome, 545
Aerobic respiration, 57
Air embolism, 386

Albumin:
  decreased in cirrhosis, 483
  defined, 479
  fluid balance, 103
Albuminuria, 562
Alcohol:
  in calorie-controlled diets, 632
  liver detoxification of, 480
  oral hypoglycemic drugs and, 414
  in peptic ulcer diet, 444
  during pregnancy, 270
Alcoholism:
  case study, 613–614
  elderly, 302
  nutrition and, 610–612
Alcohol-nutritional diseases,
    611–612
Aldosterone:
  potassium regulation, 176
  sodium, 178
Aldosteronism, primary, 521
Alimentary canal:
  defined, 435
  diagram, 436
Alkalosis, defined, 100
Allergic skin reactions to oral
    hypoglycemic drugs, 414
Alpha-tocopherol, *see* Vitamin E
    (Alpha-tocopherol)
Aluminum hydroxide (Kolantyl),
    365
Alveolar surfactant, 545
Alzheimer's disease, 612–613
Amino acid:
  catabolism, 108
  defined, 96
  essential, 97–98
  nonessential, 96–98
  sequence, 99
    normal *vs.* sickle cell, 101
Amino acid content, 109
Amino acid pool, 107

Ammonia, detoxification to urea,
    480
Anabolic steroid, 319
Anabolism, 59–60
  central vein total parenteral
    nutrition, 386
Anaerobic (glycolysis) respiration,
    57
Anemia:
  alcoholism, 611
  defined, 7
  gastrectomy, 450
  iron deficiency, 198–199
  see also specific anemias
Angina pectoris, 508
Anhydrous solutions, defined, 381
Anion, defined, 169
Anorexia:
  cancer patients, 585
  defined, 133
Anorexia nervosa:
  adolescence, 290
  defined, 256–257
Antacids:
  food-drug interactions in elderly,
    369
  nutrient absorption and, 365–366
  pancreatitis, 497
Anthropometric measurements,
    240–242
  children, 343
  Midarm Muscle Circumference, 343
  nutritional assessment, 338,
    342–343
  triceps skin fold thickness, 342
Antiarrhythmics, 530
Antibiotics, 551
  in drug history, 331
Antibody, defined, 102. *See also*
    Islet cell antibodies
Anticholinergic drugs, ulcerative
    colitis, 469

Anticonvulsants in drug history, 331
Antifungal agents, 362
Antigen, defined, 102
Antihistamine, 364–365
Antihypertensive agent:
  in drug history, 331
  summary, 529
Anti-inflammatory agent, 366
Antineoplastic agent, drug history, 331
Antioxidant defined, 136
Antipsychotic drugs, 610
Anuria, 566
Appetite:
  obesity and, 245
  of toddlers, 285–286
Arachidonic fatty acid, 73–74
Ascending colon, 464
Ascites, 483
  sodium restriction, 487
Ascorbic acid, see Vitamin C
Aseptic environment, 386
Aspartame (Nutra Sweet), in diabetic diets, 416–417
Aspiration pneumonia, tube feeding, 378
Aspirin:
  enteric coating, 362
  undernutrition in elderly, 302
Assessment for nutritional care, 9–10
  clinical care process, 337–349
    adult levels, 339
    anthropometric measurements, 338, 342–343
    historical data, 330–338
    laboratory assessment, 343–345
    physical examinations, 338
    specific high-risk patients, 337–338
Asthma, 283
Ataxia, 611
Atelectasis, 497
Atheroma, 507
Atherosclerosis, 507–519
  causative factors, 508–512
    modifiable risk factors, 508–512
    nonmodifiable biologic risk factor, 508
  risk of high-protein diet, 312
  type I diabetes, 398–399
  type II diabetes, 412
  vegetarian diet and, 25

Athletic performance:
  carbohydrates and, 313–315
  fluid and electrolytes in, 316–317
  preevent meal, 317–318
  protein and, 311–312
  weight-gain diet, 318–319
  weight-loss diet, 319
ATP (Adenosine triphosphate), 57
  phosphorus, 175
  synthesis, 57–58
    functions, 182
  thiamin, 140–141
Atrial arrhythmias, 364
Atrophy, defined, 376
Attention deficit disorders (ADD), 608
Autodigestion, 495
Autoimmunity, 395
Autosomal dominant trait, 513
Azotemia, defined, 382

Bacterial pneumonia, 547
Barrel chest, 543
Basal energy expenditure (BEE), 545
Basal metabolic rate, 191, 231–233
  age, 232
  body surface area, 231
  fasting and malnutrition, 233
  fever, 231
  hormones, 232
    and obesity, 248
  pregnancy and lactation, 232
  sex, 231
Basal region of brain, 612
Basic substance, 363
Beets, fallacies about, 14
Behavior, malnutrition and, 608
Behavior modification as treatment for obesity, 254–256
  reinforcement, 255
  stimuli, 255
Beriberi, 142
Beta cell diabetes, 394–395
Beverly Hills Diet, 251
Bile:
  deficiency, vitamin K deficiency and, 140
  defined, 479
Bile salts:
  defined, 82
  lipids and, 81
Biliary atresia, 481
Biliary obstruction, 513

Bilirubin, 480
Binder compound, calcium and, 172–173
Binge eating, 249
Biological value (BV), defined, 109
Biotin:
  body requirements, 155
  characteristics, absorption and metabolism, 153
  food sources, 155
  functions, 154
  summary, 125
  toxicity and clinical deficiency, 155
Bisacodyl (Dulcolax), 365
Blackhead, 289
Bland diet, 443
Blood acidosis, defined, 54
Blood capillary, 56
Blood glucose levels, drugs that increase, 417
Blood lipid profile, 79
Blood lipids, elevated levels, 508, 512–513
Blood pressure, hypertension and, 520
Blood testing for type I diabetes:
  fasting blood glucose/sugar (FBG/FBS), 400
  glycolsylated hemoglobin (HbA$_{1c}$), 401
  oral glucose tolerance (OGTT), 400
Blood urea nitrogen (BUN), 383
  kidney disease, 563
Blurred vision in insulin-dependent diabetes, 397
Body composition, 239–242
  anthropometric measurements, 240–242
  nutritional assessment, 338
Body frame size, 239
Body size and nutritional assessment, 338
Body surface area, 231
  burn patients, 599
Body temperature, water and maintenance of, 213
Bolus, defined, 435
Bolus feeding, 378
Bonding, emotional, 279
Bone growth and development, 175
  vitamin A, 128–129
  vitamin D, 132–133

Bottle feeding for infants, 278–281
Bowman's capsule, 560
Branched chain amino acids, hepatic coma, 489
Bread and cereal exchange lists, 622
Breast cancer, diet and, 584
Breastfeeding for infants, 278–281
Bronchial pneumonia, 545
Bronchial tree, 543
Bronchiectasis, 549
Bronchiogenic cancer, 548–549
Bronchitis, 283, 542
Buffer compound, defined, 104
Buffer system, phosphorus, 175
Bulimarexia, 257
Bulimia, 257
Burn patients, diet therapy, 599–604
  case study, 602–604
  stage 1 burn care, 600
  stage 2 burn care, 600–602
  stage 3 burn care, 602–604
Burns, small, 599

Cachexia, 585–586
Calcidiol, defined, 131
Calcification:
  defined, 133
  vitamin D deficiency and, 134
Calcitriol, 131
Calcium:
  absorption, 169, 171
    acid environment, 171
    lactose present, 171
    vitamin D, 171
  antagonists, 530
  deficiency diseases, 173–174
  food sources, 172–173
  functions, 171–172
  general characteristics, 169
  hypertension and, 521
  impaired absorption, 174
  iron absorption, 195
  requirement during lactation, 268
  requirement during pregnancy, 267
Calcium-phosphorous ratio, 171
Calipers, 241
Calorie:
  defined, 15
  energy measurement, 228
Calorie-controlled diets, supplemental food choices, 630–631

Cambridge Diet Plan, 251
Cancer patients:
  case study, 588–589
  nutritional problems and diet therapy, 585–589
Carbohydrate:
  catabolism, 57–59
  chemistry, 39
  complex, 14
  cultural differences in amounts and food sources, 60–62
  defined, 39
  digestion and absorption, 54–56
  in elderly, 298
  exchange groups and, 61–64
  food sources, 39–52
    disaccharide, 39, 44–47
    monosaccharide, 39–43
    polysaccharides, 39
    saccharide, 39
  functions, 53–54
    as energy source, 53–54
  in high-protein diet, 312
  information summary, 41
  loading, 315–316
    drawbacks, 316
  metabolism, 56–60
  myths about, 314
  physical activity and, 313–315
    as muscle fuel, 313
  in type I diabetic diet, 405–406
Carcinogenic agents, 584
Cardiotonic glycosides, 532
Cardiovascular disease:
  cost of, 507
  defined, 78
  elderly, food-drug interaction, 368
  epidemiology, 507
  lipoproteins, 79–80
Cardiovascular drugs and undernutrition in elderly, 302
Carotene, defined, 129
Case studies in nutrition, format, viii. See also specific conditions
Caseous necrosis, 547
Catabolic steroid, 331
Catabolism:
  amino acids, 108
  carbohydrates, 57–59
Cathartic drugs, 215
  nutrient absorption, 365
  undernutrition in elderly, 302

Catheter, 379
Cations, defined, 169
Cecum, 464
Celiac crisis, 455
Celiac disease, 454–456
  diet therapy, 456
  gluten-restricted diet, 456
  symptoms, 455
Celiac sprue, iron absorption, 196
Cellulose, 48–51
Central vein, defined, 379
Central vein total parenteral nutrition, 384–387
  catheter and metabolis complications, 386–387
  candidates for, 385–386
  solution and administration, 386
  transitional feeding, 387
Cephalin, 76
Cereals as first solid food, 282
Cerebrovascular accidents, see Stroke
Cheese, fallacies about, 14
Cheilosis, 144, 146
Chemically defined (elemental) diets, 377–378
Chemotherapy, side effects, 587
Chenodeoxycholic acid, 493
Children:
  anthropometry in, 343
  nutrition, 284–287
    problems, 290
  recommended food intake, 729–730
Chlorine, 180–183
  absorption, 180
  deficiency diseases, 181
  food sources, 181
  functions, 180–181
Chlorophyll, 182–183
Chlorothiazide (Diuril), 573
Chlorpropamide (Diabinase), 414
Cholecalciferol, see Vitamin D
Cholecystectomy, 493
Cholecystitis, 492
Cholecystokinin, 492
Cholelithiasis, 492
Cholesterol:
  food sources, 78, 628–629
  lipids, 71
  liver synthesis, 480
  role in atherosclerosis, 509–510
  steroid hormones, 77–78
Cholestyramine (Questran), 365, 517, 573

Choline, 612
Chromium, 204
Chromosome, defined, 394
Chronic glomerulonephritis, 564
Chronic intermittent colitis, 468
Chronic obstructive pulmonary
    disease (COPD), 368,
    542–546
  bronchitis, 542
  case study, 551–553
  diet therapy, 544–545
  emphysema, 542–544
  nutrition, 545–546
Chronic persistent hepatitis, 481
Chronic renal disease, 562
Chronic renal failure, 566–570
  case study, 573–578
  diet and drug therapy, 568–570
Chylomicrons, 79
  defined, 82
Chyme, 437–438
Cirrhosis of liver, 367, 481–488
  alcoholism, 611
  causes, 481
  dietary treatment, 484–488
  drug treatment, 488
  selenium and, 204
  symptoms, 482–484
Citric acid cycle, see Krebs cycle
Clear liquid diet, 348
Clinical care process, 329–351
  assessment, 329–349
    adult levels, 339
    anthropometric measurements,
      338, 342–343
    historical data, 330–338
    laboratory, 343–345
    physical examinations, 338
    specific high-risk patients,
      337–338
  diagnosis-related groups, 340
  evaluation, 351
  implementation, 349–351
  planning, 347–349
  summary, 330
Clofibrate (Atromid-S), 519
Clotting factors and calcium, 172
Cobalamin, see Vitamin B$_{12}$
Coenzyme, 122
Colectomy, total, 469
Colestipol (Colestid), 517, 519
Colic, 283
Colitis:
  acute fulminating, 468
  chronic continuous, 468

chronic intermittent, 468
  exacerbations, 468
Collagen:
  defined, 102
  vitamin C, 156
  zinc and, 201
Collateral channel liver, 483
Colon, see Large intestine (colon)
Colon cancer diet and, 584
Colonic diverticulosis, 465–467
  cause, 466
  diet therapy, 466
  symptoms, 466
Common cold, vitamin C and,
    159–160
Complementary protein
    supplementation, 24
Complete protein, 99
Cone, defined, 127
Confabulation, 612
Congenital lactase deficiency, 458
Congenital metabolic disorder, 283
Congestive failure, 302, 531–532
  diet therapy, 532
  drug therapy, 532
Conversion tables, 728
Convulsion, pyridoxine toxicity,
    146
Copper, 203
Cornea, 127
Cornea, 127
Coronary arteries, 508
Cor pulmonale, 542
Cotazym, 498
Cotazym-s, 498
Coxsackie B-4 viruses, 394
Creatinine, 559
Creatinine clearance, 560
  protein intake, 568
Creatinine height index, 344
Cretinism, iodine deficiency,
    200–202
Crohn's disease, 460–463
  cause, 461
  diet therapy, 461
  summary of, 463
  symptoms, 461
Cultural influence on food habits,
    10–12
  carbohydrates, 60–62
  defined, 10
  as factor in obesity, 250
Cushing's disease, 521
Cyanosis, 542
Cystic duct, 493

Cystic fibrosis, 550–551
  defined, 86, 496
  diet therapy, 497–498
  drug therapy, 498–499
    antibiotics, 551
    expectorants or mucolytic
      drugs, 551
  lungs, 497
  pancreas, 497
Cytochrome enzyme systems, 196

DDT (dichloro diphenyl
    trichloroethane), 281
Deamination, defined, 108–109
Decompensation in congestive
    heart failure, 531–532
Decubiti, 353
Dehydration:
  fluid shifting, 213
  in high-protein diet, 312
  hypertonic imbalance, 218
    diagram, 219
  steatorrhea, 85
  tube feeding, 378
Deltoid muscle, 402
Dementia, 612–613
  niacin deficiency, 150–151
Demographic nutritional
    assessment, 351
Denaturation defined, 99–100, 102
Densitometry, 240
Dental caries:
  in adolescence, 290
  defined, 39
Dental changes in elderly, 301
Deoxyribonucleic acid (DNA),
    107–108
  recombinant, 401
Depression in elderly, food-drug
    interaction, 369
Dermatitis, 76
  niacin deficiency, 150–151
Descending colon, 464
Desirable body weight, 236–239. See
    also Ideal body weight
Dextrin defined, 54
Dextrose, monohydrous vs.
    anhydrous forms, 381
Diabetes insipidus, 393
Diabetes mellitus:
  atherosclerosis, 509
  carbohydrates and, 39
  definition and prevalence, 393
  drugs that interfere with control,
    415, 417–418

elderly, food-drug interactions, 369–370
pregnancy and, 415
type I (insulin-dependent), 393–410
type II (non-insulin-dependent), 411–414
see also Insulin-dependent diabetes mellitus (IDDM); Non-insulin-dependent diabetes mellitus (NDDM)
Diabetic ketoacidosis, 398
Diabetic nephropathy, 399
Diabetic retinopathy, 399
Diagnosis-related groups, nutritional care, 340
Dialysate, 570
Dialysis:
defined, 559
diet therapy, 572
hemodialysis, 570–571
peritoneal, 571–572
treatment, 570–572
Diarrhea:
celiac disease, 455
infant, 284
iron absorption, 196
movement of water between fluid compartments, 220
niacin deficiency, 150
from tube feeding, 378
Diastolic pressure, 520
Diet:
acid ash, 573
adequacy, 20
adolescence, 287–289
atherosclerosis and, 509–512
polyunsaturated *vs.* saturated fat, 511–512
balanced, 20
food exchange system, 28–30
bland, 443
calorie-controlled for diabetics, 406
cancer and, 584–585
carbohydrates in, 313–314
clear liquid, 348
clear liquid (surgical), 595–597
for elderly, 303–304
elemental (chemical defined), 377
fad weight loss, 14
fat-controlled, 510
food guides for planning, 20–30
full liquid, 595
sample menu, 598–599

Giordano-Giovannetti, 568–570
gluten-restricted, 456
high-fat and atherosclerosis, 509
high-fiber, 348
high-potassium, 348
high-protein, moderate-fat, high carbohydrate, 485–487
hyperkinesis and, 609
initiation and nomenclature, 348–349
lactose-restricted, 460
liberal, 443
low-fat, 487, 510
40-gram fat, 494–495
low-protein, sample menu, 490
low-residue, 348
low-sodium, 348
minimum-residue, 462–463
nonrecommended, 250–252
nutrient density, 20
nutritionally balanced, 250, 252
postgastrectomy, 449
postoperative, 594–595
pregnancy and lactation, 269–270
preoperative, 594
protein-sodium-potassium-controlled for renal disease, 570
restricted bland, 438
sippy, 443
sodium-controlled, 524–527
soft, 348, 597
of toddlers, 284–286
in U.S., protein kilocalorie distribution, 115–116
variety, 20
food exchange systems, 30
vegetarian, 23–26
weight-gain, 318–319
weight-loss, 319
adaptability, 254
adequacy, 252
nutrient density, 252–253
sample menu (1500 kcal), 253
Diet-drug interactions, *see* Drug-nutrient interactions
Diet drugs or pills, 251
Dietary fiber, *see* Fiber
Dietary Goals for the U.S. (1977), 13
Dietary goals for U.S., 13–15, 115–116
Dietary habits of school-age children, 287
Diet history of patient, 331–338
analysis of data, 337
food diary, 333

food frequency record, 333–337
24-hour recall, 331–333
usual intake pattern, 333–334
Diet therapy:
acute renal failure, 567
assessment, 329–347
availability of adequate normal or modified diet, 349
burn patients, 599–604
cancer patients, 583, 586–589
celiac disease, 456
chronic obstructive pulmonary disease, 544–545
chronic renal failure, 568–570
colonic diverticulosis, 466
congestive heart failure, 532
Crohn's disease, 461–463
cystic fibrosis, 497–498
defined, 328, 547–548
diabetics:
pregnancy and, 415
sweeteners for, 416
dialysis, 572
diverticulitis, 467
dumping syndrome, 448–450
evaluation, 351
gallstones, 493–495
gastritis and acute gastritis, 440
goal of, 348
hepatic coma, 488–491
hyperlipoproteinemia, 514–517
implementation, 349–351
insulin-dependent diabetics, 405–410
lactose intolerance, 460
liver diseases, 484–488
lung cancer, 549
myocardial infarction, 530–531
non-insulin-dependent diabetes, 413
objective, 348
pancreatitis, 496
peptic ulcer, 442–453
current dietary treatment, 443–445
sample menu, 446–447
planning, 347–349
pneumonia, 547
principle and purpose, 328–329
renal calculi, 573
types of diets, 348–349
normal, 348
therapeutic, 348
ulcerative colitis, 468–469
Diffusion and digestion, 56

Digestibility:
 defined, 108
 protein, 108
Digoxin, potassium and
  magnesium imbalance,
  368
Dipeptides, defined, 105
Diplopia, 611
Disaccharide, 39, 44–47
 clinical application, 44
 current *vs.* recommended
  amounts in U.S. diets,
  60–61
 lactose, 46
 maltose, 47
 sucrose, 46
Disease, protein requirements and,
  115
Diuresis, 566
Diuretics:
 defined, 177
 hypertension, 528–530
 liver disease, 488
 nutrient excretion, 367
 renal calculi, 573
 thiazide, 529
 treating obesity with, 251
Diverticulitis, 465–467
 diet therapy, 467
 symptoms, 467
 vegetarian diet and, 25
Diverticulosis, defined, 51
DNA, *see* Deoxyribonucleic acid
  (DNA)
Dorsal plexus network, 379
Dorsum, defined, 379
Drug history of patient, 331
Drug:
 absorption:
  on empty stomach, 633
  with food or milk, 633
  nutrients that interfere,
   361–362
   increased absorption, 362,
    365–366
   decreased absorption, 361
 decrease in blood glucose levels,
  418
 defined, 360
 diabetes and, 415, 417–418
 excretion, effect of nutrients,
  363–364, 367
 food ingestion decreased,
  364–365

increase in blood glucose level,
 417
liver detoxification, 480
metabolism of nutrients, 362–363,
 366–367
Drug-nutrient interactions, 360,
 633–634
 altered drug effects, 360–364
 nutritional balance, 364–367
 elderly, 368–370
 undernutrition in, 302
Drug therapy:
 acute renal failure, 567
 chronic renal failure, 568–570
 congestive heart failure, 532
 cystic fibrosis, 498–499
  antibiotics, 551
  expectorants or mucolytic
   drugs, 551
 gall bladder disorders, 493
 hepatic coma, 489, 491
 hyperlipoproteinemia, 517, 519
 hypertension, 528–530
 lipoprotein disorders, 513–519
 liver diseases, 488
 myocardial infarction, 531
 pancreatitis, 497
 renal calculi, 573
 vitamin-mineral supplements,
  634
Dumping syndrome:
 case study, 469–472
 diagram, 448
 dietary treatment, 448–450
 gastrectomy for peptic ulcer, 445,
  448
 partial gastrectomy, 419
 sample menu, 451–452
Duodenal ulcer, 440
Duodenum, defined, 55
Dysphagia, 435
 lung cancer, 549
Dyspnea, 542

Eating disorders, 613
Eclampsia, 271
Economics, food fallacies and, 13
Eczema, 283
Edema:
 fluid shifting, 213
 hypotonic imbalance, 218
 kidney disease, 563
Edematous condition, 440
Educational goals of book, vii–viii

Eggs:
 fallacies about, 14
 not recommended for infants,
  282–283
Elbow breadth and body weight,
  240
Elderly:
 dietary planning, 303–304
 food-drug interaction, 368–370
 nutrient needs, 296–299
  carbohydrates, 298
  fat, 298
  fiber, 299
  kilocalorie, 297–298
  minerals, 299
  protein, 298
  vitamins, 299
 nutrition programs, 304–305
  undernutrition, 301–303
 nutritional problems, 300–303
  decreased wound healing, 300–301
  protein-calorie malnutrition
   (PCM), 300
 population figures, 296
"Electrolyte replacement," 314
Electrolytes:
 depletion and fat storage, 85
 kidney function, 559
 peripheral total parenteral
  nutrition, 384
 physical activity and, 316–317
Electron transport system, 58
Elemental formula for tube feeding,
  215
Emphysema, 542–544
 diagram, 544
Emulsifying agents, 76
Endotracheal tube, 545
End-stage renal disease, 568
Energy:
 calculating requirements, 234–236
 carbohydrates as source, 53–54
 defined, 228
 in diabetic diet, 406–407
 measurement of, 228–229
 requirements:
  chronic renal failure, 569
  during pregnancy, 264–265
Energy balance, 229–230
 negative, 229
 positive, 229
Energy expenditure, 231–234
 basal metabolic rate (BMR),
  231–233

physical activity, 233–234
specific dynamic effect, 234
Energy intake, 229–230
    mean heights and weights, 230
    table of recommendations, 727
Energy source, proteins as, 104–105
Enteral nutrition:
    advantages, 376
    chronic respiratory failure, 546
    defined, 376
    tube feeding, 376–377
    see also Parenteral nutrition
Enteric coating, 362
Environmental hazards and breast
        feeding, 281
Enzymatic iron, 193
Enzymes:
    activation by magnesium, 182
    zinc in, 202
Epigastric distress (pain), 369, 440
Epinephrine, defined, 59
Epithelial cells, 102
Erythrocytes, see Red blood cells
Erythromycin, enteric coating, 362
Erythropoeitin, 560
Erythropoiesis, 152
Esophageal reflux, 369
Esophageal varices, 483
Esophagotomy, 376
Esophagus, 435–437
    diagrams, 436–437
    disorders, 435, 437
    hiatal hernia, 437
Essential amino acids, 97–98
Essential fatty acid, 74, 76
Essential hypertension, 520
Essential nutrient, 20
Estimated Safe and Adequate Daily
        Dietary Intake (ESADDI),
        33
    trace minerals, 191
    vitamin K, 139
Estrogen, in adolescence, 289
Evaluation of nutritional care, 10
    clinical care process, 351
Exchange lists:
    carbohydrates, 61–64
    for diabetics, 407–410
    fat, 86–90
    glycogen loading, 315
    meal planning appendix, 619–625
    protein content and kilocalories,
        113
        sample menu, 116

sodium and potassium values,
        565
    sodium values, 522
    water content, 564
Exercise:
    for non-insulin-dependent
        diabetics, 413–414
    obesity and, 250
Exogenous insulin sources, insulin-
        dependent diabetes, 394
Expectorants, 551
Extracellular fluid, 103
Extrinsic factor, defined, 147
Exudate, 547

Fad weight loss diets, 14, 250–251
Fasting:
    basal metabolic rate, 233
    obesity and, 251
Fasting blood glucose/sugar
        tolerance test (FBG/FBS),
        400
Fasting hypoglycemia, 418–419
    treatment, 419
Fat:
    atherosclerosis and, 509–512
    carbohydrate content, 64
    decreasing use of, 511
    digestion and absorption
        problems, 85–86
    in elderly, 298
    exchange lists, 86–90, 625
        food sources, 87–88
    in high-protein diet, 312
    insulin-dependent diabetic diet,
        406
    physical activity and, 312
    storage, 84–85
Fat cell hypothesis, 244
Fat-soluble vitamins, 122–126
    summary, 123–125
Fatty acid:
    defined, 71
    essential, 74, 76
    iodine number, 71, 74
    long chain, 71
    medium chain, 71
    monounsaturated, 71
    saturated and unsaturated, 71
    short chain, 71
Fatty liver, alcoholism, 611
Fatty plaques in arteries, 507
Feingold, B. F. (Dr.), 609
Ferric iron, 157, 193

Ferritin, 193
Ferrous iron, 157, 193
Ferrous sulfate, 199
Fetal alcohol syndrome (FAS), 264
Fever and basal metabolic rate, 231
Fiber, 48–51
    atherosclerosis and, 512
    classification, 48–51
    clinical application, 50
    diabetics and, 407, 410
        adverse effects, 410
    in elderly, 299
    food sources, 51, 626–627
    functions, 49
    iron absorption and, 195
    typical meals, 50–51
    see also specific types of fiber
Fibrinogen, defined, 479
Filtrate, 560
Fistulas, 467
Flatulence, fiber and, 410
Flavin, defined, 143
Flavin adenine dinucleotide (FAD),
        59, 144
Fluid:
    burn patients, 601
    in chronic renal failure, 568
    physical activity, 316–317
Fluid balance as protein function,
        103
Fluid imbalance clinical application,
        218
Fluoride, 204
Folacin:
    body requirements, 152
    characteristics, absorption and
        metabolism, 152
    food sources, 152
    functions, 152
    metabolism altered by
        methotrexate, 367
    requirement during lactation, 267
    requirement during pregnancy,
        266–267
    summary, 125
    toxicity and clinical deficiency,
        153
Food additives, 609
Food allergies in infants, 283
Food diary, defined, 255–256
Food exchange system, 26–28
    balanced diets, 28–30
    calculation process, 28–30
    clinical application, 31–33

Food exchange system (*Continued*)
  exchange lists, 27
  see also Exchange lists
Food fad:
  defined, 13
  economics of, 13
Food fallacies, 11–13
  vs. facts, 14
  health dangers, 11–13
  high-risk patients, 11
  malnutrition, 11
Food frequency record, 333–337
Food habits:
  cultural influence, 10–12
  preschoolers, 286
Food stamp program, 305
Fortification of food, 133
Four-Food Group Plan, 20–22
  for adolescence, 289
  clinical application, 21
  diet history, 337
  modified, 23
  during pregnancy and lactation,
      269–270
  recommended servings, 22
  for toddlers, 285–286
  vegetarian diets, 23–26
Fructose:
  blood glucose levels in diabetics,
      42
  diabetic diets, 416
  monosaccharides, 43
Fruit:
  carbohydrate content, 63
  exchange lists, 621
  during pregnancy and lactation,
      269
  as solid food for infants, 282
Functional (reactive) hypoglycemia,
      418–422
  treatment, 419–422
    sample menu, 420–422

Galactose, 40
Galactosemia:
  carbohydrates and, 39
  galactose as treatment, 42
Gall bladder:
  diagram, 479
  disorders, 492–493
    diet therapy, 493–495
    drug treatment, 493
    gallstone formation and
        symptoms, 492–493
  function, 491–492

Gallstones, 492–493
Gangrene in type I diabetes, 398
Gastrectomy:
  cobalamin deficiency, 149
  diagram, 447
  dietary counseling, 453
  long-range nutritional problems,
      450, 452–453
  partial, 419
  peptic ulcer, 445, 448–453
  postgastrectomy diet, 449
Gastric acidity, chlorine and, 181
Gastric ulcer, 440
  diagram, 441
  summary, 445
Gastritis, 440
  acute, 440
  defined, 147
Gastrointestinal disease
Gastrointestinal irritation:
  elderly, food-drug interaction,
      368
  oral hypoglycemic drugs, 414
Gastrointestinal tract changes in
      elderly, 301
Gastrostomy, 376
Gene, defined, 394
Generic drugs, 360
Genetics:
  and insulin-dependent diabetes,
      394–395
  obesity and, 243–244
Giordano-Giovannetti diet, 568–570
Globules, defined, 82
Glomerular filtration rate, 560
Glomerulus, 560
Glossitis, 144
Glucagon:
  defined, 59
  insulin shock, 404
Glucose, 40
  as energy source, 53–54
  food sources, 404
  insulin shock, 404
  insulin transfer of, 396
  intravenous therapy, 42
  oxidation, 57
  as starting material for other
      compounds, 54
Glucose tolerance factor, 204
Glucostatic theory and obesity,
      245–246
Gluten:
  defined, 454
  food sources, 456

Gluten intolerance, 86
Gluten-induced enteropathy, 348
Gluten-restricted diet, 456–458
Gluten-sensitive enteropathy,
      454–456
Glyceride, 70–71
Glycogen, 47–48
  loading, 315–316
    drawbacks, 316
Glycogenesis, 59–60, 480
  potassium and, 177
Glycogenolysis, 59–60, 480
Glycosylated hemoglobin (HbA$_{1c}$),
      401
Goiter, 200
  defined, 7
Goitrogens, 200
Goodwin, James S. (Dr.), 296–297
Gout and vitamin C toxicity, 159
Grains, during pregnancy and
      lactation, 269
Granuloma, 461
Grapefruit, fallacies about, 14
Gravity-drip method of tube
      feeding, 378
Griseofulvin, 362
Gum, 48

Health, defined, 7
Health care team, 8–10
  nurse's role, 8–9
  problem-solving process, 9–10
    assessment, 9–10
    evaluation, 10
    implementation, 10
    planning, 10
Health food, defined, 8
Heartburn, 435
Height, anthropometric
      measurements, 342
Hematocrit, 198
Hemicellulose, 48
Hemochromatosis, 481
Hemodialysis, 570–571
  acute renal failure, 567
Hemoglobin:
  defined, 100
  glycosylated, 401
  iron in, 193
  normal *vs.* sickle cell sequence,
      101
Hemolysis, defined, 138
Hemolytic anemia, 139
  vitamin C toxicity, 159
Hemosiderin, 193

Hemothorax, 386
Heparin, 183
Hepatic Aid, 489
Hepatic cirrhosis, *see* Cirrhosis of
    liver
Hepatic coma, 480
    defined, 488
    diet therapy, 488–491
    drug treatment, 489, 491
Hepatic encephalopathy, 488
Hepatic vein, 483
Hepatitis, 481
    dietary treatment, 484–488
    drug treatment, 488
Hiatal hernia, 348, 435, 437
    diagram, 438
    summary, 439
High-density lipoproteins, 79
High-fiber diet, 348
    colonic diverticulosis, 466
High-potassium diet, 348
High-risk patients, food fallacies
    and, 11
Historical data on patient:
    diet history, 331–338
    drug history, 331
    medical history, 330
    subjective, 331
Hives, 283
Homeostasis in renal failure, 567
Honey *vs.* sugar, 14, 46
Hormonal changes, post-
    menopausal, 173
Hormone:
    basal metabolic rate, 232
    human chorionic gonadotropin
        and obesity, 251
    kidney function, 559
    secretion in small intestine, 454
Hospitalized patients, nutritional
    status of, 345–347
    protein-calorie malnutrition,
        345–346
Human lymphocyte antigens
    (HLA), 394
Humaturia, 562
Humulin, 401
Hunger and obesity, 245
Hydrochloric acid:
    defined, 54
    digestion and, 105
    ferrous iron, 193
Hydrochlorothiazide (HydroDiuril),
    529
Hydrogenation, defined, 71

Hydrogen transport molecule, 58
Hydrolysates, 498
Hydrolysis of lipids, 480
Hydrometry, 240
Hydrothorax, 386
Hyperactivity, 609
Hyperaldosteronism, cirrhosis, 484
Hyperalimentation:
    central vein total parenteral
        nutrition, 385
    defined, 257
Hyperammonemia, 386
    defined, 113
Hypercalcemia, 133–134, 445
Hypercholesterolemia, fiber and, 50
Hyperglycemia:
    anabolism, 59–60
    insulin treatment, 405
    warning signs, 403
Hyperkalemia:
    chronic renal failure, 569
    defined, 177
Hyperkinesis, *see* Hyperactivity
Hyperlipidemia:
    drugs and nutrient absorption,
        365
    nephrotic syndrome, 566
    vegetarian diet and, 25
Hyperlipoproteinemia:
    atherosclerosis, 512–513
    case study, 532–535
    drug treatment, 517, 519
    sample menu for type IIa,
        515–516
    sample menu for type IV,
        518–519
    summary, 513
Hypermetabolic rate, 381
Hyperosmolar hyperglycemic
    nonketotic coma (HHNK),
    411–413
Hyperparathyroidism, 573
Hyperphosphatemia, drugs and
    nutrient absorption, 365
Hyperplasia, defined, 244
Hypertension, 519–530
    acute glomerulonephritis, 563
    atherosclerosis and, 508–509
    defined, 138
    diagnosis, 520
    portal, 483
    pregnancy-induced, 271
    sodium intake, 179–180
    stepped care treatment program,
        521–530

dietary sodium restriction,
    521–528
drug therapy, 528–530
types and causes, 520–521
    essential hypertension, 520
    secondary hypertension, 521
Hyperthyroidism, 232
Hypertonic osmolality, 216–217
    clinical application, 218
    diagram, 219
Hypertrophy:
    defined, 244
    insulin injection site, 402
Hypervitaminosis A, 122
Hypoalbuminemia, defined, 114
Hypocalcemia, gastrectomy, 450
Hypochromic microcytic anemia,
    198
Hypoglycemia, 418–422
    alcoholism, 611
    fasting, 418–419
        treatment, 419
    fiber and, 50
    functional, treatment, 419–422
    insulin shock, 404–405
    oral hypoglycemic drugs, 414
    warning signs, 403
Hypoglycemic agents, 366, 414
Hypokalemia:
    defined, 177
    drug treatment of hypertension,
        529
    liver disease, 488
Hyponatremia, 312
    drugs and nutrient absorption,
        365
Hypophosphatemia, 387
    defined, 113
    phosphorus imbalance, 176
Hypothalamus, obesity and, 245
Hypothyroidism, 232
    atherosclerosis, 513
Hypotonic osmolality, 216–217
    clinical application, 218
Hypovolemic shock, 567
Hypoxia, 344

Iatrogenic malnutrition, 345–347
Ideal body weight, 236–239
    body frame size, 239
    Metropolitan height and weight
        tables, 237
    rule-of-thumb estimation,
        238–239
    U.S. average weights, 238

Ileocecal valve, 464
Ileostomy, 469
Ileum, defined, 105
Immunity, as protein function, 102
Immunologic effects of breast
        feeding, 278
Implementation of nutritional care,
        10
Inborn error of metabolism,
        283–284
Incomplete proteins, 99
Indomethacin, food-drug
        interaction, 369
Infancy:
    defined, 278
    iron deficiency anemia, 198
    nutrition, 278–284
        first foods, 278–281
        problems, 283–284
        solid foods, 281–283
Infection, susceptibility in type I
        diabetes, 399
Inferior vena cava, 483
Inflammatory bowel disease,
        467–469
Ingestion of food decreased by
        drugs, 364–365
Inorganic nutrient, 6
Insensible water loss, 567
Insulin:
    deficiency of, 396–397
    defined, 59–60
    functions, 396–397
    injection sites, 402
    pregnancy and, 415
    treatment of type I diabetics,
        401–405
        resistance, 402
        side effects, 402
        timing of, 402–404
        type and activity, 401–402
            intermediate acting, 401
            prolonged acting, 401
            rapid acting, 401
            U100 strength, 401
    zinc in, 201
Insulin-dependent diabetes mellitus
        (IDDM):
    case study, 422–424
    chronic complications, 398–399
    clinical symptoms and
        complications, 397–398
    diagnosis and monitoring,
        399–401

blood testing, 400–401
    urine testing, 399
diet therapy, 405–410
    diet composition, 405–406
    energy content, 406–407
    fiber and, 407, 410
    kilocalorie and carbohydrate
        distribution, 407
    timing of meals, 405
general characteristics, 393–394
genesis or cause, 394–397
    insulin functions and
        deficiency, 396–397
    genetic factors, 394–395
    treatment, 401–405
Insulinoma, 418
Insulin pump, 404
Insulin shock, 404–405
Intermediate-density lipoproteins,
        79
Intermittent positive-pressure
        breathing, 543
Intestinal flora, 465
Intestinal villi, 56
Intracellular fluid, 103
Intralipid solutions, 381
Intramuscular injections of vitamins
        and minerals, 149, 364
Intrauterine devices, 199
Intrinsic factor, defined, 147
Involution, uterine contractions,
        279
Iodine, 199–201
    body requirement, 200
    deficiency and excess, 200–201
    food sources, 200
    functions, 199–200
Iodine number, 71, 74
Ionization, 212
Ion transport and calcium, 172
Iron, 192–199
    absorption:
        aided by vitamin C, 157
        factors affecting, 193–196
        meat factor, 195
    chemical form, 193
    enzymatic, 193
    excretion, 193, 196
    ferric, 193
    ferrous, 193
    food sources, 196–198
    hemoglobin and myoglobin, 193
    requirement during lactation,
        267

requirement during pregnancy,
        266–267
    storage, 193
    transport, 192
    use of, 193, 196
Iron deficiency anemia, 198–199
    high-risk groups, 198
    laboratory indicators, 198
    symptoms, 198
    treatment, 199
Ischemia, 507
Islet cell antibodies, 394
Islets of Langerhans, 394
Isotonic osmolality, 216

Jaundice:
    hepatitis and, 481
    vitamin K deficiency and, 139–140
Jejunostomy, 376
Jejunum, defined, 56
Junk food, defined, 7
Juvenile diabetes, see Insulin-
        dependent diabetes
        mellitus (IDDM)
Juvenile-onset diabetes, see Insulin-
        dependent diabetes
        mellitus (IDDM)
Juvenile-onset obesity, 244

Keratin:
    defined, 100
    protein synthesis, 102
    sulfur content, 183
Keratinization, 127–128
Ketoacidosis, defined, 394
Ketones, defined, 54
Ketosis-prone diabetes, see Insulin-
        dependent diabetes
        mellitus (IDDM)
Kidney:
    chronic renal failure, 567–570
        renal failure, 566–570
    collecting duct, 562
    diagram, 561
    disease, 562–570
        acute glomerulonephritis,
            562–563
        chronic glomerulonephritis, 564
        nephrotic syndrome, 564, 566
    distal convoluted tubule, 562
    glomerular filtration, 560
    nephrons, 560–562
    proximal tubule, 562
    secretion and blood pH, 562

Kidney stones (renal calculi), 573
  defined, 134
  diet and drug therapy, 573
Kidneys:
  functions, 559–560
    endocrine, 559–560
    excretory, 559
    reabsorption, 560, 562
Kilocalorie (kcal), 21, 228
  adolescence, 288–289
  burn patients, 601
  cancer patients, 587
  elderly needs, 297–298
  hypertension and, 520
  preoperative nutrition, 593
Krebs cycle:
  defined, 59
  thiamin, 141
Kwashiorkor:
  behavior, 608
  defined, 113–114
  hospitalized patients, 346–347

Laboratory assessment of
    nutritional status, 343–345
Lactase deficiency, 456
  congenital, 458
  developmental, 459
  secondary, 459
Lactation:
  basal metabolic rate, 232
  calcium, phosphorus and vitamin
    D requirements, 268
  daily food guide, 269
  diet during, 269–270
  iron and folacin requirements,
    267
  nutritional requirements, 264–268
  protein requirements, 266
  recommended dietary
    allowances, 265–266
  vitamins and minerals during,
    268
Lacteal, defined, 82
Lacto-ovo vegetarians, 24
Lactose:
  calcium absorption, 171
  composition, 43
  defined, 46
Lactose intolerance, 456, 458–460
  cause, 458–459
  diet therapy, 460
  disaccharides, 44
  summary, 461

symptoms, 460
  tube feeding, 378
Lactulose, 489
Laennec's cirrhosis, 481–488
Large intestine (colon), 463–469
  diagram, 464
  disorders, 465–469
  fiber breakdown, 49
  functions, 464
Large-vessel disease in type I
    diabetes, 398–399
Laxative drugs:
  nutrient absorption, 365
  undernutrition in elderly, 302
Lecithin, 76
Left subclavian vein, defined, 82
Legume, 52
Lethargy, 353
Liberal diet, 443
Lignin, 48
Linoleic acid, 73–74, 76
Lipid:
  chemistry, 70–76
  defined, 70
  digestion and absorption, 82–84
    emulsification, 82
  functions, 81
  glycerides, 70–71
  hydrolysis, 480
  metabolism, 83
Lipoatrophy, insulin injection site,
    402
Lipoprotein, 78–80
  atherosclerosis and, 510–511
  cardiovascular disease, 79–80
  classification and composition, 79
  disorders, diet and drug
    treatment, 513–519
  high-density, 79
  intermediate-density, 79
  liver synthesis, 480
  low-density, 79
  very-low-density, 79
Lipostatic theory of obesity,
    245–247
Lipotropic factors in liver disease, 484
Liquefaction, 545
Liver, 479–491
  diagram, 479
  disease, 480–491
    case study, 499–501
    cirrhosis, 481–488
    hepatic coma, 488–491
    hepatitis, 481

functions, 479–480
  decomposition, 480
  detoxification, 480
  storage, 480
  synthesis, 479–480
Long chain fatty acid, 71
Long chain triglycerides, 86
Low birth weight baby, 264
Low-density lipoproteins, 79
Low-residue diet, 348
Low-sodium diet, 348
Lumen, 56
  atherosclerosis, 507
  defined, 365
Luminal effects, 365
Lung cancer (bronchiogenic
    cancer), 548–549
  diet therapy, 549
Lungs, cystic fibrosis in, 497
Lymphocytopenia, protein-calorie
    malnutrition, 300

Macrocytic anemia, cobalamin
    deficiency, 149
Magnesium, 181–183
  deficiency and effects, 183
  functions, 182
  imbalance caused by drugs,
    368
  sources, 182
Major minerals, 169–184
Malabsorption disorders, 454–463
  Crohn's disease, 460–463
  lactose intolerance, 456–460
  nontropical sprue, 454–456
Malnutrition:
  acute renal failure, 567
  basal metabolic rate, 233
  behavior and, 608
  cancer patients, 586
  defined, 7
  food fallacies and, 11
  parenteral nutrition, peripheral
    vein solution, 381
  physical signs, 341–342
  primary, alcohol and, 610
  protein-calorie (PCM), 113–115
  secondary, alcohol and, 610
Maltose, defined, 47
Mammary gland, defined, 265
Manganese, 204
Marasmic kwashiorkor in
    hospitalized patients,
    347

Marasmus:
  behavior and, 608
  defined, 113–114
  hospitalized patients, 346–347
Margarine, 71
Massive (morbid) obesity, 242
Maturity-onset diabetes of youth
    (MODY), see Non-insulin-
    dependent diabetes
    mellitus (NDDM)
Meals on Wheels program, 304
Meat:
  carbohydrate content, 64
  exchange lists, 623–624
  fat content, 86–87
Meat factor and iron absorption,
    195
Mechanical soft diet, 597
Medical history, clinical care
    process, 330
Medium chain fatty acid, defined,
    71
Medium chain triglycerides, 86
  liver disease and, 487
Megadose, defined, 13
Megaloblastic anemia, 366
Menopause, 173
Menstruation and iron deficiency
    anemia, 199
Mental disorders and vitamin
    therapy, 609–610
Metabolic acidosis, 600
Metabolic factor (internal), in
    obesity, 243–248
Metabolism, 83
  biotin, 153
  carbohydrates, 56
  cobalamin, 146–147
  defined, 56
  drugs, effect of nutrients on,
    362–363
  folacin, 152
  inborn error of, 283–284
  niacin, 149
  nutrients altered by drugs,
    366–367
  pantothenic acid, 155
  protein, 107–108
  pyridoxine, 145
  thiamin, 140
  vitamin A, 127
  vitamin D, 130–132
  vitamin E, 136
  vitamin K, 138

Metastasis, 548
Methotrexate (Amethopterin), 367
Metropolitan Life height and
    weight tables, 236–237
Microangiopathies in type I
    diabetes, 398–399
Microcytic red blood cells, 198
Midarm Muscle Circumference
    (MAMC), 343
Mid-upper-arm circumference
    percentiles, 725
Milk anemia, 285
Milk and milk products:
  carbohydrate content, 61–62
  exchange lists, 88, 619
  peptic ulcer diet, 444
  during pregnancy and lactation,
    269
  as source of galactose, 40
Milliosmole, 214
Minerals:
  in adolescence, 289
  alcoholism and, 611
  burn patients, 601
  chronic renal failure, 569
  defined, 169
  drug depletion of, 633
  in elderly, 299
  intramuscular injection, 149, 364
  major, 169–184
    summary of, 170
  preoperative nutrition, 593–594
  requirement during lactation, 268
  requirement during pregnancy,
    268
  storage by liver, 480
  trace:
    RDAs for, 203–205
    summary, 191
  see also specific minerals
Miscarriage (spontaneous abortion),
    264
Modified four-food group system,
    23
Molybdenum, 205
Monoglyceride, 82
Monohydrous solutions, defined,
    381
Monosaccharide, 39–43
  clinical application, 42
  fructose, 43
  galactose, 40
  glucose, 40
Monounsaturated fatty acid, 71

Morbid obesity, 242
Morning sickness, 270
Motility, 361
Mouth:
  digestion, 54
  starch digestion, 54
Mucolytic drugs, 551
Mucosa atrophy, 376
Mucosal effects, 365–366
Mucous membranes, defined,
    127
Muscles:
  carbohydrates, 313
  potassium and, 176
  protein and, 311–312
Mycobacterium tuberculosis, 547
Myelin sheath, 147
Myocardial infarction, 508, 530–531
  diet therapy, 530–531
  drug therapy, 531
Myoglobin (heme iron), 193

Nasogastric tube, 376
National Academy of
    Sciences–National
    Research Council, 30
National Nutrition Program, 304
Natural food, defined, 13
Necrosis, 508
Negative energy balance, 229
Neomycin sulfate, 489
Neoplasm, defined, 584
Nephron, 560–562
Nephrosis, 513
Nephrotic syndrome, 564, 566
Nerve impulses, potassium role in
    transmission, 176
Nervous system and B complex
    vitamins, 156
Niacin, 149–152
  body requirements, 150
  food sources, 150
  functions, 150
  general characteristics, absorption
    and metabolism, 149
  hyperlipoproteinemia, 519
  summary, 124
Nicotinamide, 149–152
Nicotinamide adenine dinucleotide
    (NAD), 58
Nicotinic acid, see Niacin
Night blindness:
  defined, 127
  vitamin A deficiency, 130

Nitrogen balance, negative and positive, 111
Nitrogen equilibrium, 111
Nitrogen-fixing bacteria, defined, 112
Noncaloric nutrients, defined, 122. *See also* Minerals; Vitamins
Nonessential amino acids, 96–98
Non-insulin-dependent diabetes mellitus (NDDM), 411–414
  case study, 425–426
  chromium, 204
  general characteristics, 411
  genesis or cause, 411
  symptoms or complications, 411–413
  treatment, 413–414
    dietary, 413
    exercise, 413–414
    oral hypoglycemic drugs, 414
Nonnutritive sweeteners, diabetic diets, 416–417
Nontropical sprue:
  cause, 454
  osteomalacia, 135–136
  pathophysiology, 455
Norepinephrine, 157
Normal diet, 348
Nurse, in health care team, 8–9
Nutramigen, 42
Nutrient:
  classification, 5–6
  energy nutrients, 6
  essential, 20
  inorganic, 6
  metabolism altered by drugs, 366–367
  noncaloric, 122
  organic, 6
  recommended dietary allowances, 33–34
Nutrient density, 20
  in balanced diets, 252–253
Nutrient-drug interactions, 633–634
Nutrition:
  body processes, 5
  defined, 5
  homeostasis, 5
  nutrients, 5–6
Nutritional assessment:
  example from hospital admitting notes, 352–354
  levels of, in infants and children, 731–732

Nutritional care, defined, 7
Nutritional education and counseling, 349–350
  teaching aids and materials, 350
Nutritional status:
  cultural factors, 329
  defined, 7
  economic factors, 329
  height and weight, 342
  physiological factors, 328
  psychological factors, 328
  sociological factors, 329
Nutritional terms, 7–8
Nutrition Committee of the American Academy of Pediatrics, 281
Nutrition history of infants, 733–734
"Nutrition and Your Health," 15
Nutritious, defined, 7
Nutritive sweeteners, diabetic diets, 416
Nutritive value of foods, 636–709
Nystagmus, 611

Obesity:
  in adolescence, 290
  adult-onset, 244
  body composition, 239–242
  breastfeeding and, 279
    regulatory (external) factors, 248–249
  causes, 243–249
  defined, 229, 242
  incidence, 243
  juvenile-onset, 244
  massive (morbid), 242
  metabolic factors, 243–248
    genetics, 243–244
      fat cell hypothesis, 244
    hormonal, 248
    physiological, 245–247
      glucostatic theory, 245–246
      set point theory, 245–247
      lipostatic theory, 245–247
  nonrecommended treatments, 250–252
  recommended treatments, 250, 252–256
    behavior modification, 254–256
    nutritionally balanced diet, 250, 252
    physical activity, 254–255
  regulatory (external) factors:

  lack of exercise, 250
  psychological, 248–249
  social, 250
  severe, 242
  type II diabetes and, 411
Objective body measurements, 338
Older American Act, Title VII, 304
Oliguria, 563
Omenta, 84
Opsin, defined, 127
Oral glucose tolerance test (OGTT), 400
Oral hypoglycemic drugs, 414
Orange juice, fallacies about, 14
Organically grown food, 13
  fallacies about, 14
Organic compounds, 6
Orthomolecular approach to schizophrenia, 609–610
Osmolality, 214–215
  body fluids, 215–217
  foods and beverages, 217–220
  hypertonic, 216–217
  hypotonic, 216–217
  isotonic, 216
Osmolarity, 214
Osmole unit, 214
Osmosis, 213–214
Osmotic overload, 468
Osmotic pressure, 213
  chlorine and, 181
  clinical application, 215
  fluid balance, 103
Osteomalacia:
  causes, 173–174
  vitamin D deficiency and, 134–136
Osteoporosis, 173–174
  causes, 173–174
Over-the-counter drugs, adverse nutritional outcomes, 634
Overfat, defined, 242
Overt nutritional deficiencies, 338
Overweight:
  body composition, 239–242
  defined, 229, 242
Oxalic acid:
  absorption, 196
  defined, 172–173
Oxidation, nutrients, 6
Oxytocin, 279
Oysters, fallacies about, 14

Palmar erythema, 482
Pancreas:
    diagram, 479
    disorders, 495–499
        cystic fibrosis, 497–499
        pancreatitis, 495–497
    functions, 493, 495
Pancreatic amylase, 55
Pancreatic enzyme deficiency, 86
Pancreatic powder, 498
Pancreatitis, 413, 495–497
    alcoholism, 611
    causes and symptoms, 496
    diet therapy, 496
    drug treatment, 497
Pantothenic acid:
    body requirements, 155
    characteristics, absorption and
        metabolism, 155
    food sources, 155
    functions, 155
    summary, 125
    toxicity and clinical deficiency,
        155–156
Paralytic ileus, 600
Parenteral infusion of cobalamin,
    149
Parenteral nutrition, 379–387
    cancer patients, 587
    defined, 376
    kwashiorkor, 115
    peripheral total, 383–384
    peripheral vein, 379–381
        advantages and disadvantages,
            379–381
        diagrams, 380
        solutions, 381–384
        protein-sparing, 381–383
    reasons for, 379
    total, defined, 381
    see also Total parenteral nutrition
        (TPN)
Partial gastrectomy, 419
Pauling, Linus (Dr.), 159–160, 610
Pectin, 48
Pellagra:
    niacin deficiency, 150–152
    schizophrenia, 610
Pelvic girdle, 289
Pepsin, defined, 105
Peptic ulcer, 440–453
    case study, 469–472
    cause, 440–441
    chronic, diet for, 444

complications, 445
diet therapy, 442–453
    sample menu, 446–447
duodenal, 440
gastrectomy as treatment, 445,
    448–453
gastric, 440
sites, 442
symptoms, 441–442
Peptidase enzyme, 454
Peptide bonds, 98
Peptone, defined, 105
Perforation, peptic ulcer, 445
Peripheral edema, thiamin
    deficiency, 142
Peripheral neuritis, 611
Peripheral resistance, 528
Peripheral vein, parenteral
    nutrition, 379–381
Peristalsis, defined, 54
Peristaltic contraction, 435
Peritoneal dialysis, 567, 571–572
Peritoneum membrane, 571–572
Permeability of cell membranes, 172
Pernicious anemia:
    cobalamin deficiency, 149
    gastrectomy, 452
Phagocytic cells, 480
Pharmacologic dose, 362
Pharmacologic effect, 362
Phenolphthalein, 365
Phenothiazine tranquilizer, 361
Phenylalanine, 284
Phenylalanine hydroxylase, 284
Phenylbutazone, food-drug
    interaction, 369
Phenytoin sodium (Dilantin),
    vitamin D and, 367
Phenylketonuria (PKU), 283
Phlebitis, 379
Phospholipid, 76
    chemical composition, 71
    phosphorus, 175
Phosphorus, 174–176
    absorption, 175
    chronic renal failure, 569
    food sources, 176
    functions, 175
    general characteristics, 174–175
    imbalance diseases, 176
    ration with calcium, 171
    requirement during lactation, 268
    requirement during pregnancy,
        267

Photophobia, 144
Physical activity:
    carbohydrates and, 313–315
    energy expenditure, 233–234
        various activities, 233
    fat and, 312
    fluid and electrolytes, 316–317
    lack of and obesity, 250
    time required to burn 3500 kcal,
        255
    as treatment for obesity, 254–255
Physical growth, NCHA
    percentiles, 717–724
Phytic acid:
    defined, 172–173
    iron absorption, 196
Pimples, 289
"Pink puffers," 543
Placenta, defined, 138
Placental lactogen, 415
Planning nutritional care, 10
    clinical care process, 347–349
Plaques, 78
Plateaus in weight-loss diets,
    254
Pleurisy, 496
Pneumonia, 547
Pneumothorax, 386
Polychlorinated biphenyl (PCBs),
    281
Polydipsia in insulin-dependent
    diabetes, 397
Polyphagia in insulin-dependent
    diabetes, 397
Polysaccharide, 47–52
    cellulose, 48–51
    current vs. recommended
        amounts in U.S. diets,
        60–61
    glycogen, 47–48
Polyunsaturated fatty acids,
    (PUFA), 71
    vitamin E as antioxidant, 136
Polyunsaturated oils, 512
Polyuria in insulin-dependent
    diabetes, 397
Porosity, 562
Portal hypertension, 483
Portal vein:
    defined, 82
    diagram, 482
Positive energy balance, 229
Positive nitrogen balance, 111
Postoperative diet, 594–595

Potassium, 176–178
  balance:
    chronic renal failure, 569
    as protein function, 103–104
  content in foods, 711–716
  deficiency diseases, 177–178
  diet therapy, 348
  food sources, 177
  functions, 176–177
  hypertension and, 521
  imbalance caused by drugs, 368
Potassium-40 method of
      determining body
      composition, 240
Preeclampsia, 271
Preevent meals for athletes,
      317–318
Pregnancy:
  alcohol during, 270
  basal metabolic rate, 232
  calcium requirements, 267
  daily food guide, 269
  diabetes and, 415
  diet during, 269–270
  folacin requirements, 152,
      266–267
  iron deficiency anemia, 199
  iron requirements, 266–267
  nutritional requirements, 264–268
  osteomalacia, 174
  phosphorus requirements, 267
  problems and complications,
      270–272
    hypertension, 271
    nausea and vomiting, 270
    teenage pregnancy, 271–272
  protein requirements, 266
  recommended dietary
      allowances, 265
  vitamin D requirement, 267
  vitamins and minerals during,
      268
Pregnancy-induced hypertension
      (PIH), 264, 271
Premature baby, 264
Preoperative diet, 594
Preoperative nutrition, 593–594
Preschooler, nutrition for, 286
Presenile dementia, 612
Primary aldosteronism, 521
Primary level preventive health
      care, 4
Primary malnutrition in alcoholism,
      610

Problem-oriented medical record
      (POMR), 351–354
Progesterone, 415
Prospective Payment System (PPS),
      340
Protein:
  adolescent needs, 289
  burn patients, 601
  cancer patients, 587
  chemistry, 96–102
    amino acid sequence, 99
    complete and incomplete
        proteins, 99
    denaturation, 99–100
    essential and nonessential
        amino acids, 96–98
    structure, 98
  complementary, 107–108
  complete, 107
  content in exchange groups, 113,
      116
  defined, 96
  digestibility, 108
  digestion and absorption,
      105–106
    amino acids, dipeptides and
        tripeptides, 105–106
    small intestine, 105–106
    stomach, 105–106
  disadvantages of high-protein
      diet, 311–312
  disease and, 115
  drawing of denatured, 101
  in elderly, 298
  food sources, 112–113
    during pregnancy and
        lactation, 269
  functions, 102–105
    buffer action, 104
    energy source, 104–105
    fluid balance, 103
    growth and replacement, 102
    immunity, 102
    sodium and potassium balance,
        103–104
  insulin-dependent diabetics, 406
  intake in chronic renal failure, 568
  kilocalorie distribution in U.S.
      diets, 115–116
  malnutrition in kidney disease,
      566
  metabolism, 107–108
    catabolism of amino acids, 108
    synthesis, 107

  muscle development and athletic
      performance, 311–312
  normal shape, 101
  preoperative nutrition, 593
  quality, 109–110
    amino acid content, 109
    biological value, 109
  recommended dietary allowance
      (RDA), 111–112
    age groups, 112
  requirement during lactation, 266
  requirement during pregnancy,
      266
  synthesis, 107–108
Protein-calorie malnutrition (PCM),
      113–115
  elderly, 300
    symptoms and assessment, 300
    treatment, 300
  hospitalized patients, 345–346
Protein efficiency ratio (PER),
      109–110
Protein-sparing solutions:
  crystalline amino acids, 382
  D_5W, 381
  10% fat emulsion, 382–383
Proteinuria, 271, 562
Proteoses, defined, 105
Prothrombin, 138
Pruritis vulvae, 398
P : S ratio:
  hyperlipoproteinemia, 515, 517
  table of representative foods, 710
Psychotherapeutic drugs, 281
Psychotherapy for anorexics, 257
PUFA, see Polyunsaturated fatty
      acids (PUFA)
PULMOCARE formula, 546
Pulmonary disease, elderly, food-
      drug interaction in, 368
Pulmonary therapy, 543
Pyloric obstruction, peptic ulcer,
      445
Pyloric sphincter valve, 438
Pyridoxine, 145–146
  food sources, 146
  summary, 124
  toxicity and clinical deficiency,
      146
Pyrosis, 435
Pyruvic acid metabolism, 57

"Quick-energy foods," myths
      about, 314

Quinidine intoxication, 531
Quinidine sulfate (Cin-Quin), 364
Quinone, defined, 138

Reabsorption, 560–562
Reactant, water as, 212
Reagent in urine testing, 399
Rebound scurvy:
  defined, 11
  vitamin C toxicity, 159
Recombinant DNA, 401
Recommended Dietary Allowances
      (RDA), 30, 33–34
  adult, 297
  age and sex groups, 33–34
  defined, 20
  diet history, 337
  energy intake, 229–230
    mean heights and weights, 230
  pregnancy and lactation, 265
  protein, 111–112
  trace minerals, 203–205
  U.S., 34
Red blood cells:
  folacin deficiency, 152–153
  hypochromic, 198
  macrocytic anemia, 150
  mycrocytic, 198
  phagocytic decomposition, 480
  vs. sickle cells, 100–101
  synthesis:
    B complex vitamins, 156
    increased during pregnancy,
        266–267
    vitamin C, 157
    vitamin C synthesis, 157
    vitamin E toxicity and deficiency,
        138
    vitamin K, 138–139
Reflectance photometer, 400
Reflux, 435
Regurgitation:
  hiatal hernia, 435
  tube feeding, 378
Renal calculi, see Kidney stones
      (renal calculi)
Renal failure, 566–570
  acute, 566–567
    diet and drug therapy, 567
  calcium absorption, 174
Renal osteodystrophy, 568
Renin, 560
Repletion, defined, 384
Respiratory failure, 545–546

Respiratory infections, vitamin A
      deficiency, 130
Respiratory insufficiency, 545–546
Retina, defined, 127
Retinene, 126
Retinol, see Vitamin A
R-group, 96
Rheumatoid disease in elderly,
      food-drug interaction, 369
Rhodopsin, defined, 127
Riboflavin, 143–144
  body requirements, 144
  food sources, 144
  functions, 144
  general characteristics, 143–144
  summary, 124
  toxicity and clinical deficiency,
      144
Rickets:
  clinical signs, 174
  defined, 7
  vitamin D deficiency and,
      134–135
Rod, defined, 127

Saccharin in diabetic diets, 417
Salivary amylase, 54
  chlorine and, 181
Sample menu:
  clear liquid (surgical), 596–597
  dumping syndrome, 451–452
  exchange groups, protein content
      and kilocalories, 116
  full liquid, 598–599
  functional (reactive)
      hypoglycemia, 420–422
  gluten-restricted diet, 457–458
  high-protein, moderate-fat, high-
      carbohydrate diet, 485–487
  hyperlipoproteinemia (type IIa),
      515–516
  hyperlipoproteinemia (type IV),
      518–519
  minimum-residue diet, 462–463
  peptic ulcer, 446–447
  protein, 20-gram diet, 490–491
  sodium dietary restriction,
      524–526
  weight-loss, 1500-kcal diet, 253
Satiety and obesity, 245
Saturated fatty acid, 71
  functions, 74–75
Scar tissue in liver, 482–483
Scarsdale Medical Diet, 251

Schizophrenia, 609–610
  pellagra and, 610
School-age children, nutrition,
      286–287
School lunch programs, 286–288
Sclerosis, 379
Scurvy, vitamin C prevents, 156
Sebaceous glands, 289
Sebum, 289
Secondary lactase deficiency, 459
Secondary level preventive health
      care, 4
Secondary malnutrition and
      alcoholism, 610
Select Committee on Nutrition and
      Human Needs, 60
Selenium, 204
Senate Select Committee on
      Nutrition and Human
      Needs, 13, 15
Senile dementia, 612
Sepsis, defined, 382
Septic abortion, 562
Serosa, 461
Serous fluid, 213
Serum albumin levels in protein-
      calorie malnutrition, 300
Serum glutamic oxaloacetic
      transaminase (SGOT), 481
Serum glutamic pyruvic
      transaminase (SGPT), 481
Serum transferrin test, 344
Set point theory and obesity,
      245–247
Severe obesity, 242
Short bowel, 86
Short chain fatty acid, 71
Sickle cell disease:
  clinical application, 100
  defined, 99–100, 102
Sigmoid colon, 464
Sippy diet, 443
Skin itching or infection in insulin-
      dependent diabetes, 397–398
Small calorie, see Calorie
Small intestine, 453–463
  digestion, 55–56
  functions, 453–454
  malabsorption disorders, 454–463
    Crohn's disease, 460–463
    lactose intolerance, 456–460
    nontropical sprue, 454–456
    nutrient absorption sites, 455
    protein digestion, 105–106

Small-vessel disease
(microangiopathies) in
type I diabetes, 398–399
Smoking and atherosclerosis, 509
SOAP format for progress notes,
351–352
Sodium, 178–180
absorption and excretion, 178
balance as protein function,
103–104
content in foods, 711–716
diet therapy, 348, 521–528
level in normal diet, 521–522
levels, 523
mechanism, 528
sample menu, 524–526
food sources, 178–179
functions, 178
hypertension and, 179–180, 520
intake in chronic renal failure,
568
measurement, 522
in normal diet, 521–522
Sodium-potassium pump, 104
Soft diet, 348, 597
Solute, water as, 213
Solvent, water as, 213
Sorbitol in diabetic diets, 416
Specific dynamic effect, 234
Specific heat, 213
Spermatogenesis, 319
Spider angioma, 482
Spironolactone (Aldactone):
hypertension, 529
liver disease, 488
potassium and magnesium
imbalance, 368
Spleen, defined, 156
Sprue, osteomalacia and, 174
Sputum, 547
Starch, 52
Steatorrhea, 85
osteomalacia, 174
Steroid hormone:
defined, 77–78
inactivation, 480
Sterol, 77–78
Stillborn infant, 264
Stimuli and behavior modification,
255
Stomach, 437–453
anatomy, 439
digestion, 54
disorders, 440–453

gastritis, 440
peptic ulcer, 440–453
protein digestion, 105–106
surgery, iron absorption and, 196
Storage iron, 193
Stress hormones, vitamin C and,
157
Stroke:
defined, 393
type II diabetes, 413
Study aids for nutrition, viii
Subclavian vein, central vein total
parenteral nutrition, 384
Subcutaneous adipose tissue, 84
Sucrose, defined, 46
Sugar:
contents in food groups, 64
vs. honey, 14, 46
hyperkinesis and, 609
naturally occurring, 15
Sulfonylurea drugs, 366, 414
Sulfur, 183–184
food sources, 184
functions, 183
Superior vena cava:
central vein total parenteral
nutrition, 384
thrombosis, 386
Surgery as treatment for obesity,
252
Sweet 'n' Low in diabetic diets, 417
Sympatholytics, 530
Synapse, defined, 172
Synergistic effect, 509
Synovial fluid, 213
Systemic flushing, 519
Systolic pressure, 520

Tachycardia:
defined, 178
dumping syndrome, 445
Take Off Pounds Sensibly (TOPS),
255
Tardive dyskinesia, 613
Target organ, defined, 131
Teenage pregnancy, 271–272
Teeth:
development and vitamin D
deficiency, 136
mottling due to excess fluoride,
204
Ten State Nutrition Survey, 298
Tertiary level preventive health
care, 4

Testicular degeneration, 319
Testosterone in adolescents, 289
Tetany and magnesium deficiency,
183
Tetracycline, 361
Theophylline, food-drug
interaction, 368
Therapeutic nutrition, 328. *See also*
Diet therapy
Thiamin, 140–142
body requirements, 141–142
food sources, 142
functions, 140–141
general characteristics, absorption
and metabolism, 140
summary, 124
toxicity and clinical deficiency,
142
Thiazide diuretics, 367
Thoracic cavity, 379
Threshold level, 560
Thrombosis, 379
superior vena cava, 386
Thyroid gland, 199
obesity and, 251
Thyroxine, 199
obesity and, 248
Toddlers, nutrition, 284–286
Tolazamide (Tolinase), 414
Tolbutamide (Orinase), 414
Tongue, appearance and B complex
vitamins, 156
Total iron-binding capacity, 198
Total parenteral nutrition (TPN):
central vein, 384–387
chronic respiratory failure, 546
defined, 218, 381
hepatic coma, 489
peripheral, 383–384
electrolytes and vitamins, 384
see also Enteral nutrition;
Parenteral nutrition
Toxemia, 264
as outdated term, 271
Toxicity, vitamin, 122
Trace minerals, 191–205
Transferrin (nonheme iron), 192
Transitional feeding, 387
Transport iron, 192
Transverse colon, 464
Triamterene (Dyrenium), 529
Triceps muscle, 241
skin fold thickness, 342
percentiles, 726

Tricyclic antidepressants, 369
Triglyceride:
    defined, 54, 70–71
    long chain, 86
    medium chain, 86
Triiodothyronine, 199
Trimesters of pregnancy, 265
Tripeptides, defined, 105
Tryptophan, 145
Tube feeding:
    bolus feeding, 378
    complications, 378–379
    disaccharides, 44
    elemental formula, 377
    esophagotomy, 376
    fluid restriction formula, 377
    gravity-drip method, 378
    isotonic formula, 377
    nasogastric, 376–377
    transitional feeding, 387
    see also Enteral nutrition;
        Parenteral nutrition
Tubercle, 547
Tuberculosis, 547–548
24-hour recall, 331–333
Type I diabetes, see Insulin-
        dependent diabetes
        mellitus (IDDM)
Type II diabetes, see Non-insulin-
        dependent diabetes
        mellitus (NDDM)
Tyrosine, 284

Ulcer, peptic, 440–453
Ulcerative colitis, 467–469
    cause, 468
    diet therapy, 468–469
    iron absorption, 196
    symptoms, 468
Undernutrition, elderly, 301–303
    alcoholism, 302
    decreased taste sensitivity, 301
    dental changes, 301
    drug-diet interactions, 302
    economic reasons, 303
    gastrointestinal tract changes, 301
Underweight:
    classification, 256–257
    defined, 242
U.S. RDAs, see Recommended
        Dietary Allowances (RDA)
Unproductive symptoms, 547
Unsaturated fatty acid, 71
    functions, 74–75

Urea:
    ammonia detoxification, 480
    defined, 105
    kidney function, 559
    liver synthesis, 480
Uremia, 568
Uremic syndrome, 566–568
Uric acid, kidney function, 559
Urine testing in insulin-dependent
        diabetes, 399
Usual body weight measurement,
        342
Usual intake pattern in diet history,
        333–334
Uterine contractions, 279

Vagus nerve, 443
Vasodilation, 530
    defined, 150
Vegan, defined, 23–24
Vegetable group:
    bread and starch, 64
    carbohydrate content, 63
    exchange lists, 620
    during pregnancy and lactation,
        269
    as solid food for infants, 282
Vegetarian diets, 23–26
    advantages and disadvantages,
        24–26
    lacto-ovo, 24
    vegan, 23–24
Ventilation, 542
Ventricular arrhythmias, 364
Very-low-density lipoproteins, 79
Vitamin A:
    absorption, storage, and
        metabolism, 127
    body requirements, 128–129
    for cancer patients, 587
    decreased wound healing in
        elderly, 300
    fallacies about, 14
    fat-soluble, 122
    food sources, 129
    functions, 127–128
        bone growth and development,
            128–129
        dim light vision, 127
        mucous membrane
            maintenance, 127–128
    nature and general
        characteristics, 126–127
    summary, 123

toxicity and clinical deficiency,
        129–130
    vitamin E as antioxidant, 136
Vitamin A, 126–130
Vitamin B₁, see Thiamin
Vitamin B₁₂, 146–149
    body requirements, 148
    characteristics, absorption and
        metabolism, 146–147
    deficient in breast milk, 278
    food sources, 148
    functions, 147
    summary, 124
    toxicity and clinical deficiency,
        148–149
Vitamin B₂, see Riboflavin
Vitamin B₆, see Pyridoxine
Vitamin C, 156–160
    acidic drugs and, 363–364
    body requirements, 157
    for cancer patients, 587
    characteristics, absorption and
        metabolism, 156
    decreased wound healing in
        elderly, 300
    fallacies about, 14
    food sources, 158
    functions, 156
    summary, 125
    toxicity and clinical deficiency,
        158–159
Vitamin C and the Common Cold,
        159–160
Vitamin D, 130–136
    absorption, storage and
        metabolism, 130–132
    body requirements, 133
    calcium absorption, 171
    deficiency in breastfed infants,
        278
    fat-soluble, 122
    food sources, 133
    functions, 132–133
    kidney function, 560
    nature and general
        characteristics, 130
    phenytoin sodium, 367
    requirement during lactation, 268
    requirements during pregnancy,
        267
    summary, 123
    synthesis, 132
    toxicity and clinical deficiency,
        133–136

calcification of soft tissues, 134
hypercalcemia, 133–134
kidney stones, 134
muscle spasms, 136
osteomalacia, 134–136
poor teeth development, 136
rickets, 134–135
Vitamin E (alpha-tocopherol), 136–138
absorption and metabolism, 136
body requirements, 136
fat-soluble, 122
food sources, 136–137
functions, 136
nature and characteristics, 136
toxicity and clinical deficiency, 138
summary, 123
Vitamin K, 138–140
absorption and metabolism, 138
body requirements, 138–139
fat-soluble, 122
food sources, 139
functions, 138
nature and general
characteristics, 138
summary, 123
toxicity and clinical deficiency,
139–140
Vitamins:
alcoholism and, 611
B complex, 140–156
nervous system malfunctions,
156
red blood cell synthesis, 156
tongue appearance, 156
*see also specific B complex
vitamins*
burn patients, 601
cancer patients, 587

chronic renal failure, 569
defined, 122
in elderly, 299
fat-soluble, 122–126
lipids, 81
summary, 123–125
food sources, harvesting, storing,
and cooking, 160–161
intramuscular injections, 149, 364
liver disease, 487
mental disorders and, 609–610
natural *vs.* synthetic, 14
preoperative nutrition, 593–594
requirement during lactation, 268
requirement during pregnancy, 268
storage by liver, 480
toxicity, 122
water-soluble, 122, 140–159
summary, 123–125
see also specific vitamins

Water:
children's requirements for, 735
functions, 212–213
body temperature
maintenance, 213
reactant, 212
solvent, 213
tissue lubricant, 213
transport agent, 213
movement between fluid
compartments, 213–220
osmolality, 214–215
body fluids, 215–217
osmosis, 213–214
as percentage of body weight,
211–212
as sodium source, 179

Water balance and potassium, 176
Water solubility, 82
Water-soluble vitamins, 140–159
defined, 122
summary, 123–125
Weakness in insulin-dependent
diabetes, 398
Weight:
anthropometric measurements,
342
ideal body, 236–239
table of U.S. average, 238
Weight-gain diet, 318–319
Weight loss:
breast feeding, 279
insulin-dependent diabetes,
397
Weight-loss diet, 319
Weight Watchers' groups, 255
Wernicke-Korsakoff disease,
611–612
thiamin deficiency, 142
Wernicke's syndrome, 611
Why Your Child is Hyperactive, 609
Wine, red, fallacies about, 14
Wound healing:
decrease in elderly, 300–301
with vitamin C, 156

Xerophthalmia, 130
Xylitol in diabetic diets, 416

Zinc:
decreased wound healing in
elderly, 300–301
food sources, 202–203
functions, 201–202